MINOR
EMERGENCIES

MINOR EMERGENCIES 4e

PHILIP M.
BUTTARAVOLI MD, FACEP
Emergency Physician
Emergency Department
Veteran's Administration Medical Center
West Palm Beach, FL
Adjunct Assistant Professor
Division of Emergency Medicine
Larner College of Medicine at the University of Vermont
Burlington, VT
USA

STEPHEN
LEFFLER MD, FACEP
President and Chief Operating Officer
University of Vermont Medical Center
Professor of Surgery
Division of Emergency Medicine
Larner College of Medicine at the University of Vermont
Burlington, VT
USA

R. RAMSEY
HERRINGTON MD, FACEP
Chief
Division of Emergency Medicine
Larner College of Medicine at the University of Vermont
Burlington, VT
USA

ELSEVIER

Elsevier
1600 John F. Kennedy Blvd.
Ste 1800
Philadelphia, PA 19103-2899

Notices

Practitioners and researchers must always rely on their own experience and knowledge in evaluating and using any information, methods, compounds or experiments described herein. Because of rapid advances in the medical sciences, in particular, independent verification of diagnoses and drug dosages should be made. To the fullest extent of the law, no responsibility is assumed by Elsevier, authors, editors or contributors for any injury and/or damage to persons or property as a matter of products liability, negligence or otherwise, or from any use or operation of any methods, products, instructions, or ideas contained in the material herein.

Previous editions copyrighted 2012, 2007, 2000.

Library of Congress Control Number: 2020952394

Senior Content Strategist: Charlotta Kryhl
Content Development Specialist: Grace Onderlinde
Senior Project Manager: Karthikeyan Murthy
Design: Amy Buxton
Illustration Manager: Paula Catalano
Marketing Manager: Kathleen Patton

Printed in India

Last digit is the print number: 9 8 7 6 5 4 3

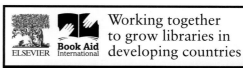

To my special partner Jennifer Stanley, an inspiration as to what vision, dedication, and perseverance, along with bottomless energy, can accomplish. She has supported me in so many ways throughout the writing of this fourth edition. I will be forever grateful.

—*Philip M. Buttaravoli*

To my wife Robyn, thank you for your ongoing support no matter what life brings our way. To Philip Buttaravoli, thank you for inviting me to be a part of the third and now fourth editions of *Minor Emergencies*.

—*Stephen Leffler*

To Drs. Phil Buttaravoli, Ruth Uphold, Steve Leffler, Ray Keller, Dave Clauss, and Peter Weimersheimer, the physician leaders in Emergency Medicine who blazed the trail of academic growth at the University of Vermont while fulfilling our clinical mission.

—*R. Ramsey Herrington*

List of Contributors

Daniel Ackil, DO, FAAEM
Assistant Professor
Division of Emergency Medicine
Larner College of Medicine at the University of
    Vermont
Burlington, VT
USA

Daniel Barkhuff, BS, MD
Assistant Professor
Division of Emergency Medicine
Larner College of Medicine at the University of
    Vermont
Burlington, VT
USA

Mark Bisanzo, MD, DTMH
Associate Professor
Division of Emergency Medicine
Larner College of Medicine at the University of
    Vermont
Burlington, VT
USA

Kevin J. Brochu, PA-C
Clinical Instructor, Larner College of Medicine
    at the University of Vermont
Physician Assistant Student Coordinator
University of Vermont Medical Center,
    Emergency Services
Clinical Preceptor, Franklin Pierce University
Community Faculty, Massachusetts College of
    Pharmacy and Health Sciences
Boston, MA
USA

Philip M. Buttaravoli, MD, FACEP
Emergency Physician
Emergency Department
Veteran's Administration Medical Center
West Palm Beach, FL
Adjunct Assistant Professor
Division of Emergency Medicine
Larner College of Medicine at the University of
    Vermont
Burlington, VT
USA

Katherine Dolbec, MD, CAQSM
Assistant Professor
Division of Emergency Medicine
Larner College of Medicine at the University of
    Vermont
Burlington, VT
USA

Kurt Eifling, MD, FAWM
Adjunct Clinical Instructor
Division of Emergency Medicine, University of
    Arkansas for Medical Sciences
Northwest Arkansas
Fayetteville, AR
USA

Deborah Governale, MMsC, PA-C
Physician Assistant in Emergency Medicine
University of Vermont Medical Center
Burlington, VT
USA

Nicholas J. Koch, MD
Director of Simulation Education
Assistant Professor
Division of Emergency Medicine
Larner College of Medicine at the University of
    Vermont
University of Vermont Medical Center
Burlington, VT
USA

Skyler Lentz, MD
Assistant Professor
Division of Emergency Medicine and Division
of Critical Care Medicine
Larner College of Medicine at the University of
Vermont
Burlington, VT
USA

Evie Marcolini, MD
Associate Professor
Emergency Medicine and Neurology
Geisel School of Medicine at Dartmouth
Hanover, New Hampshire
USA

Mariah McNamara, MD, MPH
Associate Professor
Division of Emergency Medicine
Department of Surgery
University of Vermont
Larner College of Medicine
Burlington, VT
USA

Nathaniel Moore, MBA, FAWM, PA-C
Physician Assistant in Emergency Medicine
University of Vermont Medical Center
Burlington, VT
USA

Laurel B. Plante, MD, FACEP
Assistant Professor
Division of Emergency Medicine
Larner College of Medicine at the University of
Vermont
Burlington, VT
USA

Joe Ravera, MD
Assistant Professor
Division of Emergency Medicine
Director of Pediatric Emergency Medicine
Surgery—Division of Emergency Medicine
University of Vermont Medical Center
Burlington, VT
USA

Jessica Russell, PA-C
Physician Assistant in Emergency Medicine
University of Vermont Medical Center
Burlington, VT
USA

Matthew S. Siket, MD, MS, FACEP
Associate Professor
Division of Emergency Medicine
Larner College of Medicine at the University of
Vermont
Burlington, VT
USA

Stephen J. Skinner, MD
Assistant Professor
Division of Emergency Medicine
Larner College of Medicine at the University of
Vermont
Burlington, VT
USA

Alison Sullivan, MD, MS
Assistant Professor
Division of Emergency Medicine
University of Vermont Medical Center
Burlington, VT
USA

Katherine A. Walsh, MD
Assistant Professor
Division of Emergency Medicine
Division of Emergency Department
University of Vermont Medical Center
Burlington, VT
USA

Katie M. Wells, MD, MPH
Director, International Emergency Medicine
Division Director, Diversity, Equity, and Inclusion
Assistant Professor
Division of Emergency Medicine
Larner College of Medicine at the University of
Vermont
Burlington, VT
USA

Daniel Wolfson, MD
Associate Professor
Division of Emergency Medicine
Larner College of Medicine at the University of
Vermont
Burlington, VT
USA

Foreword

Foreword to *Minor Emergencies, 4th Edition*

I could not be happier to write an introduction to the textbook *Minor Emergencies*. Diseases described here occur commonly, and most of the clinical situations presented in this book will present daily. This is the material that forms the body of an emergency medical practice. Treatment of these illnesses and injuries is the basis of an acute care practice. These are the complaints from which, if handled well, most patients recover.

During my emergency medical career, I opened the chest and crossed-clamped aortas at least 12 or 13 times. All stopped bleeding, but none of the patients lived longer than 12 hours. This is not the book for this problem. Every patient presenting with a corneal foreign body that I treated (and there were probably more than a thousand) got better. Simple, straightforward problems often can have excellent outcomes. Simple does not mean unimportant, however. Just ask the corneal foreign body patient how they felt just before and just after the topical pain medication.

In emergency medicine, as in theater acting, there are no small parts, and people who think there are do not understand the significance of their role. Patients deserve to have each complaint to be properly evaluated and treated. Proper history, correct physical examination, evaluation, and treatment are still the basis of care. To the patient and their family members doing it right always matters. To the patient's mind, there is no such thing as a minor emergency—if it is me or my family involved, I expect it to be taken seriously.

This textbook reminds us that no matter what the patient's complaint may be, calming the patient, proper evaluation, and direct approach are always best. Each medical problem discussed in this book has both psychological and physical dimensions, and both need to be addressed. The days of the omnipotent doctor are gone. Involving the patient in their care is the therapy of choice. To the patient, everything is new and frightening. Making them a partner in their care is the best technique we can use.

Gregory L. Henry, MD, FACEP
Clinical Professor
Department of Emergency Medicine
University of Michigan Medical School, Ann Arbor

Preface

Preface to the Second Edition

"Good judgment comes from experience, and a lot of that comes from bad judgment."

—Will Rogers

As a medical student at the University of Vermont in the late 1960s interested in emergency room care (this was considered peculiar at the time), I found myself disappointed that my medical education (excellent in every other way) was lacking when it came to the treatment of simple minor emergencies. I had this in mind when, in 1975, as the medical director of the emergency service at George Washington University Medical Center (and the first residency-trained emergency physician in the Washington, DC, area), I was given the opportunity to present a 1-hour lecture to their medical students on emergency medical care—"Common Simple Emergencies." (At that time, 1 hour was considered very generous for covering all of emergency medicine.)

I eventually expanded this slide show and lecture to a 6-hour series, which I presented regularly at the Georgetown University Medical Center Emergency Department. Even though there were still few published data on most of the topics covered in the lecture series, in 1985, with the help of emergency medicine attending physician Dr. Thomas Stair, I turned "Common Simple Emergencies" into a 300-page book. For the most part, the information contained within this publication was based on common practice and personal experience.

Fifteen years later, with more published data available, the book was again published under the present title and was expanded to 500 pages. The general format ("What To Do/What Not To Do") was maintained. Even with the greater volume of information, the book remained a practical guide.

Today, in stark contrast to when the original edition was published in 1985, there is a plethora of scientific data on most of the subjects covered in *Minor Emergencies*. The book has now grown to over 800 pages. In the face of the sometimes overwhelming volume of data now available, I have endeavored to continue to present these topics on minor emergencies in a manner that will still allow this larger text to be a useful and practical guide.

I have maintained the simple basic format used in the previous edition and have continued to use bold font to bring the reader's eye to the key information in each chapter. I have added red font to help identify different topics within the text. The discussions are now highlighted and compressed using small font and double columns. These changes have allowed me to make the book more complete and comprehensive, yet still allow it to remain useful at a glance.

The clinical material has all been updated, new topics have been added, and I have used evidence-based data whenever available. Many more photographs and drawings have been added (in color) to benefit the reader. In addition, I have personally reviewed the index to help ensure its usefulness and have attempted to include many identifying symptoms in the index to help users find the topic they are searching for.

I have done all of this so that you as a clinician can have more fun with your patients. When emergencies are minor, it gives you an opportunity to lighten up and enjoy the art of healing. Patients appreciate a confident clinician with a good sense of humor who can stop the pain and/or the worry, fix the problem in a compassionate way, and make them laugh through the process. This book can provide you with the information that you need to perform competently and to relax when presented with the minor emergencies that patients will always need your help with. (You will have to supply the humor.) You will be greatly rewarded for your treatment by seeing their smiling faces and hearing their expressions of gratitude after happily making them well.

Philip M. Buttaravoli, MD, FACEP

Preface to the Third Edition

To incorporate an academic element to the latest edition of *Minor Emergencies*, I have returned to my alma mater, the University of Vermont, thereby bringing the book full circle to its earliest origins. I asked Emergency Department Medical Director Stephen Leffler MD, FACEP whether he and the rest of the emergency department medical staff would be interested in updating the clinical material in *Minor Emergencies* and bringing the book into the digital age with an electronic publication that would include video displays.

Steve, along with his department staff, accepted the challenge enthusiastically.

With their involvement, this latest edition of *Minor Emergencies* should prove to be more accurate and convenient for the user. There will be periodic updates of the electronic version, and this will maintain a continuous renewal of clinical information.

The book title of this third edition has been shortened with the elimination of the subtitle "Splinters to Fractures." This subtitle was thought to be more misleading than informative, and the new abbreviated title better reflects the book's true essence.

It is my hope that this new edition will continue to provide support for all clinicians out there who are caring for the public's minor emergencies on a daily basis.

Philip M. Buttaravoli, MD, FACEP

A Note From the Authors

We have no relationships with or financial interests in any commercial companies that pertain to any of the products mentioned in this publication.

Any comments, suggestions, and/or questions can be directed to Drs. Buttaravoli and Leffler at e-med@juno.com and Stephen.Leffler@vtmednet.org under the subject heading Minor Emergencies.

Philip M. Buttaravoli, MD, FACEP
(Butter ah'voli)
Stephen Leffler, MD, FACEP

Preface to the Fourth Edition

After having won first place in the surgical division of the British Medical Association book awards, we believe there is no reason to change the basic formula for success that we created in the third edition. Over time, though, it does become necessary to inform our readers of the new developments in the field of minor emergencies.

To bring the fourth edition up to date, Dr. Leffler and I have brought Dr. Ramsey Herrington on board as an additional lead author. Dr. Herrington is the chairman of the Department of Emergency Medicine at the University of Vermont Medical Center, where he has been instrumental in establishing a new Emergency Medicine Residency Program.

The emergency physician members of this new program have been key participants in contributing to the update of the fourth edition's new and established chapters. The basic format has stayed the same, and the book should remain a practical guide for both seasoned practitioners and those health care workers who are just starting their careers in emergency medicine, urgent care, and/or family practice.

This will be the last time that I will be actively involved with the publication of *Minor Emergencies*, and I can only hope that I have helped to fill in a small niche that was initially missing from our medical education. I thank everyone who has seen the value in treating minor emergencies with the respect that they deserve.

Philip M. Buttaravoli, MD, FACEP

Acknowledgments

We have enjoyed the special opportunity to work with Nani Clansey, who has always been a delight to work with and has been most informative and supportive in the creation of this fourth edition. In addition, it has been a pleasure working with the extremely competent, efficient, and hardworking assistance of Charlotta Kryhl, Commissioning Editor, and Karthikeyan Murthy, Project Manager, at Elsevier.

Also, special thanks to the contributing emergency department medical staff at the University of Vermont who will be taking over full responsibility for updating future editions of this publication.

Contents

PART 3
Ear, Nose, and Throat Emergencies 105
■ Katie M. Wells and Deborah Governale

PART 4
Oral and Dental Emergencies 175
■ Daniel Wolfson and Nathaniel Moore

PART 5
Pulmonary and Thoracic Emergencies   245
■ Alison Sullivan and Katherine A. Walsh

PART 6
Gastrointestinal Emergencies   267
■ Daniel Ackil and Nicholas J. Koch

PART 7
Urologic Emergencies   327
■ Laurel B. Plante and Stephen J. Skinner

PART **10**
Soft Tissue Emergencies   587

■ Philip M. Buttaravoli and Kevin J. Brochu

PART **11**
Dermatologic Emergencies 703
■ Mark Bisanzo and Kurt Eifling

Appendices

Video contents

The videos can be accessed through the Elsevier eBook (details on inside front cover), and via QR codes in the chapters.

PART 1

Neurologic and Psychiatric Emergencies

■ Evie Marcolini ■ Matthew S. Siket

Acute Dystonic Drug Reaction

Presentation

The patient with a dystonic reaction to a neuroleptic or other agent typically presents to the emergency department (ED) or urgent care center with posturing, facial grimacing and involuntary muscle movements, and/or difficulty speaking. Pain is minimal, if at all. The jaw, tongue, lip, throat, and neck muscles are frequently involved. Hyperextension and lateral deviation of the neck along with upward gaze is a classic presentation (Fig. 1.1). Often no history is available. The patient may not be able to speak, may not be aware of taking any phenothiazines or butyrophenones (e.g., Haldol that has been used to cut heroin), may not admit to using an illicit drug or psychotropic medication, or may not make the connection between the symptoms and drug use (e.g., one dose of Compazine given to treat nausea or vomiting). The drugs that are most likely to produce a classic dystonic reaction are prochlorperazine (Compazine), haloperidol (Haldol), chlorpromazine (Thorazine), promethazine (Phenergan), and metoclopramide (Reglan), but the list is long and includes some common agents such as benzodiazepines and antihistamines. Acute dystonia usually presents with one or more of the following types of symptoms:

Buccolingual—protruding or pulling sensation of the tongue

Torticollis—twisted neck or facial muscle spasm

Oculogyric—roving or deviated gaze

Tortipelvis—abdominal rigidity and pain

Opisthotonic—severe hyperextension of entire spinal column

Acute dystonia can resemble partial seizures, the posturing of psychosis, or the spasms of tetanus, strychnine poisoning, or electrolyte imbalance.

More chronic neurologic side effects of phenothiazines, including the restlessness of akathisia, tardive dyskinesia, and parkinsonism, do not usually respond as dramatically to drug treatment as does acute dystonia. Onset of oculogyric crisis and torticollis reactions usually

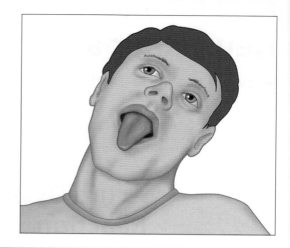

Fig. 1.1 Patient with dystonic drug reaction.

occurs within a few minutes or hours but may occur 12 to 24 hours after treatment with a high-potency neuroleptic such as haloperidol.

What to Do

✓ **Maintain a high degree of suspicion** for involvement of an offending drug even when the patient does not volunteer such an exposure. Do the required detective work to reveal any chance of the intake of one of the suspected drugs.

When such a suspicion is confirmed:

○ **Administer 1 to 2 mg of benztropine (Cogentin) intravenously (IV)/intramuscularly (IM) or 25 to 50 mg of diphenhydramine (Benadryl) IV/IM,** and watch for improvement of the dystonia over the next 5 minutes. Usually the medication begins to work within 2 minutes of IV administration, and the symptoms completely resolve within 15 minutes. **This step is both therapeutic and diagnostic.** Benztropine produces fewer side effects (mostly drowsiness) and may be slightly more effective, but diphenhydramine is more likely to be available in the ED or urgent care center.

✓ Benztropine may be given to children older than 3 years of age at the dose of 0.02 to 0.05 mg/kg IV, IM, or orally. Diphenhydramine may be given to pediatric patients age 2 to 11 years at 1 to 2 mg/kg IM/IV every 6 to 8 hours as needed, max dosing 50 mg/dose and up to 300 mg/day; orally for patients less than 6 years old is not recommended; 6 to 12 years, 25 mg or 5 to 10 mL orally every 4 to 6 hours.

✓ **Instruct the patient to discontinue use of the offending drug** and arrange for follow-up if medications must be adjusted. **If the culprit is long acting, prescribe benztropine 1 to 2 mg orally twice a day × 2 to 3 days for adults, or diphenhydramine 25 mg orally every 6 hours for 24 to 72 hours to prevent a relapse.**

✓ **Pediatric patients should be admitted for monitoring if a long-acting agent has been ingested.**

What Not to Do

❌ Do not immediately begin a comprehensive diagnostic workup. It may not be necessary. If findings are typical, administer benztropine or diphenhydramine first to see if symptoms completely resolve.

❌ Do not confuse dystonia with tetanus, seizures, stroke, psychosis, meningitis, or dislocation of the mandible. None of these will resolve with IV benztropine or diphenhydramine.

❌ Do not persist with treatment if the response is questionable or there is no response. Continue with the workup to find another cause for the dystonia (e.g., tetanus, seizures, hypomagnesemia, hypocalcemia, alkalosis, neuromuscular disease).

❌ Do not use a benzodiazepine to relieve the dystonia. Recognize that a benzodiazepine may resolve spasms from many agents, but it will not help to diagnose a neuroleptic agent as the cause.

Discussion

Dystonic reactions have been reported in 10% to 60% of patients treated with a neuroleptic medication, most commonly when patients just start or increase the dose of the drug or the drug is administered too rapidly through the IV route. Patients with a family history of dystonia, patients with recent use of cocaine or alcohol, younger patients, male patients, and patients already being treated with agents such as fluphenazine or haloperidol are at higher risk for a dystonic reaction.

Dystonia is idiosyncratic, not the result of a drug overdose. The extrapyramidal motor system depends on excitatory cholinergic and inhibitory dopaminergic neurotransmitters, the latter being susceptible to blockage by phenothiazine and butyrophenone medications. Anticholinergic medications restore the excitatory–inhibitory balance. **One IV dose of benztropine or diphenhydramine is relatively innocuous, rapidly diagnostic, and probably justified to be used as an initial step in the treatment of any patient with a dystonic reaction.** IM administration may take as long as 30 minutes before an effect is seen.

Suggested Readings

Jhee, S. S. (2003). Delayed onset of oculogyric crisis and torticollis with intramuscular haloperidol. *Annals of Pharmacotherapy, 37,* 1434–1437.

Lee, A. S. (1979). Treatment of drug-induced dystonic reactions. *Journal of the American College of Emergency Physicians, 8,* 453–457.

Marano, M., di Biase, L., Salomone, G., et al. (2016). The clinical course of a drug-induced acute dystonic reaction in the emergency room. *Tremor and Other Hyperkinetic Movements, 6,* 436. PMID 28105387.

Heat Illness

(Heat Syncope, Heat Cramps, Heat Exhaustion)

Presentation

Heat illnesses comprise a spectrum of illnesses resulting from failure of the body's normal thermoregulatory mechanisms after exposure to excessive heat. Most heat-related illness is mild; however, severe hyperthermia associated with heat stroke, neuroleptic malignant syndrome, or serotonin syndrome is a severe, life-threatening condition and should not be overlooked.

The milder forms of heat-related illness include heat syncope (or presyncope), or heat cramps. These illnesses are usually found after prolonged exposure to excessive heat and humidity in patients who are unable to remove themselves from the situation.

Heat syncope is postural syncope or presyncope related to excessive heat exposure.

Heat cramps are painful muscle cramps after vigorous exertion in hot environments (often several hours later) in the calves, thighs, and/or shoulders.

Heat exhaustion is a slightly more severe form of heat illness, but is easily treated with hydration and cooling. Elderly patients (without air-conditioning on a hot, humid day), workers, or athletes (exerting themselves in a hot climate while taking in an inadequate amount of fluid) may be more symptomatic, with fatigue, weakness, lightheadedness, headache, nausea, and vomiting in addition to orthostatic symptoms and painful muscle spasms. **The patient may have a normal temperature (but generally >38 °C), or the temperature may be elevated to 40 °C (104 °F), with tachycardia, clinical evidence of dehydration, and (often, especially with exertion) profuse sweating. Mental status is normal.**

Another minor form of heat stress is heat edema, which occurs in elderly individuals and consists of swelling of the feet and ankles in response to extreme heat. Miliaria, also known as heat rash or prickly heat, is common in hot and humid climates and presents with small, red, pruritic papules that result from plugging of sweat gland ducts.

The severe forms of heat-related illness, such as heat stroke, are characterized by alteration in mental status associated with hyperthermia (temperature >40.5 °C). Neuroleptic malignant syndrome and serotonin syndrome are not typically classified as heat-related illnesses but present with severe hyperthermia and altered mental status and can be easily confused with heat stroke.

What to Do

✓ **Assess and monitor all patients with minor heat illness for the development of heat stroke.** This is a much more serious form of heat illness, **accompanied by a core temperature** of greater than 40 °C and altered mental status that can lead to delirium, seizures, or coma.

✅ **Remove patients with any form of heat illness from the hot environment. Clothing should be removed to promote cooling, and a temperature obtained (rectally, if possible).**

✅ Obtain a careful history from the patient or witnesses, with special attention to the type and length of heat exposure, recent hydration and nutrition, any underlying medical problems, and any medications being used that might predispose the patient to developing heat illness.

✅ Perform a physical examination, noting abnormal vital signs, signs of associated medical illness, evidence of dehydration, and/or diaphoresis.

✅ **For heat syncope or presyncope, remove the patient from the source of heat, allow patient to rest, and administer oral or intravenous rehydration.** Evaluate for any injury resulting from a fall, and **all potentially serious causes of syncope should be considered** (see Chapter 11).

✅ **For isolated heat cramps**, provide muscle stretching and massage, and administer an oral electrolyte solution (0.5 tsp table salt in 1 quart of water) or intravenous normal saline for rapid relief.

✅ **For heat exhaustion, provide intravenous rehydration with normal saline or a glucose-in-hypotonic saline solution, such as D5 in .45% sodium chloride (1 L over 30 minutes). Obtain serum sodium, potassium, glucose, magnesium, calcium, and phosphorus levels, as well as hematocrit, blood urea nitrogen, and creatinine levels. Correct electrolyte abnormalities appropriately.** Avoid rapid correction of hypernatremia, as this can cause cerebral edema.

✅ **With temperature above 40 °C, and normal mental status, spray or sponge the patient with tepid or warm water (to prevent shivering) and then fan to enhance evaporation and cooling.** Refrigerated gel packs or ice packs may be applied to the forehead, neck, axillae, and groin. Ice water immersion is most effective for rapid cooling but poorly tolerated in most patients (especially elderly patients).

✅ **If not treated properly, heat exhaustion may evolve to heatstroke, a major medical emergency that may lead to cardiac arrhythmias, rhabdomyolysis, serum chemistry abnormalities, disseminated intravascular coagulation, irreversible shock, and death.** Core or rectal temperature monitoring, physical examination, and laboratory analysis should provide the correct diagnosis.

✅ **When a mild form of heat illness responds successfully to treatment**, with vital signs returning to normal and symptoms relieved, the patient may be discharged with instructions on how to avoid future episodes and advised to continue adequate fluid intake over the next 24 to 48 hours. Elderly and mentally ill patients and their caregivers should be encouraged to maintain adequate fluid intake to prevent recurrence. Those who must work in a hot environment with high humidity should be encouraged to acclimate themselves over several weeks. Successive increments in the level of work performed in a hot environment result in adaptations that eventually allow a person to work safely at levels of heat that were previously intolerable or life threatening.

✅ Elderly patients and their caretakers, as well as parents of small children, should be educated about high-risk situations and instructed about putting limits on activity during hot and humid days.

✅ **Admission should be considered for any patient who presents with altered mental status, heat stroke, or altered electrolytes and elderly patients who have chronic medical problems, significant electrolyte abnormalities, or risk for recurrence. All patients who are treated but do not have a complete resolution of their symptoms over several hours should also be admitted.**

What Not to Do

❌ Do not do a comprehensive laboratory workup on young, healthy patients with minimal symptoms or minor heat-related illness.

❌ Do not use pharmacologic agents that are designed to accelerate cooling. None have been found to be helpful. The role of antipyretic agents in heat illness has not been evaluated.

❌ Do not continue therapeutic cooling techniques after the temperature reaches 38.5 °C. Beyond this point, continued active cooling may result in hypothermia.

❌ Do not recommend salt tablets to prevent heat illness. Fluid losses during exercise are much greater than electrolyte losses.

❌ Do not overlook the possibility of neuroleptic malignant syndrome and serotonin syndrome with patients who have recently begun taking neuroleptic drugs or serotonergic agents.

Discussion

Hyperthermia, defined as a core temperature above 40 °C, may present with sweating, flushing, tachycardia, fatigue, lightheadedness, headache, and paresthesia, progressing to weakness, muscle cramps, oliguria, nausea, agitation, hypotension, syncope, confusion, delirium, seizures, and coma. Mental status changes and core temperature distinguish potentially fatal heat stroke from heat exhaustion.

Control of thermoregulation resides within the hypothalamus, which stimulates cutaneous vasodilation and sweating through the autonomic nervous system in response to elevation of blood temperature. Blood flow to the skin may increase 20-fold. Cooling normally occurs by transfer of heat from the skin by radiation, convection, and evaporation. As the ambient temperature exceeds the body's temperature, a rise in body temperature may occur in response to radiation and convection of heat from the environment. When the humidity rises, the body's ability to cool through evaporation is diminished.

Dehydration and salt depletion impair thermoregulation by reducing the body's ability to increase cardiac output needed to shunt heated blood from the core circulation to the dilated peripheral circulation. Cardiovascular disease and use of medications that impair cardiac function can also result in increased susceptibility to heat illness.

Although athletes are commonly thought to be most at risk for heat illness, children and the elderly, poor, and socially isolated are particularly vulnerable.

Compared with adults, children produce proportionately more metabolic heat, have a greater surface area-to-body mass ratio (which causes a greater heat gain from the environment on a hot day), and have a lower sweating capacity, which reduces their ability to dissipate heat through evaporation. These facts emphasize the importance of monitoring heat exposure in children. A fatal event can occur within 20 minutes if normal heat loss mechanisms become overwhelmed. Every year, children left unattended in parked motor vehicles die from heat stroke.

Both children and young adults (most often athletes and laborers) are vulnerable to exertional heat illness, where there has been intense strenuous activity in a hot, humid environment. Elderly, chronically ill, or sedentary adults, as well as children, are vulnerable to nonexertional heat illness. Environmental

Discussion continued

conditions, along with a predisposition for impaired thermoregulation, lead to heat illness in these patients. The elderly and infirm may have diminished cardiac output, a decreased ability to sweat, and decreased ability to vasoregulate. Medications may predispose them to heat illness because of mitigating effects on cardiac output (beta blockers) or on sweating (anticholinergics) or because of volume depletion (diuretics). Nonexertional heat illness may be indolent in its onset and may be associated with significant volume depletion.

Heatstroke is a serious form of heat illness. Treatment, especially aggressive cooling procedures and fluid replacement, must begin immediately to help ensure survival. Morbidity and mortality are directly associated with the duration of elevated core temperature. More intensive evaluation and treatment are required for these patients than is covered in this chapter. The most serious complications of heat stroke are those falling within the category of multiorgan dysfunction syndrome. They include encephalopathy, rhabdomyolysis, acute renal failure, acute respiratory distress syndrome, myocardial injury, hepatocellular injury, intestinal ischemia or infarction, pancreatic injury, and hemorrhagic complications, especially disseminated intravascular coagulation, with pronounced thrombocytopenia.

Suggested Readings

American Academy of Pediatrics. (2000). Climatic heat stress and the exercising child and adolescent. *Pediatrics*, *106*(1 Pt 1), 158–159.

Bouchama, A., & Knochel, J. P. (2002). Heat stroke. *New England Journal of Medicine*, *346*, 1978–1988.

Cheshire, W. P. (2016). Thermoregulatory disorders and illness related to heat and cold stress. *Autonomic Neuroscience: Basic and Clinical*, *196*, 91–104.

Wexler, R. K. (2002). Evaluation and treatment of heat-related illnesses. *American Family Physician*, *65*(2307–2314), 2319–2320.

Hyperventilation

Presentation

The patient presenting with hyperventilation syndrome typically appears anxious and exhibits shortness of breath with an inability to fill the lungs adequately. The patient also may have palpitations, dizziness, intense anxiety, fear, chest or abdominal pain, tingling or numbness around the mouth and fingers, and possibly even flexor spasm of the hands and feet (carpopedal spasm) (Fig. 3.1). The patient's respiratory volume is increased, which may be apparent as increased respiratory rate, increased tidal volume, or frequent sighing. The remainder of the physical examination is unremarkable. The patient's history may reveal a precipitating emotional cause or prior similar events. The patient may experience alternating periods of hypoventilation or brief periods of apnea as the body tries to allow carbon dioxide (CO_2) levels to drift back up to the normal range. If this occurs, the pattern is usually abrupt onset of transient apnea without a drop in O_2 saturation, immediately preceded and followed by profound hyperventilation.

What to Do

✓ Perform a brief physical examination, specifically evaluating mental status and listening to breath sounds. Evaluate for evidence of toxins, leg swelling, or other risk factors for pulmonary emboli such as tachycardia or fever.

✓ **Measure pulse oximetry,** which should be between 98% and 100%, and utilize end-tidal capnometry to guide treatment.

✓ **Calm and reassure the patient.** Evaluate the patient's ability to follow instructions, and encourage deep, slow breathing. If possible, determine the trigger, if any, to help address the etiology of the event.

✓ **If the patient cannot voluntarily reduce ventilatory rate and volume**, **breathing through a length of tubing** (Fig. 3.2) **or a reservoir bag with supplemental oxygen may be utilized.** This will allow the patient to continue moving a large quantity of air but will provide air rich in carbon dioxide (CO_2), allowing the blood partial CO_2 (PCO_2) to rise toward normal. **Administration of 50 to 100 mg of hydroxyzine (Vistaril) intramuscularly (IM) or lorazepam (Ativan) 1 to 2 mg sublingually (SL), IM, or intravenously (IV) often helps to calm the patient, resulting in a reduced respiratory effort.**

✓ **If these symptoms cannot be reversed and respiratory effort cannot be reduced in this manner within 15 to 20 minutes, confirm the diagnosis by obtaining arterial blood gas measurements to rule out metabolic acidosis or hypoxia indicative of underlying disease.**

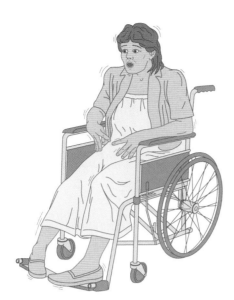

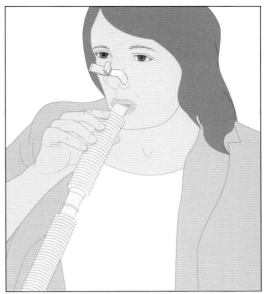

Fig. 3.1 The patient experiences anxiety and shortness of breath and feels as though she is unable to fill her lungs, leading to carpopedal spasm.

Fig. 3.2 Instruct the patient to breathe through a length of tubing to increase the percentage of inspired CO_2.

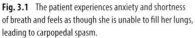 Reexamine the patient after hyperventilation is controlled. If possible, identify the psychological stressor that prompted the episode.

Ensure that the patient understands the hyperventilation syndrome and knows some strategies for breaking the cycle next time. Arrange for follow-up with a primary care physician.

What Not to Do

Do not overlook the true medical emergencies, including pneumothorax, asthma, chronic obstructive pulmonary disease (COPD), pneumonia, pulmonary embolus, hyperthyroidism, diabetic ketoacidosis, liver disease, salicylate overdose, sepsis, uremia, substance abuse, sympathomimetic toxidrome, myocardial infarction, congestive heart failure (CHF), and stroke, which also may present with hyperventilation.

Do not use the traditional method of breathing into a paper bag to increase the concentration of inspired CO_2. This increases the potential for inadvertently causing hypoxia and is no longer considered to be appropriate therapy.

Do not do an extensive laboratory and imaging study workup when the history and physical examination are convincingly consistent with psychogenic hyperventilation syndrome. However, be suspicious of an organic cause when the patient has risk factors or does not improve as expected.

Discussion

The acute respiratory alkalosis of hyperventilation causes transient imbalances of calcium, potassium, and other ions, with the net effect of increasing the irritability and spontaneous depolarization of excitable muscles and nerves. Patients with a first-time event of hyperventilation syndrome are the most likely to visit the emergency department, urgent care center, or physician's office, and this is an excellent time to educate them about its

pathophysiology and the prevention of recurrence. Patients who have repeated episodes may be experiencing panic attacks, which can be addressed with cognitive therapy or a mild benzodiazepine.

During recovery after hyperventilation, the transition from hypocapnia to normocapnia is associated with hypoventilation. Be aware that patients may experience significant hypoxemia after hyperventilation.

Suggested Readings

Callaham, M. (1989). Hypoxic hazards of traditional paper bag rebreathing in hyperventilating patients. *Annals of Emergency Medicine, 18*, 622–628.

Chin, K., Ohi, M., Kita, H., et al. (1997). Hypoxic ventilatory response and breathlessness following hypocapnic and isocapnic hyperventilation. *Chest, 112*, 154–163.

Demeter, S. L., & Cordasco, E. M. (1986). Hyperventilation syndrome and asthma. *American Journal of Medicine, 81*, 989–994.

Saisch, S. G. N., Wessely, S., & Gardner, W. N. (1996). Patients with acute hyperventilation presenting to an inner-city emergency department. *Chest, 110*, 952–957.

Psychogenic Nonepileptic Attack

(Dissociative Convulsions)

Presentation

The patient with psychogenic nonepileptic attack (PNEA), also known as psychogenic nonepileptic seizure (PNES), typically presents with the appearance of having tonic-clonic seizure activity or can develop this during a visit.

There may be a history of sexual abuse, eating disorders, depression, substance abuse, anxiety disorders, or personality disorders, and the episode may be preceded by a stressful event. The terminology "pseudoseizure" or "hysterical seizure" is outdated and considered counterproductive as it may give the patient the perception that medical professionals consider this faked or voluntary behavior. Head turning from side to side and pelvic thrusting are common with PNEA, and it may be difficult to determine initially whether the patient is manifesting a true epileptic seizure.

A patient with true seizures usually has abdominal contractions but lacks corneal reflexes, whereas a patient with PNEA usually has corneal reflexes but lacks abdominal contractions. The patient's general color and vital signs are normal, without any evidence of airway obstruction. Consciousness is often partially preserved and sometimes regained very quickly after the convulsive period with PNEA. Commonly, the patient is fluttering the eyelids or resists having the eyes opened. With eyelids closed, a patient with rapid (saccadic) eye movements is awake. On the other hand, a patient with slow, roving eye movements may have a depressed level of consciousness. Tearfulness during the event argues against epileptic seizure (ES). Ictal eye closure is a highly reliable indicator for PNES, while ictal eye opening is generally an indicator of ES.

With PNEA, there is typically no fecal or urinary incontinence, self-induced injury, or lateral tongue biting. Most true seizures are accompanied by a postictal state of disorientation and altered level of arousal and responsiveness. During an epileptic seizure, the plantar response is often extensor, whereas during a PNEA event it is usually flexor.

Noxious stimuli are not reliable in discriminating between PNEA and epileptic seizure. The remainder of the physical examination should be unremarkable.

What to Do

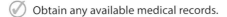 Obtain any available medical records.

Perform a complete physical examination, including a full set of vital signs and O$_2$ saturation. Patients under the stress of real illness or injury can manifest unusual behavior that may be misinterpreted as seizurelike activity.

✅ **Check glucose with a bedside finger stick.**

✅ **Monitor vital signs frequently.**

✅ **When there is significant emotional stress involved, administer a mild tranquilizing agent, such as hydroxyzine pamoate (Vistaril), 50 to 100 mg intramuscularly (IM), or lorazepam (Ativan), 1 to 2 mg intravenously (IV) or IM.**

✅ **Consider obtaining a drug screen** and ask if the patient is safe at home, or has been abused in any way. **In women, consider ordering a pregnancy test.**

✅ **If an epileptic seizure is questionable, verify with a lactate level or blood gas analysis, which should show metabolic acidosis with a true epileptic seizure.**

✅ **When the patient becomes more responsive,** reassess, obtain a complete history, and offer follow-up care, including psychological support, if appropriate. PNEA is commonly associated with sexual abuse, eating disorders, depression, substance abuse, anxiety disorders, and personality disorders.

✅ **If the patient is not awake, alert, and oriented after about 15 minutes, begin a more comprehensive medical workup.** Illnesses to consider include Guillain-Barré syndrome, myasthenia gravis, electrolyte disorders, hypoglycemia, hyperglycemia, renal failure, occult neoplasm, dysrhythmias, systemic infection, toxins, and other neurologic disorders.

What Not to Do

❌ Do not accuse the patient of faking a seizure. Even if the activity is not an epileptic seizure, it is neither voluntary nor is it within the patient's ability to physically control.

❌ Do not attempt to discriminate between PNEA and epileptic seizure with painful stimuli, or by dropping a patient's hand onto the face. These are not discriminatory and may reinforce the patient's history of personal abuse and mistrust of medical professionals.

❌ Do not administer anticonvulsants when PNEA is suspected.

❌ Do not routinely perform extensive workups or become overly aggressive by intubating these patients.

❌ Do not release the patient who has not fully recovered. Instead, the patient must be fully evaluated for an underlying medical problem, which may require hospital admission.

Discussion

PNEA is more common in women than men. In most cases, this represents an involuntary manifestation of psychosocial distress. Antagonizing the patient often prolongs the condition, whereas ignoring the patient seems to take the spotlight off the peculiar behavior, allowing the patient to recover. Some psychomotor or complex partial seizures are difficult to diagnose because of dazed confusion or fuguelike activity and might be labeled as PNEA. The patient might require an electroencephalogram (EEG), administered during sleep, and deserves a referral to a neurologist.

Epilepsy is a common disorder. Psychogenic nonepileptic attack (PNEA) is one of the epilepsy mimics. Video EEG is now the gold standard tool that differentiates between epileptic seizures (ES) and PNEA. Oxygen saturation (SaO_2) and ictal vital signs, including heart rate (HR), respiration rate (RR), body temperature, systolic blood pressure (SBP), and diastolic blood pressure, show crucial changes during ES and PNEA.

The key to successful treatment is earning the trust of the patient to help encourage evaluation and treatment by a behavioral health specialist. This starts with recognizing the patient's symptoms as involuntary and respecting the patient as having true disease that requires a coordinated effort by the larger medical community.

Suggested Readings

Badry, R. (2020). Changes in vital signs during epileptic and psychogenic nonepileptic attacks: A video-EEG study. *Journal of Clinical Neurophysiology*, *37*(1), 74–78.

Benbadis, S. R. (2004). Photo quiz: The value of tongue laceration in the diagnosis of blackouts. *American Family Physician*, *70*, 1757–1758. http://www.aafp.org/afp/20041101/photo.html.

Bounds, J. A. (2007). Ictal eye closure is a reliable indicator for psychogenic nonepileptic seizures. *Neurology*, *68*(12). https://doi.org/10.1212/01.wnl.0000259662.87864.f9.

Dula, D. J., & DeNaples, L. (1995). Emergency department presentation of patients with conversion disorder. *Academic Emergency Medicine*, *2*, 120–123.

Glick, T. H., Workman, T. P., & Gaufberg, S. V. (2000). Suspected conversion disorder: Foreseeable risks and avoidable errors. *Academic Emergency Medicine*, *7*, 1272–1277.

Kaufman, K. R. (2004). Pseudoseizures and hysterical stridor. *Epilepsy and Behavior*, *5*, 269–272.

Reuber, M., Baker, G. A., Smith, D. F., et al. (2004). Failure to recognize psychogenic nonepileptic seizures may cause death. *Neurology*, *62*, 834–835.

Tolchin, B., Martino, S., & Hirsch, L. (2019). Treatment of patients with psychogenic nonepileptic attacks. *JAMA*, *321*(20), 1967–1968.

Viarasilpa, T., Panyavachiraporn, N., Osman, G., et al. (2019). Intubation for psychogenic non-epileptic attacks: Frequency, risk factors, and impact on outcome. *Seizure*, *76*, 17–21.

Idiopathic Facial Paralysis (Bell Palsy)

Presentation

The patient with Bell palsy can present with any of the following signs or symptoms: sudden onset of facial numbness; a feeling of fullness or swelling; periauricular pain; muscular facial asymmetry; an irritated, dry, or tearing eye; drooling; or changes in hearing or taste. Symptoms can develop over several hours or days. Often there will have been a viral illness 1 to 3 weeks earlier, or there may have been another trigger such as stress, fever, dental extraction, or cold exposure. Initial presentation typically includes an isolated partial or complete unilateral facial paralysis in an otherwise alert patient (Fig. 5.1). It is notable that if the forehead paralysis is bilateral, the diagnosis of central cause (stroke) must be considered.

What to Do

✅ Perform a thorough neurologic examination of the cranial and upper cervical nerves and limb strength, noting which nerves are involved and whether unilaterally or bilaterally. **Ask the patient to wrinkle the forehead, close the eyes forcefully, smile, puff the cheeks, and whistle, observing closely for facial asymmetry. Central or cerebral lesions result in relative sparing of the forehead** because of cross-innervation of the orbicularis oculi and frontalis muscles. Check for tearing, eyelid closure, hearing, and, when practical, taste. Observe for corneal desiccation. Examine the ear canal and pinna for herpetic vesicles and the tympanic membrane for signs of otitis media or cholesteatoma.

✅ **Patients with facial paralysis accompanied by acute otitis media, chronic suppurative middle-ear disease, mastoiditis, otorrhea, or otitis externa require emergent otolaryngologic consultation.**

✅ Facial weakness progressing to paralysis over weeks to months, progressive twitching, or facial spasm suggests a neoplasm affecting the facial nerve.

✅ When facial paralysis is associated with pulsatile tinnitus and hearing loss, suspect a glomus tumor or cerebellar pontine angle tumor.

✅ Diplopia, dysphagia, hoarseness, facial pain, or hypesthesia suggests involvement of cranial nerves other than the seventh and calls for neurologic consultation with early magnetic resonance imaging (MRI).

✅ If there is a history of head trauma, obtain a computed tomography (CT) scan of the head (including the skull base) or an MRI to rule out a temporal bone fracture.

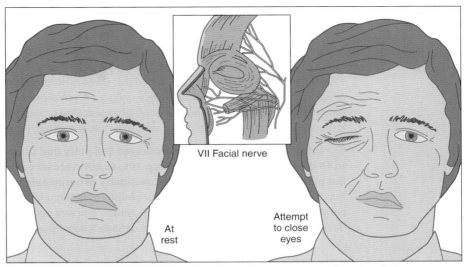

VII Facial nerve

At rest

Attempt to close eyes

Fig. 5.1. Partial or complete unilateral facial paralysis that includes one side of the forehead in Bell palsy.

✓ MRI with contrast of the skull can reveal lesions, even of small dimensions, inside the temporal bone and at the cerebellopontine angle.

✓ **When the findings are consistent with Bell palsy and when there are no absolute contraindications to steroid use, begin therapy with prednisone, 60 mg once daily for 5 days and tapering by 10 mg per day afterward.** Prednisone is the only treatment shown to reduce the risk for long-term sequelae of Bell palsy.

✓ Although there is only controversial data to support its efficacy—but because the most widely accepted cause of a true Bell palsy, at present, is a neuropathy induced by herpes simplex virus—**when a patient presents within 7 to 10 days of the onset of acute paresis (or paralysis) and symptoms are severe and no other cause is suspected, it is reasonable to prescribe a 10-day course of either acyclovir (Zovirax), 400 mg five times per day, or 5 days of the more expensive valacyclovir (Valtrex), 500 mg twice daily.** There is some evidence to suggest that treatment within 3 days of the onset of symptoms with combined acyclovir and prednisone therapy may be most beneficial. Again, this is most likely to have the most gain in patients with a complete lesion because they have a higher risk for prolonged facial weakness or other sequelae.

✓ **If the cornea is dry or likely to become dry or injured as a result of the patient's inability to produce tears and blink, protect it by patching. If patching is not necessary, recommend that the patient wear eyeglasses, apply methylcellulose artificial tears regularly during the day, and use a protective bland ointment or tape the eyelid shut at night.**

✓ When there is a history of a tick bite or rash that is consistent with erythema migrans in areas where Lyme disease is endemic, a doxycycline, 100 mg once daily for 14 days, is indicated. Amoxicillin, 500 mg three times a day for 14 to 21 days, is usually substituted for pregnant women. Cefuroxime, 500 mg twice daily for 14 to 21 days, and azithromycin, 500 mg once daily for 5 days, have also been used successfully but are generally less effective.

✅ If the cause appears to be herpes zoster varicella or shingles of the facial nerve (e.g., grouped vesicles on the tongue), acyclovir or valacyclovir should still be effective (see Chapter 172). If the geniculate ganglion is involved (i.e., Ramsay Hunt syndrome, with vesicles in or around the ear, decreased hearing, severe otalgia, encephalitis, meningitis), the patient may require hospitalization for intravenous (IV) treatment. The prognosis of Ramsay Hunt syndrome is much worse than that of Bell palsy, with only 10% recovering normal function.

✅ **Inform the patient with uncomplicated Bell palsy that symptoms may progress for 7 to 10 days. Of patients with Bell palsy, 70% to 80% recover completely within a few weeks, but patients should be aware of the possibility of permanent facial weakness.** Be aware that prognosis is linked to the severity of symptoms. Although most (94%) patients with a partial paralysis recover fully, approximately 40% with a complete paralysis at the time of presentation have some residual weakness. Provide for definite follow-up and reevaluation.

What Not to Do

❌ Do not overlook alternative causes of facial palsy that require different treatment, such as cerebrovascular accidents and cerebellopontine angle tumors (which usually produce weakness in limbs or defects of adjacent cranial nerves), multiple sclerosis (which usually is not painful, spares taste, and often produces intranuclear ophthalmoplegia), and polio (which presents as fever, headache, neck stiffness, and palsies).

❌ Do not order a CT scan unless there is a history of trauma or the symptoms are atypical and include such findings as vertigo, central neurologic signs, or severe headache.

❌ Do not immediately assume that all unilateral facial paralysis is idiopathic facial paralysis. Bell palsy is not likely in patients who report gradual onset of facial paralysis over several weeks or facial paralysis that has persisted for 3 months or more. These patients require further evaluation by a neurologist or an otolaryngologist.

Discussion

Idiopathic nerve paralysis is a common malady, affecting 1 in 60 persons over the course of a lifetime, especially diabetic or pregnant patients and those between the ages of 15 and 45 years. Up to 10% of patients have a recurrence on the ipsilateral or contralateral side. The facial nerve is responsible for facial muscle innervation; lacrimal, nasal, and submandibular gland innervation; taste for the anterior two-thirds of the tongue; and sensation of the external auditory canal, pinna, and tympanic membrane. Although Bell palsy was described classically as a pure facial nerve lesion, and physicians have tried to identify the exact level at which the nerve is compressed, the most common presenting complaints are related to trigeminal nerve involvement. The mechanism is probably a spotty demyelination of several nerves at several sites caused by reactivated herpes simplex virus. Genetic, metabolic, autoimmune, vascular, and nerve entrapment etiologies have been proposed without definitive proof. **Corticosteroids have been shown to improve recovery, and antivirals have demonstrated improved recovery only in severe cases. Eye protection is important for every patient.**

Suggested Readings

Adour, K. K., Ruboyianes, J. M., Von Doersten, P. G., et al. (1996). Bell's palsy treatment with acyclovir and prednisone compared with prednisone alone: A double-blind, randomized, controlled trial. *Annals of Otology, Rhinology & Laryngology, 105*, 371–378.

Almeida, J. R., et al. (2014). Management of Bell palsy: Clinical practice guideline. *Canadian Medical Association Journal, 186*(12), 917–922.

Austin, J. R., Peskind, S. P., Austin, S. G., et al. (1993). Idiopathic facial nerve paralysis: A randomized double-blind controlled study of placebo versus prednisone. *The Laryngoscope, 103*, 1326–1333.

Baringer, J. R. (1996). Herpes simplex virus and Bell's palsy (editorial). *Annals of Internal Medicine, 124*, 63–65.

Baumgarten, K. L., Lopez, A. A., & Pankey, G. A. (1999). Rash, Bell's palsy, and back pain following a flu-like illness. *Infectious Medicine, 16*(370–372), 378–379.

Becelli, R. (2003). Diagnosis of Bell palsy with gadolinium magnetic resonance imaging. *Journal of Craniofacial Surgery, 14*, 51–54.

Grogan, P., & Gronseth, G. (2003). Practice parameter: Steroids, acyclovir, and surgery for Bell's palsy (an evidence-based review). Report of the quality standards subcommittee of the American Academy of Neurology. *Neurology, 56*, 830–836.

Hato, N., Matsumoto, S., Kisaki, H., et al. (2003). Efficacy of early treatment of Bell's palsy with oral acyclovir and prednisolone. *Otology & Neurotology, 24*, 948–951.

Murakmi, S., Mizobuchi, M., Nakashiro, Y., et al. (1996). Bell's palsy and herpes simplex virus: Identification of viral DNA in endoneural fluid and muscle. *Annals of Internal Medicine, 124*, 27–30.

Ronthal, M. (2011). *Bell's palsy: Prognosis and treatment.* UptoDate. http://www.uptodate.com.

Smith, G. N., et al. (2020). Committee Opinion No. 399: Management of tick bites and Lyme disease during pregnancy. *Journal of Obstetrics and Gynaecology (Canada), 42*(5), 644–653.

Stankiewicz, J. A. (1987). A review of the published data on steroids and idiopathic facial paralysis. *Otolaryngology-Head and Neck Surgery, 97*, 481–486.

Migraine Headache

Presentation

Migraine headache is one of the most disabling neurologic disorders, with a lifetime prevalence of 33% in women and 13% in men worldwide. In a third of cases, patients will have an aura, which can manifest with visual phenomena or paresthesias, typically in the hand or oral area. The headache is typically moderate to severe and can be associated with other symptoms such as photophobia, phonophobia, neck pain, nausea, emesis, and cutaneous allodynia. The headache is typically unilateral, throbbing, and worsened by movement, and it commonly lasts 1 to 24 hours or more.

Basilar-type migraine may be associated with fully reversible dysarthria, vertigo, tinnitus, decreased hearing, double vision, or ataxia. Unlike other headaches, migraines are especially likely to wake the patient in the morning. There may be a family or personal history of similar headaches, and onset during the patient's teens or 20s is common. Primary headaches, which include migraine, tension-type headache, and cluster headache, are benign; these headaches are usually recurrent and not caused by organic disease. Secondary headaches are caused by underlying organic diseases, ranging from sinusitis to subarachnoid hemorrhage.

What to Do

✅ **Treatment of migraine headache depends on timing.** Patients can take preventative treatment, such as beta blockers, antidepressants, calcium channel blockers, angiotensin-converting enzyme inhibitors, or antiseizure medication such as valproic acid. These are of variable effectiveness, and patients can also use alternative methods such as cognitive behavioral therapy or relaxation training to mitigate the occurrence of migraines.

✅ At the onset of headache, **patients can take a variety of simple analgesics, such as ibuprofen or acetaminophen, but should be warned against using these medications too often, thereby creating a medication-overuse headache.**

✅ If the migraine is moderate to severe in nature, **triptans such as sumatriptan (Imitrex), subcutaneously, 1 to 6 mg (may repeat in 1 hour), or intranasally, 1 to 2 sprays (may repeat after 2 hours); intranasal zolmitriptan (Zomig Nasal Spray), 2.5 mg (may repeat every 2 hours up to 10 mg); or any of the oral triptan agents have been shown to be very effective and are considered first-line agents.**

✅ If the patient has already used a triptan **and presents with a persistent headache, there are many options, including diphenhydramine (Benadryl), 25 to 50 mg IV, ketorolac (Toradol), 30 mg IV, magnesium (an IV infusion of magnesium sulfate), 1 to 2 g in a 10%**

solution over 5 to 10 minutes, and/or any of the antiemetics, barring any contraindications individual to the patient. With cost in mind, migraine headaches (and similar recurrent primary headache syndromes, with or without nausea and vomiting) are usually treated successfully with IV prochlorperazine (Compazine), 10 mg (0.15 mg/kg up to 10 mg for pediatric migraine headaches), or metoclopramide (Reglan), 10 mg, with or without a bolus of saline to counteract vasodilatation and orthostasis. To help prevent mental and motor restlessness (akathisia), administer diphenhydramine (Benadryl), 12 to 25 mg IV, along with the prochlorperazine or metoclopramide.

✅ If the patient has not taken a triptan, dihydroergotamine (D.H.E. 45) may be used.

✅ Opioids specifically are contraindicated in migraine as they have been shown to perpetuate medication-overuse headaches and opioid-induced hyperalgesia, even with brief administration.

✅ Intranasal 4% lidocaine (Xylocaine) is also an option for resistant migraine. Use a 1-mL syringe. Have the patient lie supine with the head hyperextended 45 degrees and rotated 30 degrees toward the side of the headache, and drip 0.5 mL (10 drops) of the lidocaine solution into the ipsilateral nostril over 30 seconds. The patient should remain in this position for 30 minutes. If the headache is bilateral, repeat on the other side. Another technique is to take 4% lidocaine jelly, apply it to a long cotton pledget, and slide it down the nasal canal using bayonet forceps, posterior to the middle turbinate on the side of the headache. The clinician should be aware that the evidence for the effectiveness of intranasal lidocaine in the acute treatment of migraine is inconsistent.

✅ Clinicians must consider medication efficacy, potential side effects, and potential medication-related adverse events when prescribing acute medications for migraine.

✅ If there are persistent changes in mental status, fever, or stiff neck, or on neurologic examination focal findings such as diplopia or unilateral hyperreflexia, paresthesias, weakness, or ataxia, consider CT, lumbar puncture (LP), or both to rule out intracranial pathology or infection as the cause of the so-called migraine.

✅ Other danger signals that should trigger a more intensive diagnostic workup, looking for secondary disorders, include hyperacute onset of a new severe headache ("the worst ever"); a progressive history of seizures; onset with exertion, cough, bending, or sexual intercourse; onset during pregnancy (cerebral venous thrombosis); and the presence of a systemic malignant disease, infection, compromised immune system, any new neurologic findings, or papilledema on funduscopic examination.

✅ In patients who are older than age 50 years, consider the possibility of temporal arteritis and obtain an erythrocyte sedimentation rate (ESR). If temporal arteritis is present, there may be jaw claudication and tenderness over the temporal artery.

✅ Instruct the patient to return to the emergency department or clinic if there is any change in or worsening of the usual migraine pattern and make arrangements for medical follow-up.

✅ First-time migraine attacks warrant a thorough elective neurologic evaluation to establish the diagnosis.

✅ Long-term prophylaxis may include nonprescription plain magnesium gluconate (200–400 mg three times a day), antidepressants, calcium channel antagonists, nonsteroidal anti-inflammatory drugs (NSAIDs), beta blockers, or anticonvulsants. Lifestyle changes, such as eliminating caffeine, smoking, and certain food triggers, may also be indicated.

What Not to Do

(X) Do not begin a comprehensive laboratory workup with neuroimaging when the patient presents with a typical benign primary headache with no neurologic deficits.

(X) Do not administer medications containing ergotamine, caffeine, or barbiturates. They are not recommended for continual prophylaxis. They are not effective when used in this manner, and withdrawal from these drugs may actually produce headaches.

(X) Do not fail to provide a definite follow-up appointment, especially for first attacks.

(X) Do not fail to consider the possibility of meningitis, subarachnoid hemorrhage, glaucoma, or stroke; conditions that may deteriorate rapidly if undiagnosed. Patients with subarachnoid hemorrhage who have normal mental status on presentation are at highest risk for misdiagnosis. Do not talk yourself out of doing a CT/LP in any patient with sudden onset (hyperacute) of the worst headache ever just because the patient looks good or has a normal examination.

Discussion

Unilateral pain is even more characteristic of migraine than is the aura. (Migraine is a corruption of the hemicrania continua.) The pathophysiology is probably unilateral cerebral vasospasm (producing the neurologic symptoms of the aura), followed by vasodilation (producing the headache). Neurologic symptoms may persist into the headache phase, but the longer they persist, the less likely it is that they are caused by the migraine. Cluster headaches and other trigeminal-autonomic cephalalgias are characterized by trigeminal activation coupled with parasympathetic activation. These headaches are intermittent, short lasting, sharp, excruciating, and unilateral, accompanied by lacrimation and rhinorrhea. Attacks occur in clusters lasting from 7 days to 1 year, and during the pain, patients are usually agitated and restless. The treatment of an attack is usually the same as that for migraines.

Acute migraine headaches are self-limited and respond well to placebos, and therefore several different therapies are effective. No single drug or class of drug has clearly emerged as the best treatment for acute migraine. The wide variability in patient needs and responses means that many agents will continue to play important roles. Although butalbital-containing compounds are often used to treat migraine, their use should be limited because of the risk of overuse and consequent medication overuse headache and withdrawal problems.

Be cautious in the use of ergot or serotonin agonists to treat any patient who has angina, focal weakness, or sensory deficits. It is possible to precipitate ischemia of the brain or heart in such patients by using preparations that act by causing vasoconstriction. Sumatriptan should not be administered to postmenopausal women, men older than 40 years, and patients with vascular risk factors such as hypertension, hypercholesterolemia, obesity, diabetes, smoking, or a strong family history of vascular disease. Sumatriptan also should not be used within 24 hours of administration of an ergotamine-containing medication.

Fortunately, new options for the acute treatment of migraine attacks are currently in development. As new acute medications become available, it will be important for health care professionals to be aware of current patterns and limitations to medication use and to tailor their approach for migraine treatment to the individual patient, including identifying the appropriate use/combination of acute and preventive pharmacologic and nonpharmacologic treatments.

Discussion continued

Patients with aneurysms or arteriovenous malformations can present clinically as migraine patients. If there is something different about the severity or nature of this headache, consider the possibility of a subarachnoid hemorrhage. Headaches that are always on the same side and in the same location are very suspicious for an underlying structural lesion (e.g., aneurysm, arteriovenous malformation).

To help reassure patients, it can be noted that isolated headache was the first and only clinical symptom in just 8.2% of patients with an intracranial tumor.

Opioids are commonly requested for headache but dangerous in migraine as they can induce hyperalgesia, prevent reversal of migraine central sensitization, and decrease the effectiveness of triptans, which are otherwise a mainstay.

Suggested Readings

Aukerman, G., Knutson, D., & Miser, W. F. (2002). Management of the acute migraine headache. *American Family Physician*, *66*, 2123–2130 2140–2141.

Becker, W. J. (2015). Acute migraine treatment in adults. *Headache*, *55*(6), 778–793.

Brousseau, D. C., Duffy, S. J., Anderson, A. C., et al. (2004). Treatment of pediatric migraine headaches: A randomized, double-blind trial of prochlorperazine versus ketorolac. *Annals of Emergency Medicine*, *43*, 256–262.

Cameron, J. D., Lane, P. L., & Speechley, M. (1995). Intravenous chlorpromazine vs intravenous metoclopramide in acute migraine headache. *Academic Emergency Medicine*, *2*, 597–602.

Charles, A. (2017). The pathophysiology of migraine: Implications for clinical management. *The Lancet Neurology*, *17*, 1–9.

Clinch, C. R. (2001). Evaluation of acute headaches in adults. *American Family Physician*, *63*, 685–692.

Coppola, M., Yealy, D. M., & Leibold, R. A. (1995). Randomized, placebo-controlled evaluation of prochlorperazine versus metoclopramide for emergency department treatment of migraine headache. *Annals of Emergency Medicine*, *26*, 541–546.

Corbo, J., Esses, D., Bijur, P. E., et al. (2001). Randomized clinical trial of intravenous magnesium sulfate as an adjunctive medication for emergency department treatment of migraine headache. *Annals of Emergency Medicine*, *38*, 621–627.

Demirkaya, S., Dora, B., et al. (2001). Efficacy of intravenous magnesium sulfate in the treatment of acute migraine attacks. *Headache*, *41*, 171–177.

Dodick, D. W. (2018). Migraine. *Lancet*, *391*, 1315–1330.

Drotts, D. L., & Vinson, D. R. (1999). Prochlorperazine induces akathisia in emergency patients. *Annals of Emergency Medicine*, *34*, 469–475.

Ferrari, M. D., et al. (2001). Oral triptans (serotonin 5-HT 1B/1D agonists) in acute migraine treatment: A meta-analysis of 53 trials. *Lancet*, *358*, 1668.

Frank, L. R., Olson, C. M., Shuler, K. B., et al. (2004). Intravenous magnesium for acute benign headache in the emergency department. *Canadian Journal of Emergency Medicine*, *6*, 327–332.

Huff, J. S. (1998). What is a migraine, anyway, and when is it gone? *Academic Emergency Medicine*, *5*, 561–562.

Hutchinson, S., Lipton, R. B., Ailani, J., et al. Characterization of acute prescription migraine medication use. *Mayo Clinic Proceedings*, *95*(4), 709–718.

Kabbouche, M. A., Vockell, A. B., LeCates, S. L., et al. (2001). Tolerability and effectiveness of prochlorperazine for intractable migraine in children. *Pediatrics*, *107*, e62.

Kao, L. W., Kirk, M. A., Evers, S. J., et al. (2003). Droperidol, QT prolongation, and sudden death: What is the evidence? *Annals of Emergency Medicine*, *41*, 546–558.

Klapper, J. A., & Stanton, J. (1993). Current emergency treatment of severe migraine headaches. *Headache*, *33*, 560–562.

Lipton, R. B., Bigal, M. E., Steiner, T. J., et al. (2004). Classification of primary headaches. *Neurology*, *63*, 427–435.

Maizels, M., Scott, B., Cohen, W., et al. (1996). Intranasal lidocaine for treatment of migraine. *Journal of the American Medical Association*, *276*, 319–321.

Marmura, M. J., Silberstine, S. D., & Schwedt, T. J. (2015). The acute treatment of migraine in adults: The American Headache Society evidence assessment of migraine pharmacotherapies. *Headache*, *55*(1), 3–20.

Matchar, D. B. (DATE). Acute management of migraine. Paper presented at the 55th Annual Meeting of the American Academy of Neurology, Honolulu, Hawaii.

Mauskop, A., Altura, B. T., Cracco, R. Q., et al. (1996). Intravenous magnesium sulfate rapidly alleviates headaches of various types. *Headache*, *36*, 154–156.

Miner, J. R., Fish, S. J., Smith, S. W., et al. (2001). Droperidol vs prochlorperazine for benign headaches in the emergency department. *Academic Emergency Medicine*, *8*, 873–879.

Salomone, J. A., Thomas, R. W., Althoff, J. R., et al. (1994). An evaluation of the role of the ED in the management of migraine headaches. *American Journal of Emergency Medicine*, *12*, 134–137.

Seim, M. B., March, J. A., & Dunn, K. A. (1998). Intravenous ketorolac vs intravenous prochlorperazine for the treatment of migraine headaches. *Academic Emergency Medicine*, *5*, 573–576.

Silvers, S. M., Simmons, B., Wall, S., et al. (2002). Clinical policy: Critical issues in the evaluation and management of patients presenting to the emergency department with acute headache. *Annals of Emergency Medicine*, *39*, 108–122.

Tabata bai, R. R., & Swadron, S. P. (2016). Headache in the emergency department: Avoiding misdiagnosis of dangerous secondary causes. *Emergency Medicine Clinics of North America*, *34*, 695–716.

Tepper, S. (2012). Opioids should not be used in migraine. *Headache*, *52*(Suppl. 1), 30–34.

Vinson, D. R. (2002). Treatment patterns of isolated benign headache in US emergency departments. *Annals of Emergency Medicine*, *39*, 215–222.

Vinson, D. R., & Drotts, D. L. (2001). Diphenhydramine for the prevention of akathisia induced by prochlorperazine: A randomized, controlled trial. *Annals of Emergency Medicine*, *37*, 125–131.

Weaver, C. S., Jones, J. B., & Chisholm, C. D. (2004). Droperidol vs. prochlorperazine for the treatment of acute headache. *Journal of Emergency Medicine*, *26*, 145–150.

Adult Seizures

Presentation

The patient with seizure may present in full tonic-clonic seizure or may have experienced a seizure witnessed by others. Seizure may be preceded by an aura or have sudden onset without warning. Most patients presenting with seizure have a preexisting seizure disorder, and the most common etiology of seizure is noncompliance with medication. Two of the most telling physical exam findings of a patient who has had a seizure include incontinence and lateral tongue biting, but the lack of these signs does not rule out seizure.

What to Do

✓ Many seizures are self-limiting, but if a patient is actively seizing, prepare to administer a benzodiazepine, usually lorazepam (Ativan), either intravenously (IV) or intramuscularly (IM). Observe the seizure activity for patterns, such as eye deviation and/or focal/unilateral presentation.

✓ First-line agents and dosing include the following:

○ **1–4 mg IV lorazepam (Ativan)**
○ 5–10 mg IV/IM/PR diazepam (Valium) max 5 mg/min (max dose 30 mg)
○ 1–5 mg IV/IM/PR midazolam (Versed)

✓ **With a prolonged seizure resistant to initial agents, loading with phenytoin (Dilantin) or fosphenytoin (Cerebyx) is recommended to prevent recurrence of seizures. Give phenytoin, 18 to 20 mg/kg IV over 30 minutes, at less than 50 mg/min. (The patient should be on cardiac monitoring during administration, and a Dilantin level should be sent first if the patient is thought to be taking the drug.)** Alternatively, give fosphenytoin, 15 to 20 PE/kg IV or IM at a maximum IV rate of 150 PE (phenytoin sodium equivalents)/min with an initial maintenance dose of 4 to 6 PE/min. (Although much more expensive than phenytoin, fosphenytoin can be given more quickly over 15 minutes, or, if IV access is absent, this drug can be given IM; it does not have the tissue toxicity of extravasated phenytoin if IV access is questionable.)

✓ **If the patient is still seizing, third-line agents are indicated, including barbiturates, valproate, levetiracetam, and/or propofol in the setting of endotracheal intubation.**

✓ **Status epilepticus** is defined as a generalized tonic-clonic seizure in an adult that lasts more than 5 minutes or intermittent convulsions, without recovery of baseline level of consciousness between seizures.

✅ **In all cases of status epilepticus, check the patient's blood glucose level by performing a quick finger stick test and administering IV glucose if the level is below normal.**

✅ **If the patient arrives in the postictal phase**, examine thoroughly for injuries and signs of systemic disease that can provoke seizures. Elevated temperature can be a sign of meningitis or encephalitis. Nuchal rigidity strongly suggests either central nervous system (CNS) infection or subarachnoid hemorrhage. Record a complete neurologic examination. Repeat the neurologic examination periodically, looking for findings suggestive of focal brain disease.

✅ **If the patient is indeed recovering**, you may be able to obviate much of the diagnostic workup by waiting until the patient is lucid enough to give a history. **Postictal inability to arouse may last 10 minutes after a generalized tonic-clonic seizure, with confusion typically lasting less than 30 minutes.**

✅ **If the patient arrives awake and oriented after a presumed seizure**, corroborate the history through witness accounts or the presence of injuries, such as a scalp laceration, a bitten tongue, or the presence of urinary or fecal incontinence.

✅ **Consider other etiologies of altered mental status if there is no typical postictal recovery period.**

✅ Investigate for alcohol or substance abuse; withdrawal from alcohol, benzodiazepines, or barbiturates can provoke seizures.

✅ **If the patient has a history of seizure disorder or is taking anticonvulsant medications**, determine current and past frequency of seizures. Look for evidence of and reasons for noncompliance, such as loss of insurance or ability to obtain medications.

✅ **If the seizure is clearly related to alcohol withdrawal, give 2 mg of IV lorazepam (Ativan) and ascertain why the patient reduced consumption of alcohol.** Support the patient's attempt to abstain or detoxify with resources as possible.

✅ **If a patient is demonstrating signs of delirium tremens**, such as tremors, tachycardia, and hallucinations, withdrawal should be medically supervised and treated with benzodiazepines. Initial treatment with IV lorazepam has been shown to produce a significant reduction in the risk for recurrent seizures related to alcohol.

✅ Because many alcoholics are malnourished, emergency department physicians will often presumptively treat alcohol withdrawal symptoms with an IV infusion containing glucose, 100 mg of thiamine, 2 g of magnesium, 1 mg of folic acid, and multivitamins, even though there is no convincing evidence that this regimen is of any true benefit in isolated alcohol withdrawal. However, **thiamine has been shown to be beneficial in preventing coma and death as a result of Wernicke encephalopathy in patients presenting with altered mental status.** Administration of thiamine and vitamins is inexpensive and has very few side effects. Given this, it is advisable to treat alcoholic patients presenting with acute delirium for both alcohol withdrawal and thiamine deficiency.

✅ **If the seizure is a new event, obtain a serum glucose level (to confirm a rapid bedside test result) as well as serum electrolyte concentrations (sodium, calcium, magnesium), renal function tests, hepatic function tests (if liver impairment is suspected), complete** blood cell count (if infection is suspected), and urine toxicology screen (if drugs of abuse are suspected). In women of childbearing age, test for pregnancy.

✓ **With new-onset seizures, a brain computed tomography (CT) scan should be performed to rule out intracranial hemorrhage, ischemic stroke, or tumor. Magnetic resonance imaging (MRI) is the gold standard in evaluating seizure disorders and should be obtained when available.**

✓ **Lumbar puncture should be performed when** fever, persistent altered mental status, or nuchal rigidity indicates a possibility of meningitis or encephalitis. Suspicion of subarachnoid hemorrhage should also prompt lumbar puncture, even when head CT scans are normal. A lumbar puncture should also be performed on immunocompromised patients.

✓ **About 50% of all patients with a new onset of seizure require hospitalization.** Most of these patients can be identified by abnormalities evident on physical examination, head CT scan, toxicology studies, or the other tests mentioned earlier.

✓ **If the patient has an established seizure disorder, blood tests are not routinely needed when the patient has a single breakthrough seizure. Anticonvulsant drug levels should be checked when toxicity or noncompliance is suspected.** The dose should be adjusted to keep the level above the breakthrough point. Finding a level below the reported therapeutic range should not prompt a dose increase in a patient who has been seizure free for a prolonged period. Neuroimaging and lumbar puncture are unnecessary unless there are new findings to cause suspicion for tumor, intracranial hemorrhage, or CNS infection.

✓ **A neurologist should be consulted before antiepileptic drug treatment is initiated for brief new-onset seizures.** Many neurologists think it is in the patient's best interest to withhold long-term anticonvulsant therapy until a second seizure occurs. The neurologist may want to make a detailed evaluation of, and counsel the patient regarding, risk for seizure recurrence, the advantages and disadvantages of anticonvulsant therapy, and the psychosocial effect of another seizure. **Patients with a single, brief, uncomplicated seizure, a normal neurologic examination, no comorbidity, and no known structural brain disease need not be started on any antiepileptic drug prior to outpatient referral.**

✓ **High risk for recurrence** is present when there is a history of brain insult, when an electroencephalogram (EEG) demonstrates epileptiform abnormalities, and when MRI demonstrates a structural lesion.

✓ **Patients with generalized seizures should be advised to avoid dangerous situations. They should not swim without supervision and not work at heights. Driving should also be restricted until an appropriate seizure-free period has elapsed, in consultation with a neurologist.**

What Not to Do

✗ Do not forget to check blood glucose at the bedside.

✗ Do not fail to be aggressive with the administration of benzodiazepines in the initial phase of treatment. The most common mistake is underdosing or waiting too long. The longer a seizure persists, the greater the risk of status epilepticus.

✗ Do not fail to consult neurology early if the seizure is not aborted with first-line agents.

Do not stick anything in the mouth of a seizing patient. The ubiquitous padded throat sticks may be nice for a patient to hold and to bite on at the first sign of a seizure, but they do nothing to protect the airway and are ineffective when the jaw is clenched.

 Do not fail to assume an alcoholic cause. Ethanol abusers sustain more head trauma and seizure disorders than the population at large.

 Do not treat alcohol withdrawal seizures with phenobarbital or phenytoin. Both are ineffective (and unnecessary because the problem is self-limiting) and can themselves produce withdrawal seizures.

 Do not fail to consider a psychogenic nonepileptic seizure attack (PNEA) in the differential diagnosis and treat appropriately. Do not attempt to apply a noxious stimulus to rule out epileptic seizure. If this is PNEA, it will stop spontaneously, and appropriate management should be instituted (see Chapter 4).

 Do not release a patient who has persistent neurologic abnormalities before a head CT scan or specialty consultation has been obtained.

 Do not allow a patient who experienced a seizure to drive home.

Discussion

Seizures are time-limited paroxysmal events that result from abnormal, involuntary, rhythmic neuronal discharges in the brain. Except for rare instances, seizures are not predictable and can occur at inconvenient or dangerous times. Seizures are usually short, lasting less than 5 minutes, but can be preceded by a prodromal phase and followed by a long postictal phase, during which there is a gradual return to baseline.

Epilepsy is a disease characterized by spontaneous recurrence of unprovoked seizures. Provoked seizures result from transient alterations in brain metabolism in an otherwise normal brain. Some factors that can trigger such seizures are hypoglycemia, hyponatremia, hypocalcemia, alcohol and medication withdrawal, meningitis, encephalitis, stroke, and certain toxins.

The new terminology for seizures divides them into two classes: generalized seizures and partial seizures. With generalized seizures, there is a complete loss of consciousness at onset of the seizure. Partial seizures are characterized by retained consciousness because they begin in a limited brain region. Partial seizures can secondarily generalize.

There are seven types of generalized seizures, which start throughout the entire cortex at the same time and therefore cause loss of consciousness. They are the following:

1. Generalized tonic-clonic (grand mal) seizures with a tonic phase of whole-body stiffening, followed by a clonic phase of repetitive contractions

2. Tonic seizures, which consist of only the stiffening phase

3. Clonic seizures, which consist of only the repetitive contractions

4. Myoclonic seizures, characterized by brief, lightninglike muscular jerks

5. Absence (petit mal) seizures, which are manifested as brief (1–10 seconds) episodes of staring and unresponsiveness (These seizures, unlike complex partial seizures, are rarely found in adults, are very brief, do not produce postictal confusion, and occur very frequently [up to 100 per day].)

6. Atypical absence seizures, which are similar to absence seizures but last longer and often include more motor involvement

7. Atonic seizures, characterized by sudden loss of muscle tone and subsequent falling or dropping to the floor unprotected (drop attacks) (These seizures must be differentiated from syncope [see Chapter 11].)

Partial seizures are divided into simple and complex. In simple partial seizures, only one neurologic

Discussion continued

modality is affected during the seizure. The resulting symptoms depend on the area of the brain cortex from which the seizure arises. Motor (focal) seizures may produce clonic hand movements. Sensory, autonomic, and psychiatric symptoms may be expressed as visual phenomena, olfactory sensations (usually unpleasant), déjà vu phenomena, and formed hallucinations or memories. These auras are merely simple partial seizures.

Complex partial seizures (psychomotor or temporal lobe seizures) are associated with alteration, but not loss, of consciousness. The patient is awake and staring blankly but is not responsive to external stimuli. These seizures may be accompanied by automatism (repetitive, purposeless movements, such as lip smacking and chewing, hand wringing, patting, and rubbing) and last 30 to 50 seconds. They are followed by postictal confusion and occur weekly to monthly.

The age of the patient is associated with the probable underlying cause of a first seizure and therefore is a factor in disposition. In patients age 12 to 20 years, the seizure is probably idiopathic, although other causes are certainly possible. In the 40-year-old patient experiencing a first seizure, neoplasm, posttraumatic epilepsy, and withdrawal must be excluded. In the 65-year-old patient experiencing a first seizure, cerebrovascular insufficiency must also be considered. With elderly patients, the possibility of an impending stroke, in addition to the other possible causes, should be kept in mind during treatment and workup.

Also, patients should be discharged for outpatient care only if there is full recovery of neurologic function, should possibly be given a full loading dose of phenytoin, and should make clear arrangements for follow-up or return to the emergency department if another seizure occurs. An EEG can usually be done electively, except in cases of status epilepticus. A toxic screen may be needed to detect the many drug overdoses that can present as seizures, including amphetamines, cocaine, isoniazid, lidocaine, lithium, phencyclidine, phenytoin, and tricyclic antidepressants.

Suggested Readings

D'Onofrio, G., Rathlev, N. K., Ulrich, A. S., et al. (1999). Lorazepam for the prevention of recurrent seizures related to alcohol. *New England Journal of Medicine, 340*, 915–919.

Eisner, R. F., Turnbull, T. L., Howes, D. S., et al. (1986). Efficacy of a "standard" seizure workup in the emergency department. *Annals of Emergency Medicine, 15*, 33–39.

Foreman, B., & Hirsch, L. J. (2012). Epilepsy emergencies: Diagnosis and management. *Neurology Clinics, 30*, 11–41.

Henneman, P. L., DeRoos, F., & Lewis, R. J. (1994). Determining the need for admission in patients with new-onset seizures. *Annals of Emergency Medicine, 24*, 1108–1114.

Huff, J. S., et al. (2014). Clinical policy: Critical issues in the evaluation and management of adult patients presenting to the emergency department with seizures. *Annals of Emergency Medicine, 63*, 437–447.

Jagoda, A., & Gupta, K. (2011). The emergency department evaluation of the adult patient who presents with a first-time seizure. *Emergency Medicine Clinics of North America, 29*, 41–49.

Shneker, B. F., & Fountain, N. B. (2003). Epilepsy. *Disease a Month, 49*, 426–478.

Towne, A. R., & DeLorenzo, R. J. (1999). Use of intramuscular midazolam for status epilepticus. *Journal of Emergency Medicine, 17*, 323–328.

Seizures (Convulsions, Fits), Febrile and Pediatric

Presentation

Frightened parents bring in their young child who has just had a first-ever generalized seizure with jerking tonic-clonic movements and loss of consciousness (LOC), followed by a period of postictal obtundation that gradually resolves within 30 minutes. The patient has completely recovered by the time the child is brought to your attention. The parents describe their child becoming cyanotic with breathing difficulty, unresponsiveness, and jerking eye movements during the seizure. The child may be found to have a fever, and there may be a family history of febrile seizures. A vaccination with diphtheria and tetanus toxoids and whole-cell pertussis vaccine may have been administered earlier in the day or 1 to 2 weeks following a measles, mumps, and rubella vaccination.

What to Do

In the Afebrile Child

✓ **Begin by assessing the ABCs** (airway, breathing, and circulation). Ensure hemodynamic and airway stability in your primary survey, then perform a full secondary survey.

✓ **Obtain a history of possible precipitating factors** such as trauma or toxin/drug ingestion. Inquire into recent condition(s) and medical history as well as any family history of seizure disorders.

✓ **Have witnesses describe the event in detail,** including the type of motor and eye movements, changes in breathing and skin color, and whether there was complete LOC or incontinence. Determine the duration of the seizure and the length of the postictal period.

✓ **Perform a physical examination** that includes evaluation of pupil size and reactivity, and a targeted neurologic examination, including funduscopy to look for retinal hemorrhage, which would suggest intentional injury. After the patient has experienced full recovery from the postictal state, the physical examination should be entirely normal.

✓ **Routine laboratory testing other than a screening glucose is usually not needed in children older than 6 months of age,** unless there is a history of illness, vomiting or diarrhea, or suspected ingestion.

✓ **Infants younger than 6 months of age are at particularly high risk of hypoglycemia;** fingerstick glucose testing should be performed as soon as possible. Serum sodium, calcium, and magnesium levels should also be tested to exclude electrolyte disturbance. Toxicology screening should be considered if there is suspicion of toxin exposure.

✓ **A computed tomography (CT) scan should be obtained if** there are findings of head trauma, a first-time focal (partial) seizure, continuous seizure activity lasting longer than 5 minutes, focal postictal deficits not rapidly resolving (Todd paralysis), persistently altered level of consciousness, sickle cell disease, bleeding disorders, malignancy, or human immunodeficiency virus (HIV) infection. **For most children, immediate neuroimaging is not indicated.**

✓ **Children who have one isolated unprovoked seizure**—for whom there is no suspicion of trauma, infection, or intoxication—and who have returned to their baseline state may be discharged with appropriate medical follow-up. Antiepileptic drugs (AEDs) are not prescribed.

✓ **Parents should be appropriately reassured and informed that 60% of such children never have a recurrence.** Discharge instructions should describe what to do if the seizure recurs.

✓ **If continuous seizure activity persists for more than 5 minutes, consider bag-valve-mask ventilation or intubation if there is significant respiratory compromise. Intravenous access should be placed, and a bedside glucose test performed.**

✓ **If the patient is hypoglycemic,** 0.5 to 1 g/kg of glucose should be given as a bolus (2 mL/kg of 25% dextrose in water or, in neonates, 5 mL/kg of 10% dextrose in water).

✓ **Treatment of status epilepticus should be approached similarly in pediatric and adult patients. First-line treatment should be in the form of a benzodiazepine. Preferred agents vary, depending on the route of administration:**

- ○ **With intravenous (IV) or intraosseous (IO) access:**
  - — Give lorazepam (Ativan), 0.1 mg/kg IV over 2 to 5 minutes; may repeat in 5 to 10 minutes up to a 4-mg dose (recommended treatment), or
  - — Give diazepam (Valium), 0.2 to 0.5 mg/kg IV every 15 to 30 minutes to a maximum 5-mg dose.
- ○ **Without IV or IO access:**
  - — Give lorazepam, 0.1 mg/kg per rectum up to a 4-mg dose, or
  - — Give diazepam gel (Diastat), 0.5 mg/kg per rectum up to a 10-mg dose, or
  - — Give midazolam (Versed), 0.1 to 0.2 mg/kg IM or IN × 1 up to a 10-mg dose.

✓ **If status epilepticus persists following one to two doses of a benzodiazepine,** then administer an anti-epileptic drug (AED). Note the doses for the recommended agents are generally the same (20 mg/kg) and have a longer duration of action. These are second-line agents and include the following:

- ○ Phenytoin (Dilantin), 20 mg/kg IV at less than 1 mg/kg/min up to 1000 mg
- ○ Fosphenytoin (Cerebyx), 20 mg/kg PE (phenytoin sodium equivalents) up to 1000 mg at less than 3 mg/kg/min (safety and efficacy not established for pediatric patients)
- ○ Phenobarbital, 10 to 20 mg/kg IV up to 1000 mg at less than 1 to 2 mg/kg/min
- ○ Valproate sodium (Depakote), 20 to 40 mg/kg IV over 10 min; 20 mg/kg can be given as a second dose if the patient is still seizing. Goal blood level is 100 mcg/mL and max dose is 3000 mg.
- ○ Levetiracetam (Keppra), 20 to 60 mg/kg with a maximum dose of 4500 mg over 15 minutes

✅ **Refractory status epilepticus is a life-threatening emergency and should be managed with medications that are deeply sedating and suppress overall brain activity. Intubation should generally be considered at this point.** Agents include:

- ⭕ Ketamine, 2 mg/kg bolus, followed by 0.5 to 1 mg/kg/hour
- ⭕ Midazolam (Versed), 0.1 mg/kg bolus, followed by 0.1 mg/kg/hour
- ⭕ Pentobarbital, 2 to 5 mg/kg bolus, followed by 0.5 mg/kg/hour
- ⭕ Propofol, 1 to 2 mg/kg bolus, followed by 20 mcg/kg/min

In the Febrile Child

✅ A careful history and physical examination should be done to identify a possible source of the fever and to rule out any evidence of trauma.

✅ **Children between the ages of 6 months and 5 years who have simple febrile seizures** (generalized, lasting <5 minutes and occurring only once in a 24-hour period) carry few risks for complications and do not require any routine diagnostic studies.

✅ Children with fever should be evaluated for urinary tract infection.

✅ **Lumbar puncture should be performed to exclude meningitis in patients whose level of consciousness has not returned to baseline; who have a bulging fontanel, a positive Kernig or Brudzinski sign, photophobia, severe headache, or pretreatment with antibiotics; or who are lethargic or irritable.**

✅ **Children who are younger than 6 months of age** should be evaluated for metabolic abnormalities, underlying neurologic disorders, meningitis, and encephalitis.

✅ **Antipyretics have not been found to be effective in preventing the recurrence of febrile seizures.** Benzodiazepines are also probably of no practical benefit when used for prophylaxis and may have other untoward effects.

✅ **There is no evidence that children with simple febrile seizures have any difference in cognitive outcomes than children without such seizures, and although these seizures appear frightening they are generally harmless.** Parents should be reassured and given written, detailed information about febrile seizures and then referred back to their primary care physician for follow-up.

✅ **Febrile seizures that are focal, last more than 10 minutes, or recur within 24 hours are complex febrile seizures that require a more intensive investigation and are associated with a greater risk for later epilepsy.**

What Not to Do

❌ Do not routinely perform a lumbar puncture on an afebrile child who has returned to normal mental status and has no meningeal signs or concern for central nervous system (CNS) infection.

❌ Do not do routine laboratory testing on children who are older than 6 months of age who have not been ill without vomiting or diarrhea and where there is no suspicion of a toxic ingestion.

❌ Do not start AEDs on patients with simple febrile seizures or first-time, unprovoked, uncomplicated seizures.

Discussion

Seizures are classified as either focal or generalized. Generalized seizures can be of several types: absence, atonic, tonic-clonic, tonic, myoclonic, or infantile spasms. Focal seizures were previously classified as partial/simple partial if consciousness is preserved or complex partial if LOC is impaired. Focal seizures may exhibit Jacksonian spread or "march" along the homunculus as the network of excitable neurons expands and lead to secondary generalization.

Nonepileptic episodes may be mistaken for seizures and include syncope (which may include a brief seizure with immediate awakening), breath-holding spells (which usually occur with crying until there is a noiseless state of expiration, color change, LOC, and postural tone with occasional body jerking and urinary incontinence), and night terrors (in which a child age 2 to 6 years awakens suddenly within 4 hours of falling asleep, appears frightened or confused, cries, and becomes diaphoretic, tachycardic, and tachypneic and then falls asleep and is amnestic regarding the event the following morning). Other disorders that can mimic seizures include migraine headaches (which can be accompanied by an aura, motor dysfunction, and clouding of consciousness), brief resolved unexplained event (BRUE) (which are episodes characterized by some combination of infant apnea, color change, choking, gagging, and loss of muscle tone), and psychogenic nonepileptic attack (most commonly occurring in teenage girls and usually consisting of bilateral, thrashing motor activity and rarely result in injury) (see Chapter 4).

Febrile seizures are defined as those that occur in children 6 months to 5 years of age who have fever but do not have evidence of intracranial infection or known seizure disorder.

Because most febrile seizures occur during the first 24 hours of illness, the seizure is the first sign of a febrile illness in approximately 25% to 50% of cases. Although children with febrile seizures have high mean temperatures (39.8 °C), they are not at high risk for serious bacterial illness.

Most clinicians now define status epilepticus to be continuous or repetitive seizure activity for longer than 5 minutes. Because almost all seizures stop within 5 minutes, AED therapy should be initiated for any patient with a seizure lasting longer than 5 minutes. Seizure duration of longer than 1 hour, especially with hypoxia, has been associated with permanent neurologic injury.

Overall, the risk for recurrent febrile seizures is increased in younger patients (<12 months old) with a first-time febrile seizure, patients with lower temperatures (<40 °C) on presentation of their first seizure, patients with shorter duration of fever before the seizure (<24 hours), and patients with a family history of febrile seizures.

In the general population, the risk for development of epilepsy by the age of 7 years is approximately 1%. Children who have had one simple febrile seizure have a slightly higher risk for developing epilepsy. Children who were younger than 12 months of age at their first simple febrile seizure or those who have had several simple febrile seizures have a 2.4% risk for developing epilepsy. The risk for developing epilepsy increases to 30 to 50 times that of the general population in patients who have had one or more complex febrile seizures, particularly seizures with focal features, or in a child with abnormal neurologic development.

Suggested Readings

Abend, N. S., & Loddenkemper, T. (2015). Pediatric status epileptic management. *Current Opinions in Pediatrics, 6,* 668–674.

Brophy, G. M., Bell, R., Claassen, B. R., et al. (2012). Guidelines for the evaluation and management of status epilepticus. *Neurocritical Care, 1,* 3–23.

El Radhi, A. S. (2003). Do antipyretics prevent febrile convulsions? *Archives of Disease in Childhood, 88,* 641–642.

Freedman, S. B., & Powell, E. C. (2003). Pediatric seizures and their management in the emergency department. *Clinical Pediatric Emergency Medicine, 4,* 195–206.

Shah, S. S., Alpern, E. R., Zwerling, L., et al. (2002). Low risk of bacteremia in children with febrile seizures. *Archives of Pediatric and Adolescent Medicine, 156,* 469–472.

Trainor, J. L., Hampers, L. C., Krug, S. E., et al. (2001). Children with first-time simple febrile seizures are at low risk of serious bacterial illness. *Academic Emergency Medicine, 8*, 781–787.

Valencia, I., Sklar, E., Blanco, F., et al. (2003). The role of routine serum laboratory tests in children presenting to the emergency department with unprovoked seizures. *Clinical Pediatrics, 42*, 511–517.

Warden, C. R., Zibulewsky, J., Mace, S., et al. (2003). Evaluation and management of febrile seizures in the out-of-hospital and emergency department settings. *Annals of Emergency Medicine, 41*, 215–222.

Tension-Type (Muscle Contraction) Headache

Presentation

The patient complains of a dull, steady (nonpulsating) pain, described as a pressing, tightening, squeezing, or constricting band, located bilaterally anywhere from the eyes to the occiput, perhaps including the neck or shoulders. Often the headache is a bilateral tightness or sensation of pressure around the temples. Most commonly, the headache develops near the end of the day or after some particularly stressful event. The severity should progress gradually and not achieve maximum intensity within seconds to minutes of onset. There is usually no photophobia, nausea, or vomiting, although photophobia and phonophobia can occur (but not both), and the patient may have a loss of appetite. These headaches may also be associated with fatigue. Tension-type headache pain can last from 30 minutes to several days and can be continuous in severe cases. It is classified as infrequent episodic (<1 day per month), frequent episodic (1–14 days per month), or chronic (>15 days per month, occurring with or without muscle spasm). The pain may improve with rest or administration of nonsteroidal anti-inflammatory drugs (NSAIDs), acetaminophen, or other medications. The physical examination should be unremarkable, except for possible cranial or posterior cervical muscle spasm or tenderness and difficulty relaxing.

What to Do

✓ **Obtain a thorough history** by gathering a detailed description about the character and onset of symptoms. Did the pain begin abruptly and reach maximum intensity within seconds to minutes? Was there loss of consciousness at onset? Was the pain precipitated by exertion or trauma? Have there been other neurologic symptoms? Is this pain different from any other previously experienced headache? Knowing whether the character of the headache is similar to other prior headaches is more valuable than knowing if this presenting headache is the worst of the patient's life.

✓ **Perform a thoughtful physical examination** that includes both the screening and focused components of a neurologic exam. Assess for focal neurologic deficits and differentiate positive (irritative) symptoms from negative (ablative) symptoms as discussed later.

✓ **Screen patients for concerning red flag features** that should raise suspicion for dangerous secondary causes of headache and often warrant additional diagnostic workup, including neuroimaging.

○ Sudden onset headache that achieves maximum intensity within seconds to minutes suggests a thunderclap headache, which is frequently associated with dangerous causes

- ○ Altered mental status or focal neurologic deficits

- ○ New-onset headache noted in a patient of older age (>50 years) or with known pregnancy, malignancy, coagulopathy, or immunocompromised state

- ○ Fever and/or neck stiffness

- ○ Acute vision loss

✓ **When neuroimaging is indicated,** a noncontrast computed tomography (NCCT) scan of the head is most often the initial test of choice. This should be expedited in patients exhibiting any red flag signs or symptoms; however, **most patients presenting with a headache or with signs/symptoms of a tension-type headache do not require any imaging.** Occasionally, patients with concerning headache symptoms and a normal NCCT may still warrant additional imaging (either with magnetic resonance imaging [MRI] or a CT or MR angiogram or venogram).

✓ **If the headache is accompanied by fever and stiff neck or change in mental status,** infectious causes, including bacterial meningitis and encephalitis, should be considered and a lumbar puncture (LP) performed.

✓ **If there is a history or suspicion of head injury, especially in elderly patients or those on anticoagulants or with a bleeding diathesis,** obtain a CT scan to rule out an intracranial hemorrhage. Chronic alcoholic patients should be presumed to have a higher risk for coagulopathy in these circumstances.

✓ **If the temporal arteries are tender,** check for visual defects, jaw claudication, myalgias, and an elevated erythrocyte sedimentation rate, which accompany temporal arteritis.

✓ **If there is a history of recent dental work or grinding of the teeth, tenderness anterior to the tragus, or crepitus on motion of the jaw,** suspect arthritis of the temporomandibular joint.

✓ **Finally, after checking for all other causes of headache, palpate the temporalis, occipitalis, and other muscles of the calvarium and neck** to look for areas of tenderness and spasm that sometimes accompany muscle tension headaches. **Watch for especially tender trigger points** (Fig. 9.1) **that may resolve with gentle pressure, massage, or trigger-point injection (see** Chapter 121**). Such trigger-point injection may completely relieve symptoms within 5 to 10 minutes. Pain relief helps to make the diagnosis more certain.**

✓ **If a benign headache syndrome is suspected** and there are no contraindications, prescribe anti-inflammatory analgesics (e.g., ibuprofen, naproxen), recommend rest, and have the patient try applying cool compresses and massaging any trigger points. If NSAIDs are contraindicated, acetaminophen may also be effective.

✓ Arrange for follow-up. Instruct the patient to return to the emergency department or contact primary care physician if symptoms change or worsen.

What Not to Do

(X) Do not skip performing and documenting a careful history and physical examination in these patients. While patients with acute headaches may be very uncomfortable, a thoughtful history and thorough exam are key to ensuring diagnostic accuracy and resource allocation.

(X) Do not presume benign causes such as tension headache, migraine, or sinusitis without substantiated evidence on history and exam. Patients with a history of migraines may still present with dangerous secondary causes, and premature closure should be avoided especially if there are new or uncharacteristic features or other red flag signs/symptoms.

(X) Do not ignore new neurologic symptoms. The presence of new focal neurologic deficits or altered mental status should be thoroughly explored, and a reassuring NCCT does not exclude all dangerous pathology.

(X) Do not obtain neuroimaging in patients with recurrent headaches with a normal neurologic exam and no concerning red flag features, or if being performed solely for reassurance in patients not suspected of having a dangerous diagnosis.

(X) Do not discharge the patient without providing follow-up instructions. Many serious illnesses begin with minor cephalgia, and patients may postpone necessary early follow-up care if they believe that they were definitively diagnosed on their first visit.

(X) Do not prescribe opiates or barbiturates for benign headache syndromes. More effective treatments with less addictive potential exist, and controlled substances should be reserved for patients who fail these treatments or are unable to take them. This stance is supported by multiple academic societies and endorsed by the Choosing Wisely campaign.

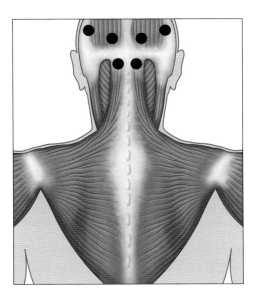

Fig. 9.1 Tension headache trigger points.

Discussion

Headaches are common and usually benign, but any headache brought to medical attention deserves a thorough evaluation. Screening tests are of little value; a complete history and physical examination are required.

Tension-type headache is not a diagnosis of exclusion but a specific diagnosis. (*Tension* refers to muscle spasm more than life stress.) Although tension-type headaches are common, the pathophysiology and likely mechanism remain unclear. The cause of these headaches is most likely multifactorial, including myofascial factors and heightened sensitivity of nerve fibers, both centrally and peripherally. Tension-type headache is frequently lumped in with migraine, as both are considered benign primary headache syndromes. Because they share some features, it is often difficult to distinguish one from the other. In fact, there seems to be support for the theory that tension-type headache and migraine are distinct entities, as well as for the suggestion that these disorders are the extremes of a continuum.

Focal tenderness over the greater occipital nerves (C2, C3) can be associated with an occipital neuralgia or occipital headache and can be secondary to cervical radiculopathy resulting from cervical spondylosis. This tends to occur in older patients and should not be confused with tension headache.

Neurologic symptoms are distinguished by positive (irritative) phenomena and negative (ablative) phenomena. Positive symptoms include the addition of an abnormal symptom such as pain, tingling, visual floaters, flashing lights, etc. These are distinct from negative symptoms, which describe the loss of a normal function or sensation, such as focal weakness, sensory loss, or vision loss. When evaluating neurologic complaints, including headache, positive symptoms are more suggestive of migraine, whereas negative symptoms may suggest a cerebrovascular cause such as stroke.

Thunderclap headaches should always be given careful attention. With rare exception, these patients warrant neuroimaging, typically starting with a NCCT since it is widely available and rapid. Thunderclap headaches are primarily concerning for subarachnoid hemorrhage (SAH), but other causes of abrupt and severe headache should be considered, including but not limited to venous sinus thrombosis, cervical artery dissection, vasoconstriction, stroke, and pituitary apoplexy.

Modern CT scanners are very sensitive for detecting intraparenchymal and subarachnoid blood, though the sensitivity declines over time, especially for small, subtle bleeds. Recent studies support that NCCT alone is sufficiently sensitive for excluding SAH if performed within 6 hours of symptom onset and a lumbar puncture may not be necessary. Patients with a very high pretest probability or with a limited scan (older generation CT or images impaired from motion artifact, etc.) or if symptoms have been ongoing for more than 6 hours should still undergo a lumbar puncture to exclude SAH.

When a lumbar puncture is performed, the presence or absence of xanthrochromia is considered the gold standard for the confirmation/exclusion of subarachnoid blood. This may take up to 12 hours to appear and may disappear after 2 weeks. Comparing the total red blood cell (RBC) count in tubes 1 and 4 is often used to determine subarachnoid versus traumatic blood, but no absolute number of RBCs in tube 4, or percent of decline from tube 1 to 4, is universally agreed upon as diagnostic. Lumbar puncture should also be performed when bacterial meningitis or encephalitis is being considered. Opening pressure is also generally indicated for patients with headache undergoing a lumbar puncture, especially if papilledema is noted on fundoscopy, as this may suggest idiopathic intracranial hypertension (IIH), formerly known as pseudotumor cerebri.

A CT/MR angiogram may be considered as a follow-up or alternative to lumbar puncture when SAH is suspected to exclude aneurysmal rupture. However, this may lead to the discovery of an unruptured incidental aneurysm, which is present in approximately 2% to 3% of the population. A CT/MR angiogram is also indicated if cerebral vasoconstriction is considered. A CT or MR venogram is the test of choice for sinus thrombosis.

Other causes of headache include carbon monoxide exposure from wood-burning heaters, fevers and viral myalgias, caffeine withdrawal, hypertension, glaucoma, tic douloureux (trigeminal neuralgia), and intolerance of foods containing nitrite, tyramine, or xanthine.

Suggested Readings

Cady, R. K., & Schreiber, C. P. (2002). Sinus headache or migraine? Considerations in making a differential diagnosis. *Neurology*, *58*(9 Suppl. 6), S10–S14.

Dodick, D. W. (2010). Pearls: Headache. *Seminars in Neurology*, *30*(1), 74–81.

Edlow, J. A. (2018). Managing patients with nontraumatic, severe, rapid-onset headache. *Annals of Emergency Medicine*, *71*, 400–408.

Edlow, J. A., & Caplan, L. R. (2000). Avoiding pitfalls in the diagnosis of subarachnoid hemorrhage. *New England Journal of Medicine*, *342*(1), 29–36.

Edlow, J. A., & Fisher, J. (2012). Diagnosis of subarachnoid hemorrhage: Time to change the guidelines? *Stroke*, *43*(8), 2031–2032.

Edlow, J. A., Malek, A. M., & Ogilvy, C. S. (2008). Aneurysmal subarachnoid hemorrhage: Update for emergency physicians. *Journal of Emergency Medicine*, *34*(3), 237–251.

Edlow, J. A., Panagos, P. D., Godwin, S. A., et al. (2008). Clinical policy: Critical issues in the evaluation and management of adult patients presenting to the emergency department with acute headache. *Annals of Emergency Medicine*, *52*(4), 407–436.

Goldstein, J. N., Camargo, C. A., Jr., Pelletier, A. J., et al. (2006). Headache in United States emergency departments: Demographics, work-up and frequency of pathological diagnoses. *Cephalalgia*, *26*(6), 684–690.

Loder, E., Weizenbaum, E., Frishberg, B., et al. (2013). Choosing wisely in headache medicine: The American Headache Society's list of five things physicians and patients should question. *Headache*, *53*(10), 1651–1659.

Mark, D. G., Hung, Y. Y., Offerman, S. R., et al. (2013). Nontraumatic subarachnoid hemorrhage in the setting of negative cranial computed tomography results: External validation of a clinical and imaging prediction rule. *Annals of Emergency Medicine*, *62*(1), 1–10.

Meurer, W. J., Walsh, B., Vilke, G. M., et al. (2016). Clinical guidelines for the emergency department evaluation of subarachnoid hemorrhage. *Journal of Emergency Medicine*, *50*(4), 696–701.

Perry, J. J., Sivilotti, M. L. A., Sutherland, J., et al. (2017). Validation of the Ottawa subarachnoid hemorrhage rule in patients with acute headache. *Canadian Medical Association Journal*, *189*(45), e1379–e1385.

Perry, J. J., Stiell, I. G., Sivilotti, M. L., et al. (2011). Sensitivity of computed tomography performed within six hours of onset of headache for diagnosis of subarachnoid haemorrhage: Prospective cohort study. *BMJ*, *343*, d4277.

Rinkel, G. E., Djibuti, M., Algra, A., et al. (1998). Prevalence and risk of rupture of intracranial aneurysms. *Stroke*, *29*, 251–256.

Schwedt, T. J., Matharu, M. S., & Dodick, D. W. (2006). Thunderclap headache. *The Lancet Neurology*, *5*(7), 621–631.

Tabatabai, R. R., & Swadron, S. P. (2016). Headache in the emergency department: Avoiding misdiagnosis of dangerous secondary causes. *Emergency Medicine Clinics of North America*, *34*(4), 695–716.

Vergouwen, M. D., & Rinkel, G. J. (2013). Clinical suspicion of subarachnoid hemorrhage and negative head computed tomographic scan performed within 6 hours of headache onset—no need for lumbar puncture. *Annals of Emergency Medicine*, *61*(4), 503–504.

Trivial, Minimal, and Minor Head Trauma

(Concussion)

Presentation

A patient presents after a fall from standing with a head strike. There was no loss of consciousness, but a small laceration is noted on the occiput with surrounding swelling, described by bystanders as a "goose egg." The patient complains of a dull headache and transient nausea and drowsiness. There was no seizure, vomiting, amnesia, or alteration in mental status and the patient exhibits no focal neurologic deficits on examination.

Head trauma is a common chief complaint of adult and pediatric patients presenting to the emergency department (ED), accounting for over 1.5 million visits annually, the majority of which are for minor injuries.

Trivial or minimal head injuries occur after a slight impact of a lightweight blunt object (such as a small stick) or when the calvarium is bumped against a hard surface (such as the underside of a cabinet). The forehead and occiput are common sites of impact.

Minor head injuries are common after motor vehicle accidents, sports-related injuries, and assaults. There is usually a more forceful impact, and patients may exhibit signs or characteristic **symptoms of concussion** (retrograde amnesia with or without loss of consciousness, dizziness, nausea, feeling "dazed" or "foggy," and decreased awareness of surroundings). Over the ensuing days, patients may exhibit irritability, sensitivity to light/noise, and sleep disturbances.

The term *concussion* is synonymous with mild traumatic brain injury (TBI) and is commonly used to describe the constellation of clinical symptoms after a head injury. TBI occurs as a result of sudden motion of a viscoelastic brain in a rigid cranial vault. This causes tissue strains, such as cortical contusions and compressive hematomas, as well as cellular excitotoxic injury and neuroinflammation. Accurately differentiating minor from major TBI is an important skill of the emergency clinician.

What to Do

✅ **Corroborate and record the history as given by witnesses if able.** Ascertain why the patient was injured (e.g., Was there a seizure or sudden weakness?) and rule out particularly dangerous types of head trauma. For example, a blow inflicted with a heavy pointed blunt object such as a brick or a hammer is at high risk of causing a depressed skull fracture, and a pedestrian who has been struck by a vehicle or who is victim of a violent assault is at high risk of having a serious intracranial lesion.

✅ **Begin your physical assessment** with the ABCs (airway, breathing, and circulation) and calculate the Glasgow Coma Scale (GCS). TBI is considered mild with a GCS of 13 to 15, moderate with a GCS of 9 to 12, and severe if GCS is 8 or below.

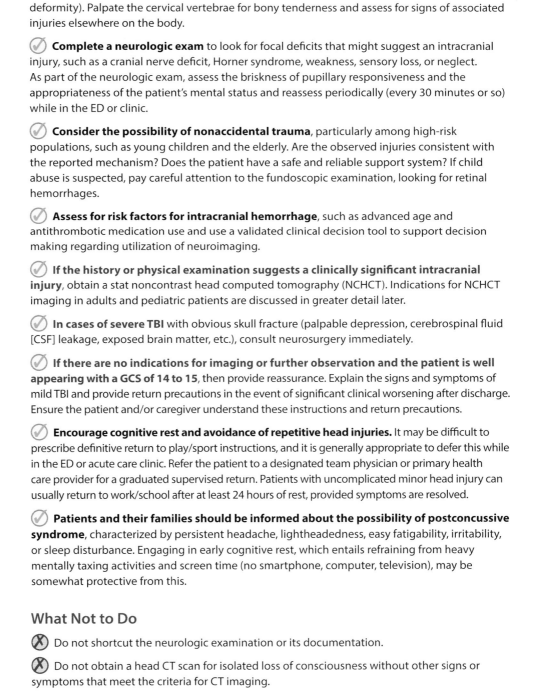

✓ Complete a thorough secondary survey and focus special attention on the head and neck. Assess for signs of skull fracture (battle sign, racoon eyes, hemotympanum, or palpable bony deformity). Palpate the cervical vertebrae for bony tenderness and assess for signs of associated injuries elsewhere on the body.

✓ **Complete a neurologic exam** to look for focal deficits that might suggest an intracranial injury, such as a cranial nerve deficit, Horner syndrome, weakness, sensory loss, or neglect. As part of the neurologic exam, assess the briskness of pupillary responsiveness and the appropriateness of the patient's mental status and reassess periodically (every 30 minutes or so) while in the ED or clinic.

✓ **Consider the possibility of nonaccidental trauma**, particularly among high-risk populations, such as young children and the elderly. Are the observed injuries consistent with the reported mechanism? Does the patient have a safe and reliable support system? If child abuse is suspected, pay careful attention to the fundoscopic examination, looking for retinal hemorrhages.

✓ **Assess for risk factors for intracranial hemorrhage**, such as advanced age and antithrombotic medication use and use a validated clinical decision tool to support decision making regarding utilization of neuroimaging.

✓ **If the history or physical examination suggests a clinically significant intracranial injury**, obtain a stat noncontrast head computed tomography (NCHCT). Indications for NCHCT imaging in adults and pediatric patients are discussed in greater detail later.

✓ **In cases of severe TBI** with obvious skull fracture (palpable depression, cerebrospinal fluid [CSF] leakage, exposed brain matter, etc.), consult neurosurgery immediately.

✓ **If there are no indications for imaging or further observation and the patient is well appearing with a GCS of 14 to 15**, then provide reassurance. Explain the signs and symptoms of mild TBI and provide return precautions in the event of significant clinical worsening after discharge. Ensure the patient and/or caregiver understand these instructions and return precautions.

✓ **Encourage cognitive rest and avoidance of repetitive head injuries.** It may be difficult to prescribe definitive return to play/sport instructions, and it is generally appropriate to defer this while in the ED or acute care clinic. Refer the patient to a designated team physician or primary health care provider for a graduated supervised return. Patients with uncomplicated minor head injury can usually return to work/school after at least 24 hours of rest, provided symptoms are resolved.

✓ **Patients and their families should be informed about the possibility of postconcussive syndrome**, characterized by persistent headache, lightheadedness, easy fatigability, irritability, or sleep disturbance. Engaging in early cognitive rest, which entails refraining from heavy mentally taxing activities and screen time (no smartphone, computer, television), may be somewhat protective from this.

What Not to Do

✗ Do not shortcut the neurologic examination or its documentation.

✗ Do not obtain a head CT scan for isolated loss of consciousness without other signs or symptoms that meet the criteria for CT imaging.

Discussion

There is no universal agreement on the definition of a concussion. One of the most popular working definitions is a trauma-induced alteration in mental status that may or may not be accompanied by a loss of consciousness. Its pathophysiologic basis remains a mystery. It is unclear whether concussion is associated with lesser degrees of diffuse structural change seen in severe TBI or if the entire mechanism is caused by reversible functional changes.

The fundamental role of the clinician in the head-injured patient is to ensure stability and differentiate mild from moderate and severe TBI. Used in conjunction with a focused neurologic examination, the GCS is a reliable tool to grade the severity of a TBI. Generally, a GCS of 13 to 15 is considered mild, though there is some debate as to whether a GCS of 13 should be considered mild or moderate.

Accurately selecting which head-injured patients warrant NCHCT imaging can be aided by the use of a clinical decision rule, such as the Canadian CT Head Rule (CCHR), New Orleans Criteria (NOC), or the NEXUS II Criteria. Comparison of these decision tools is provided in Table 10.1.

A NCHCT is generally indicated for patients of advanced age after even a seemingly minor head strike. Known physiologic changes with aging may make the geriatric brain more susceptible to injury. Reduction in overall brain mass increases the space between the brain and the skull, which increases the risk for shearing and tearing of the bridging vessels. This also allows expansion of intracranial pressure and the classic symptoms expected with this pathophysiology. The use of an antithrombotic agent (antiplatelet and/or anticoagulant) magnifies this risk.

Minor head injuries are common in the pediatric population, and the vast majority can be managed without the need for neuroimaging. The presence of neurologic deficits, an impaired mental status, signs of skull fracture, or penetrating injury warrant emergency imaging. When imaging is obtained, a NCHCT is preferred over skull radiographs (which are insensitive for intracranial abnormalities) and magnetic resonance imaging (MRI) (which is often not feasible emergently and often requires procedural sedation). The decision to obtain a NCHCT in a pediatric

patient should be made carefully, weighing the potential benefits against the risk of exposure to ionizing radiation. **Decision rules such as the Pediatric Emergency Care Applied Research Network (PECARN) algorithm can help support ED clinician decision making around imaging in pediatric head trauma.** When there is no abnormality in mental status, no clinical signs of skull fracture, no history of vomiting, no headache, or no scalp hematoma (in children ≤2 years of age), careful observation at home is an acceptable approach, with reevaluation and CT scanning for persistent or worsening symptoms. Children who are awake, alert, and asymptomatic (except when child abuse is suspected in children ≤2 years of age) do not require special imaging.

The PECARN pediatric head CT rule is unique in that the absence of symptoms identified a subset of patients that generally do not require imaging. This differs from most rules in which the presence of a criteria is an indication for imaging. The predictors of clinically significant TBI used in the PECARN rules are listed in Table 10.2.

Adult and pediatric patients with a reassuring assessment and, if indicated, reassuring imaging, can generally be safely discharged home and advised to rest. Some patients may warrant a short period of observation to assess for signs of clinical worsening. Following discharge, patients should be encouraged to engage in cognitive rest for 24 to 48 hours to theoretically lower the incidence of postconcussion syndrome, though there is a paucity of strong evidence supporting this. Postconcussion syndrome is a poorly understood phenomenon with symptoms that may include chronic headaches, dizziness, sleep disturbance, and psychological and/or cognitive changes. Gradually returning to normal mental and physical activities is a reasonable prescription.

Athletes should not be advised to return to play when still symptomatic and all patients should be strongly cautioned against risking any further head injuries. Second impact syndrome is a rare emerging phenomenon caused by a second head injury while the brain is recovering from an initial TBI. Since irreversible neurologic injury can occur from rapid cerebral edema, it is best avoided by gradually returning to sport under appropriate medical supervision.

TABLE 10.1 **Comparison of Clinical Decision Rules for Imaging in Adult Patients With Head Injury**

| Item | Clinical Decision Rule | | |
	NOC	NEXUS II	CCHR
Age cutoff (only applicable to patients below this age)	60	65	65
GCS requirement	15	15	13–15
Traumatic signs	Visible trauma above the clavicles	Skull fracture Scalp hematoma	Suspected open or depressed skull fracture Signs of basilar skull fracture
Neuro signs/Sx	Seizure	Neuro deficit	Seizure GCS <15 2 hours postinjury
Symptoms	Headache Vomiting Amnesia	Abnormal behavior Vomiting (persistent)	Vomiting >1 Amnesia >30 min prior to injury
High-risk comorbidities		Coagulopathy	Blood thinner use
Intoxication	Drug or alcohol		

CCHR, Canadian Head CT Rule; *GCS,* Glasgow Coma Scale; *NEXUS II,* National Emergency X-Radiography Utilization Study; *NOC,* New Orleans Criteria for head trauma

TABLE 10.2 **Clinical Predictors Used in the PECARN Rule. Applicable to Patients With a GCS of 15. Note the Absence of Any of These Criteria Has a High Negative Predictive Value**

Age <2 years old	Age >2 and <18 years old
Altered mental status	Altered mental status
Nonfrontal scalp hematoma	Loss of consciousness
Loss of consciousness >5 seconds	Signs of skull fracture
Severe mechanism of injury	History of vomiting
Palpable skull fracture	Severe mechanism of injury
Abnormal behavior	Severe headache

PECARN, Pediatric Emergency Care Applied Research Network

Suggested Readings

Bergman, D. A. (1999). The management of minor closed head injury in children. *Pediatrics*, *104*, 1407–1415.

Borczuk, P. (1995). Predictors of intracranial injury in patients with mild head trauma. *Annals of Emergency Medicine*, *25*, 731–736.

Collins, M. W., Lovell, M. R., & McKeag, D. B. (1999). Current issues in managing sports-related concussion. *Journal of the American Medical Association*, *282*, 2283–2285.

Cook, L. S., Levitt, M. A., Simon, B., et al. (1994). Identification of ethanol-intoxicated patients with minor head trauma requiring computed tomography scans. *Academic Emergency Medicine*, *1*, 227–234.

Davis, R. L., Hughes, M., Gubler, D., et al. (1995). The use of cranial CT scans in the triage of pediatric patients with mild head injury. *Pediatrics*, *95*, 345–349.

Hall, P., Adami, H. O., Trichopoulos, et al. (2004). Effect of low dose of ionizing radiation in infancy on cognitive function in adulthood: Swedish population-based cohort. *BMJ*, *328*, 19.

Haydel, M. J., Preston, C. A., Mills, T. J., et al. (2000). Indications for computed tomography in patients with minor head injury. *New England Journal of Medicine*, *343*, 100–105.

Holmes, J. F., Baier, M. E., Derlet, R. W., et al. (1997). Failure of the Miller criteria to predict significant intracranial injury in patients with a Glasgow Coma Scale Score of 14 after minor head trauma injury. *Academic Emergency Medicine*, *4*, 788–792.

Jagoda, A. S., Bazarian, J. J., Bruns, J. J., et al. (2008). Clinical policy: Neuroimaging and decisionmaking in adult mild traumatic brain injury in the acute setting. *Annals of Emergency Medicine*, *52*, 714–748.

Kupperman, N., Holmes, J. F., Dayan, P. S., et al. (2009). Pediatric emergency care applied research network (PECARN). Identification of children at very low risk of clinicaly-important brain injuries after head trauma: A prospective cohort study. *Lancet*, *374*, 1160–1170.

Madden, C., Witzke, D. B., Sanders, A. B., et al. (1995). High-yield selection criteria for cranial computed tomography after acute trauma. *Academic Emergency Medicine*, *2*, 248–253.

McCrory, P. R., & Berkovic, S. F. (2001). Concussion: The history of clinical and pathophysiological concepts and misconceptions. *Neurology*, *57*, 2283–2289.

Miller, E. C., Derlet, R. W., & Kinser, D. (1996). Minor head trauma: Is computed tomography always necessary? *Annals of Emergency Medicine*, *27*, 290–294.

Miller, E. C., Holmes, J. F., Derlet, R. W., et al. (1997). Utilizing clinical factors to reduce head CT scan ordering for minor head trauma patients. *Journal of Emergency Medicine*, *15*, 453–457.

Mitchell, K. A., Fallat, M. E., Raque, G. H., et al. (1994). Evaluation of minor head injury in children. *Journal of Pediatric Surgery*, *29*, 851–854.

Mower, W. R., Hoffman, J. R., Herbert, M., et al. Developing a decision instrument to guide computed tomographic imaging of blunt head injury patients. *The Journal of Trauma*, 59, 954–959.

Palchak, M. J. (2003). A decision rule for identifying children at low risk for brain injuries after blunt head trauma. *Annals of Emergency Medicine*, *42*, 492.

Poirier, M. P. (2003). Concussions: Assessment, management, and recommendations for return to activity. *Clinical Pediatric Emergency Medicine*, *4*, 179–185.

Reynolds, F. D. (2003). Time to deterioration of the elderly, anticoagulated, minor head injury patient who presents without evidence of neurologic abnormality. *The Journal of Trauma*, *54*, 492–496.

Rubin, D. M., Christian, C. W., Bilaniuk, L. T., et al. (2003). Occult head injury in high-risk abused children. *Pediatrics*, *111*, 1382–1386.

Schunk, J. E., Rogerson, J. D., & Woodward, G. A. (1996). The utility of head computed tomographic scanning in pediatric patients with normal neurologic examinations in the emergency department. *Pediatric Emergency Care*, *12*, 160–165.

Schutzman, S. A., & Greenes, D. S. (2001). Pediatric head trauma. *Annals of Emergency Medicine*, *37*, 65–74.

Shackford, S. R., Wald, S. L., Ross, S. E., et al. (1992). The clinical utility of computed tomographic scanning and neurologic examination in the management of patients with minor head injuries. *The Journal of Trauma*, *33*, 385–394.

Stiell, I. G., Wells, G. A., Vandemheen, K., et al. (1997). Variation in ED use of computed tomography for patients with minor head injury. *Annals of Emergency Medicine*, *30*, 14–22.

Stiell, I. G., Wells, G. A., Vandemheen, K., et al. (2001). The Canadian CT head rule for patients with minor head injury. *Lancet*, *357*, 1391–1396.

Vasovagal or Neurocardiogenic or Neurally Mediated Syncope

(Faint, Swoon)

Presentation

The patient experiences a brief loss of consciousness, preceded by a feeling of lightheadedness, a sense of warmth and nausea, and the awareness of passing out. This may or may not be accompanied by weakness and diaphoresis. In addition, the patient may or may not experience ringing in the ears or a sensation of tunnel vision.

First, there is a period of sympathetic tone, with increased pulse and blood pressure, in anticipation of some stressful incident, such as bad news, an upsetting sight, or a painful procedure. Immediately after or during the stressful occurrence, there is a precipitous drop in sympathetic tone and/or surge in parasympathetic tone, resulting in peripheral vasodilatation or bradycardia, or both, leading to hypotension and causing the victim to lose postural tone, fall down, and lose consciousness.

Once the patient is in a horizontal position, normal skin color, normal pulse, and consciousness return within seconds. This time period may be extended if the patient is maintained in an upright sitting position.

Transient bradycardia and a few myoclonic limb jerks or tonic spasms (syncopal convulsions) may accompany vasovagal syncope, but there are no sustained seizures, incontinence, lateral tongue biting, palpitations, dysrhythmias, or injuries beyond a minor contusion or laceration resulting from the fall. Ordinarily, the victim spontaneously revives within a brief period of time, suffers no sequelae, and can recall the events leading up to the faint.

The whole process may transpire in an emergency department or a clinic setting, or a patient may have fainted elsewhere, in which case the diagnostic challenge is to reconstruct what happened to rule out other causes of syncope.

What to Do

✅ **To prevent potential fainting spells in an Emergency Department or clinic,** arrange for anyone anticipating an unpleasant experience to sit or lie down prior to the offensive event.

✅ **If an individual faints,** catch the patient to avoid injury in the fall, lay the patient supine on the floor or stretcher for 5 to 10 minutes, protect the airway, record several sets of vital signs, and be prepared to proceed with resuscitation if the episode becomes more than a simple vasovagal syncopal episode.

✅ **If a patient is brought in after fainting elsewhere,** obtain a detailed history. Ask about the setting, precipitating factors, descriptions given by several eyewitnesses, and sequence of recovery. Look for evidence of painful stimuli (i.e., phlebotomy), emotional stress, or other unpleasant experiences such as the sight of blood.

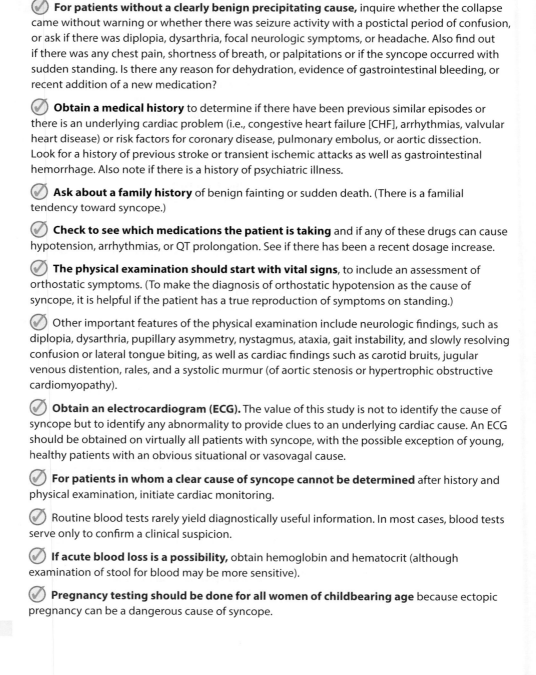 **Consider other benign precipitating causes** such as prolonged standing (especially in the heat), recent diarrhea and dehydration, or Valsalva maneuver during urination, defecation, or cough.

Determine if there were prodromal symptoms consistent with benign neurocardiogenic syncope such as lightheadedness, nausea, and diaphoresis.

For patients without a clearly benign precipitating cause, inquire whether the collapse came without warning or whether there was seizure activity with a postictal period of confusion, or ask if there was diplopia, dysarthria, focal neurologic symptoms, or headache. Also find out if there was any chest pain, shortness of breath, or palpitations or if the syncope occurred with sudden standing. Is there any reason for dehydration, evidence of gastrointestinal bleeding, or recent addition of a new medication?

Obtain a medical history to determine if there have been previous similar episodes or there is an underlying cardiac problem (i.e., congestive heart failure [CHF], arrhythmias, valvular heart disease) or risk factors for coronary disease, pulmonary embolus, or aortic dissection. Look for a history of previous stroke or transient ischemic attacks as well as gastrointestinal hemorrhage. Also note if there is a history of psychiatric illness.

Ask about a family history of benign fainting or sudden death. (There is a familial tendency toward syncope.)

Check to see which medications the patient is taking and if any of these drugs can cause hypotension, arrhythmias, or QT prolongation. See if there has been a recent dosage increase.

The physical examination should start with vital signs, to include an assessment of orthostatic symptoms. (To make the diagnosis of orthostatic hypotension as the cause of syncope, it is helpful if the patient has a true reproduction of symptoms on standing.)

Other important features of the physical examination include neurologic findings, such as diplopia, dysarthria, pupillary asymmetry, nystagmus, ataxia, gait instability, and slowly resolving confusion or lateral tongue biting, as well as cardiac findings such as carotid bruits, jugular venous distention, rales, and a systolic murmur (of aortic stenosis or hypertrophic obstructive cardiomyopathy).

Obtain an electrocardiogram (ECG). The value of this study is not to identify the cause of syncope but to identify any abnormality to provide clues to an underlying cardiac cause. An ECG should be obtained on virtually all patients with syncope, with the possible exception of young, healthy patients with an obvious situational or vasovagal cause.

For patients in whom a clear cause of syncope cannot be determined after history and physical examination, initiate cardiac monitoring.

Routine blood tests rarely yield diagnostically useful information. In most cases, blood tests serve only to confirm a clinical suspicion.

If acute blood loss is a possibility, obtain hemoglobin and hematocrit (although examination of stool for blood may be more sensitive).

Pregnancy testing should be done for all women of childbearing age because ectopic pregnancy can be a dangerous cause of syncope.

✓ **A head computed tomography (CT) scan should only be obtained in patients with focal neurologic symptoms and signs or new-onset seizure activity or to rule out hemorrhage in patients with head trauma or headache.**

✓ **Admit patients with any of the following to the hospital:**

○ A history of congestive heart failure or ventricular arrhythmias

○ Associated chest pain or other symptoms compatible with acute coronary syndrome, aortic dissection, or pulmonary embolus

○ Evidence of significant congestive heart failure or valvular heart disease on physical examination

○ ECG findings of ischemia, arrhythmia (either bradycardia or tachycardia), prolonged QT interval, or bundle branch block (BBB)

○ Concomitant conditions that require inpatient treatment

✓ **Consider admission for patients with syncope and any of the following:**

○ Age >60 years

○ History of coronary artery disease or congenital heart disease

○ Family history of unexpected sudden death

○ Exertional syncope in younger patients without an obvious benign cause for the syncope

○ A complaint of shortness of breath

○ A hematocrit of <30%

○ An initial systolic blood pressure of <90 mmHg or severe orthostatic hypotension

✓ **Patients not requiring admission** should be referred to an appropriate follow-up physician and should be instructed to avoid precipitating factors, such as extreme heat, dehydration, postexertional standing, alcohol, and certain medications. It is also reasonable to recommend an increase in salt and fluid intake to decrease syncopal episodes in the younger patient.

✓ **Referral for tilt-table testing** is appropriate when there has been recurrent, unexplained syncope without evidence of organic heart disease or after a negative cardiac workup.

✓ **After full recovery, explain to patients with classic vasovagal syncope** that fainting is a common physiologic reaction and that, in future recurrences, they can recognize the early lightheadedness and prevent a full swoon by lying down or sitting and putting their head between the knees.

✓ **Consider restricting unprotected driving, swimming, and diving for those with severe and recurrent episodes of vasovagal syncope without a trigger.**

What Not to Do

✗ Do not allow family members to stand while being given bad news, do not allow parents to stand while watching their children being sutured, and do not allow patients to stand while being given shots or undergoing venipuncture.

(X) Do not traumatize the fainting victim by using ammonia capsules, slapping, or dousing with cold water.

(X) Do not obtain a head CT scan unless there are focal neurologic symptoms and signs, unless there has been true seizure activity, or unless you have an indication to rule out intracranial hemorrhage.

(X) Do not refer patients for EEG studies unless there were witnessed tonic-clonic movements and postevent confusion.

(X) Do not obtain routine blood tests unless there is a clinical indication based on the history and physical examination.

(X) Do not refer patients with obvious vasovagal syncope for tilt-table testing.

(X) Do not routinely discharge high-risk cardiogenic syncope such as those with a history of coronary artery disease, congestive heart failure, or ventricular dysrhythmia; patients who complain of chest pain; patients who have physical signs of significant valvular heart disease, congestive heart failure, stroke, or focal neurologic disorder; or patients who have electrocardiographic findings of ischemia, bradycardia, tachycardia, increased QT interval, or BBB.

Discussion

Syncope is defined as a transient loss of consciousness and muscle tone. It is derived from the Greek word *synkoptein*, "to cut short." Presyncope is described as "the feeling that one is about to pass out."

Most commonly, the cause of syncope in young adults is vasovagal or neurocardiogenic. Observation of the sequence of stress, relief, and fainting makes the diagnosis, but, better yet, the whole reaction can usually be prevented. Although most patients suffer no sequelae, vasovagal syncope with prolonged asystole can produce seizures and rare incidents of death. The differential diagnosis of loss of consciousness is extensive; therefore loss of consciousness should not immediately be assumed to be caused by vasovagal syncope.

Several triggers may induce neurally mediated syncope, including emotional stress (anxiety; an unpleasant sight, sound, or smell) or physical stress, such as pain, hunger, dehydration, illness, anemia, and fatigue. In adolescents, symptoms of syncope may be related to the menstrual cycle or be associated with starvation in patients with eating disorders. Situational triggers include cough, micturition, and defecation.

Orthostatic hypotension is the second most common cause of syncope after neurocardiogenic syncope and is most frequently seen in the elderly. There are many causes of orthostatic hypotension,

the most common of which are hypovolemia (vomiting, diarrhea, hemorrhage, pregnancy) and drugs (antihypertensives, angiotensin-converting enzyme [ACE] inhibitors, diuretics, and phenothiazines).

Neurologic causes of syncope include seizures, transient ischemic attacks, and migraine headaches, as well as intracranial hemorrhage.

Cardiac-related syncope is potentially the most dangerous form of syncope. Patients with known cardiac disease who also experience syncope have a significantly increased incidence of cardiac-related death. The patients at risk have ischemic heart disease, most significantly congestive heart failure, congenital heart disease, and valvular heart disease (particularly aortic valvular disorder) or are taking drugs that produce QT prolongation or are known to induce torsades de pointes (i.e., amiodarone, tricyclics, selective serotonin-reuptake inhibitors [SSRIs], phenothiazines, macrolides, quinolones, and many antifungals—becoming very dangerous in combination with one another).

Brugada syndrome is a rare but potentially lethal familial dysrhythmic syndrome characterized by an ECG that shows a partial right BBB with elevation of ST segments in leads V_{1-3}, which have a peculiar down sloping with inverted T waves (Fig. 11.1).

(Continued)

Discussion continued

Danger signs for cardiac-related syncope include sudden onset without warning or syncope—preceded by palpitations as well as associated chest pain, shortness of breath—and illicit drug use. Other danger signs are postexertional syncope (think about fixed cardiac lesions) and syncope that occurred while the patient was seated or lying down.

Several risk scores have been developed to help identify those at highest risk of short-term morbidity following a syncopal event. The Canadian Syncope Risk Score (https://www.mdcalc.com/canadian-syncope-risk-score) was recently validated and differentiates patients into very low, low, medium, high, and very high risk categories. The presence of vasovagal symptoms, history of heart disease, elevated blood pressure, troponin, and ECG findings all factor into the decision aid.

Other serious causes of syncope that should be considered (and are usually accompanied by discreet signs and symptoms) are aortic dissection and rupture, pulmonary embolism, ectopic pregnancy with rupture, and carotid artery dissection.

Elderly patients have a higher percentage of underlying cardiovascular, pulmonary, and cerebrovascular disease, and therefore syncope in the elderly is more often associated with a serious problem than it is in younger patients. Myocardial infarction, transient ischemic attack, and aortic stenosis are examples of this. Carotid sinus syncope (secondary to tight collars, head turning, and shaving among others) is almost exclusively a disease of the elderly. If suspected, carotid sinus massage can confirm the diagnosis but should not be attempted if the patient has carotid bruits, ventricular tachycardia, or recent stroke or myocardial infarction. Arrhythmias, particularly bradyarrhythmias, are also more common in the elderly. For these reasons, elderly patients more often require hospitalization for monitoring and further diagnostic testing.

It should also be appreciated that elderly patients are more prone to abnormal responses to common benign situational stresses, including postural changes, micturition (exacerbated by prostatic hypertrophy in men), coughing (especially in patients with chronic obstructive pulmonary disease), and defecation associated with constipation. These abnormal responses are compounded by the effects of underlying illnesses and medications, including anticholinergics, antihypertensives (including eye drops with beta-blocker activity), and central nervous system (CNS) depressants.

Often, no single cause of syncope in the elderly can be identified. Patients improve after several small changes; however, including discontinuance of unnecessary medications, avoidance of precipitating events, and the use of support stockings or fludrocortisone (Florinef acetate), 0.05 to 0.4 mg by mouth once daily (usual: 0.1 mg by mouth once daily), for postural hypotension (off label).

(Continued)

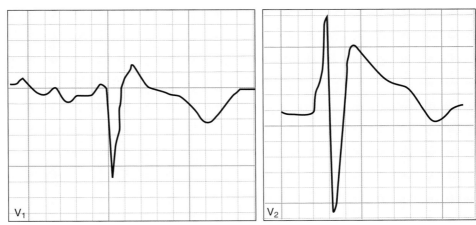

Fig. 11.1. Brugada syndrome (V_1 and V_2).

Discussion continued

Tilt-table testing has become a common component of the diagnostic evaluation of syncope. The accuracy of tilt testing is unknown, and a positive tilt test only diagnoses a propensity for neurocardiogenic events. Despite these limitations, referral for tilt-table testing can be useful in patients with recurrent, unexplained syncope and a suspected neurocardiogenic cause (a patient having typical vasovagal symptoms) but without a clear precipitant; in patients without cardiac disease or in whom cardiac testing has been negative; and in patients in whom testing clearly reproduces the symptoms.

Many pharmacologic agents have been used in the treatment of recurrent neurocardiogenic syncope. The relatively favorable natural history of neurocardiogenic syncope, with a spontaneous remission rate of 91%, makes it difficult to assess the efficacy and necessity of these drugs.

Psychiatric evaluation is recommended in young patients with recurrent, unexplained syncope without cardiac disease who have frequent episodes associated with many varied prodromal symptoms as well as other complaints.

Suggested Readings

Alegria, J. R., Gersh, B. J., & Scott, C. G. (2003). Comparison of frequency of recurrent syncope after beta-blocker therapy versus conservative management for patients with vasovagal syncope. *The American Journal of Cardiology*, *92*, 82–84.

Farwell, D. J. (2004). Does the use of syncope diagnostic protocol improve the investigation and management of syncope? *Heart*, *90*, 52.

Feinberg, A. N., & Lane-Davies, A. (2002). Syncope in the adolescent. *Adolescent Medicine*, *13*, 553–567.

Graham, D. T., Kabler, J. D., & Lunsford, L. (1961). Vasovagal fainting: A diphasic response. *Psychosomatic Medicine*, *6*, 493–507.

Lin, J. T. Y., Ziegler, D. K., Lai, C. W., et al. (1982). Convulsive syncope in blood donors. *Annals of Neurology*, *11*, 525–528.

Linzer, M., Yang, E. H., Estes, M., et al. (1997). Diagnosing syncope. I. Value of history, physical examination, and electrocardiography. *Annals of Internal Medicine*, *126*, 989–996.

Linzer, M., Yang, E. H., Estes, M., et al. (1997). Diagnosing syncope. II. Unexplained syncope. *Annals of Internal Medicine*, *127*, 76–86.

Massin, M. M., Bourguignont, A., & Coremans, C. (2004). Syncope in pediatric patients presenting to an emergency department. *The Journal of Pediatrics*, *145*, 223–228.

Quinn, J. V., McDermott, D., Stiell, I. G., et al. (2006). Prospective validation of the San Francisco syncope rule to predict patients with serious outcomes. *Annals of Emergency Medicine*, *47*, 448–454.

Quinn, J. V., Stiell, I. G., McDermott, D. A., et al. (2004). Derivation of the San Francisco syncope rule to predict patients with short-term serious outcomes. *Annals of Emergency Medicine*, *43*, 224–232.

Sarasin, F. P. (2002). Prevalence of orthostatic hypotension among patients presenting with syncope in the ED. *American Journal of Emergency Medicine*, *20*, 497–501.

Schnipper, J. L., & Kapoor, W. N. (2001). Cardiac arrhythmias: Diagnostic evaluation and management of patients with syncope. *Medical Clinics of North America*, *85*, 423–456.

Theopistou, A., Gatzoulis, K., & Economou, E. (2001). Biochemical changes involved in the mechanism of vasovagal syncope. *The American Journal of Cardiology*, *88*, 376–381.

Thiruganasambandamoorthy, V., Kwong, K., Wells, G. A., et al. (2016). Development of the Canadian Syncope Risk Score to predict serious adverse events after emergency department assessment of syncope. *Canadian Medical Association Journal*, *188*(12), e289–e298.

Thiruganasambandamoorthy, V., Sivilotti, M. L. A., Le sage, N., et al. (2020). Multicenter emergency department validation of the Canadian syncope risk score. *JAMA Internal Medicine*, *180*(5), 737–744.

Dizziness and Vertigo

Presentation

The patient presents with a complaint of dizziness, which may be abrupt or gradual in onset. The symptoms may be reported in many different ways, such as lightheadedness, disequilibrium, room-spinning vertigo, imbalance, wooziness, or incoordination. The patient may have persistent symptoms associated with severely debilitating nausea and hence be reluctant to engage in an examination or provocative maneuvers. However, differentiating benign from dangerous causes of dizziness can be challenging, and a careful history and physical examination are key to accurate diagnosis and management.

What to Do

✅ Avoid the classic paradigm of distinguishing causes of dizziness by the symptom quality such as lightheadedness or vertigo. This parochial approach is prone to diagnostic error, as the term *dizziness* means different things to different people.

✅ **Instead of focusing on the type of dizziness, obtain a thoughtful history that focuses on the timing, triggers, and associated symptoms.** Were the symptoms abrupt in onset? Has the course been episodic or persistent? If episodic, was there a precipitating trigger such as turning the head to one side or sitting/standing up? Are associated symptoms present that might suggest a specific diagnosis (e.g., palpitations and shortness of breath may suggest a cardiac dysrhythmia).

✅ **Assess for focal neurologic symptoms by performing a thorough neurologic examination.** Assess the cranial nerves and cerebellar function. **Posterior circulation stroke is uncommon but is the most likely type of stroke to be misdiagnosed.** Is there visual field loss, ataxia, loss of balance or coordination? A complete neurologic examination assessing for subtle focal deficits is of paramount importance.

✅ **During your physical examination, take your time examining the eyes. Assess for nystagmus** by having the patient visually follow your finger as it moves a few degrees to the left and then to the right (not to extremes of gaze) (Fig. 12.1), and note whether there are more than the normal two to three beats of nystagmus before the eyes are still. Determine the direction of the nystagmus (horizontal, vertical, or rotatory) and whether fixating the patient's gaze reduces the nystagmus (usually a peripheral finding).

✅ **Examine ears for cerumen, foreign bodies, otitis media, and hearing loss.** Ideally, check for speech discrimination. (Can the patient differentiate between the words *kite, flight, right*?) Abnormalities may be a sign of an acoustic neuroma.

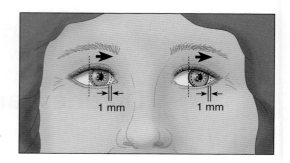

Fig. 12.1 The eye should only move a few degrees to the left or right when examining for nystagmus.

✅ Complete the remainder of the physical examination and avoid anchoring or premature closure. Dizziness is a nonspecific symptom and requires a broad differential diagnosis.

✅ **If the patient describes triggered episodes of dizziness, determine the precipitant (most likely head turning or change in position from laying to standing). Provocative maneuvers such as the Dix-Hallpike test can be used to confirm a diagnosis of posterior canal benign paroxysmal positional vertigo (BPPV). Note that provocative maneuvers should only be performed in patients clearly describing triggered, episodic dizziness.**

✅ **Once the laterality is confirmed, a canalith repositioning maneuver such as the Epley maneuver can be attempted to alleviate the symptoms (see later).**

✅ **If the patient describes acute and sustained dizziness, then differentiate central from peripheral causes (i.e., stroke from vestibular neuronitis). This can be performed using a careful neurologic examination that includes the Head Impulse, Nystagmus, and Test of Skew (HINTS) battery of tests.** (See YouTube description: https://www.youtube.com/watch?v=VwmrjYuvqtQ&ab_channel=Medmastery.)

✅ **If a central cause is suspected,** then obtain neuroimaging, preferably a diffusion-weighted magnetic resonance imaging (MRI) of the brain (without gadolinium), and/or consult neurology.

✅ **If the patient's symptoms are suggestive of a peripheral cause,** then prescribe a vestibular suppressant. **When a vestibular diagnosis (vestibular neuronitis or labyrinthitis) is suspected,** focus on alleviating symptoms such as nausea. If there are no contraindications (e.g., glaucoma), transdermal scopolamine (Transderm Scōp) can be applied for 3 days. Some authors recommend hydroxyzine (Vistaril, Atarax), and others suggest that corticosteroids (methylprednisolone [Solu-Medrol], prednisone) may improve recovery in patients with vestibular neuronitis. If not responding, the patient may require hospitalization for further parenteral treatment and evaluation.

✅ **When BPPV is suspected (brief, triggered events of severe vertigo typically lasting <1 minute provoked by head turning and resolving with the head remaining still) and no concerning signs or symptoms are present, perform a Dix-Hallpike (formerly Nylen-Barany) maneuver** (Fig. 12.2) to confirm the diagnosis and determine which ear is involved.

✅ **To perform the Dix-Hallpike maneuver,** have the patient sit up for at least 30 seconds, then lie back, and quickly hang the head over the end of the stretcher, with the head turned 45 degrees to the right. Wait 30 seconds for the appearance of torsional nystagmus or the

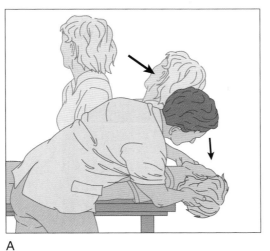
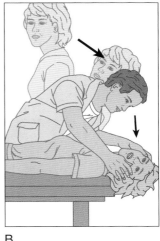

A   B

Fig. 12.2 (A) The patient's head is 30 degrees below horizontal. With the head turned to the right, quickly lower the patient to the supine position. (B) Repeat with the patient's head turned to the left.

sensation of vertigo. Repeat the maneuver on the other side. **When this maneuver produces positional nystagmus after a brief latent period lasting less than 30 seconds, it indicates benign paroxysmal positional vertigo. The ear that is down when the greatest symptoms of nystagmus are produced is the affected ear, which can be treated using canalith-repositioning maneuvers.** An equivocal test is not a contraindication to performing canalith-repositioning maneuvers.

⊘ To prevent nausea and vomiting when these symptoms are not tolerable for the patient, premedicate with an antiemetic. **These maneuvers can be performed quickly at the bedside, thereby moving semicircular canal debris to a less sensitive part of the inner ear (utricle). This can produce rapid results, often providing much satisfaction to both patient and clinician.**

⊘ **The most well studied of these maneuvers is the Epley maneuver (See Video 12.1).** With the patient seated, the patient's head is rotated 45 degrees toward the affected ear. The patient is then tilted backward to a head-hanging position, with the head kept in the 45-degree rotation. The patient is held in this position (same as the Dix-Hallpike position with the affected ear down) until the nystagmus and vertigo abate (at least 20 seconds, preferably up to 3–4 minutes). The head is then turned 90 degrees toward the unaffected ear and kept in this position for at least another 20 seconds, preferably up to 3 to 4 minutes. With the head remaining turned, the patient is then rolled onto the side of the unaffected ear. This may again provoke nystagmus and vertigo, but the patient should again remain in this position for at least 20 seconds, preferably up to 3 to 4 minutes. Finally, the patient is moved to the seated position, and the head is tilted down 30 degrees, allowing the canalith to fall into the utricle. This position is also held for at least 20 seconds, preferably up to 3 to 4 minutes (Fig. 12.3).

⊘ All discharged patients should be encouraged to closely follow up in the outpatient setting and provided with strict return precautions. They can also be given instructions on how to reposition the canalith at home if this is a repeating event and no concerning risk factors are present.

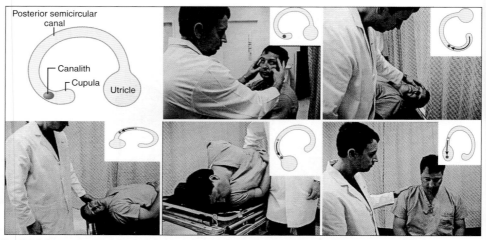

Fig. 12.3. Epley maneuver. (Top, *left to right*) The first window is a legend for the *inset,* which is a simplified representation of a posterior semicircular canal. This figure shows the Epley canalith-repositioning maneuver for the left semicircular canal. The patient's head is turned 45 degrees toward the affected ear, with the patient holding the physician's arm for support. The patient is then lowered to a supine position. The patient's head remains turned 45 degrees and should hang off the end of the bed. (Bottom) In the third position, the patient's head is rotated to face the opposite shoulder. Next, the patient is rolled onto the side, taking care to keep the head rotated. The patient is now returned to a seated position with the head tilted forward. (Adapted from Koelliker, P., Summers, R., & Hawkins, B. [2001]. Benign paroxysmal positional vertigo. *Annals of Emergency Medicine, 37,* 392–398. With permission from The American College of Emergency Physicians.)

What Not to Do

(X) Do not rely on differentiating the type of dizziness by distinguishing lightheadedness from vertigo. This is an error-prone approach, since the term *dizziness* means different things to different people. Instead focus on timing and triggers.

(X) Do not expect to determine the exact cause of dizziness for all patients who present for the first time. Make every reasonable attempt to determine whether the origin is benign or potentially serious, and then make the most appropriate disposition.

(X) Do not attempt provocative maneuvers if the patient is symptomatic with nystagmus at rest. Persistent symptoms are inconsistent with BPPV, which is the only indication for doing such provocative maneuvers.

(X) Do not give long-term vestibular suppressant medications to patients with BPPV unless you are unable to perform repositioning maneuvers and the patient's symptoms are severe.

(X) Do not make the diagnosis of Meniere disease (endolymphatic hydrops) without the triad of paroxysmal vertigo, sensorineural deafness, and low-pitched tinnitus, along with a feeling of pressure or fullness in the affected ear that lasts for hours to days. With repeat attacks, a sustained low-frequency sensorineural hearing loss and constant tinnitus develop.

(X) Do not obtain laboratory testing or neuroimaging studies in patients with classic BPPV. When neuroimaging is indicated, MRI should be favored over CT due to its superior sensitivity for detecting posterior circulation stroke. Most causes of dizziness can be determined through obtaining a complete patient history and clinical examination.

Discussion

Dizziness is a nonspecific symptom. Classically, vertigo is used to describe an illusion of motion, usually rotational, of the patient or the patient's surroundings, whereas lightheadedness suggests feeling faint or presyncopal. However, these symptom descriptions often overlap, and relying on the description of the type of dizziness experienced may lead to diagnostic error. A more accurate and consistent approach focuses on the timing and triggers of the symptoms. Differentiating acute and sustained dizziness, for example, from triggered or episodic dizziness is much more likely to produce distinct and appropriate potential causes. The ATTEST pneumonic is a helpful way to approach dizziness systematically and avoid misdiagnosis. This stands for **A**ssociated symptoms, **T**iming, **T**riggers, **E**xam **S**igns and **T**esting.

When symptoms are acute in onset and sustained, acute vestibular syndrome (AVS) should be presumed. Causes of AVS can be either central (stroke) or peripheral (vestibular neuronitis) in etiology. Patients with peripheral AVS should exhibit horizontal and unidirectional nystagmus with neutral gaze that becomes more pronounced when looking to one side and dissipates when looking to the other side.

The vestibular nerve is unique among the cranial nerves in that the neurons in this nerve, on each side, are firing spontaneously at 100 spikes/sec with the head still. With sudden loss of input from one side, there is a strong bias into the brainstem from the intact side. This large bias in neural activity causes nystagmus. The direction of the nystagmus is labeled according to the quick phase, but the vestibular deficit is actually driving the slow phase of nystagmus.

Vestibular neuritis is preceded by a common cold 50% of the time. The prevalence of vestibular neuritis peaks at 40 to 50 years of age. Vestibular neuritis is probably similar to Bell palsy and is thought to represent a reactivated dormant herpes infection in the Scarpa ganglion within the vestibular nerve. Viral labyrinthitis can be diagnosed if there is associated hearing loss or tinnitus at the time of presentation, but the possibility of an acoustic neuroma should be kept in mind, especially if the vertigo is mild.

The nystagmus should NOT be direction changing in peripheral AVS. Nystagmus is one part of the HINTS exam, which stands for **H**ead **I**mpulse, **N**ystagmus, and **T**est of **S**kew. This battery of three tests can outperform MRI in the early detection of posterior

stroke when performed and interpreted correctly. The Head Impulse Test (HIT) assesses the vestibule-ocular reflex, which is the best way to test unilateral vestibular nerve function in awake patients. It is performed by quickly rotating the patient's head (10–15 degrees) from center to lateral or lateral to center, while the patient is visually fixated on a central point, such as the examiner's nose. The faster the head is moved, the easier the test is to interpret. An abnormal finding occurs when the patient loses focus on the central target and a corrective saccade is noted. Observation of this finding is highly suggestive of a peripheral cause of AVS. The test of skew is also called the alternating cover test and is performed by quickly covering and uncovering one eye at a time with the patient fixated on a central target and observing for a vertical (up and down) correction. Noting this hypertropia/hypotropia is specific for a central lesion and suggests stroke as a cause of AVS. Taken together, the HINTS exam is concerning for a central cause of dizziness if any one component is not reassuring. This includes not observing a saccade on HIT, seeing anything other than horizontal, unidirectional nystagmus, or observing an abnormal test of skew. For this reason, it is imperative that the HINTS exam only be performed in patients who are actively symptomatic from AVS. Any patient with AVS and a concerning HINTS exam or new focal neurologic deficit should raise concern for a possible brainstem or cerebellar stroke. Diffusion-weighted (DW) MRI is the diagnostic gold standard for these patients and is strongly preferred to CT scan when feasible. CT of the brain is not adequate to rule out ischemic stroke. Prior to discharge of any patient suspect of having peripheral AVS, a trial of ambulation should be attempted. Generally, a peripheral vestibular lesion produces unidirectional postural instability with preserved walking, whereas an inferior cerebellar stroke often causes severe postural instability and falling when walking is attempted. Regardless, newly nonambulatory patients should probably not be discharged.

When dizziness is episodic, it should be determined if episodes occur spontaneously or are triggered. Precipitants typically include head turning (which suggests BPPV) or standing up (which suggests orthostasis). Provocative testing is indicated when a trigger is identified. When episodes occur spontaneously, careful attention to detail in the patient's history is important. This group can be particularly challenging to diagnose, since

(continued)

Discussion continued

many have resolved symptoms at the time of their evaluation. Considerations include transient ischemic attack (TIA) if focal deficits were described, vestibular migraine when accompanied by an aura or headache, Meniere disease in cases associated with tinnitus and hearing loss, and numerous nonneurologic causes such as cardiac dysrhythmia. The appropriate diagnostic workup for patients with spontaneous episodic dizziness depends on the suspected differential. Generally, a 12-lead electrocardiogram (ECG) is reasonable, and bloodwork is commonly obtained. While neurovascular imaging is typically not needed when migraine or Meniere disease is suspected, patients at risk of TIA should have both brain and vessel imaging performed.

While the majority of causes of dizziness are benign, this chief complaint is best approached with caution and a high degree of vigilance. While posterior strokes are relatively uncommon, they are frequently missed on initial presentation and the consequences can be deadly. Careful attention to detail in history-taking and a thoughtful and thorough neurologic examination are your best allies.

Suggested Readings

Edlow, J. A. (2016). A new approach to the diagnosis of acute dizziness in adult patients. *Emergency Medical Clinics of North America*, *34*(4), 717–742.

Edlow, J. A. (2018). Managing patients with acute episodic dizziness. *Annals of Emergency Medicine*, *5*, 602–610.

Edlow, J. A. (2019). The timing-and-triggers approach to the patient with acute dizziness. *Emergency Medicine Practice*, *21*(12), 1–24.

Epley, J. M. (1995). Positional vertigo related to semicircular canalithiasis. *Otolaryngology-Head and Neck Surgery*, *112*, 154–161.

Froehling, D. A., Silverstein, M. D., Mohr, D. N., et al. (1994). Does this patient have a serious form of vertigo? *Journal of the American Medical Association*, *271*, 385–388.

Halmagyi, G. M., & Curthoys, I. S. (1988). A clinical signs of canal paresis. *Archives of Neurology*, *45*(7), 737–739.

Herr, R. D., Zun, L., & Matthews, J. J. (1989). A directed approach to the dizzy patient. *Annals of Emergency Medicine*, *18*, 664–672.

Hotson, J. R., & Baloh, R. W. (1998). Acute vestibular syndrome. *New England Journal of Medicine*, *339*, 680–685.

Kattah, J. C., Talkad, A. V., Wang, D. Z., et al. (2009). HINTS to diagnose stroke in the acute vestibular syndrome: Three-step bedside oculomotor examination more sensitive than early MRI diffusion-weighted imaging. *Stroke*, *40*(11), 3504–3510.

Kim, J. S., & Zee, D. S. (2014). Clinical practice. Benign paroxysmal positional vertigo. *New England Journal of Medicine*, *370*(12), 1138–1147.

Koelliker, P., Summers, R. L., & Hawkins, B. (2001). Benign paroxysmal positional vertigo: Diagnosis and treatment in the emergency department. *Annals of Emergency Medicine*, *37*, 392–398.

Marill, K. A., Walsh, M. J., & Nelson, B. K. (2000). Intravenous lorazepam versus dimenhydrinate for treatment of vertigo in the emergency department: A randomized clinical trial. *Annals of Emergency Medicine*, *36*, 310–319.

Newman-Toker, D. E. (2016). Missed stroke in acute vertigo and dizziness: It is time for action, not debate. *Annals of Neurology*, *79*(1), 27–31.

Radtke, A., van Brevern, M., Tiel-Wilck, K., et al. (2004). Self-treatment of benign paroxysmal positional vertigo: Semont maneuver versus Epley procedure. *Neurology*, *63*, 150–152.

Ravid, S., Bienkowski, R., & Eviatar, L. (2003). A simplified diagnostic approach to dizziness in children. *Pediatric Neurology*, *29*, 317–320.

Siket, M., & Edlow, J. (2020). Vertigo and dizziness. In A. Mattu, & S. Swadron (Eds.), *CorePendium*. Burbank, CA: CorePendium LLC. https://www.emrap.org/corependium/chapter/rec4hVWEPJ9LZSiDx/Vertigo-and-Dizziness.

Stewart, K., Whelan, D., & Banerjee, A. (2017). Are cervical collars a necessary post-procedure restriction in patients with benign paroxysmal positional vertigo treated with particle repositioning manoeuvres? *International Journal of Surgery*, *47*, S8–S8.

Strupp, M., Zingler, V. C., Arbusow, V., et al. (2004). Methylprednisolone, valacyclovir, or the combination for vestibular neuritis. *New England Journal of Medicine*, *351*, 354–361.

Tusa, R. J. (2001). Vertigo. *Neurology Clinics*, *19*, 23–55.

Weakness

Presentation

An older patient, complaining of isolated "weakness" or an inability to perform the usual activities or care for oneself, comes to an acute care clinic or emergency department (ED), often brought in by family members.

What to Do

✅ Obtain as much of the history as possible. Speak to available family members or friends, as well as the patient, and ask for details. Are there any new medications or dosage increases that can produce weakness (also consider toxins)? Is the patient weak before certain activities (suggests depression)? Is the weakness located in the limb girdles (suggests polymyalgia rheumatica when there is symmetric joint pain or painful myopathy)? Is the weakness mostly in the distal muscles (suggests neuropathy)? Is the weakness caused by repetitive actions (suggests myasthenia gravis)? Is the weakness unilateral, with slurring of speech or confusion (suggests stroke)?

✅ **Obtain a thorough medical history and complete physical examination,** including a review of symptoms (e.g., headaches, weight loss, cold intolerance, change in appetite or bowel habits, urinary symptoms), with a full set of vital signs; also include testing for strength of all muscle groups (graded on a scale of 1–5), deep tendon reflexes, and neurologic status. Perform a complete neurologic exam, including having the patient stand and walk if possible. Perform a rectal examination for occult stool blood. **Obtain a head computed tomography (CT) scan if there is an unexplained change in mental status or there are abnormal neurologic findings. Obtain a magnetic resonance imaging (MRI) or CT with contrast if a structural cord lesion is suspected.**

✅ **Have a low threshold to obtain laboratory tests that include serum glucose, a complete blood count, electrolytes, cardiac enzymes, a 12-lead electrocardiogram (ECG), and urinalysis.** Consider thyroid studies and possibly a sedimentation rate. Consider hypoxia, hypercarbia, myocardial infarction, anemia, infection, diabetes, uremia, polymyalgia rheumatica, hyponatremia, or hypokalemia and hyperkalemia, which are the most common causes of reported weakness. Tests determining serum phosphate, and calcium levels may also be valuable.

- ○ Weakness is frequently the only complaint in elderly patients with acute myocardial infarction. Weakness or fatigue is the most common atypical complaint for women with acute myocardial infarction.
- ○ Weakness is one of the most common complaints in the elderly with acute urinary tract infection.

What Not to Do

(X) Do not presume a benign cause of new-onset weakness, especially if focal or localizing to one side.

(X) Do not overly focus on rare causes without first excluding more common and emergent conditions. It is appropriate to limit the urgent care or ED evaluation of weakness to acutely intervenable conditions and refer ongoing evaluation of chronic and nonemergent conditions to the patient's primary health care provider.

Discussion

The complaint of weakness is nonspecific and can be diagnostically challenging in the emergency department or acute care clinic. Commonly, patients with nonlocalizing, nonspecific weakness have a very broad differential diagnosis. New-onset focal weakness, somnolence, or failure to thrive should never be presumed as minor and should be evaluated promptly.

Subjective or perceived generalized weakness is quite different from new-onset objective and measurable neuromuscular weakness. Differentiating causes of fatigue and malaise from neurologic causes such as Guillain-Barre syndrome (GBS), myasthenia gravis, Lambert-Eaton myasthenic syndrome, and transverse myelitis is important. Other rare causes such as botulism, hypokalemic periodic paralysis, and tick paralysis are potentially deadly and can be easily missed.

Patients with GBS typically experience progressive ascending bilateral leg weakness without sensory loss and associated with loss of deep tendon reflexes. Symptoms can rapidly progress to involve respiratory failure requiring emergent airway management if not detected and managed promptly. Diagnosis is made by lumbar puncture showing elevated protein levels and managed with intravenous immunoglobulin (IVIG) and/or plasmapheresis. Airway monitoring is imperative

and assessing a blood gas, forced vital capacity (FVC), and negative inspiratory force (NIF) at the first sign of respiratory involvement is encouraged.

Myasthenic crisis can present with generalized weakness and also progresses to respiratory collapse. Proximal and large muscle weakness is common, and cranial nerve abnormalities, such as ptosis, are often detected on exam. Myasthenia is often precipitated by medications and is treated similarly to GBS with IVIG and/or plasmapheresis. Assessing FVC and NIF with close airway monitoring is indicated in these patients as well.

Acute-onset focal localizing weakness should be considered stroke until proven otherwise. Peripheral causes such as nerve impingement (consider compressive neuropathy of the radial nerve from prolonged direct pressure of the upper medial arm or axilla, aka Saturday night palsy) may also cause focal weakness as a specific peripheral nerve distribution, but providers are cautioned against anchoring too early on this diagnosis.

When no cause of weakness is uncovered and the patient's physical examination and diagnostic workup are reassuring, consider other nonphysiologic causes. Depression and somatization may present with generalized weakness, though these are best considered diagnoses of exclusion.

Suggested Readings

Frohman, E. M., & Wingerchuk, D. M. (2010). Clinical practice. Transverse myelitis. *New England Journal of Medicine*, *363*(6), 564–572.

Ganti, L., & Rastogi, V. (2016). Acute generalized weakness. *Emergency Medicine Clinics of North America*, *34*(4), 795–809.

Krishnan, C., & Kerr, D. A. (2005). Idiopathic transverse myelitis. *Archives of Neurology*, *62*(6), 1011–1013.

Smith, D. E., & Siket, M. S. (2010). High-risk chief complaints III: Neurologic emergencies. *Emergency Medicine Clinics of North America*, *38*(2), 523–537.

Willison, H. J., Jacobs, B. C., & van Doorn, P. A. (2016). Guillain-Barré syndrome. *Lancet*, *388*(10045), 717–727.

PART 2

Ophthalmologic Emergencies

■ Daniel Barkhuff ■ Skyler Lentz

CHAPTER

Conjunctivitis

(Pink Eye)

14

Presentation

Conjunctivitis is the most common diagnosis in patients with a red eye and discharge, but not all red eyes are the result of conjunctivitis. With bacterial conjunctivitis the patient complains of a red, irritated eye and perhaps a gritty or foreign-body sensation; a thick, purulent discharge that continues throughout the day; and crusting or matting of the eyelids on awakening (Fig. 14.1). It is most often unilateral. With viral conjunctivitis, the complaint may be of a similar discomfort or burning, with clear tearing, preauricular lymphadenopathy, or symptoms of upper respiratory tract infection (Fig. 14.2). On the other hand, with allergic conjunctivitis, the main complaint may be itching, with minimal conjunctival injection, seasonal recurrence, and cobblestone hypertrophy of the tarsal conjunctivae or bubblelike chemosis of the conjunctiva covering the sclera (Fig. 14.3). Ocular symptoms are usually accompanied by nasal symptoms, and there may be other allergic events in the patient's history that support the diagnosis of ocular allergy.

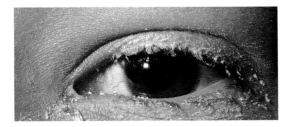

Fig. 14.1 Bacterial conjunctivitis. (Adapted from Palay, D. H., & Krachmer, J. H. [2005]. *Primary care ophthalmology* [2nd ed.]. St. Louis, MO: Mosby.)

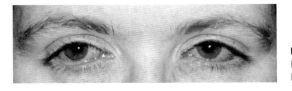

Fig. 14.2 Viral conjunctivitis. (Adapted from Palay, D. H., & Krachmer, J. H. [2005]. *Primary care ophthalmology* [2nd ed.]. St. Louis, MO: Mosby.)

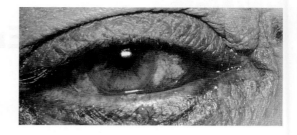

Fig. 14.3 Allergic conjunctivitis. (Adapted from Palay, D. H., & Krachmer, J. H. [2005]. *Primary care ophthalmology* [2nd ed.]. St. Louis, MO: Mosby.)

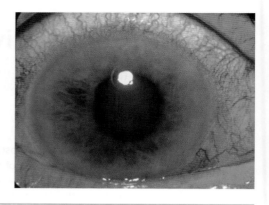

Fig. 14.4 Ciliary flush. (Attributed, unmodified from Jonathan Trobe MD. https://commons.wikimedia.org/wiki/File:Acute_Angle_Closure-glaucoma.jpg.)

Examination discloses generalized injection of the conjunctiva, with thinning out toward the cornea. (Localized inflammation suggests some other diagnosis, such as presence of a foreign body, an inverted eyelash, episcleritis, or a viral or bacterial ulcer.)

Vision and pupil reactions should be normal, and the cornea and anterior chamber should be clear. Any discomfort should be temporarily relieved by the instillation of topical anesthetic solution.

If few symptoms are present on awakening but discomfort worsens during the day, dry eye is probable. Eye opening during sleep, which leads to corneal exposure and drying, results in ocular redness and irritation that is worse in the morning.

Physical and chemical conjunctivitis caused by particles, solutions, vapors, and natural or occupational irritants that inflame the conjunctiva should be evident from the history.

Deep pain, pain not relieved by topical anesthetic, severe pain of sudden onset, photophobia, vomiting, decreased vision, and injection that is more pronounced around the limbus (ciliary flush) (Fig. 14.4) suggest more serious involvement of the cornea or the globe's internal structures (e.g., corneal ulcer, keratitis, acute angle–closure glaucoma, uveitis) and demand early or immediate ophthalmologic consultation.

What to Do

✓ **Instill proparacaine or tetracaine (Alcaine, Ophthaine, Ophthetic) anesthetic drops to allow a more comfortable examination and to help determine whether the patient's discomfort is limited to the conjunctiva and cornea.** If there is no pain relief, the pain comes from deeper eye structures.

✅ **Examine the eye,** including assessment of visual acuity (correct for any refractive error and record results) and pupil reaction and symmetry, inspection for foreign bodies, estimation of intraocular pressure by palpating the globe above the tarsal plate, and examination with a slit lamp (when available), and fluorescein staining and ultraviolet or cobalt blue light to assess the corneal epithelium.

✅ Ask about and look for signs of any rash, arthritis, or mucous membrane involvement, which could point to Stevens-Johnson syndrome, Kawasaki syndrome, reactive arthritis syndrome, or some other syndrome that can present with conjunctivitis.

✅ **For bacterial conjunctivitis, instruct the patient to begin therapy by applying warm or cool compresses (for comfort and cleansing) every 4 hours, followed by instillation of ophthalmic antibiotic solutions, such as trimethoprim plus polymyxin B (Polytrim) 10 mL, 1 to 2 drops every 2 to 6 hours;** azithromycin 1% (AzaSite) 2.5 mL, 1 drop twice a day for 2 days, then 1 drop once daily for 5 more days; or **ciprofloxacin 0.3% solution (Ciloxan) 5 mL, 1 to 2 drops every 2 to 4 hours;** or instillation under the lower lid of topical antibiotic ointments (which transiently blur vision and may be cosmetically unacceptable), such as erythromycin 0.5% (Ilotycin), bacitracin–polymyxin B (Polysporin), or tobramycin 0.3% (Tobrex), 3.5 g each, with oral analgesics as needed. Consider sending culture from eye for antimicrobial sensitivities and take careful history regarding possible sexually transmitted disease exposure. No clinical sign or symptom can adequately distinguish all viral from bacterial infections. Therefore, if it is unclear whether the problem is viral or bacterial, it is safest to treat it as bacterial.

✅ Continue therapy for approximately 5 days or for at least 24 hours after all signs and symptoms have cleared. It should be noted that several studies suggest that bacterial conjunctivitis is self-limiting and will resolve without any antibiotics in most patients. Therefore it is reasonable to use the less expensive topical preparations on the less severe cases (i.e., polymyxin B/trimethoprim–generic). No evidence exists demonstrating the superiority of any topical antibiotic agent.

✅ Spread to the other eye may occur without stringent hygiene; instruct patients in hygiene and potential need to institute treatment in the other eye if symptoms occur.

✅ **With contact lens wearers (in whom *Pseudomonas* is more likely to be a problem), it is more justifiable to use a fluoroquinolone (i.e., moxifloxacin [Vigamox] 0.5% solution 3 mL, 1 to 2 drops three times a day, or gatifloxacin [Zymar] 0.3% solution 5 mL, 1 to 2 drops every 2 hours when awake, then taper to 1 to 2 drops four times a day). Instruct the patient not to wear their contacts until redirected by their ophthalmologist or until symptoms have completely resolved for more than 24 hours.**

✅ **For mild to moderate viral and chemical conjunctivitis, apply cold compresses and weak topical vasoconstrictors, such as naphazoline 0.1% (Naphcon), every 3 to 4 hours,** unless the patient has a shallow anterior chamber that is prone to acute angle–closure glaucoma with mydriatics. Inform the patient or parents about the self-limited nature of most cases and the lack of benefits (with some risk for complications) from topical antibiotics. You could reassure them further by offering a delayed prescription that they could get filled if the symptoms have not resolved after 5 days. If necessary, provide mild systemic analgesics. Educate the patient and family about proper hygiene. Infected individuals should be counseled to wash hands frequently and use separate towels, and to avoid close contact with others during the period of contagion.

✅ **For allergic conjunctivitis, apply cold compresses and prescribe ketotifen fumarate 0.025% (Zaditor [over the counter]) or azelastine hydrochloride 0.05% (Optivar), 1 drop** twice a day. These are H_1-antihistamines and mast cell stabilizers. The antihistaminic effect of ketotifen occurs within minutes after administration and has a duration of up to 12 hours. **Combining this topical therapy with systemic antihistamines may give the maximal symptomatic relief.** Topical corticosteroid drops provide dramatic relief, but prolonged use increases the risk for opportunistic viral, fungal, and bacterial corneal ulceration; cataract formation; and glaucoma. **When a steroid is required, loteprednol (Alrex) 0.2% suspension, 1 drop four times a day, reportedly does not cause cataract or glaucoma.** Ophthalmologic consultation is recommended. If a severe contact dermatitis is suspected, a short course of oral prednisone is indicated (see Chapter 162).

✅ If the problem is dry eye (keratoconjunctivitis sicca), treat with artificial tear drops (Refresh Tears, Lacri-Lube, Gen Teal). If chlorine from a swimming pool is causing chronic red eye (athletes and recreational swimmers), using a nonsteroidal antiinflammatory drug (NSAID) eye drop (ketorolac [Acular] 0.5%, 1 drop four times a day) may provide some comfort, but swimming goggles are the best solution.

✅ Instruct the patient to follow up with an ophthalmologist if the infection does not completely resolve within 2 days. Obtain earlier consultation if there is any involvement of the cornea or iris, impaired vision, light sensitivity, inequality in pupil size, or other signs of corneal infection, iritis, or acutely increased intraocular pressure. In addition, refer patients who have had eye surgery, have a history of herpes simplex keratitis, or wear contact lenses to an ophthalmologist.

✅ Return to school or daycare should parallel behavior in the common cold.

What Not to Do

❌ Do not fail to get an ophthalmologic consultation when there is loss of vision, abnormal pupillary response, history of eye trauma, voluminous purulent discharge, recurrent conjunctivitis, or immunocompromise.

❌ Do not fail to consider the possibility of sexual abuse in children with gonococcal conjunctivitis.

❌ Do not forget to wash hands and equipment after examining the patient; herpes simplex or epidemic keratoconjunctivitis (Fig. 14.5) can be spread to clinicians and other patients. For viral forms of conjunctivitis, do not forget to instruct the patient regarding the contagious nature of the disease and the importance of handwashing and use of separate towels and pillows for 10 days after the onset of symptoms.

❌ Do not use ophthalmic neomycin because of the high incidence of hypersensitivity reactions.

❌ Do not patch an infected eye; this interferes with the cleansing function of tear flow.

❌ Do not use topical antiviral drugs for simple cases of viral conjunctivitis. They are of no benefit.

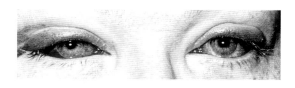

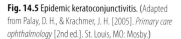 **Fig. 14.5** Epidemic keratoconjunctivitis. (Adapted from Palay, D. H., & Krachmer, J. H. [2005]. *Primary care ophthalmology* [2nd ed.]. St. Louis, MO: Mosby.)

Ⓧ Do not give steroids without arranging for ophthalmologic consultation, and never give steroids if a herpes simplex infection is suspected.

Ⓧ Do not make a diagnosis of conjunctivitis unless visual acuity is normal and there is no evidence of corneal involvement, iritis, or acute glaucoma.

Discussion

Warm or cool compresses are soothing for all types of conjunctivitis. Antibiotic drops and ointments should be reserved for when bacterial infection is likely. Neomycin-containing ointments and drops should probably be avoided because allergic sensitization to this antibiotic is common. Any corneal ulceration found with fluorescein staining requires ophthalmologic consultation. Most viral and bacterial conjunctivitis hosts will resolve spontaneously, with the possible exception of *Staphylococcus, Meningococcus,* and *Gonococcus* organism infections, which can produce destructive sequelae without treatment.

Most bacterial conjunctivitis in immunocompetent hosts is caused by *Streptococcus pneumoniae, Haemophilus influenzae, Staphylococcus aureus,* or *Moraxella catarrhalis.* Routine conjunctival cultures are seldom of value, but the Gram method should be used to stain and culture **any copious yellow-green, purulent exudate that is abrupt in onset and quickly reaccumulates after being wiped away** (findings with both *Neisseria gonorrhoeae* and *N. meningitidis*). *N. gonorrhoeae* infection confirmed by Gram-negative intracellular diplococci requires immediate ophthalmologic consultation and treatment with IM ceftriaxone (also treat sexual partners) as well as topical antibiotics. Corneal ulceration, scarring, and blindness can occur in a matter of hours.

Chlamydial conjunctivitis will usually present with lid droop, mucopurulent discharge, photophobia, and preauricular lymphadenopathy. Small, white, elevated conglomerations of lymphoid tissue can be seen on the upper and lower tarsal conjunctiva, and 90% of patients have concurrent genital infection. In adults,

doxycycline, 100 mg orally twice a day for 7 days or azithromycin (Zithromax), 1 g by mouth × 1 dose, plus topical tetracycline (Achromycin Ophthalmic Ointment) 1%, every 3–4 hours for 3 weeks should control the infection. (Also treat sexual partners.) Although it is somewhat difficult to culture, *Chlamydia* can be confirmed by monoclonal immunofluorescent antibody testing from conjunctival smears or by polymerase chain reaction (PCR) testing.

Newborn conjunctivitis requires special attention and culture of any discharge as well as immediate ophthalmologic consultation. The pathogens of greatest concern are *N. gonorrhoeae, C. trachomatis,* and herpes simplex virus (HSV). *N. gonorrhoeae* infections usually begin 2 to 4 days after birth, whereas *C. trachomatis* infections start 3 to 10 days after birth. If conjunctivitis is noted on the first day of life, this is more likely to be a reaction to silver nitrate prophylaxis.

Epidemic keratoconjunctivitis is a bilateral, painful, highly contagious conjunctivitis usually caused by an adenovirus (serotypes 8 and 19). The eyes are extremely erythematous, sometimes with subconjunctival hemorrhages. There is copious watery discharge and preauricular lymphadenopathy. Treat the symptoms with analgesics, cold compresses, and, if necessary, corticosteroids (loteprednol [Alrex], 0.2% suspension, 1 drop four times a day). Because the infection can last as long as 3 weeks and may result in permanent corneal scarring, provide ophthalmologic consultation and referral. Patients should be instructed on handwashing with soap, changing pillowcases, and not sharing household items. Patients should also be told to avoid communal activities (work, school, daycare) for 10 to 14 days or

Discussion continued

while there is a discharge, to avoid infecting others. These patients should also avoid wearing contact lenses. Nondisposable contacts should be sterilized, and patients with disposable contacts should use new lenses after 14 days.

Herpes simplex conjunctivitis is usually unilateral. Symptoms include a red eye, photophobia, eye pain, and blurred vision with a foreign-body sensation. There may be periorbital vesicles, and a branching (dendritic) pattern with bulbar terminal endings of fluorescein staining confirms the diagnosis. Treat with trifluridine 1% (Viroptic), 1 drop every 2 hours nine times daily, then reduce dose to 1 drop every 4–6 hours after reepithelialization for another 7 to 14 days (maximum 21 days of treatment). In addition, instill 1 cm vidarabine (Vira-A) ointment five times daily at 3-hour intervals up to 21 days. Also give acyclovir, 800 mg orally five times daily for 7 to 10 days, or valacyclovir (Valtrex), 1 g twice a day for 7 to 10 days. Analgesics and cold compresses will help provide comfort. Cycloplegics, such as homatropine

5% (1 to 2 drops two to three times a day), may help control pain resulting from iridocyclitis. Topical corticosteroids are contraindicated because they can extend duration of the infection. Because corneal herpetic infections frequently leave a scar, ophthalmologic consultation is required.

Herpes zoster ophthalmicus is shingles of the ophthalmic branch of the trigeminal nerve, which innervates the cornea and the tip of the nose. It begins with unilateral neuralgia, followed by a vesicular rash in the distribution of the nerve. Ophthalmic consultation is again required (because of frequent ocular complications), but topical corticosteroids may be used. Prescribe systemic acyclovir (Zovirax), 800 mg every 4 hours (five times daily) for 7 to 10 days, or valacyclovir (Valtrex), 1 g by mouth three times a day for 7 to 10 days. Topical antivirals are not beneficial.

Chronic and/or recalcitrant conjunctivitis may be indicative of an underlying malignancy, such as sebaceous or squamous cell carcinoma.

Suggested Readings

Abramaian, F. M. (2002). Outbreak of bacterial conjunctivitis at a college—New Hampshire, January-March 2002. *Annals of Emergency Medicine*, *40*, 524–527.

American Academy of Ophthalmology Cornea/External Disease Panel. (2018). *Preferred practice pattern guidelines: Conjunctivitis*. Retrieved from http://www.aao.org/preferred-practice-pattern/conjunctivitis-ppp-2018.

Azari, A., & Barney, N. (2013). Conjunctivitis: A systematic review of diagnosis and treatment. *Journal of the American Medical Association*, *310*(16), 1721–1729.

Bremond-Gignac, D., Mariano-Kurkdjian, P., et al. (2010). Efficacy and safety of azithromycin 1.5% eye drops for purulent bacterial conjunctivitis in pediatric patients. *The Pediatric Infectious Disease Journal*, *29*, 3.

David, S. P. (2002). Should we prescribe antibiotics for acute conjunctivitis? *American Family Physician*, *66*, 1649–1651.

Kowalski, R. P., Karenchak, L. M., & Romanowski, E. G. (2003). Infection disease: Changing antibiotic susceptibility. *Ophthalmology Clinics of North America*, *16*, 1–9.

Rose, P. W., Harnden, A., Brueggemann, A. B., et al. (2005). Chloramphenicol treatment for acute infective conjunctivitis in children in primary care. *Lancet*, *366*, 37–43.

Schiebel, N. (2003). Use of antibiotics in patients with acute bacterial conjunctivitis. *Annals of Emergency Medicine*, *41*, 407–409.

Shaikh, S., & Ta, C. N. (2002). Evaluation and management of herpes zoster ophthalmicus. *American Family Physician*, *66*, 1723–1730.

Sheikh, A. (2003). Use of antibiotics in patients with acute bacterial conjunctivitis. *Annals of Emergency Medicine*, *41*, 407.

Yaphe, J., & Pandher, K. S. (2003). The predictive value of the penlight test for photophobia for serious eye pathology in general practice. *Family Practice*, *20*, 425–427.

Contact Lens Complications 15

Presentation

A patient who wears hard, impermeable, or rigid gas-permeable contact lenses comes to the emergency department in the early morning complaining of severe eye pain after they have left their lenses in for longer than the recommended time period. Extended-wear soft contact lenses can cause a similar syndrome when worn for days or weeks and have become contaminated with bacteria and/or irritants. The patient may not be able to open their eyes for examination because of pain and blepharospasm. They may have obvious corneal injury, with signs of iritis and conjunctivitis, or may have no findings visible without fluorescein staining.

What to Do

✅ **Instill topical anesthetic drops such as proparacaine (Alcaine, Ophthaine) to provide comfort for examination.**

✅ Perform a history, including contact lens care habits and a complete eye examination. A complete examination includes best-corrected visual acuity, assessment of pupil reflexes, examination with funduscopy, and inspection of conjunctival sacs. Use a slit lamp if available.

✅ With a bright-light examination, note whether there are any hazy areas or ulcerations on the cornea.

✅ **Instill fluorescein dye** (use a single-dose dropper or wet a dye-impregnated paper strip and touch it to the tear pool in the lower conjunctival sac), have the patient blink, and examine the eye under cobalt blue or ultraviolet light, looking for the green fluorescence of dye bound to dead areas of absent corneal epithelium. Rinse out the dye afterward.

✅ When a corneal defect is visualized, sketch the area of corneal injury on the patient record.

✅ **Contact lens–induced acute red eye (CLARE)** can occur with extended-wear contact lenses and has been defined as **an acute onset of a red eye associated with corneal infiltrates.** Typically, symptoms of ocular discomfort, foreign-body sensation, and redness are noted on awakening. These findings are usually unilateral, and, on examination, conjunctival injection, mild chemosis, and peripheral corneal infiltrates are seen. The corneal epithelium overlying the infiltrates may be intact, or a mild punctate keratopathy may be present. **Treatment consists of discontinuation of contact lens use until complete resolution has occurred. There is apparently no medical therapy indicated for this condition, but it would be considered reasonable and prudent to initiate the same treatment as that provided for superficial punctate keratitis.**

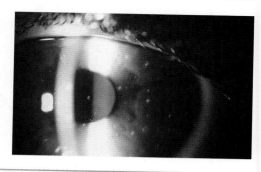

Fig. 15.1 General appearance of superficial punctate keratitis under slit-lamp examination. (Adapted from Yanoff, M., & Duker, J. S. (2004). *Ophthalmology* (2nd ed.). St. Louis, MO: Mosby.)

When the symptoms consist of a mild burning, a foreign-body sensation, and/or dryness, and examination with fluorescein staining shows mild punctate uptake (**superficial punctate keratitis**) (Fig. 15.1), **treatment consists of discontinuation of lens use and the instillation of fluoroquinolone drops to cover *Pseudomonas*—ciprofloxacin 0.3% (Ciloxan), 1 to 2 drops every 1 to 6 hours (use more frequently for the first 2 to 3 days). Prescribe analgesics (e.g., naproxen, ibuprofen, oxycodone) as needed, and administer the first dose if appropriate.**

Instruct the patient to avoid wearing his lenses until cleared by the ophthalmologist and to seek ophthalmologic follow-up within 1 day.

When patients complain of severe pain, irritation, photophobia, and tearing associated with infiltrates, corneal inflammation, and epithelial defects, they are at high risk for the most serious complication of contact lens wear (**microbial keratitis**) (Fig. 15.2). The most commonly cultured organisms are Gram negative, particularly *Pseudomonas aeruginosa,* but fungal organisms are also possible. The more severe the symptoms, the larger the corneal epithelial defect (>1.5 mm); the more central its location, the greater potential morbidity, with resultant risk of permanent loss of vision. **These patients demand prompt ophthalmologic consultation, along with the initiation of treatment with appropriate topical antibiotics (i.e., a combination of either fortified cefazolin or vancomycin (*Staphylococcus* coverage) and fortified tobramycin or gentamicin.** Suspected microbial ulcers must be scraped and cultured and a Gram stain performed. Contact lens care solutions and the contact lens case should also be cultured along with the ulcer if possible. **Patients with less severe cases can be treated with moxifloxacin (Vigamox), 0.5% solution, 3 mL, 1 to 2 drops every 2 hours when awake or gatifloxacin (Zymar), 0.3% solution, 5 mL, 1 to 2 drops every 2 hours when awake, then taper to 1 to 2 drops four times a day.** Ophthalmologic consultation with next-day follow-up is still very important.

In the presence of minimal signs of inflammation in a patient with significant pain that is out of proportion to the findings, consider the possibility of *Acanthamoeba* keratitis. Later in the disease process this can present as a ring-shaped corneal infiltration (Fig. 15.3). This form of infection from overwearing of a soft lens can damage the eye rapidly and may require excision and hospitalization.

What Not to Do

Do not discharge a patient with topical anesthetic ophthalmic drops for continued administration; they may potentiate serious injury.

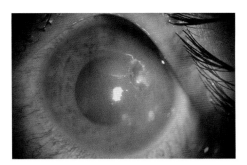

Fig. 15.2 Microbial keratitis. Intraepithelial infiltration of the cornea by *Pseudomonas* organisms in a hydrophilic contact lens wearer. (Adapted from Yanoff, M., & Duker, J. S. (2004). *Ophthalmology* (2nd ed.). St. Louis, MO: Mosby.)

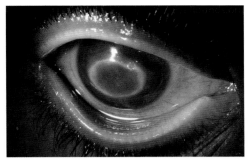

Fig. 15.3 *Acanthamoeba* keratitis. Corneal ring infiltrate. (EyeRounds.org University of Iowa.)

Ⓧ Do not let a patient reuse contaminated or infected lenses.

Ⓧ Do not patch eyes damaged by contact lens abrasions or early ulcerative keratitis.

Ⓧ Do not prescribe antibiotic ointments that do not provide prophylaxis against *Pseudomonas* organisms (e.g., erythromycin, sulfas).

Ⓧ Do not use drops or ointments containing steroids without an ophthalmologist's recommendation.

Discussion

Hard or rigid gas-permeable contact lenses and extended-wear soft lenses left in place too long deprive the avascular corneal epithelium of oxygen and nutrients that are normally provided by the tear film. This produces diffuse ischemia, which can cause an increase in bacterial binding to the corneal epithelium. Soft lenses can absorb chemical irritants, allergens, bacteria, and amoebas if they soak in contaminated cleaning solution. Allergic reactions (see Chapter 14) are hypersensitivity reactions that occur after repeated exposure to a sensitizing antigen. In the past, thimerosal was a common offender, but sorbate and benzalkonium chloride are likely causes now.

Patient-related factors—such as alteration of the recommended wearing or replacement schedules and noncompliance with recommended contact lens care regimens for economic reasons, convenience, or in error—contribute to contact lens–related complications.

Studies have shown that the major risk for infection with conventional contact lenses is overnight wear.

The risk for infection is still five times greater with extended-wear contact lenses compared with that for daily wear. Initial results of studies looking at silicone hydrogel contact lenses (Pure Vision) worn for extended periods are encouraging in that they appear to result in a lower incidence of microbial keratitis than seen with the standard extended-wear lenses.

There are millions of contact lens wearers in the United States. Adverse reactions range from minor transient irritation to corneal ulceration and infection that may result in permanent loss of vision caused by corneal scarring. *Pseudomonas* organism infection is most commonly associated with contact lens–related microbial keratitis. Thus the management of these cases should differ from the routine care of mechanical corneal abrasions that are not caused by contact lens wear. Occlusive patching and corticosteroid medications favor bacterial growth and are therefore not generally recommended for initial treatment in the setting of contact lens use.

Suggested Readings

Alipour, F., Khaheshi, S., Soleimanzadeh, M., Heidarzadeh, S., & Heydarzadeh, S. (2017). Contact lens-related complications: A review. *Journal of Ophthalmic & Vision Research*, *12*(2), 193–204. https://doi.org/10.4103/jovr.jovr_159_16

Cope, J. R., Konne, N. M., Jacobs, D. S., et al. (2018). Corneal infections associated with sleeping in contact lenses—six cases, United States, 2016–2018. *MMWR Morbidity & Mortality Weekly Report*, *67*(32), 877–881.

Donshik, P. C. (2003). Extended wear contact lenses. *Ophthalmology Clinics of North America*, *16*, 79–84.

Schein, O. D. (1993). Contact lens abrasions and the nonophthalmologist. *American Journal of Emergency Medicine*, *11*, 606–608.

Suchecki, J. K., Donshik, P., & Ehlers, W. H. (2003). Contact lens complications. *Ophthalmology Clinics of North America*, *e16*, 471–484.

CHAPTER 16

Corneal Abrasion

Presentation

The patient may complain of eye pain or a sensation of the presence of a foreign body after direct ocular trauma. The patient may have abraded the cornea while inserting or removing a contact lens. Removal of a corneal foreign body produces some corneal abrasion, but corneal abrasion can occur without any identifiable trauma. There is often excessive tearing, blurred vision, and photophobia. Often the patient cannot open their eye for the examination because of pain and blepharospasm. Abrasions are occasionally visible during side lighting of the cornea. Conjunctival inflammation can range from minimal to severe conjunctivitis with accompanying iritis.

What to Do

✓ **Instill topical anesthetic drops to eliminate any pain or blepharospasm and thereby permit examination (e.g., proparacaine [Ophthetic], tetracaine [Pontocaine]).**

✓ Perform a complete eye examination (including assessment of best-corrected visual acuity, funduscopy, anterior chamber bright-light examination, and inspection of conjunctival sacs for a foreign body).

✓ **Perform the fluorescein examination** by wetting a paper strip impregnated with dry, orange fluorescein dye and touching this strip into the tear pool inside the lower conjunctival sac. After the patient blinks, darken the room and examine the eye under cobalt-blue filtered or ultraviolet light. (The red-free light on the ophthalmoscope does not work.) **Areas of denuded or dead corneal epithelium will fluoresce greenish blue or aqua and confirm the diagnosis** (Fig. 16.1).

✓ If a foreign body is present, remove it and irrigate the eye as discussed in Chapter 18.

✓ **When a corneal abrasion is present, treat the patient with antibiotic drops for 3 to 5 days, such as trimethoprim plus polymyxin B (Polytrim), 10 mL, 1 drop every 2–6 hours, while awake.** Some physicians prefer ophthalmic ointment preparations, which may last longer but tend to be messy and blur the vision. If ointment is preferred, erythromycin 0.5%, 3.5 g, or polymyxin B/bacitracin, 3.5 g, applied inside the lower lid (ribbon of 1 to 2 cm) four times a day is effective and least expensive. **In patients who wear contact lenses or who were injured by organic material (such as a tree branch), an antipseudomonal antibiotic (e.g., ciprofloxacin [Ciloxan] 0.3%, 1 to 2 drops every 1–6 hours, or ofloxacin [Ocuflox] 0.3%, 1 to 2 drops every 1–6 hours, should be used. Contact lens wearing may be discontinued until the abrasion is healed (see "Bandage" contact lens below).**

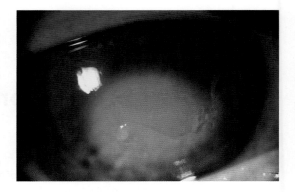

Fig. 16.1 Corneal epithelial abrasion showing fluorescein uptake. (From Goldman, L., & Ausiello, D. (2004). *Cecil textbook of medicine* (22nd ed.). Philadelphia, PA: Elsevier.)

Artificial tears or gel may provide symptomatic relief.

Analgesic nonsteroidal antiinflammatory drug (NSAID) eye drops of diclofenac (Voltaren), 0.1%, 5 mL, or ketorolac (Acular), 0.5%, 5 mL, 1 drop instilled four times a day, provide pain relief and do not inhibit healing. When the diagnosis of an uncomplicated corneal abrasion is certain and the pain is significant, it is now considered to be reasonable to give the patient the bottle of tetracaine drops (0.5-1%) used on the initial exam, to take home to be self-administered every 45-60 minutes for 24-48 hours to relieve their pain. They must be warned against rubbing or injuring their eye while it is completely insensitive and informed as to the importance of getting follow-up if there is any continued discomfort when stopping the drops after 48 hours.

If iritis is present (as evidenced by consensual photophobia or, in severe cases, an irregular pupil or miosis and a limbic flush in addition to conjunctival injection), consult the ophthalmologic follow-up physician about starting treatment with topical mydriatics and steroids (see Chapter 21).

Even when there are no signs of iritis, one instillation of a short-acting cycloplegic, such as cyclopentolate 1% (Cyclogyl), will relieve any pain resulting from ciliary spasm.

Although not likely to be available to the non–contact lens user, **a soft, disposable "bandage" contact lens (e.g., NewVue, Acuvue) in combination with antibiotic and NSAID drops can provide further comfort as well as the ability to see out of the affected eye.** As with any contact lens worn overnight, there is probably an increased risk for infectious keratitis, so this should be provided after a consultation with an ophthalmologist.

Prescribe analgesics as needed, and administer the first dose when appropriate. Most abrasions heal without significant long-term complications; therefore pain relief should be our primary concern with uncomplicated abrasions. This treatment of pain should be guided by an individual patient's age, concomitant illness, drug allergy, ability to tolerate NSAIDs, potential for opioid abuse, and employment conditions, such as driving and machine operation.

Warn the patient that some of the pain will return when the local anesthetic wears off.

Make an appointment for ophthalmologic or primary care follow-up to reevaluate the abrasion the next day. If the abrasion has not fully healed, the patient should be evaluated again 3 to 4 days later, even if they feel well.

✓ **For a corneal laceration with avulsed corneal tissue visible on exam, consultation with an ophthalmologist is recommended urgently, as removal of partially avulsed tissue will improve both comfort and healing.**

✓ Instruct patients about the importance of wearing eye protection. This is particularly needed for persons in high-risk occupations (e.g., miners, woodworkers, metalworkers, landscapers) and those who participate in certain sports (e.g., hockey, lacrosse, racquetball). Other preventive measures include keeping the fingernails of infants and children clipped short and removing objects such as low-hanging tree branches from the home environment.

What Not to Do

✕ Do not undertreat pain, but balance the need for analgesia with best-practice guidelines for prescribing opioids. The aforementioned treatments may not provide adequate analgesia, and supplementation with oral NSAIDs or short course of opioid medication may be necessary for 1 day.

✕ Do not miss anterior chamber hemorrhage or other significant eye trauma that is likely to cause immediate visual impairment.

✕ Do not use a soft contact lens if bacterial conjunctivitis, ulcer, or abrasions caused by contact lens overwear are present.

✕ Do not routinely use an eye patch. Although eye patching traditionally has been recommended in the treatment of corneal abrasions, studies now show that patching does not help healing or pain, interferes with binocular vision, and may even hinder corneal repair.

Discussion

Corneal abrasions constitute a loss of the superficial epithelium of the cornea (see Fig. 16.1). They are generally painful because of the extensive innervation in the affected area. Healing is usually complete in 1 to 2 days unless the abrasions are deep, there is extensive epithelial loss, or there is underlying ocular disease (e.g., diabetes). Larger abrasions that involve more than half of the corneal surface may take 4 to 5 days to heal. Scarring will occur only if the injury is deep enough to penetrate the collagenous layer.

Fluorescein binds to corneal stroma and dead or denuded epithelium but not to intact corneal epithelium. Collections of fluorescein elsewhere—pooling in conjunctival irregularities and in the tear film—are not pathologic findings.

The traditional use of eye patching has been shown to be unnecessary for both corneal reepithelialization and pain relief. Prophylactic antibiotic treatment is used because concomitant infection can cause slower healing of corneal abrasions; however, there is no strong evidence for their use.

Pain is the main symptom and should be treated adequately. Topical and oral NSAIDs are both good options. However, topical NSAIDs may be expensive and have not clearly been shown to be superior to oral NSAIDs but may have a role in those with a contraindication to oral NSAIDs (e.g. gastric ulcer or chronic kidney disease). Some patients may require a short course of opioid medication after weighing the risks and benefits.

Continuous instillation of topical anesthetic drops (e.g., proparacaine [Ophthetic], tetracaine [Pontocaine]) is controversial in the literature, with some suggesting a short course of diluted topical anesthetic to be safe, but this practice is not unanimously recommended due to concern that it may impair healing, inhibit protective reflexes, permit further eye injury, and even cause sloughing of the corneal epithelium. The most recent literature is more reassuring that with short term use, and good patient education, there is minimal risk of such complications.

With small, superficial abrasions, ophthalmologic follow-up is not required if the patient is completely asymptomatic within 12 to 24 hours. **With deep or larger abrasions** or with any worsening symptoms or persistent discomfort,

Discussion continued

ophthalmologic follow-up is necessary within 24 hours because of the risk for corneal infection or ulceration. Ophthalmologic follow-up is also required for **recurrent corneal erosions**—repeated spontaneous disruptions of the corneal epithelium. This can occur in corneal tissue weakened by abrasion months or years earlier. Symptoms are the same as those for corneal abrasions but occur spontaneously on awakening and opening the eyes or after simply rubbing the eyes. Lesions usually are found near the original abrasion. Immediate consultation is recommended for penetrating injury, corneal ulcer, vision loss, inability to remove foreign body, or evidence of hypopyon (pus in anterior chamber) or hyphema (blood in anterior chamber).

Patients who wear contact lenses should also be reevaluated in 24 hours and again 3 to 4 days later, even if they feel well. Hard and soft contact lenses can abrade the cornea and cause a diffuse keratitis or corneal infiltrates and ulcers (see Chapter 15).

In follow-up examination of corneal abrasions, inspect the base of the corneal defect, ensuring that it is clear. If the base of the abrasion becomes hazy, it may indicate the early development of a corneal ulcer and demands immediate ophthalmologic consultation.

Suggested Readings

Arbour, J. D., Brunette, I., Boisjoly, H. M., et al. (1997). Should we patch corneal erosions? *Archives of Ophthalmology*, *115*, 313–317.

Boyd, B. M., & Snyder, R. (2018). Tetracaine challenges old dogma for emergency department management of corneal abrasion pain and beckons a definitive study. *Annals of Emergency Medicine*, *71*(6), 779–782.

Campanile, T. M., St. Clair, D. A., & Benaim, M. (1997). The evaluation of eye patching in the treatment of traumatic corneal epithelial defects. *Journal of Emergency Medicine*, *15*, 769–774.

Carley, F. (2001). Mydriatics in corneal abrasion. *Journal of Accident and Emergency Medicine*, *18*, 273.

Flynn, C. A., D'Amico, F., & Smith, G. (1998). Should we patch corneal abrasions? A meta-analysis. *Journal of Family Practice*, *47*, 264–270.

Kaiser, P. K., & Pineda, R. (1997). A study of topical nonsteroidal anti-inflammatory drops and no pressure patching in the treatment of corneal abrasions. *Ophthalmology*, *104*, 1353–1359.

Kirkpatrick, J. (1993). No eye pad for corneal abrasions. *Eye*, *7*, 468–471.

Le Sage, N., Verreault, R., & Rochette, L. (2001). Efficacy of eye patching for traumatic corneal abrasions: A controlled clinical trial. *Annals of Emergency Medicine*, *28*, 129–134.

Michael, J. G., Hug, D., & Dowd, M. D. (2002). Management of corneal abrasion in children: A randomized clinical trial. *Annals of Emergency Medicine*, *40*, 67–72.

Salz, J. J., Reader, A. L., Schwartz, L. J., et al. (1994). Treatment of corneal abrasions with soft contact lenses and topical diclofenac. *Journal of Refractive Corneal Surgery*, *10*, 640–646.

Shipman, S., Painter, K., et al. (2020). Short-Term topical tetracaine is highly efficacious for the treatment of pain caused by corneal abrasions: A double-blind randomized clinical trial. *The Annals of Emergency Medicine*, *SO196-0644* (20), 30739. http://bit.ly/3st0Pni

Swaminathan, A., Otterness, K., Milne, D., et al. (2015). The safety of topical anesthetics in the treatment of corneal abrasions: A review. *Journal of Emergency Medicine*, *49*(5), 810–815.

Szucs, P. A., Nashed, A. H., Allegra, J. R., & Eskin, B. (2000). Safety and efficacy of diclofenac ophthalmic solution in the treatment of corneal abrasions. *Annals of Emergency Medicine*, *35*, 131–137.

Wakai, A., Lawrenson, J. G., Lawrenson, A. L., et al. (2017). Topical non-steroidal anti-inflammatory drugs for analgesia in traumatic corneal abrasions. *Cochrane Database of Systematic Reviews*, *5*(5), CD009781. https://doi.org/10.1002/14651858.CD009781.pub2

Weaver, C. S., & Terrell, K. M. (2003). Update: do ophthalmic nonsteroidal anti-inflammatory drugs reduce the pain associated with simple corneal abrasion without delaying healing? *Annals of Emergency Medicine*, *41*, 134–140.

Wipperman, J. L., & Dorsch, J. N. (2013). Evaluation and management of corneal abrasions. *American Family Physician*, *87*(2), 114–120.

Floaters

Presentation

Patients may present with a complaint of acute monocular floaters or flashes of light. Floaters can be described as gray or dark "blobs" or "worms" in the visual field and are caused by the interference of light moving through the vitreous (Fig. 17.1). "Flashes" are flashes of white light caused by traction on the retina from the shrinking of vitreous jelly. The most common cause of acute visual floaters is a posterior vitreous detachment. The incidence of posterior vitreous detachment increases with age as the vitreous liquifies, shrinks, and contracts over time. The resulting traction and change in vitreous contour can cause the appearance of floaters and flashes. The differential diagnoses to consider are a retinal detachment, retinal tear, vitreous hemorrhage, migraine with aura, and cerebrovascular causes.

A migraine aura involves usually binocular rather than monocular visual changes that are typical of a primary ocular problem. More rarely occipital strokes can cause visual changes, but this is generally also binocular. In a patient with a transient monocular vision loss with vascular risk factors or symptoms of giant cell arteritis, amaurosis fugax should be considered. A retinal tear or detachment often causes visual impairment but should not be transient. A full retinal tear usually presents with partial monocular loss of visual field described as a "shadow" or "dark curtain." A retinal detachment requires urgent referral to an ophthalmologist and is important to identify. A vitreous hemorrhage can present as monocular vision loss, dark streaks in the vision, or hazy vision. A posterior vitreous detachment, vitreous hemorrhage, and retinal detachment can sometimes be identified by bedside ultrasound.

What to Do

✓ Perform a best-corrected visual acuity examination; examine the cornea and anterior chamber, and perform a **careful ophthalmoscopic and funduscopic exam to look for vitreous hemorrhage** (Fig. 17.2) **or perform a slit lamp exam to visualize the anterior chamber and look for retinal pigment (sometimes called "tobacco dust") that suggests a retinal tear** (Fig. 17.3). The funduscopic exam may reveal a pale area of retina suggestive of a retinal detachment (Fig. 17.4). Consider using a short-acting mydriatic such as tropicamide (antimuscarinic) and/or phenylephrine to dilate the pupil for an optimal retinal exam.

✓ **Perform a pupillary exam, as a relative afferent pupillary defect can suggest a retinal tear affecting the macula.**

✓ **Perform an ocular ultrasound** (Fig. 17.5) looking for retinal detachment (Fig. 17.6) or retinal debris that might suggest hemorrhage. Use the linear ultrasound probe, and place a plastic dressing over the eye so the ultrasound gel does not enter and irritate the eye. A retinal

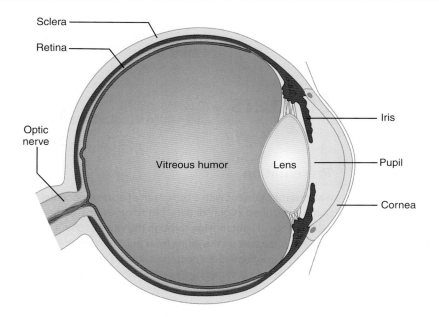

Fig. 17.1 Anatomy of the eye.

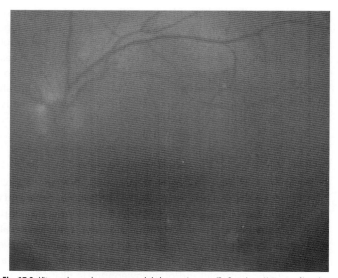

Fig. 17.2 Vitreous hemorrhage seen on ophthalmoscopic exam. (EyeRounds.org University of Iowa.)

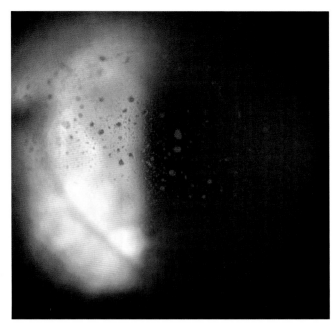

Fig. 17.3 Pigmented cells on slit lamp exam; "tobacco dust" suggestive of pigment release from a full-thickness retinal tear. (EyeRounds.org University of Iowa.)

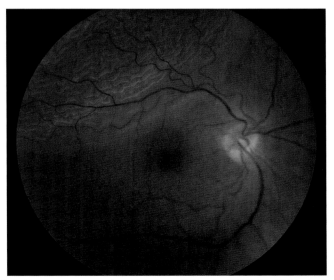

Fig. 17.4 Retinal detachment m upper portion, with rippling and lighter color. (© 2013. Sohn, EH. University of Iowa.)

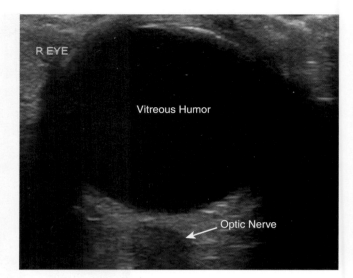

Fig. 17.5 Normal ocular ultrasound with clear anechoic *(black)* vitreous and the posterior shadow of the optic nerve. (Image courtesy Joe Ravera, MD and annotated by Skyler Lentz, MD.)

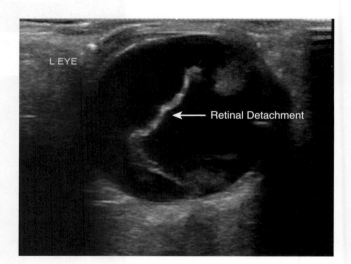

Fig. 17.6 Ocular ultrasound with retinal detachment seen as a hyperechoic membrane that does not cross the optic nerve and appears to be tethered near the optic nerve. (Image courtesy Joe Ravera, MD and annotated by Skyler Lentz, MD.)

detachment appears as a nonmobile reflective membrane not crossing the optic nerve or attached to the optic nerve, whereas a vitreous hemorrhage will be ill defined and mobile. A posterior vitreous detachment (PVD) will be a thin, mobile reflective line not connected to the optic nerve or crossing the optic nerve (Fig. 17.7).

✅ **Check visual fields in each eye. Patients with a monocular visual field defect should be referred to ophthalmology the same day, as this suggests a retinal detachment.**

✅ **Any associated subjective or objective vision loss or diminished vision on visual acuity exam should be discussed emergently with ophthalmology, as this may suggest a retinal tear or detachment and risks permanent visual impairment.**

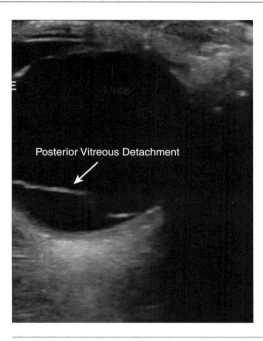

Fig. 17.7 Ocular ultrasound with a posterior vitreous detachment seen as a hyperechoic membrane. (Image courtesy Joe Ravera, MD and annotated by Skyler Lentz, MD.)

✓ **Those with no visual defect** and a suspected uncomplicated PVD should be seen within about 1 week.

✓ **Floaters or flashes without visual impairment and lack of exam finding suggestive of retinal tear or retinal detachment suggest uncomplicated posterior vitreous detachment and can be referred to ophthalmology in about 1 week while counseling to return for vision loss.**

✓ Ask about headache and prior migraine with aura history. A **migraine** usually has binocular symptoms of scintillating scotomata (see Chapter 6). An **ophthalmic migraine** has a similar visual disturbance that is sometimes described as a blind spot followed by a chain of jagged flashing lights that migrate to the periphery of the visual field. This episode lasts for approximately 10 to 20 minutes but is not associated with a headache or other migraine symptoms such as nausea.

✓ Perform a thorough neurologic exam and ask about neurologic symptoms that may suggest a cerebrovascular cause.

✓ **On exam a vitreous hemorrhage or vitreous pigment increases the likelihood of retinal tear and should be discussed with ophthalmology urgently.**

✓ **An identified retinal tear or retinal detachment seen on ultrasound or ophthalmoscopic exam should be discussed and referred to ophthalmology immediately.**

✓ **If a thorough ocular exam is performed and a primarily ocular cause is not found, consider cerebrovascular causes such as central retinal artery occlusion or amaurosis fugax, among others.**

What Not to Do

Ⓧ Do not forget to perform visual acuity, fundoscopic, and visual field exams; consider ocular ultrasound.

Ⓧ Do not mistake a retinal detachment for an uncomplicated PVD. Any monocular visual field loss or vision loss should be considered a retinal detachment and discussed or referred emergently to an ophthalmologist.

Ⓧ Do not forget to consider cerebrovascular causes if a primary ocular problem is not discovered to explain the symptoms or if there are any new neurologic symptoms.

Discussion

The most common cause of acute visual floaters is posterior vitreous detachment. The incidence of PVD increases with age. The vitreous shrinks over time and can detach from the retina. This causes floaters by interfering with the light passing through the normal eye anatomy (see Fig. 17.1). The vitreous detachment causes traction on the retina that sometimes leads to a tear or eventual retinal detachment over the next several weeks. If an uncomplicated PVD is suspected and there is no vision loss, pupillary defect, visual field loss, vitreous hemorrhage, or vitreous pigment, follow-up is not emergent. There is roughly a 3.4% 6-week incidence of retinal tear following diagnosis of PVD, so these patients should be seen by an ophthalmologist within about 1 week for a detailed retinal exam. If there is visual field loss or subjective vision loss, then this suggests a retinal detachment, and emergent ophthalmologic consultation is recommended. Similarly, if a retinal detachment or tear is noted by ophthalmoscopic or ultrasound, emergent consultation is advised to prevent permanent visual impairment.

If a primary ocular etiology of the visual changes is not found after a thorough history and eye exam, then other diagnoses should be considered. A migraine can present with visual aura, usually binocular. In those with vascular risk factors, cerebrovascular causes should be considered such as amaurosis fugax (temporary loss of vision in one eye). A retinal detachment should not be transient. The patient should be asked about giant cell arteritis (GCA) symptoms (e.g., temporal headache or jaw claudication), as untreated GCA may cause vision loss. A central retinal artery occlusion should also be considered. In this case a pale retina or cherry-red spot may be seen on funduscopic exam along with the absence of an alternative explanation for vision loss such as a retinal detachment.

If a cerebrovascular cause is suspected, consider advanced neurovascular imaging and a neurology consultation.

Suggested Readings

Avila, J. (2016). *Ultrasound of the retinal vs. vitreous detachment*. EM:RAP Productions https://www.youtube.com/watch?v=gNLTZipajwM.

Dawood, S., & Skondra, D. (2017). Monocular floaters and flashes. *Disease-a-Month, 63*(3), 80–87.

Hollands, H., Johnson, D., Brox, A., et al. (2009). Acute-onset floaters and flashes: Is this patient at risk for retinal detachment? *Journal of the American Medical Association, 302*(20), 2243–2249.

Johnson, D., & Hollands, H. (2012). Acute-onset floaters and flashes. *Canadian Medical Association Journal, 184*(4), 431.

Foreign Body, Conjunctival

Presentation

Low-velocity projectiles, such as windblown dust particles, can be retained in the tear film, the upper tarsal plate, or in a conjunctival sac. The patient will feel a foreign-body sensation but may not be very accurate in locating the foreign body by sensation alone. On examination, normally occurring white papules inside the lids can be mistaken for foreign bodies, and transparent foreign bodies can be invisible in the tear film (until outlined by fluorescein dye) after orbit radiographs are obtained.

What to Do

✓ **Ensure that the mechanism of injury did not include high-velocity debris (e.g., hammering metal on metal, drilling, grinding, or exposure to explosive forces).**

✓ **Instill topical anesthetic drops** (proparacaine [Ophthaine, Alcaine, Ophthetic] or tetracaine [Pontocaine]). This should relieve discomfort and any uncontrollable blepharospasm.

✓ Perform a best-corrected visual acuity examination and funduscopy; examine the cornea, anterior chamber, and tear film with a bright light (best done with a slit lamp), and then examine the conjunctival sacs.

✓ To examine the lower sac, pull the lower lid down with your finger while the patient looks up (Fig. 18.1).

✓ **To examine the upper sac, hold the proximal portion of the upper lid down with a cotton-tipped swab while pulling the lid out and up by its lashes, everting most of the lid, as the patient looks down. Push the cotton swab downward to help turn the upper conjunctival sac inside out** (Fig. 18.2A–C) (See Video 18.1). The stiff tarsal plate usually keeps the upper lid everted after the swab is removed as long as the patient continues looking downward. Looking up will reduce the lid to its usual position.

✓ **A loose foreign body usually will adhere to a moistened swab lightly touched to the surface of the conjunctiva and is thereby removed** (see Fig. 18.2D and E), **or it can be washed out by copious irrigation with saline.** Occasionally the foreign body will have to be rubbed off of the inside of the lid with the moistened swab.

✓ **Perform a fluorescein examination** to disclose any corneal abrasions caused by the foreign body. These vertical scratches occur when the lid closes over a coarse object and should be treated as described in Chapter 16.

✓ Follow with a brief saline irrigation to remove possible remaining fragments.

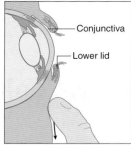

Fig. 18.1 The patient looks up while the lid is pulled down.

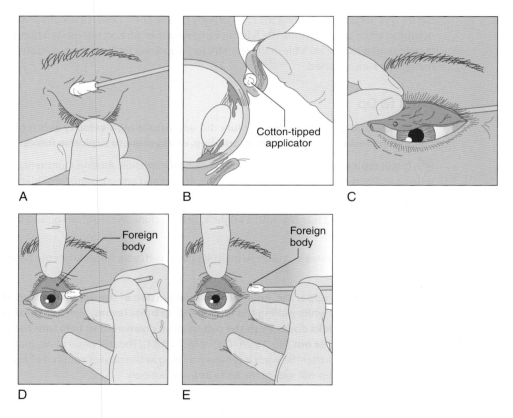

Fig. 18.2 (A) A cotton-tipped applicator is placed above the upper lid. (B) Lid eversion with the patient looking downward. (C) Push down on the applicator to reveal a foreign body hidden under the tarsal plate. (D, E) The moistened applicator touches the foreign body, lifting it away.

What Not to Do

(X) Do not overlook a foreign body lodged in the deep recesses of the upper conjunctival sac.

(X) Do not overlook an eyelash that has turned in and is rubbing on the surface of the eye. Sometimes a lash may be sticking out of the inferior lacrimal punctum. Extract any such lashes.

(X) Do not overlook an embedded or penetrating foreign body. Maintain a high index of suspicion with high-velocity injuries or when there is periorbital tissue damage. Radiography or computed tomography (CT) examination should be performed for suspected metallic intraocular foreign bodies, whereas magnetic resonance imaging (MRI) should be obtained to rule out a nonmetallic object. Use of bedside ultrasound may also be useful in locating corneal foreign bodies and intraocular foreign bodies.

(X) Do not overlook a corneal abrasion. Fluorescein staining will uncover these superficial lesions.

Discussion

Good first aid (providing copious irrigation, pulling the upper lid down over the lower lid, and avoiding rubbing of the eyes) will take care of most ocular foreign bodies. The history of **injury with a high-velocity fragment**, such as a metal shard chipped off from a hammer or chisel, should raise suspicion of a penetrating foreign body, and radiographs or CT scans should be obtained. CT scan of the orbits has the highest sensitivity in identifying metal foreign objects.

The signs associated with an intraocular foreign body can be extremely subtle, causing only slight erythema and local discomfort. Visual acuity often is markedly decreased, but normal visual acuity is possible. There may be **conjunctival chemosis, hyphema, localized cataract, or an iris injury with resultant pupil deformity**. MRI should be used to locate radiolucent objects such as wood or plastic but should never be used to image magnetic

foreign bodies. Ultrasound can be used to detect an intraocular foreign body, but it is not sensitive enough to be the only imaging modality to rule out a foreign body.

Techniques for conjunctival foreign-body removal can also be applied to locating a **displaced contact lens** (see Chapter 24); be aware, however, that fluorescein dye absorbed by soft contact lenses fades slowly.

When eyelids become glued shut with cyanoacrylate (Crazy Glue or Super Glue), it is usually impossible to perform a complete eye examination or even gently separate the eyelids. Simply apply an antibacterial ointment and, if more comfortable for the patient, patch the eye. Spontaneous opening will occur in 1 to 2 days, and a more thorough examination can be performed at that time if any discomfort persists.

Suggested Reading

Shiver, S. A., Lyon, M., Blaivas, M., et al. (2005). Detection of metallic ocular foreign bodies with handheld sonography in a porcine model. *Journal of Ultrasound in Medicine, 24,* 1341–1346.

Foreign Body, Corneal

CHAPTER 19

Presentation

Patients often present after eye injury from falling or airborne particles such as rust, particles from metal grinding, windblown grit, and wood or masonry from construction sites. The patient will complain of a foreign-body sensation and tearing and, possibly over time, will develop constant pain, redness, and photophobia (posttraumatic iritis). Moderate-velocity to high-velocity foreign bodies (fragments chipped from a chisel when struck by a hammer or spray from a grinding wheel) can be superficially embedded on the corneal surface or lodged deep in the corneal stroma, the anterior chamber, or even the vitreous. Superficial foreign bodies may be visualized by simple sidelighting of the cornea or by slit-lamp examination. Deep foreign bodies may be visible on funduscopy only as moving shadows, with a slight or invisible puncture in the sclera.

What to Do

✓ **Instill topical anesthetic drops** (proparacaine [Ophthaine, Alcaine, Ophthetic] or tetracaine [Pontocaine]). This should relieve discomfort and any uncontrollable blepharospasm.

✓ Perform a best-corrected visual acuity examination, funduscopy (looking for shadows), and bright-light anterior chamber examination (slit lamp is best); check pupil symmetry and anterior chamber cell/flare (for iritis) and conjunctivae (for loose foreign bodies).

✓ **Under magnification, a superficial corneal foreign body (usually metal or grit, but occasionally a tiny paint chip or plastic) will be seen adherent to the corneal surface.** Often it is embedded within the corneal epithelium. With iron particles, there will be a halo of particulate debris and rustlike discoloration within the surrounding epithelial tissue (Fig. 19.1).

✓ **With more serious punctures** through the anterior corneal surface penetrating into the anterior chamber, leakage of intraocular fluid from the puncture site might be seen. Streaming of fluorescein dye in this scenario is called the **Seidel sign.** Such a perforation requires immediate ophthalmologic intervention and application of a protective eye shield as well as elevation of the head of the bed and appropriate analgesia.

✓ **If there is any suspicion of a penetrating intraocular foreign body, because there was a high-velocity mechanism of injury, obtain special orbital radiographs or computed tomography (CT) scans to locate it or rule it out.** At present, CT scans are considered the gold standard and have the highest accuracy in diagnosis and localization. The physician should request 3-mm sections through the orbit, unless a foreign body was seen on plain radiography, in which case 6-mm sections are acceptable. **Magnetic resonance imaging**

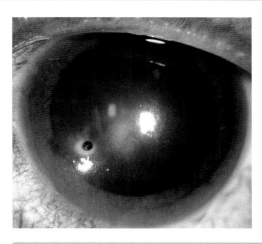

Fig. 19.1 Small iron-containing corneal foreign body. (Adapted from Palay, D. A., & Krachmer, J. H. (2005). *Primary care ophthalmology* (2nd ed.). St. Louis, MO: Mosby.)

(MRI) should be used to locate a nonmetallic object (e.g., plastic or wood) if not seen on other imaging. MRI should never be used if a magnetic foreign body is suspected. If an intraocular foreign body is discovered, immediate ophthalmologic consultation and intervention must be obtained. Any intraocular foreign body can lead to infection and endophthalmitis, a serious condition that can lead to loss of the eye.

✅ **A loosely embedded corneal foreign body might be removed by touching it with a moistened swab,** as shown in Chapter 18, but **if the object is firmly embedded, it will have to be scraped off (under magnification, preferably with a slit lamp) with an ophthalmic spud or an 18-gauge needle** (Fig. 19.2). Some emergency physicians recommend using a small needle for scraping to minimize the possibility of a corneal perforation, but with a tangential approach the larger needle is less likely to cause harm.

✅ Give the patient an object to fixate on so that they will keep their eye still; brace your hand on their forehead or cheek and approach the eye tangentially so that no sudden motion can cause a perforation of the anterior chamber with the needle. **Removal of the foreign body leaves a defect that should be treated as a corneal abrasion** (see Chapter 16).

✅ **If a rust ring is present, it may appear that a foreign body still remains adherent to the cornea after it has been picked away** (Fig. 19.3). **Use the needle to continue scraping away this rust-impregnated corneal epithelium. A corneal burr, if available, is preferable for this task** (Fig. 19.4). This mechanical burr should be held in the same tangential manner as the needle, as described earlier. The operator's hand should also be braced against the side of the patient's face.

✅ If the extent of the corneal defect is unclear, perform an additional fluorescein examination.

✅ Any large corneal infiltrate or corneal ulcer or significant anterior chamber reaction should be managed as a bacterial keratitis (see Chapter 15).

✅ **Finish treatment with further irrigation to loosen possible remaining fragments and with instillation of drops of a mydriatic (homatropine 5%) when photophobia and signs of iritis are present** (see Chapter 21).

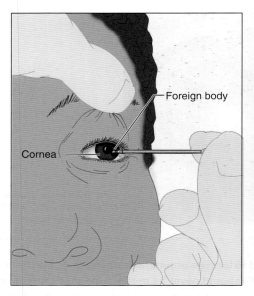
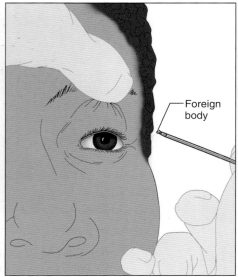

Fig. 19.2 Removing a corneal foreign body with an 18-gauge needle.

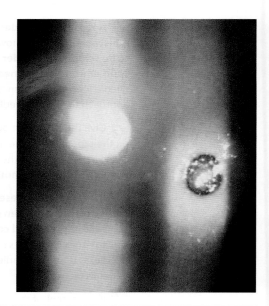

Fig. 19.3 Iron-containing corneal foreign body after removal with a residual rust ring. (Adapted from Marx, J., Hockberger, R., & Walls, R. (2006). *Rosen's emergency medicine* (3rd ed., vol 6). St. Louis, MO: Mosby.)

✓ **Instill and prescribe a nonsteroidal antiinflammatory drug (NSAID) ophthalmologic analgesic drop (diclofenac [Voltaren], 0.1%, 5 mL, or ketorolac [Acular], 0.5%, 5 mL, 1 drop four times daily while awake).**

✓ **Provide for antibiotic eye drops or ointment (polymyxin B/trimethoprim [Polytrim], 10 mL, 1 drop every 2 to 6 hours while awake, or polymyxin B/bacitracin, 3.5 g, applied inside the lower lid [ribbon of 1 to 2 cm] four times a day while awake).**

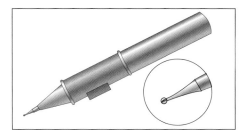

Fig. 19.4 Battery-operated corneal burr for rust ring removal.

(✓) **Oral analgesic medications such as NSAIDs should also be provided.** The first dose should be given before the patient is discharged from the medical facility.

(✓) With deep central corneal foreign bodies, the patient should be advised of the possibility of unavoidable scar formation and subsequent vision impairment. This conversation should be documented.

(✓) **Make an appointment for ophthalmologic follow-up in 1 to 2 days to evaluate for complete healing or any residual corneal staining.**

What Not to Do

(✗) Do not use MRI when there is a suspected magnetic intraocular foreign body.

(✗) Do not overlook a foreign body lodged deep inside the globe; the delayed inflammatory response can lead to blindness or even loss of the eye.

(✗) Do not leave an iron corneal foreign body in place without arranging for early ophthalmologic follow-up the next day.

(✗) Do not allow a patient to leave without ophthalmologic consultation when there is diffuse or focal corneal opacity, abnormal shape of the pupil, evidence of infection (e.g., hypopyon), or significant loss of visual acuity.

(✗) If homatropine was instilled, do not forget to tell the patient that they will have blurred near vision and an enlarged pupil for 12 to 24 hours.

Discussion

Superficial corneal foreign bodies are much more common than deeply embedded corneal foreign bodies. Sometimes the foreign body may not be present at the time of the eye examination. It may have spontaneously dislodged, leaving only the resultant rust ring and/or punctate corneal abrasion with pain and possible photophobia.

Generally, superficial foreign bodies that are removed soon after the injury leave no permanent scarring or visual defect. The deeper the injury, the more the corneal stroma is involved; the longer the time interval between the injury and treatment, the greater the likelihood of complications. If infection develops, the prognosis will also worsen. Keep a high suspicion for an intraocular foreign body if there is a projectile mechanism.

Suggested Reading

Mueller, J., & McStay, C. (2008). Ophthalmologic procedures in the emergency department. *Emergency Medicine Clinics of North America, 26*, 1.

Hordeolum

(Stye)

Presentation

The patient complains of redness, nodular swelling, and pain in the eyelid, perhaps at the base of an eyelash (stye or external hordeolum) or deep within the lid (meibomitis, meibomianitis, or internal hordeolum, which is best appreciated with the lid everted) and perhaps with conjunctivitis and purulent drainage. In some cases, the complaint may be that of generalized edema and erythema of the lid (cellulitis). There may be a history of similar problems.

Examination most commonly reveals a localized tender area of swelling, often with a pointing eruption on either the internal or the external side of the eyelid (Fig. 20.1).

What to Do

✅ Examine the eye, including assessment of best-corrected visual acuity and inversion of the lids (see Chapter 18 for technique). No corneal or intraocular disease should be found.

✅ **Show the patient how to instill antibiotic drops or ointment (e.g., polymyxin B/trimethoprim [Polytrim], 10 mL, 1 drop every 2 to 6 hours; or polymyxin B/bacitracin, 3.5 g, ribbon of 1 to 2 cm lower lid four times a day) into the lower conjunctival sac every 2 to 6 hours.**

✅ **Instruct the patient to apply warm tap water compresses for approximately 15 minutes four times a day.**

✅ **If there are signs of spreading infection (e.g., tender lid edema and erythema with or without preauricular lymphadenitis), provide appropriate systemic antibiotic coverage (e.g., cephalexin [Keflex], 500 mg every 6 hours; dicloxacillin [Dynapen], 500 mg every 6 hours; or amoxicillin/clavulonic acid 875mg/125 mg twice a day for 7 days). Consider coverage for methicillin-resistant *Staphylococcus aureus* (MRSA) in patients with a history of MRSA infection (e.g., doxycycline, 100 mg twice a day, trimethoprim-sulfamethoxazole twice a day, or clindamycin three or four times a day, depending on local MRSA sensitivities, for 7 days).**

✅ Instruct the patient to consult an ophthalmologist or return to the emergency department (ED) or clinic if the problem is not clearly resolving in 2 days or if it gets any worse. Tell them not to squeeze the stye because this may spread the infection into surrounding tissues. Also let them know that frequent recurrences are common.

✅ **If the abscess does not spontaneously drain or resolve in 2 days and if it is pointing, it may be incised with the tip of a No. 11 scalpel blade or 18-gauge needle. Drainage should be accomplished by making a small puncture at the point of maximum tissue thinning, where underlying pus is visible.** Again, instruct the patient to continue using warm compresses and then to consult an ophthalmologist or return to the ED or clinic if the problem is not clearly resolving in 2 days or if it gets any worse.

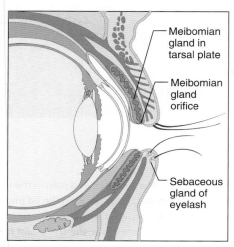 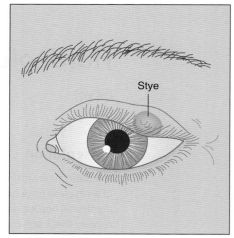

Fig. 20.1 Stye of sebaceous gland (gland of Zeiss).

What Not to Do

❌ Do not overlook orbital or periorbital cellulitis, which is a severe infection and requires aggressive systemic antibiotic treatment and possibly imaging.

❌ Do not culture drainage from a stye unless MRSA is suspected. Eye cultures are usually of little clinical value, and they are costly.

❌ Do not make deep incisions along the lid or eyelash margins. This can lead to lid deformity or abnormal eyelash growth.

Discussion

The terminology describing the two types of hordeolum has become confusing. Meibomian glands run vertically within the tarsal plate, open at tiny puncta along the lid margin, and secrete oil to coat the tear film. The glands of Zeiss and Moll are the sebaceous glands opening into the follicles of the eyelashes. Either type of gland can become occluded and superinfected (*S. aureus* is the causative pathogen in 90% to 95% of cases), producing meibomianitis (internal hordeolum) or a stye (external hordeolum). The immediate care for both acute infections is the same.

Recurrence may be due to a chronic underlying problem with rosacea, which may require additional dermatologic treatments.

A chronic granuloma of the meibomian gland is called a chalazion; it is painless, will not drain, and requires excision.

Most hordeola eventually point and drain by themselves. Therefore warm soaks (four times a day for 15 minutes) are the mainstays of treatment. When lesions are pointing, surgical drainage speeds the healing process.

If the patient appears to have diffuse cellulitis of the lid, fever, and/or painful or restricted extraocular movements, posterior extension (creating an orbital cellulitis) should be suspected. Such cases must be managed aggressively with intravenous antibiotics and immediate subspecialty consultation.

Suggested Reading

Carlisle, R. T., & Digiovanni, J. (2015). Differential diagnosis of the swollen red eyelid. *American Family Physician, 92*(2), 106–112.

Iritis
(Acute Anterior Uveitis)

Presentation

The patient usually complains of the onset over hours or days of unilateral eye pain, blurred vision, and photophobia. He may have noticed a pink eye for a few days, suffered mild to moderate trauma during the previous day or two, or experienced no overt eye problems. There may be tearing but usually no discharge. Eye pain is not markedly relieved after instillation of a topical anesthetic. On inspection of the junction of the cornea and conjunctiva (the corneal limbus), a circumcorneal injection, which on closer inspection is a tangle of fine ciliary vessels, is visible through the white sclera. This limbal blush or ciliary flush is usually the earliest sign of iritis. A slit lamp with 10× magnification may help with identification, but the injection is usually evident merely on close inspection. As the iritis becomes more pronounced, the iris and ciliary muscles go into spasm, producing an irregular, poorly reactive, constricted pupil and a lens that will not focus. The slit-lamp examination should demonstrate white blood cells or light reflection from a protein exudate in the clear aqueous humor of the anterior chamber (cells and flare) (Fig. 21.1).

What to Do

✅ **Using topical anesthesia, perform a complete eye examination that includes best-corrected visual acuity assessment, pupil reflex examination, funduscopy, slit-lamp examination of the anterior chamber (including pinhole illumination to bring out cells and flare), and fluorescein staining to detect any corneal lesion (See Video 21.1).**

✅ Shining a bright light in the normal eye should cause pain in the symptomatic eye **(consensual photophobia).** Visual acuity may be decreased in the affected eye.

✅ **Attempt to ascertain the cause of the iritis.** (Is it generalized from a corneal insult, trauma or conjunctivitis, a late sequela of blunt trauma, infectious, or autoimmune?) Approximately 50% of patients have idiopathic uveitis that is not associated with any other pathologic syndrome. Idiopathic iritis should be suspected when there is acute onset of pain and photophobia in a healthy individual who does not have systemic disease or comorbid autoimmune disease.

✅ **When a patient presents with a first occurrence of unilateral acute anterior uveitis and the history and physical examination are unremarkable, there is no need for any diagnostic workup for systemic disease. With recurrent or bilateral acute uveitis, with or without suspicious findings historically or on physical examination, a diagnostic workup should be initiated at the time of the visit or by the ophthalmologist on follow-up. Unless history and physical examination indicate otherwise, a thoughtful diagnostic workup should be initiated to narrow the broad differential; this could include a complete blood**

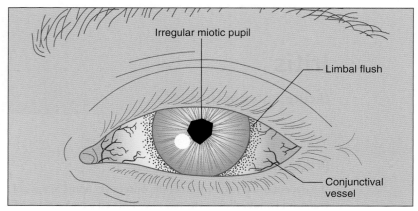

Irregular miotic pupil

Limbal flush

Conjunctival vessel

A

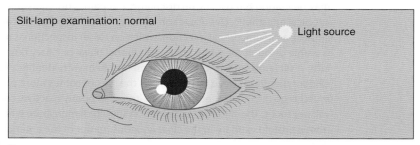

Slit-lamp examination: normal

Light source

B

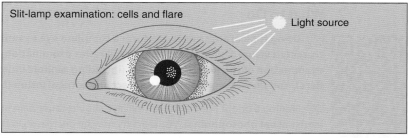

Slit-lamp examination: cells and flare

Light source

C

Fig. 21.1 (A) Early signs of iritis. (B) Normal reflection of pinhole light from the cornea and iris. (C) Cells and flare from iritis in highlight appear similar to what is seen when a light beam is projected through a dark, smoky room.

count (CBC), an erythrocyte sedimentation rate (ESR), a Lyme titer, Venereal Disease Research Laboratory test (VDRL), liver function tests, antinuclear antibodies (ANA), and chest radiograph, among others.

When possible, **determine intraocular pressure,** which may be normal or slightly decreased in the acute phase because of decreased aqueous humor production. An elevated pressure should alert you to the possibility of acute glaucoma.

✓ **Explain to the patient the potential severity of the problem;** this is no routine conjunctivitis, but a process that can develop into blindness. You can reassure them that the prognosis is good with appropriate treatment.

✓ **Arrange for ophthalmologic follow-up within 24 hours, with the ophthalmologist agreeing to the treatment as follows:**

○ **Dilate the pupil and paralyze ciliary accommodation with 1% cyclopentolate (Cyclogyl) drops,** which will relieve the pain of the muscle spasm and keep the iris away from the lens, where miosis and inflammation might cause adhesions (posterior synechiae). **For a more prolonged effect (homatropine is the agent of choice for uveitis), instill a drop of homatropine 5% (Isopto Homatropine) before discharging the patient.**

○ **Suppress the inflammation with topical steroids, such as 1% prednisolone (Inflamase, Pred Forte), 1 drop four times a day.**

✓ Newer formulations of corticosteroids, such as loteprednol 0.2% (Alrex) or 0.5% (Lotemax), 5 mL, 1 drop four times a day, may reduce the risk for raising intraocular pressure, but they also appear to be less efficacious in reducing inflammation.

✓ **Prescribe oral pain medicine if necessary, including nonsteroidal antiinflammatory drugs (NSAIDs) if tolerated.**

✓ **Ensure that the patient is seen the next day for follow-up.**

What Not to Do

✗ Do not let the patient shrug off this "pink eye" and neglect to obtain follow-up, even if they are feeling better, because of the real possibility of permanent visual impairment.

✗ Do not give antibiotics or antivirals unless there is evidence of a bacterial or viral infection.

✗ Do not overlook a possible penetrating foreign body as the cause of the inflammation.

✗ Do not assume the diagnosis of acute iritis until other causes of red eye have been considered and ruled out.

✗ Avoid dilating an eye with a shallow anterior chamber thereby precipitating acute angle–closure glaucoma (Fig. 21.2).

Discussion

Physical examination should focus on visual acuity; presence of pain; location of redness; shape, size, and reaction of the pupil; and intraocular pressure if it can be obtained safely. If a slit lamp is available, the diagnosis can be made more definitively.

Uveitis is defined as inflammation of one or all parts of the uveal tract. Components of the uveal tract include the iris, the ciliary body, and the choroids. Uveitis may involve all areas of the uveal tract and can be acute or chronic; however, it is the acute form—confined to the iris and anterior chamber (iritis) or the iris, anterior chamber, and ciliary body (iridocyclitis)—that is most commonly seen in an emergency department (ED) or urgent care facility.

Iritis (or iridocyclitis) represents a potential threat to vision and requires emergency treatment and expert follow-up. The inflammatory process in the anterior eye can opacify the anterior chamber, deform the iris

(continued)

Discussion—continued

or lens, scar them together, or extend into adjacent structures. Posterior synechiae can potentiate cataracts and glaucoma. Treatment with topical steroids is the mainstay of therapy for acute anterior uveitis, but this therapy can backfire if the process is caused by an infection (especially herpes keratitis); therefore the slit-lamp examination looking for typical dendritic lesions is especially useful. Topical steroids alone can also contribute to cataract formation as well as the development of glaucoma, so this treatment should be directed by an ophthalmologist.

Iritis is most commonly idiopathic and may have no apparent cause, may be related to recent trauma, or may be associated with an immune reaction. In addition to association with infections such as

herpes, Lyme disease, and microbial keratitis, uveitis is found in association with autoimmune disorders such as ankylosing spondylitis, Behçet syndrome, reactive arthritis syndrome (conjunctivitis, urethritis, and polyarthritis), psoriatic arthritis, sarcoid, juvenile arthritis, and inflammatory bowel disease and in association with underlying malignancies.

Sometimes an intense conjunctivitis or keratitis (see Chapters 14 and 15) may produce some sympathetic limbal flush, which will resolve as the primary process resolves and requires no additional treatment. A more definite, but still mild, iritis may resolve with administration of cycloplegics and may not require steroids. All of these conditions, however, mandate ophthalmologic consultation and follow-up.

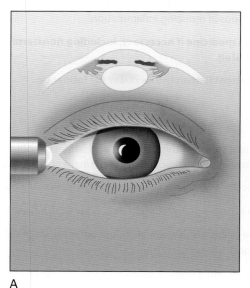 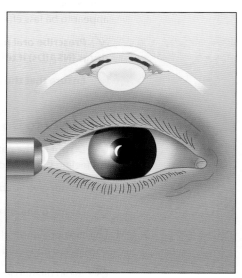

Fig. 21.2 (A) Normal iris. (B) Domed iris casts a shadow. The shallow anterior chamber is prone to acute angle–closure glaucoma if the pupil is dilated.

Suggested Readings

Au, Y. K., & Henkind, P. (1981). Pain elicited by consensual pupillary reflex: A diagnostic test for acute iritis. *Lancet, 2*, 1254–1255.

Patel, H., & Goldstein, D. (2003). Pediatric uveitis. *Pediatric Clinics of North America, 50*, 125–136.

Powdrill, S. (2010). Ciliary injection: A differential diagnosis for the patient with acute red eye. *Journal of the American Academy of Physician Assistants, 23*, 50–54.

Prete, M., Dammacco, R., Fatone, M. C., et al. (2016). Autoimmune uveitis: Clinical, pathogenetic, and therapeutic features. *Clinical and Experimental Medicine, 16*, 125.

Periorbital and Conjunctival Edema

Presentation

The patient is frightened by facial distortion and itching that appeared either spontaneously or up to 24 hours after being bitten by a bug or coming in contact with some irritant. One or both eyes may be involved. The patient may have been rubbing their eyes; however, an allergen or chemical irritant may cause periorbital edema long before a reaction, if any, is evident on the skin of the hand (e.g., occurring in the context of petting an animal then rubbing one's eyes).

There may be minimal to marked generalized conjunctival swelling (chemosis), giving the sensation of fullness under the eyelid, but there is little injection (Fig. 22.1). In extreme cases, this chemosis may appear as a large, watery bubble (watch-glass chemosis), which may be frightening to the patient but is quite harmless. Tenderness and pain should be minimal or absent, but pruritus may at times be intense. There should be little or no erythema of the skin, no photophobia, no pain with extraocular movements, and no fever. Visual acuity should be normal, there should be no fluorescein uptake over the cornea, and the anterior chamber should be clear.

What to Do

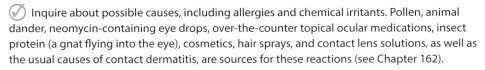 Inquire about possible causes, including allergies and chemical irritants. Pollen, animal dander, neomycin-containing eye drops, over-the-counter topical ocular medications, insect protein (a gnat flying into the eye), cosmetics, hair sprays, and contact lens solutions, as well as the usual causes of contact dermatitis, are sources for these reactions (see Chapter 162).

After completing a full eye examination, reassure the patient that this condition is not as serious as it looks.

Have the patient thoroughly wash their face as soon as it is practical to do so.

Prescribe hydroxyzine (Atarax) or diphenhydramine (Benadryl), 25 to 50 mg every 6 hours, or a nonsedation antihistamine (e.g., loratadine, fexofenadine, cetirizine) for mild to moderate periorbital swelling and a course of steroids, 3 to 5 days (prednisone, 20 to 40 mg once daily) for more severe cases.

Ophthalmic drops are soothing and reduce swelling when the conjunctiva is involved and avoid the systemic effects of antihistamines. **Prescribe olopatadine 0.1% (Patanol), ketotifen fumarate 0.025% (Zaditor) [now over the counter], or azelastine hydrochloride 0.05% (Optivar), 1 drop twice daily. These are H_1-antihistamines and mast-cell stabilizers and should be prescribed for 1 week, then as needed thereafter.**

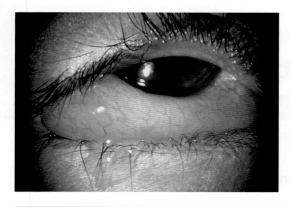

Fig. 22.1 Spontaneous swelling and itching are common symptoms of periorbital and conjunctival edema. This represents an allergic conjunctivitis with chemosis secondary to an airborne allergen. (Adapted from Palay, D. H., & Krachmer, J. H. (2005). *Primary care ophthalmology* (2nd ed.). St. Louis, MO: Mosby.)

✓ **A short course of a topical steroid agent (loteprednol 0.02% [Alrex] or 0.05% [Lotemax], 1 drop four times a day) should be reserved for the more severe cases and in consultation with an ophthalmologist. This may be used for up to 1 week.**

✓ Instruct the patient to apply cool compresses to reduce swelling and discomfort. Artificial tears may be soothing.

✓ Warn the patient about the potential signs of infection.

What Not to Do

✗ Do not apply heat; heat causes an increase in swelling and pruritus.

✗ Do not confuse this condition with orbital or periorbital cellulitis, either of which is a serious infection manifested by pain, heat, and fever. Orbital cellulitis is more posterior, involves the ocular muscles (which causes painful extraocular movements), and calls for intravenous (IV) antibiotic therapy and hospital admission.

Discussion

The dramatic swelling that often brings a patient to the emergency department (ED) or the family doctor occurs because there is loose connective tissue surrounding the orbit. Fluid quickly accumulates when a local allergic response leads to release of histamine from mast cells, which causes increased capillary permeability, resulting in dramatic eyelid and periorbital swelling. The insect envenomation, allergen, or irritant responsible may be located some distance away from the affected eye, on the scalp or face, but the loose periorbital tissue is the first to swell. If the swelling is due to contact dermatitis (e.g., poison ivy) and the allergen is bound to the skin, oral steroids should be continued for 10 to 14 days until the skin renews itself (see Chapters 162 and 184). Supportive care with oral or topical antihistamines can help with symptoms.

Suggested Reading

Bilkhu, P. S., Wolffsohn, J. S., Naroo, S. A., et al. (2014). Effectiveness of nonpharmacologic treatments for acute seasonal allergic conjunctivitis. *Ophthalmology, 121*(1), 72–78.

Periorbital Ecchymosis

CHAPTER 23

(Black Eye)

Presentation

The patient has suffered blunt trauma to the eye, most often resulting from a blow, a fall, a sports injury, or a car accident, and is alarmed because of the swelling and discoloration. Family or friends may be more concerned than the patient about the appearance of the eye. There may be an associated subconjunctival hemorrhage, but the remainder of the eye examination should be normal, and there should be no palpable bony deformities, diplopia, or subcutaneous emphysema (Fig. 23.1).

What to Do

✅ **Determine, as well as possible, the specific mechanism of injury.**

✅ **Perform a complete eye examination,** including a bright-light examination to rule out an early hyphema (blood in the anterior chamber) or an abnormal pupil; a funduscopic examination to rule out a retinal detachment (bedside ultrasound can be useful for this as well), vitreous hemorrhage, or dislocated lens; and a fluorescein stain to rule out corneal abrasion. Best-corrected visual acuity testing should always be performed and, with an uncomplicated injury, is expected to be normal. **All patients with visual loss, severe pain, proptosis, pupil irregularity, or new visual floaters should have further workup and be referred to an ophthalmologist immediately.**

✅ **Obtain imaging when a blowout fracture is suspected.** Test extraocular eye movements, looking especially for restriction of eye movement or diplopia on upward gaze, and check sensation over the infraorbital nerve distribution. Paresthesia in the distribution of the infraorbital nerve suggests a fracture of the orbital floor. Enophthalmos usually is not observed, although it is part of the classic textbook triad associated with a blowout fracture. Subcutaneous emphysema is a recognized complication of orbital wall fracture.

✅ **Symmetrically palpate the supraorbital and infraorbital rims as well as the zygoma, feeling for the type of deformity that would be encountered with a displaced tripod fracture (See Video 23.1).** A unilateral deformity will be obvious if your thumbs are fixed in a midline position while you use your index fingers to palpate the patient's facial bones, both left and right, simultaneously (Fig. 23.2).

✅ **When there is a substantial mechanism of injury or if there is any clinical suspicion of an underlying fracture, obtain a computed tomography (CT) scan of the orbit and the**

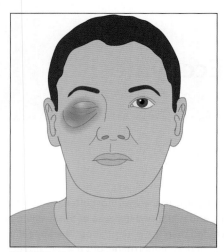

Fig. 23.1 Blunt trauma to the eye.

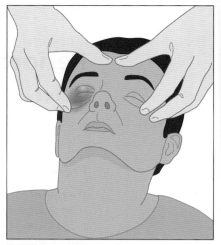

Fig. 23.2 Proper hand placement for symmetrically palpating the supraorbital and infraorbital rims.

brain if a serious traumatic brain injury is suspected. CT scans are more sensitive than plain radiographs and allow visualization of subtle fractures of the orbit and small amounts of orbital air.

✓ If a significant injury is discovered, consult an ophthalmologist or facial surgeon. Patients with a hyphema should see an ophthalmologist within 24 hours. The patient should be instructed to rest with their head elevated and avoid nose blowing or sneezing. A protective metal shield should be placed over the eye, and the patient should be instructed to refrain from taking aspirin or nonsteroidal antiinflammatory drugs (NSAIDs). Hospital admission is not required.

✓ **Consider the possibility of abuse;** when suspected, obtain the appropriate consultations and make the appropriate referrals.

✓ **When a significant injury has been ruled out, reassure the patient that the swelling will subside, and that the discoloration may spread and will take 1 to 2 weeks to clear. Acetaminophen should be sufficient for analgesia.**

✓ **Instruct the patient to follow up with an ophthalmologist if there is any problem with vision or if pain develops after the first few days.** Rarely, traumatic iritis, retinal tears, or vitreous hemorrhage may develop later, secondary to blunt injury.

✓ **With sports-related injuries,** recommend protective eyewear made of polycarbonate. Polycarbonate lenses are available in prescription and nonprescription lenses in a sturdy sports frame.

What Not to Do

🚫 Do not order unnecessary radiographs. For minor injuries, if the eye examination is normal and there are no palpable deformities, radiographs and CT scans are unnecessary.

🚫 Do not ignore the finding of bilateral deep periorbital ecchymoses (raccoon eyes), especially if caused by head trauma remote to the eye. This may be the only sign of a basilar skull fracture and warrants imaging.

Discussion

Black eyes are usually nothing more than uncomplicated facial contusions. Patients become upset about them because they are so near to the eye, because they produce such noticeable facial disfigurement, and because the patient may seek retaliation against the person who hit him. Nonetheless, serious injury or abuse must always be considered and appropriately ruled out before the patient is discharged.

The extent of ocular damage depends on the size, hardness, and velocity of the blunt object causing the injury. A direct blow to the globe from a blunt object smaller than the eye's orbital opening is more likely to cause injury to internal ocular structures (e.g., iris injury, ruptured globe, hyphema, retinal hemorrhage, retinal detachment, and vitreous hemorrhage). Injury by a blunt object larger than the orbital opening exerts force on the floor of the orbit or the medial wall, which is more likely to result in fractures of the thin bones (e.g., blowout fracture).

Sudden orbital swelling or inflation immediately after nose blowing is caused by air being forced from a paranasal sinus (most often the maxillary) to the orbit through a fracture, which may act as a one-way valve, increasing the orbital pressure and potentially leading to a compressive optic neuropathy.

Suggested Readings

Cook, T. (2002). Ocular and periocular injuries from orbital fractures. *Journal of the American College of Surgeons*, *195*, 831–834.

Corrales, G., & Curreri, A. (2009). Eye trauma in boxing. *Clinics in Sports Medicine*, *28*, 591–607.

Rodriguez, J. O., Lavina, A. M., & Agarwal, A. (2003). Prevention and treatment of common eye injuries in sports. *American Family Physician*, *67*, 1481–1488.

Removal of Dislocated Contact Lens

Presentation

The patient may know that the lens has dislocated into one of the recesses of the conjunctiva and complains only of the loss of refractory correction, or they may have lost track of the lens completely, in which case the eye is a logical place to look first. Pain and blepharospasm suggest a corneal abrasion, perhaps resulting from the patient's attempts to remove an absent lens that was thought to still be in place.

What to Do

✓ **If pain and blepharospasm are a problem, topically anesthetize the eye.**

✓ **Pull back the eyelids as if looking for conjunctival foreign bodies, invert the upper lid, and, if necessary,** instill fluorescein dye (a last resort with soft lenses, which absorb the dye tenaciously and ruin the contact lens).

✓ **If the lens is loose, slide it over the cornea, and let the patient remove it in the usual manner. Irrigation may loosen a dry, stuck lens.**

✓ **For a more adherent hard lens, use a commercially available suction cup lens remover. Soft lenses may be pinched between the fingers, or a commercially available rubber pincer can be used** (Fig. 24.1). **Another option is to take a Morgan irrigation lens attached to a 5-mL syringe filled with 2 mL of normal saline. Flush the Morgan lens with the saline, place the lens over the contact, aspirate on the syringe to produce suction, and remove the Morgan lens and the contact lens together from the conjunctival sac** (Fig. 24.2).

✓ Complete the eye examination, including best-corrected visual acuity assessment and bright-light and fluorescein examination. Treat any corneal abrasion with antipseudomonal topical antibiotics and further care as explained in Chapter 16.

✓ Instruct the patient to refrain from wearing the lens until all symptoms have abated for 24 hours and to see an ophthalmologist if there are any problems.

What Not to Do

✗ Do not give up on locating a missing lens too easily. Lost lenses have been excavated from under scar tissue in the conjunctival recesses years after they were first dislocated.

✗ Do not omit examination with fluorescein stain for fear of ruining a soft contact lens. The dye may take a long time to elute out, but it is most important to find the dislocated lens.

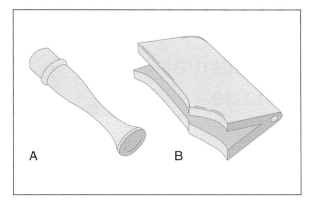

Fig. 24.1 (A) Rubber suction cup used for extracting hard lenses. (B) Rubber pincer used for extracting soft lenses.

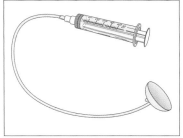

Fig. 24.2 Morgan lens attached to a 5-mL syringe.

Discussion

The deepest recess in the conjunctiva is under the upper lid, but lenses can lodge anywhere; in extremely rare cases, lenses have perforated the conjunctival sac and migrated posterior to the globe. Be sure to evert the upper conjunctival sac by pushing down with a cotton-tipped applicator (see C hapter 18). Search thoroughly for the missing lens, though often no lens can be found because it was missing from the start through actual loss or forgetfulness.

Subconjunctival Hemorrhage

Presentation

This condition may occur spontaneously or may follow minor trauma, coughing, vomiting, straining at stool, or exercising heavily. There is no pain or visual loss, but the patient may be frightened by the appearance of the affected eye and have some sensation of superficial fullness or discomfort. Often a friend or family member is frightened by the appearance and insists that the patient see a physician. This hemorrhage usually appears as a bright red area covering part of the sclera but contained by the conjunctiva (Fig. 25.1). Hemorrhage may cover the whole visible globe, sparing only the cornea.

What to Do

✓ **Look for associated trauma or other signs of a potential bleeding disorder, including overmedication with anticoagulants.** A history of significant trauma or evidence of recurrent hemorrhage or bleeding from other sites (e.g., hematuria, melena, ecchymosis, epistaxis) warrants a careful evaluation for ocular trauma or a bleeding diathesis.

✓ **Perform a complete eye examination** that includes (1) best-corrected visual acuity assessment, (2) conjunctival inspection, (3) examination of the anterior chamber, (4) extraocular movement testing, (5) fluorescein staining, and (6) funduscopic examination.

✓ **Reassure the patient that there is no serious eye damage; explain that the blood may continue to spread, but the redness should resolve in 2 to 3 weeks.**

What Not to Do

✗ Do not do an extensive hematologic workup for isolated subconjunctival hemorrhage in healthy patients who are not taking anticoagulants.

✗ Do not neglect to warn the patient that the redness may spread during the next 2 days. If the patient is not warned, they may return, alarmed by the reported "growing hemorrhage."

✗ Do not ignore any significant finding discovered during the history or complete eye examination. The patient should have an otherwise benign ocular exam. Penetrating injuries, lacerations, and ruptured globes also present with subconjunctival hemorrhage, obscuring the damage beneath.

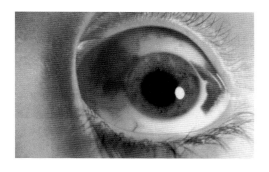

Fig. 25.1 A bright red area covering part of the sclera. (From Marx, J., Hockberger, R., & Walls, R. (2006). *Rosen's emergency medicine* (6th ed.). St. Louis, MO: Mosby.)

Discussion

Subconjunctival hemorrhage represents one of the most common eye disorders. The incidence increases markedly in patients over 50 years of age. A major risk factor is hypertension. Subconjunctival hemorrhage has also been shown to be associated with anticoagulant therapy, including low-dose heparin and warfarin, with an incidence of 1.5% to 5%.

Although this condition looks serious, it is usually caused by a harmless leak in a superficial conjunctival blood vessel resulting from trivial trauma or a sudden Valsalva maneuver or coughing. Patients only need to be reassured that, although it appears to be serious, this is a minor problem that will resolve spontaneously over time without any eye damage. Recurrent hemorrhage or evidence of other bleeding sites should prompt referral and evaluation for vasculitis, clotting disorder, or other systemic process. In infants, vitamin C deficiency and abusive trauma should always be considered.

Suggested Readings

Incorvaia, C., Costagliola, C., & Parmeggiani, F. (2002). Recurrent episodes of spontaneous subconjunctival hemorrhage in patients with factor XIII Val34Leu mutation. *American Journal of Ophthalmology*, *134*, 927–929.

Nguyen, T. M., & Phelan, M. P. (2013). Subconjunctival hemorrhage in a patient on dabigatran (Pradaxa). *American Journal of Emergency Medicine*, *31*(2), 455 e3–e5.

Rajvanshi, P., & McDonald, G. (2001). Subconjunctival hemorrhage as a complication of endoscopy. *Gastrointestinal Endoscopy*, *53*, 251–253.

Salmon, J. F. (2020). *Kanski's clinical ophthalmology* (9th ed.). London: Elsevier Limited.

Sodhi, P. K., & Jose, R. (2003). Subconjunctival hemorrhage: The first presenting clinical feature of idiopathic thrombocytopenic purpura. *Japanese Journal of Ophthalmology*, *47*, 316–318.

Ultraviolet Keratoconjunctivitis

(Welders or Tanning Bed Burn)

Presentation

The patient arrives in the emergency department (ED) or clinic complaining of severe, intense, burning eye pain, usually bilateral, beginning 6 to 12 hours after a brief exposure without eye protection to a high-intensity ultraviolet (UV) light source, such as a sunlamp or welder's arc. The eye examination shows conjunctival injection and tearing; fluorescein staining may be normal or may show diffuse superficial uptake (discerned as a punctate keratopathy under slit-lamp examination). The patient may also have first-degree burns on their skin.

What to Do

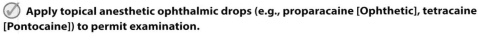 **Apply topical anesthetic ophthalmic drops (e.g., proparacaine [Ophthetic], tetracaine [Pontocaine]) to permit examination.**

Perform a complete eye examination, including best-corrected visual acuity assessment, funduscopy, anterior chamber bright-light examination, fluorescein staining, and conjunctival sac inspection. There may be mild visual impairment.

Prescribe cold compresses, rest, and analgesics (e.g., acetaminophen, ibuprofen, naproxen) to control pain. As always, balance the need for analgesia with the harm associated with prescription of opiates (e.g., oxycodone, hydrocodone).

Provide lubricating ophthalmic ointment (erythromycin 0.5%, 3.5 g; or polymyxin B/bacitracin, 3.5-g tube applied inside the lower lid [ribbon of 1 to 2 cm] four times a day), or, if drops are preferred, polymyxin B/trimethoprim (Polytrim), 10 mL, 1 drop every 2 to 6 hours. However, no evidence supports this practice. **Use of a bland ointment (e.g., Lacri-Lube) may be all that is required to reduce pain.**

Where available, prescribe analgesic nonsteroidal antiinflammatory drug (NSAID) eye drops (diclofenac [Voltaren] 0.1%, 5 mL; or ketorolac [Acular] 0.5%, 5 mL, 1 drop four times a day).

Administration of a short-acting cycloplegic drop (e.g., cyclopentolate 1%) may help relieve the pain of reflex ciliary spasm.

Warn the patient that pain will return when the local anesthetic wears off but that the oral medication and topical NSAID prescribed should provide some relief. Symptoms should resolve after 24 to 36 hours. Medications can be stopped after symptoms resolve. Be aware that there is reassuring evidence that short term use (24-48 hours) of topical anesthetics such as tetracaine can be safely used at home by the patient for complete pain relief when required. (See chapter 16)

✓ **Patients should be instructed on the use of proper eye protection before being discharged.**

What Not to Do

✗ Do not use the traditional eye patches. These dressings have been found to be of no value and might actually delay reepithelialization. Moreover, some patients find the loss of sight (with bilateral patches) and depth perception (in the case of single-eye patching) to be unacceptable and wearing the patches to be more uncomfortable than going without them.

Discussion

The history of exposure to a welder's arc torch or other source of UV light exposure may be difficult to elicit from an unsuspecting patient because of the long asymptomatic interval (6 to 12 hours after a brief exposure). This requires a high level of suspicion on the part of the examiner along with persistent, focused questioning.

Longer exposures to lower-intensity UV light sources may be more obvious and resemble a sunburn.

Healing should be complete in 12 to 24 hours with the resolution of pain. If the patient continues to experience discomfort for longer than 48 hours, an ophthalmologist should be consulted.

Other sources of UV phototoxicity can be found in scientific research and manufacturing technology. Several epidemic outbreaks of UV keratoconjunctivitis have been reported as the result of exposure to UV light from broken high-intensity mercury vapor lamps, such as those found in community gymnasiums. **Another common source of UV phototoxicity is the intense sunlight exposure found in water sports and sunny snow conditions (known to the layperson as** snow blindness**).**

Suggested Reading

Kirschke, D. L., Jones, T. F., Smith, N. M., et al. (2004). Photokeratitis and UV-radiation burns associated with damaged metal halide lamps. *Archives of Pediatric and Adolescent Medicine, 158,* 372–376.

PART 3

Ear, Nose, and Throat Emergencies

■ Katie M. Wells ■ Deborah Governale

Cerumen Impaction

(Earwax Blockage)

Presentation

The patient may complain of "wax in the ear," a "stuffed-up" sensation, pain, itching, decreased hearing, tinnitus, dizziness, hearing aid malfunction, ear drainage, or ear odor. Symptoms may be sudden in onset if the patient put a cotton-tipped applicator down the ear canal or placed something like mineral oil into the ear canal in an attempt to soften the wax. On physical examination, there is often dark brown, thick, dry, or pasty cerumen, frequently packed down against the eardrum (where it does not occur normally), obscuring visualization of the ear canal and the tympanic membrane.

What to Do

✓ **When excessive cerumen causes symptoms such as those listed or prevents examination of the canal and tympanic membrane, it should be removed.** Also consider removing in patients who are unable to report symptoms, such as small children and cognitively impaired patients.

✓ **There are three options for cerumen removal:** (1) cerumenolytic agents, (2) irrigation, and (3) manual removal. These methods may be used alone or in combination.

✓ **There is no clear evidence in the literature that one method of removing cerumen impaction is superior,** thus the treatment method used should depend on the available resources, experience of the treating clinician, potential harms based on the specific patient, and shared decision making.

✓ **Irrigation and manual removal** can increase risk of infection in immunocompromised or diabetic patients. Canal trauma can lead to hemorrhage or hematoma in patients on anticoagulants.

✓ **Cerumenolytics and irrigation** should be avoided if tympanic membrane (TM) injury is suspected or tympanostomy tubes are in place.

✓ **Approximately 1/1000 irrigations has a complication.** Complications include canal laceration, pain, dizziness, vertigo, syncope, TM perforation, bleeding, transient hearing loss, and subsequent development of otitis externa.

✅ **For difficult cases or patients with known or suspected TM perforation,** consider referral to an otolaryngologist (ENT), who has access to a microscope with better visualization and fine tools to delicately remove wax.

Procedure for Cerumenolytic Application

Cover the patient with a waterproof drape. Have the patient lie so that the affected ear is facing up. Gently instill your cerumenolytic agent to fill the external auditory canal (EAC). Leave the agent there for 5 to 10 minutes, then have the patient turn the head to let gravity drain the canal. If the cerumen is still impacted, you can repeat or move to another technique. A Cochrane review concluded that no specific cerumenolytic was superior, and none was superior to saline or water, but that most agents led to some clearing of cerumen. **Cerumenolytic options include water, saline, hydrogen peroxide, mineral oil, olive oil, sodium bicarbonate, acetic acid, triethanolamine, carbamide peroxide, and docusate. Some cerumenolytics can cause side effects, such as local irritation of the canal or allergic reaction, usually local.**

Procedure for Irrigation

✅ First, explain the procedure to the patient, who must be able to cooperate to prevent any accidental trauma. **Ask about the possibility of eardrum perforation or myringotomy tubes, which are contraindications to irrigation.** Instill warm (body temperature) water into the canal and let it sit for a few minutes .

✅ Cover the patient with a waterproof drape and have him hold a basin or thick towel below the ear.

✅ **Fill a syringe with body-temperature water. Syringes between 5 mL and 10 mL may be used when fit with a short (1-cm), soft-tubing catheter** (Fig. 27.1). A large-gauge butterfly catheter with the needle cut off can be used. Try to avoid using an angiocath with the needle removed because the ridged sharp plastic is much more likely to cause an injury.

✅ **Aim along the anterosuperior wall of the external canal while pulling the pinna posteriorly to straighten out the canal (do not occlude the whole canal), and irrigate quickly, with pressure, to produce a jet lavage. Do not insert the tip of the tubing past the lateral one-third of the EAC, usually less than 8 mm in an adult. Use a more gentle irrigation pressure on small children. This irrigation usually needs to be repeated multiple times before the wax is finally flushed out (See Video 27.1).**

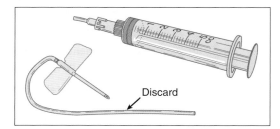

Discard

Fig. 27.1 Syringe (5 mL) with short, soft catheter.

✅ Intermittently reexamine the ear to determine if the wax has been adequately cleared. If so, grossly test the patient's hearing. If not, continue irrigating or use another technique.

Procedure for Manual Removal

✅ Warn the patient about potential discomfort or minor bleeding. Do not probe blindly into the canal. Perform manual removal under direct vision using an otoscope or using a headlamp. **Manual removal can be accomplished with a curette (metal or plastic), probe, spoon, hook, forceps, or suction.**

✅ **After irrigation or manual removal, a final rinse with an acetic acid otic solution (VoSol Otic) may help prevent secondary otitis.** This may be particularly important in older, diabetic, or immunocompromised patients.

What Not to Do

❌ Do not irrigate an ear in which there is suspected or known tympanic membrane perforation or a myringotomy tube.

❌ Do not irrigate the ear with cold (or hot) solutions. This may cause severe vertigo with nausea and vomiting.

❌ Do not leave pooled water in the canal, which can lead to external otitis.

❌ Do not recommend or allow patient to use ear candling, which can lead to severe burns and has not been shown to be effective.

Discussion

Cerumen acidifies the ear canal with lysozymes, thereby inhibiting bacterial and fungal growth. It is also hydrophobic and repels water from the ear, further protecting it from infection.

Cerumen is produced by the sebaceous glands of the hair follicles in the outer one-third of the ear canal, and it naturally migrates outward along these hairs. One of the problems associated with ear swabs is that they can push wax inward, away from these hairs, and against the eardrum where the wax can then stick and harden. Cerumen is most likely to become impacted when it is pushed against the eardrum by these cotton-tipped applicators, hairpins, or other objects that people put down their

ear canals, and by hearing aids. Less common causes of cerumen impaction include overproduction of earwax and an abnormally shaped ear canal.

Advise patients that the best method of cleaning the external ear is to wipe the outer opening of the canal with a washcloth covering the patient's finger. Instruct them not to enter the ear canal itself. They can use cerumenolytic agents at home as long as there are no contraindications such as tympanostomy tubes, other TM perforation, or other history of ear pathology that would require talking with their otolaryngologist first. **If a patient does not improve with cerumen removal, seek alternate causes of the symptoms.**

Suggested Readings

Burton, M. J., & Doree, C. J. (2007). Ear drops for the removal of ear wax (Cochrane review). *The Cochrane Library*, *2*.

Robbins, B. (2004). Randomized clinical trial of docusate, triethanolamine polypeptide, and irrigation in cerumen removal in children. *Journal of Pediatrics*, *145*, 138–139.

Roland, P., Smith, T. L., Schwartz, R. L., et al. (2008). Clinical practice guideline: Cerumen impaction. *Otolaryngology–Head and Neck Surgery*, *139*, S1–S21.

Roland, P. S., Easton, D. A., Gross, R. D., et al. (2004). Randomized, placebo-controlled evaluation of Cerumenex and Murine earwax removal products. *Archives of Otolaryngology—Head and Neck Surgery*, *130*, 1175–1177.

Schwartz, S. R., Magit, E., et al. (2017). Clinical practice guideline (update): Earwax (cerumen impaction). *Otolaryngology–Head and Neck Surgery*, *156*(Suppl. 1), S1–S29.

Singer, A. J., Sauris, E., & Viccellio, A. W. (2000). Cerumenolytic effects of docusate sodium: A randomized, controlled trial. *Annals of Emergency Medicine*, *36*, 228–232.

Epistaxis

(Nosebleed)

Presentation

Patients may arrive in the emergency department (ED) or urgent care center with active bleeding from their nose or spitting up blood that is draining into their throat from a nasal source. There may be a report of minor trauma, such as sneezing, nose blowing, or nose picking. On occasion, the hemorrhage has stopped, but the patient is concerned because the bleeding has been recurrent or the bleeding was copious. In rare instances, the bleeding may be brisk requiring resuscitation. Bleeding is most commonly present at the anterior aspect of the nasal septum, within Kiesselbach plexus or from the inferior turbinate. Sometimes, especially with posterior epistaxis, a specific bleeding site cannot be determined. This chapter refers to the care of patients with epistaxis who do not require resuscitation or have airway compromise.

What to Do

✅ **Controlling significant hemorrhage should always take precedence over obtaining a detailed history or visualization of the specific bleeding site.**

✅ **Have the patient maintain compression on the nostrils** by pinching with a gauze sponge while all equipment and supplies are being assembled at the bedside. If the patient is unable to pinch the nostrils, a compression device can be made by taping two tongue blades together at one end and placing the other end across the soft portion of the nose, or commercially available nasal clips may be used.

✅ Use of a headlight with a focused beam will allow you to have both hands free for examination and manipulation while ensuring good lighting and visualization.

✅ **Have the patient sit upright.** If necessary, provide anxiolysis with medication such as lorazepam or midazolam. Cover the patient and yourself to protect clothing. Follow universal precautions by using gloves and wearing protective eyewear and a surgical mask.

✅ Many providers instill one to two sprays of a vasoconstrictor, such as oxymetazoline or phenylephrine, in the affected naris during initial nasal compression. Resolution of many nosebleeds occurs with this intervention alone. It is recommended that you also apply an anesthetic agent to allow for comfortable inspection and intervention.

✅ **Prepare a solution to anesthetize and vasoconstrict the nasal mucosa. This can consist of lidocaine and phenylephrine (the ingredients in Co-phenylcaine), 4% lidocaine with epinephrine, or 0.05% oxymetazoline (Afrin) with an anesthetic agent (See Video 28.1).**

✅ **Form two elongated cotton pledgets (using one-fourth of a cotton ball for each pledget), and soak them in the prepared solution.**

✅ **Instruct the patient to vigorously blow any clots from the nose (Fig. 28.1), and then quickly inspect for a bleeding site using the nasal speculum and Frazier suction tip (or other thin suction tip). Be sure to orient the nasal speculum vertically to avoid pain and allow clear visualization of the septum. Clear out any clots or foreign bodies.** The bleeding may be too brisk to identify a bleeding site at this time; therefore inspection may be delayed until vasoconstriction has slowed the hemorrhage.

✅ **Insert the medicated cotton pledgets as far back as possible into both nostrils (or one nostril, if the bleeding source is evident) using the bayonet forceps** (Fig. 28.2).

✅ Allow the patient to relax with the pledgets in place for approximately 15 to 20 minutes, applying pressure either manually or with a device as described earlier.

✅ **During this lull**, inquire about the patient's history of nosebleeds and other medical problems. Ask about recent trauma, moisture content of the home or work environment (such as a dry heat source in the winter), symptoms of viral or allergic rhinitis, the pattern of this nosebleed (timing, frequency, severity), which side the bleeding seems to be coming from, use of any blood-thinning medications or intranasal products (legal or illegal). Cocaine and over-the-counter nasal steroid sprays are the most commonly used products that increase risk for epistaxis. Often, no cause for the bleeding can be identified, but when there is diffuse oozing, multiple bleeding sites, or recurrent bleeding, or if the patient is taking an anticoagulant, a hematologic evaluation should be considered (complete blood count [CBC] and international normalized ratio [INR]) and referral for consideration of other underlying diseases such as hereditary hemorrhagic telangiectasia, Von Willebrand, or other bleeding dyscrasias.

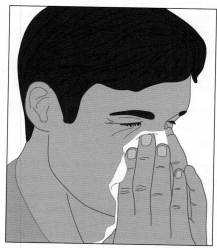

Fig. 28.1 The patient must blow the clots from his nose prior to the insertion of medicated cotton pledgets.

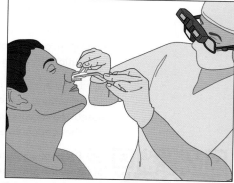

Fig. 28.2 Insertion of medicated cotton pledgets.

✅ **In many cases, active bleeding will stop with the use of a vasoconstrictor alone. The cotton pledgets can be removed and the nasal cavity inspected using the nasal speculum and head lamp.** Gently inserting the nasal speculum and spreading the naris vertically will permit visualization of most anterior bleeding sources. If bleeding continues, insert another pair of medicated cotton pledgets, and repeat this procedure with more prolonged nasal compression.

✅ **Although infrequent, there are times when the patient is hemorrhaging so briskly that tamponade with a balloon catheter should be used without complete inspection, topical anesthesia, or attempted cautery.**

✅ **If the bleeding point can be located and the bleeding is not too brisk, attempt to cauterize a 0.5-cm area of mucosa around the bleeding site with a silver nitrate stick, starting proximally, and then cauterize the site itself.** Silver nitrate requires a relatively bloodless surface. Apply the cautery for 10 seconds or less (Fig. 28.3). Do not apply cautery to both sides of the septum as this can lead to septal necrosis.

✅ **If the bleeding stops with cauterization, observe the patient for 15 to 30 minutes.** The cauterized area can then be covered with absorbable gelatin foam (Gelfoam), oxidized cellulose (Surgicel), or antibiotic ointment.

✅ **If there is ongoing bleeding and a source cannot be located or if bleeding continues after cauterization, nonabsorbable or absorbable packing may be used.**

✅ **The two most common nonabsorbable packings are the sponge and the balloon.** The sponge is made of hydroxylated polyvinyl acetate, is compressed, and expands into a soft sponge when wet (**Merocel sponge,** Medtronic, Minneapolis, MN; **Rhino Rocket**, Shippert Medical, Centennial, CO).

✅ **The balloon consists of an inflatable tube covered with a mesh of hemostatic carboxymethyl cellulose hydrocolloid (Rapid Rhino,** Arthro Care, Austin, TX).

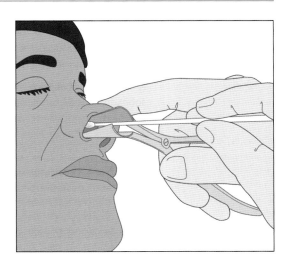

Fig. 28.3 Cauterize mucosa with a silver nitrate stick.

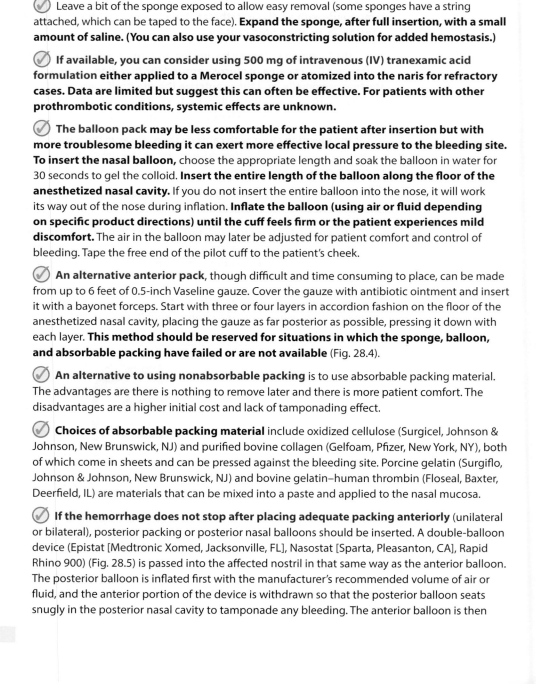 There are short and long varieties of the sponge and balloon, as well as balloons with anterior and posterior compartments. Longer packs can be used for patients suspected of posterior bleeding.

To use the Merocel sponge, coat it lightly with antibiotic ointment to provide some lubrication, and insert along the floor of the nasal cavity into the already anesthetized nose. If you are having trouble fitting the Merocel sponge, it can be trimmed.

Leave a bit of the sponge exposed to allow easy removal (some sponges have a string attached, which can be taped to the face). Expand the sponge, after full insertion, with a small amount of saline. (You can also use your vasoconstricting solution for added hemostasis.)

If available, you can consider using 500 mg of intravenous (IV) tranexamic acid formulation either applied to a Merocel sponge or atomized into the naris for refractory cases. Data are limited but suggest this can often be effective. For patients with other prothrombotic conditions, systemic effects are unknown.

The balloon pack may be less comfortable for the patient after insertion but with more troublesome bleeding it can exert more effective local pressure to the bleeding site. To insert the nasal balloon, choose the appropriate length and soak the balloon in water for 30 seconds to gel the colloid. Insert the entire length of the balloon along the floor of the anesthetized nasal cavity. If you do not insert the entire balloon into the nose, it will work its way out of the nose during inflation. Inflate the balloon (using air or fluid depending on specific product directions) until the cuff feels firm or the patient experiences mild discomfort. The air in the balloon may later be adjusted for patient comfort and control of bleeding. Tape the free end of the pilot cuff to the patient's cheek.

An alternative anterior pack, though difficult and time consuming to place, can be made from up to 6 feet of 0.5-inch Vaseline gauze. Cover the gauze with antibiotic ointment and insert it with a bayonet forceps. Start with three or four layers in accordion fashion on the floor of the anesthetized nasal cavity, placing the gauze as far posterior as possible, pressing it down with each layer. This method should be reserved for situations in which the sponge, balloon, and absorbable packing have failed or are not available (Fig. 28.4).

An alternative to using nonabsorbable packing is to use absorbable packing material. The advantages are there is nothing to remove later and there is more patient comfort. The disadvantages are a higher initial cost and lack of tamponading effect.

Choices of absorbable packing material include oxidized cellulose (Surgicel, Johnson & Johnson, New Brunswick, NJ) and purified bovine collagen (Gelfoam, Pfizer, New York, NY), both of which come in sheets and can be pressed against the bleeding site. Porcine gelatin (Surgiflo, Johnson & Johnson, New Brunswick, NJ) and bovine gelatin–human thrombin (Floseal, Baxter, Deerfield, IL) are materials that can be mixed into a paste and applied to the nasal mucosa.

If the hemorrhage does not stop after placing adequate packing anteriorly (unilateral or bilateral), posterior packing or posterior nasal balloons should be inserted. A double-balloon device (Epistat [Medtronic Xomed, Jacksonville, FL], Nasostat [Sparta, Pleasanton, CA], Rapid Rhino 900) (Fig. 28.5) is passed into the affected nostril in that same way as the anterior balloon. The posterior balloon is inflated first with the manufacturer's recommended volume of air or fluid, and the anterior portion of the device is withdrawn so that the posterior balloon seats snugly in the posterior nasal cavity to tamponade any bleeding. The anterior balloon is then

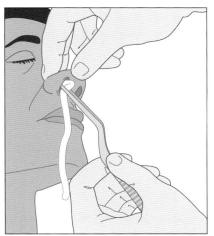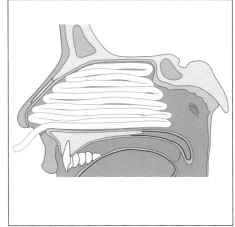

Fig. 28.4 Packing the nasal cavity with ribbon gauze.

inflated to prevent the posterior balloon from becoming unseated and possibly obstructing the airway and to address any concurrent anterior bleeding.

✓ **If a commercial posterior balloon device is not available,** a 12-Fr Foley catheter may be used. Insert the catheter into the affected nasal cavity until the balloon is well into the posterior nasal cavity. Inflate the balloon with 5 to 7 mL of saline. Pull the partially inflated balloon anteriorly until it is snug against the posterior turbinates. Finish inflating the balloon with another 5 to 7 mL saline. If there is pain or displacement of the soft palate, remove some of the saline from the balloon. Secure the Foley anteriorly by placing an umbilical clamp over the catheter as it exits the nose. Make sure to pad the nose tissue under the umbilical clamp with gauze to prevent pressure necrosis. An anterior Vaseline gauze pack may then be inserted if necessary.

✓ **If the bleeding cannot be controlled with all the measures described, YOU NEED HELP!** Contact an otolaryngologist (ENT) or transfer the patient to a hospital with ENT care. The specialist may use electrocautery, transpalatal injection of vasoconstrictors, endoscopic cautery, surgical ligation, or embolization procedures. While the patient is awaiting specialist care, you must ensure hemodynamic stability using IV fluids or blood, if needed.

✓ **If, on the other hand, as will most commonly occur, the bleeding has stopped with your interventions, observe the patient for 15 to 30 minutes. If there is no further bleeding from the nares or seen in the posterior pharynx, vital signs are stable and pain is controlled, the patient may be discharged.** If the hemorrhage is suspected to have been large, determine that the patient is not symptomatically orthostatic, and check hemoglobin and hematocrit before discharging.

✓ **If a nonabsorbable pack was inserted, the patient can be sent home on a regimen of antibiotics for 4 to 5 days to possibly prevent a secondary sinusitis and septal abscess and to reduce the risk of toxic shock syndrome.** The data for prophylactic antibiotic use are poor and there is concern for more risk from side effects than benefits of decreased infection. Consider antibiotics if the patient is diabetic or otherwise immunocompromised or if the ENT group to which you refer patients prefers this approach. Choices of antibiotics

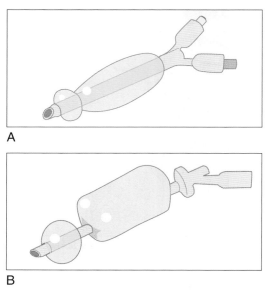

A

B

Fig 28.5 Double-balloon devices. (A) Epistat. (B) Nasostat.

include cephalexin (Keflex), amoxicillin/clavulanate (Augmentin), clindamycin (Cleocin), and trimethoprim/sulfamethoxazole (Bactrim).

✓ **The nonabsorbable packs should be removed in 2 to 5 days.** Packs for minor bleeds may be removed early; in bleeds that are difficult to control or in patients on anticoagulants, packs should be kept in the full 5 days.

✓ **Warn the patient about not sneezing with the mouth closed, bending over, straining, or picking the nose. Provide detailed printed instructions regarding home care.**

✓ **Patients with simple nosebleeds can be referred to their primary care doctor for removal of the packing or for a recheck. If the patient has frequent recurring bleeding, a posterior bleed is noted or suspected, or there is concern for a nasal abnormality causing the bleeding, the patient should be referred to an ENT specialist.**

✓ **If pain is a problem,** first consider adjusting balloon pressure if this is possible without causing recurrent bleeding. Next, acetaminophen should be suggested, but aspirin and other nonsteroidal medications should be avoided.

✓ **When removing a compressed cellulose sponge pack, soften it with 1 to 2 mL of water or saline and wait 5 minutes,** thereby reducing trauma, pain, and the incidence of rebleeding.

What Not to Do

✗ Do not waste time trying to locate a bleeding site if brisk bleeding is obscuring your vision in spite of vigorous suctioning. Have the patient blow out any clots and insert the medicated cotton pledgets immediately or go directly to anterior packing.

(X) Do not order routine clotting studies unless there is persistent or recurrent bleeding, use of anticoagulants, or other evidence of an underlying bleeding disorder.

(X) Do not cauterize or place a painful device in the nose before providing adequate topical anesthesia unless rapid hemorrhage requires it.

(X) Do not use an inadequate amount of gauze packing (if this method is chosen). It will only serve as a plug in the anterior nares rather than a hemostatic pack.

(X) Do not discharge a patient as soon as the bleeding stops; observe the patient for 15 to 30 minutes. Posterior epistaxis typically stops and starts cyclically.

(X) Do not discharge a patient with bilateral nasal packs. Due to the potential risk of airway compromise, these patients should be admitted for observation.

(X) Do not send home elderly patients or those with cardiac problems or chronic respiratory disease without first checking their oxygen saturation. These patients are at risk for desaturation and may also need admission.

Discussion

Epistaxis (Greek for "nosebleed") affects people in all age groups but is most common and more troublesome in the elderly. Children tend to bleed secondary to nose picking; adolescents may bleed secondary to facial trauma. Epistaxis in the middle-age patient may be a harbinger of neoplastic disease. Nosebleeds in the elderly are generally the result of underlying vascular fragility often in combination with blood-thinning medications.

Nosebleeds are more common in winter, no doubt reflecting the low, ambient humidity indoors and outdoors and the increased incidence of upper respiratory tract infections. In most cases, anterior bleeding is clinically obvious. In contrast, posterior bleeding may be asymptomatic or may present insidiously as nausea, hematemesis, anemia, hemoptysis, or melena.

Causes of epistaxis are numerous; dry nasal mucosa, nose picking, and vascular fragility are the most common causes, but others include trauma, foreign bodies, blood dyscrasias, nasal or sinus neoplasm or infection, septal deformity or perforation, atrophic rhinitis, hereditary hemorrhagic telangiectasis, and angiofibroma. Epistaxis that results from minor blunt trauma in healthy individuals rarely requires any intervention and will spontaneously subside with head elevation alone and avoidance of any nasal manipulation. (Always inspect for a possible septal hematoma.)

Previously there were concerns about a nasopulmonary reflex causing arterial oxygen pressure to drop, thus causing problems for those with cardiac problems or chronic obstructive pulmonary disease (COPD). Subsequent research has shown that posterior packing does not lead to clinically relevant changes in cardiac or pulmonary function.

High blood pressure may make epistaxis more difficult to control. While hypertension is often present with epistaxis, it is rarely the precipitating cause and it is often just the consequence of the accompanying emotional upset. Specific antihypertensive therapy is rarely required and should be avoided in the setting of significant hemorrhage.

Use of medications, including but not limited to aspirin, nonsteroidal anti-inflammatory drugs (NSAIDs), warfarin, heparin, enoxaparin, ticlopidine, dipyridamole, clopidogrel, ticagrelor, apixaban, and rivaroxaban, not only predisposes patients to epistaxis but also makes treatment more difficult.

Hereditary hemorrhagic telangiectasia most commonly presents with frequent epistaxis. This condition is an autosomal dominant disorder marked by formation of arteriovenous malformations and telangiectasia frequently

(Continued)

Discussion continued

affecting the nasal mucosa. Onset of symptoms is usually at puberty and progressively worsens with age. Blood dyscrasias can be found in patients with lymphoproliferative disorders, immunodeficiency, systemic disease, or alcohol abuse. Thrombocytopenia can lead to spontaneous mucous membrane bleeding, with platelet counts of $10,000/mm^3$ to $20,000/mm^3$.

Platelet deficiency can be the result of chemotherapy agents, malignancies, hypersplenism, disseminated intravascular coagulopathy (DIC), and drugs, among other disorders. Platelet dysfunction can be seen in liver failure, kidney failure, and vitamin C deficiency as well as in patients taking aspirin and NSAIDs.

Von Willebrand disease is the most common clotting factor abnormality that can result in frequent, recurring nosebleeds. Factor VIII deficiency (hemophilia A) and factor IX deficiency (hemophilia B) are also common primary coagulopathies.

One study of chronic nosebleeds in children showed that a third of these patients can be expected to have a coagulation disorder. The single best predictor of coagulopathy is family history. Patients who present with frequent nosebleeds or posterior epistaxis should follow up with an ENT specialist for a complete nasopharyngeal examination and consideration of further workup.

Suggested Readings

Herkner, H., Laggner, A., Müllner, M., et al. (2000). Hypertension in patients presenting with epistaxis. *Annals of Emergency Medicine, 35*, 126–130.

Kucik, C. J., & Clenney, T. (2005). Management of epistaxis. *American Family Physician, 71*, 305–311.

Manes, P. (2010). Evaluating and managing the patient with nosebleeds. *Medical Clinics of North America, 94*, 903–912.

Pringle, M. B., Beasley, P., & Brightwell, A. P. (1996). The use of Merocel nasal packs in the treatment of epistaxis. *Journal of Laryngology and Otology, 110*, 543–546.

Roberts, J. R., & Hedges, J. R. (DATE). *Clinical procedures in emergency medicine* (3rd ed.). Philadelphia, PA: WB Saunders.

Singer, A. J., Blanda, M., Cronin, K., et al. (2005). Comparison of nasal tampons for the treatment of epistaxis in the emergency department: A randomized controlled trial. *Annals of Emergency Medicine, 45*, 134–139.

Thaha, M. A. (2000). Routine coagulation screening in the management of emergency admission for epistaxis: Is it necessary? *Journal of Laryngology and Otology, 114*, 38–40.

Tunkel, D. E., et al. (2020). Clinical practice guideline: Nosebleed (epistaxis) executive summary. *Otolaryngology— Head and Neck Surgery, 162*(1), 8–25.

Vaiman, M., Segal, S., & Eviatar, E. (2002). Fibrin glue: Treatment for epistaxis. *Rhinology, 40*, 88–91.

Viducich, R. A., Blanda, M. P., & Gerson, L. W. (1995). Posterior epistaxis: Clinical features and acute complications. *Annals of Emergency Medicine, 25*, 592–596.

Foreign Body, Ear

Presentation

Children may present after placing small objects such as a bead, a small stone, folded paper, or a bean in their ear. At times, the history is not revealed, and the child simply presents with a purulent discharge, pain, bleeding, or hearing loss. Adults also occasionally present with foreign bodies (FBs) in the auditory canal, often the result of trying to remove earwax. A panic-stricken patient may arrive complaining of "a bug crawling around" in the ear. There may be severe pain if the object or insect has scratched or stung the canal or tympanic membrane (TM).

What to Do

✓ Use an otoscope to inspect the ear canal while pulling up and back on the pinna to help straighten the ear canal, thereby providing a better view.

✓ **If the object is a button battery, has sharp edges, is against the TM, is very tightly wedged, or when there is concern for TM or middle ear injury**, consider consulting an otolaryngology (ENT) specialist prior to attempting removal.

✓ **If there is a live insect in the patient's ear, begin by filling the canal with a liquid to kill the insect. Mineral oil or 2% lidocaine works well.** (Sterile 2% lidocaine would be most appropriate if there is a myringotomy tube in place or any other opening of the TM.) Instill lidocaine 2% is the preferred agent if pain control is needed. Instruct the patient to lie on the side, and then drip the liquid into the canal while pulling lightly downward on the pinna and pushing on the tragus to remove air bubbles (Fig. 29.1). Leave this in place for 5 to 10 minutes.

✓ **With the exceptions of FBs listed earlier that require ENT evaluation, water irrigation is an effective removal technique.** This can be accomplished with a syringe and scalp vein needle tubing that has been cut short (1 cm) (Fig. 29.2). Tap water at body temperature can be used to flush out the FB. Direct the stream along the wall of the canal and around the object, thereby flushing it out (Fig. 29.3).

✓ **If a hard or spherical object remains tightly wedged in the canal, attempt to roll the FB out by getting behind it with a right-angle nerve hook, ear curette, or wire loop.** Use of these tools should be done under direct visualization through an ear speculum. The patient's head should be firmly stabilized to prevent sudden movements. Whenever an instrument is used in the ear canal, warn the patient and/or parents beforehand that there may be a small amount of bleeding and pain because of the delicate lining of the ear canal (Figs. 29.5 and 29.6).

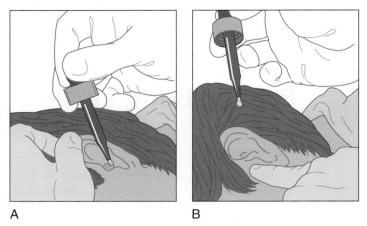

A   B

Fig. 29.1 Drop mineral oil into the ear canal and squeeze out any air bubbles to kill any bug or insect in the ear.

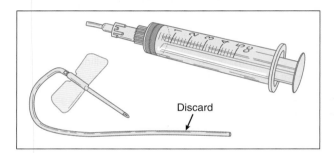

Discard

Fig. 29.2 A short, soft catheter on a 5-mL syringe is safe and effective for irrigating a loose foreign body out of the ear canal. *Note*: Discard needle and most of the tubing before use.

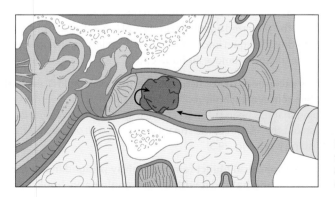

Fig. 29.3 When irrigating a foreign body out of the ear, direct the stream of warm water toward an opening between the foreign body and the canal wall.

☑ **An alternative removal technique is to place one or two drops of cyanoacrylate or other tissue adhesive on the end of the wooden shaft of a cotton swab. (Use the cotton end for irregular FBs.)** Hold the wet glue against the foreign object until it hardens (approximately 30 seconds to 1 minute), then extract the FB from the canal. Coating the canal with ointment can prevent accidental glue adherence to the external auditory canal (EAC).

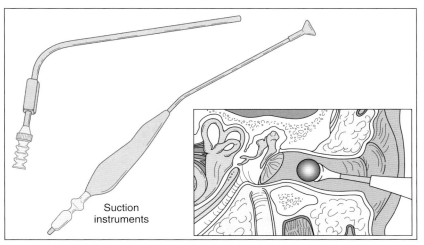

Fig. 29.4 Various suction tips can be used to pull out a loose foreign body within the ear canal.

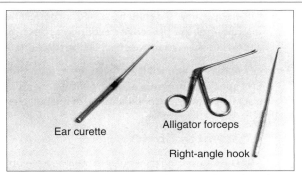

Fig. 29.5 The right-angle hook is best suited for removing hard objects from the ear, whereas alligator forceps work best on soft objects.

☑ **If the object is light and moves easily**, you can attempt to suction it out with a standard metal suction tip or (if available) a specialized flexible tip, by making an effective vacuum seal on the FB (Fig. 29.4).

☑ **A small magnet or iron-containing metallic FB** can be removed by touching a pacemaker magnet to a metal forceps and then, at the same time, touching the forceps to the FB, withdrawing all of the magnetized objects together.

☑ **For grasping soft objects, such as cotton, paper, and certain insects (after they have been killed), alligator forceps are good (Fig. 29.6). Some beads may have a hole or knob amenable to grasping with alligator forceps as well.**

☑ **When the FB is a button battery or when there is an obvious infection or uncontrolled pain, there should be no delay in removing the FB from the canal.** With button batteries, do not irrigate or instill liquids into the ear canal, because on contact with moist tissue the alkaline battery is capable of producing current that leads to liquefactive necrosis extending into deep tissues within hours. Be careful not to crush the battery. **After removal of a battery, irrigate the canal to remove any alkali residue.**

119

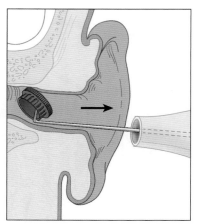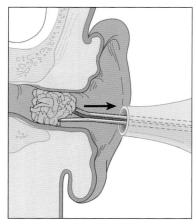

Fig. 29.6 The various metal instruments that can be used to remove foreign bodies from an ear canal.

✅ **At any time, if a child becomes uncooperative, especially when using metal instruments, use procedural sedation as described in Appendix E.** Ketamine sedation appears to have a positive effect on the success rate of FB removal in children.

✅ **If the FB cannot be removed safely with the abovementioned techniques, consult an ENT specialist urgently or emergently depending on the situation.** If after removal there is evidence of infection or perforation of the TM, referral to an ENT specialist is also appropriate.

What Not to Do

❌ Do not use a rigid instrument to remove an object from an uncooperative patient's ear without procedural sedation. An unexpected movement might cause serious injury to the middle ear.

❌ Do not attempt to remove a large bug or insect without killing it first. Many are well equipped to lodge themselves in the ear canal when alive.

❌ Do not attempt to irrigate a canal filled with a bean or other object that may swell with hydration. Irrigation with isopropyl alcohol will not cause swelling.

❌ Do not attempt to remove a large or hard object with bayonet or similar forceps. The bony canal will slowly close the forceps as they are advanced, and the object will be pushed farther into the canal. Alligator forceps are designed for use in the canal, but even they will push a large, hard FB farther into the ear.

Discussion

The external ear canal narrows at the junction of the cartilaginous segment and the bony segment, and then at the isthmus of the bony segment. Most FBs are found at these two narrow loci. The cross section of the canal is elliptic; therefore the physician can usually find an opening around a circular foreign object in which to place an instrument or for water to get behind when irrigating.

When the FB within the ear canal is a cyanoacrylate adhesive (Super Glue, Dermabond), it can be removed more easily after 48 hours when desquamation occurs. If the glue adheres to the TM, an ENT referral may be most prudent.

On telephone consultation, patients can be instructed to use cooking or baby oil, or ethyl or isopropyl alcohol, instilled into the ear canal, to kill an insect at home. It can then be removed at a subsequent office visit.

Complications of FB removal from the ear canal include trauma to the skin of the canal, canal hematoma, otitis externa, TM perforation, or ossicular dislocations and, rarely, facial nerve palsy.

Suggested Readings

Antonelli, P. J., Ahmadi, A., & Prevatt, A. (2001). Insecticidal activity of common reagents for insect foreign bodies of the ear. *Laryngoscope, 111*, 15–20.

Bressler, K., & Shelton, C. (1993). Ear foreign-body removal: A review of 98 consecutive cases. *Laryngoscope, 103*, 367–370.

Brown, L., Denmark, T. K., Wittlake, W. A., et al. (2004). Procedural sedation use in the ED: Management of pediatric ear and nose foreign bodies. *American Journal of Emergency Medicine, 22*, 310–314.

Brunskill, A. J., & Satterthwaite, K. (1994). Foreign bodies. *Annals of Emergency Medicine, 24*, 757.

Heim, S., & Maughan, K. (2007). Foreign bodies in the ear, nose, and throat. *American Family Physician, 76*, 1185–1189.

Leffler, S., Cherney, P., & Tandberg, D. (1993). Chemical immobilization and killing of intra-aural roaches: An in-vitro comparative study. *Annals of Emergency Medicine, 22*, 1795–1798.

McLaughlin, R., Ullah, R., & Heylings, D. (2002). Comparative prospective study of foreign body removal from external auditory canals of cadavers with right angle hook or cyanoacrylate glue. *Emergency Medicine Journal, 19*, 43–45.

O'Toole, K., Paris, P. M., Stewart, R. D., et al. (1985). Removing cockroaches from the auditory canal: Controlled trial. *New England Journal of Medicine, 312*, 1197.

Schulze, S. L., Kerschner, J., & Beste, D. (2002). Pediatric external auditory canal foreign bodies: A review of 698 cases. *Otolaryngology—Head and Neck Surgery, 127*, 73–78.

Skinner, D. W., & Chui, P. (1986). The hazard of button-sized batteries as foreign bodies in the nose and ear. *Journal of Laryngology and Otology, 100*, 1315–1319.

Foreign Body, Nose

Presentation

Children frequently present after inserting foreign bodies (FBs) into their nares. They may report the FB, or the event may be observed. Sometimes, however, the history is obscure, and the child presents with local pain; a purulent, unilateral nasal discharge; epistaxis; a nasal voice change; or foul breath. The most commonly encountered nasal FBs are beans, peanuts or other foodstuffs, beads, toy parts, pebbles, paper wads, and eraser tips. Most FBs can be seen on direct visualization using a nasal or otoscope speculum. These objects usually lodge on the floor of the nose just below the inferior turbinate or immediately anterior to the middle turbinate.

What to Do

✅ **There are various techniques available for removal of nasal FBs.** These include suction, air pressure, ear curettes, curved hooks, alligator forceps, bayonet forceps, balloon catheters, irrigation, and glue. The choice will depend of the shape, makeup, and depth of the FB as well as the age and cooperation of the patient.

✅ **Before attempting removal techniques in an uncooperative patient,** consider use of sedation. Be aware of the higher risk of aspiration of the FB when sedation is used.

✅ Because of the potential for spraying of body fluids from the nose, always practice universal precautions and wear appropriate eye and splash protection.

✅ Before any of the removal procedures, explain in detail what you are about to do to the patient and/or parent. Advise that the procedure will be a little uncomfortable, may cause some bleeding, and that there is a small risk the FB body could be aspirated.

✅ **After initial inspection with a nasal speculum and bright light, suction out any discharge, and instill vasoconstrictive and anesthetizing medication either by atomizing it or by inserting a small cotton pledget soaked in the medication. Vasoconstriction can be achieved with medications such as 0.25% phenylephrine or 0.05% oxymetazoline (Afrin). Tetracaine and lidocaine are most commonly used to provide topical anesthesia and can be combined with the vasoconstricting agent.**

✅ Be careful to avoid pushing the FB posteriorly when inserting the pledget. Remove the pledget after 5 to 10 minutes. If you cannot safely insert a pledget, drip or spray the same solution into the nose.

✅ **After vasoconstriction, some FBs can be blown out of the nose by a cooperative patient or suctioned out using Frazier tip suction. Further suctioning success may be** obtained by placing a piece of soft plastic tubing over the end of the suction tip, which allows more flexibility to form a seal with the FB. Placing water-soluble lubrication on the end of this tubing will also help achieve a better vacuum seal.

In infants and children who will not blow their nose on command, a parent may blow a sharp puff of air into the child's mouth while holding the opposite nostril closed. A tight-fitting Ambu mask over the mouth but excluding the nose and a bag-valve device is an alternative means for producing the positive pressure required to force the FB out of the nose.

Another air pressure technique is to place oxygen tubing, running at 10 to 15 L/min, into the contralateral nostril to the FB (Beamsley Blaster) (Fig. 30.1). This technique, along with the other positive-pressure ones, reduces the risk of forcing the FB posteriorly, thereby reducing the risk of aspiration. These methods may not work as well for FBs that have produced edema or infection.

Alligator forceps may be used to remove cloth, cotton, or paper FBs. Pebbles, beans, and other hard FBs are most easily grasped using bayonet forceps.

If an object cannot be grasped, it may be rolled out of the nose by using an ear curette or right-angle ear hook to get behind it. After sliding the tool past the FB, twist until it catches the FB and then pull anteriorly. A soft-tipped hook can be made by bending the tip of a metal Calgiswab to a 90-degree angle.

A less intrusive approach is to bypass the FB with a lubricated 5-Fogarty biliary balloon probe or small Foley catheter, passing the catheter past the foreign body before inflating the balloon with 1 mL of air and gently pulling the catheter and FB out of the nose (Fig. 30.2). A commercially available FB remover, the Katz extractor (InHealth Technologies, Carpinteria, CA), may offer an easier balloon catheter technique.

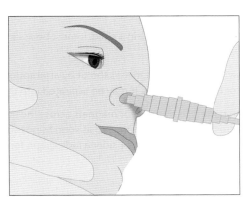

Fig. 30.1 Beamsley Blaster technique.

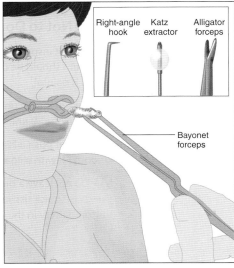

Fig. 30.2 Remove foreign bodies with bayonet forceps, right-angle hook, Katz extractor, or alligator forceps.

✅ **One can also try the glue technique. After drying the exposed surface of the FB, a drop of cyanoacrylate (Super Glue, Dermabond) can be applied to the cotton end of a regular cotton-tipped applicator, which is then touched to the FB, held there for 1 minute, and used to pull the attached FB out of the nose.**

✅ **Button batteries can cause serious local damage through liquefaction necrosis and should be removed quickly.** Button batteries of all sizes have a distinctive double contour on radiographs; therefore, with a high index of suspicion, radiographs can help assist with an uncertain diagnosis.

✅ **Earring magnets that become stuck together across the nasal septum** must also be removed as soon as possible because of the risk for pressure necrosis leading to septal perforation. Ideally, the septum should be lubricated. Using the balloon catheter technique bilaterally, both magnets should be removed simultaneously to prevent a lone magnet from dropping back into the nasopharynx and being aspirated.

✅ **Bleeding**, which will often occur during FB removal, can usually be stopped by reinsertion of a cotton pledget soaked in the topical solution used prior to the procedure or with brief direct pressure.

✅ **Small, particulate material may be irrigated from the nasal cavity by insertion of an irrigation syringe into one nostril while the patient sits up, leans forward, and repeats "eng" as you irrigate. The "eng" sound will close the back of the throat during irrigation. Slowly flush the debris out the opposite nostril** (Fig. 30.3).

✅ **After FB removal**, inspect the nasal cavity again, checking for additional objects. Always look in the other nostril, and it may be wise to check the ears.

✅ **If a FB cannot be located** but is suspected, or if attempts to remove a visible FB have failed, an otolaryngology (ENT) consultation is warranted.

What Not to Do

❌ Do not inspect the nasal cavity by opening the nasal speculum in the horizontal plane. The speculum should be opened in the vertical plane and not pressed against the nasal septum, which is painful.

❌ Do not ignore unilateral nasal discharge in a child. It must be assumed to be caused by the presence of a FB until proven otherwise.

❌ Do not push a FB down the back of a patient's throat by attempting to remove a large, solid, smooth FB with alligator or bayonet forceps. It may be aspirated into the trachea.

❌ Do not leave a button battery in the nose or magnets across the nasal tissue. These objects can cause quick tissue necrosis and must be removed as soon as possible. If you suspect a button battery in the nose but cannot find it, consider a radiograph for confirmation.

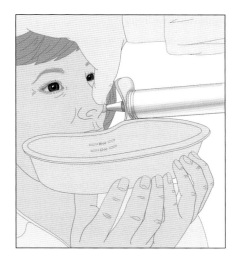

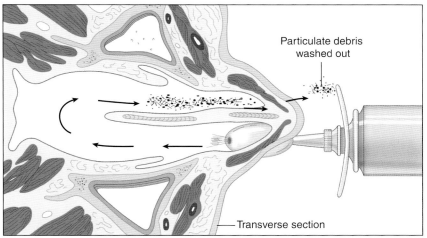

Fig. 30.3 Nasal irrigation.

Discussion

The symptoms produced by a nasal FB will vary with its size, composition, location, and the length of time it has been present. Most nasal FBs can be removed easily and safely by emergency clinicians. There is generally no need for emergent intervention. There is time available to provide procedural sedation, if necessary, as well as to assemble all supplies and instruments necessary to help ensure the success of this procedure. Because nasal FBs have different sizes, shapes, and locations within the nares, the emergency clinician should be familiar with several removal techniques.

The mucous membrane lining the nasal cavity allows the tactical advantage of vasoconstriction and topical anesthesia. The patient who has unsuccessfully attempted to blow an FB out of the nose may be successful after instillation of a vasoconstrictive solution.

If a patient has swallowed a foreign body that was pushed back into the nasopharynx, this is usually harmless if it is not a button battery or more than one magnet, and the patient and parents can be reassured (see Chapter 73). If the object has been aspirated into the tracheobronchial tree, it may produce coughing and wheezing, and bronchoscopy under anesthesia is required for retrieval.

Suggested Readings

Backlin, S. A. (1995). Positive-pressure technique for nasal foreign body retrieval in children. *Annals of Emergency Medicine, 25*, 554–555.

Brown, L., Denmark, T. K., Wittlake, W. A., et al. (2004). Procedural sedation use in the ED: Management of pediatric ear and nose foreign bodies. *American Journal of Emergency Medicine, 22*, 310–314.

Heim, S., & Maughan, K. (2007). Foreign bodies in the ear, nose, and throat. *American Family Physician, 76*, 1185–1189.

Lin, V. Y., Daniel, S. J., & Papsin, B. C. (2004). Button batteries in the ear, nose, and upper aerodigestive tract. *International Journal of Pediatric Otorhinolaryngology, 68*, 473–479.

Navitsky, R. C., Beamsley, A., & McLaughlin, S. (2002). Nasal positive-pressure technique for nasal foreign body removal in children. *American Journal of Emergency Medicine, 20*, 103–104.

Ngo, A., Ng, K. C., & Sim, T. P. (2005). Otorhinolaryngeal foreign bodies in children presenting to the emergency department. *Singapore Medical Journal, 46*, 172–178.

Noorily, A. D., Noorily, S. H., & Otto, R. A. (1995). Cocaine, lidocaine, tetracaine: Which is best for topical nasal anesthesia? *Anesthesia and Analgesia, 81*, 724–727.

Foreign Body, Throat

Presentation

Patients may present with the sensation of a foreign body (FB) stuck in their throat. They typically can still feel a sensation in the throat, especially (and perhaps painfully) when swallowing. They may be able to precisely localize the FB sensation above the thyroid cartilage (which implies the possibility of a FB in the hypopharynx that may be visible) or may only vaguely localize the sensation to the suprasternal notch (which could imply a FB anywhere in the esophagus).

Those with dentures, particularly full dentures, are more likely to swallow a bone because of reduced sensitivity and reduced ability to completely masticate. Fish bones, which are usually long, are commonly caught in the oropharynx, particularly at the region of the tonsils and the tonsillar pillars. Fish bones often may be grasped and extracted as long as they can be visualized.

A FB lodged in the tracheobronchial tree usually stimulates coughing and wheezing. Obstruction of the esophagus by a FB produces drooling and prevents the patient from swallowing secretions. An infant who refuses to eat or who has trouble handling buccal secretions should be evaluated for a FB.

This chapter refers to the care of the patient who has no evidence of airway involvement or esophageal obstruction.

What to Do

✓ Establish exactly what, if anything, was swallowed, when, and the progression of symptoms. Patients can usually accurately tell if an FB is on the right or left side.

✓ Examine the anterior neck for tenderness, masses, or subcutaneous emphysema (suggests perforation). Percuss and auscultate the chest. A FB sensation in the throat can be produced by a pneumothorax, pneumomediastinum, or esophageal disease, all of which may show up on a chest radiograph if history or exam suggest these.

✓ **Inspect the hypopharynx using a good light or headlamp mirror and tongue depressor, paying special attention to the base of the tongue, tonsils, and vallecula, where FBs are likely to lodge.** Place the tongue depressor at the middle third of the tongue and press firmly downward to give good exposure without making the patient gag. You can also maximize visibility and exposure, without making the patient gag, by holding the tongue out (use a washcloth or 4 × 4-inch gauze for traction), taking care not to lacerate the frenulum of the tongue on the lower incisors, and then instruct the patient to raise the soft palate by "panting like a dog."

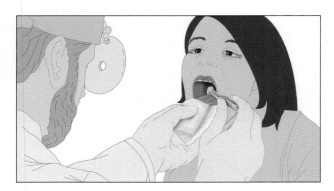

Fig. 31.1 Carefully grasp and remove any foreign body that can be seen in the throat.

✅ This may be accomplished without topical anesthesia, but **if the patient tends to gag, the soft palate and posterior pharynx can be anesthetized with any topical anesthetic such as spraying with Cetacaine, HurriCaine, or 10% lidocaine.** Some patients may continue to gag even with the topical anesthesia.

✅ **If the object can be seen directly, carefully grasp and remove it with bayonet or curved forceps** (Fig. 31.1). **Objects at the base of the tongue or in the hypopharynx may require a mirror, indirect laryngoscope, or fiberoptic nasopharyngoscopy for visualization.** Small fish bones are frequently difficult to see. They may be overlooked entirely except for their tips, or they may only appear to be threads of mucus.

✅ **If the symptoms are mild and a FB cannot be visualized, test the patient's ability to swallow using a small cup of water followed by soft food such as a piece of soft bread. If the patient can swallow liquids and solids without difficulty, they may be safely discharged.** They should be instructed to seek follow-up care as soon as possible if the pain worsens, fever develops, or if breathing or swallowing is difficult. They should be seen by an otolaryngologist (ENT) or return to the emergency department (ED) or clinic if they are not better within 48 hours. Educate patients that, in most cases, no object is found, and the FB sensation may only be due to a scratch in the throat that will resolve spontaneously.

✅ **If symptoms are severe or the patient cannot tolerate soft food or liquids yet no object is seen on direct visualization, fiberoptic nasopharyngoscopy is preferred; if unavailable, however, computed tomography (CT) scanning can reveal most significant FBs.**

✅ **If an FB is discovered on imaging studies but cannot be visualized on physical examination, obtain an ENT consultation.**

✅ **If the ENT evaluation of the hypopharynx is negative and the pain is persistent (especially pain localized to the suprasternal notch), consider that the FB may be in the esophagus and perhaps consult a gastroenterologist. Maintain a high level of suspicion when a chicken bone may have been swallowed.**

✅ **An impacted button battery represents a true emergency and requires rapid removal, because leaking alkali produces liquefactive necrosis.** Button batteries of all sizes have a distinctive double contour on radiography.

✅ **A tablet composed of irritating medicine,** if swallowed without adequate liquid, may stick to the mucosa of the pharynx or esophagus and cause an irritating ulcer with a FB sensation. The pill, having dissolved, will no longer be present.

What Not to Do

❌ Do not assume a FB is absent just because the pain disappears after a local anesthetic is applied.

❌ Do not assume a negative plain radiograph rules out the presence of a fish bone, as it is often not visible.

❌ Do not order a barium swallow to evaluate suspected fish bone impactions. The results are unreliable or misleading, and barium makes subsequent examinations of a coated esophagus more difficult.

❌ Do not reassure the patient that there is no FB if it has not been completely ruled out. Explain that although you think there is a low probability that a FB exists, careful follow-up needs to be obtained if symptoms do not completely resolve.

❌ Do not overlook the possibility of preexisting pathologic conditions discovered incidentally during swallowing.

❌ Do not attempt to remove a FB from the throat blindly by using a finger or instrument, because the object may be pushed farther down into the airway and obstruct it or may cause damage to surrounding structures.

Discussion

During swallowing, as the base of the tongue pushes a bolus of food posteriorly, any sharp object hidden in that bolus may become embedded in the tonsil, the tonsillar pillar, the pharyngeal wall, or the tongue base itself. Symptomatic patients are convinced that they have a bone stuck in their throat, although in most patients no bone is found and the symptoms resolve spontaneously. In two studies, approximately 25% of the patients with symptoms of an embedded fish bone had no demonstrable pathologic findings, and their symptoms resolved in 48 hours. Only 20% had an embedded fish bone, and most of these were easily identified and removed on the initial visit.

All patients who complain of a FB in the throat should undergo a thorough evaluation. Even relatively smooth or rounded objects that remain impacted in the esophagus have the potential to cause serious problems. A fish bone can perforate the esophagus in only a few days, and chicken bones carry even greater risk for serious injuries, such as neck abscess, mediastinitis, and esophageal-carotid artery fistula.

Globus sensation is the feeling of a lump or tightness in the throat, without underlying structural or mucosal abnormality. The initial workup is the same as that for any FB sensation in the throat, and the patient can be referred for further workup as needed.

Suggested Readings

D'Agostino, J. (2010). Pediatric airway nightmares. *Emergency Medical Clinics of North America*, *28*, 119–126.

Digoy, P. (2008). Diagnosis and management of upper aerodigestive tract foreign bodies. *Otolaryngology Clinics of North America*, *41*, 485–496.

Haliloglu, M., Ciftci, A. O., Oto, A., et al. (2003). CT virtual bronchoscopy in the evaluation of children with suspected foreign body aspiration. *European Journal of Radiology*, *48*, 188–192.

Heim, S., & Maughan, K. (2007). Foreign bodies in the ear, nose, and throat. *American Family Physician*, *76*, 1185–1189.

Lue, A. J., Fang, W. D., & Manolidis, S. (2000). Use of plain radiography and computed tomography to identify fish bone foreign bodies. *Otolaryngology—Head and Neck Surgery*, *123*, 435–438.

Laryngotracheobronchitis

(Croup)

Presentation

A child, most often between the ages of 6 months and 3 years (peak incidence 1–2 years, rarely seen >6 years), arrives with a characteristic barking cough that sounds very much like the bark of a seal. The patient may arrive with reports of having significant difficulty breathing in the middle of the night. There is usually a prodrome of low-grade fever and symptoms of a mild upper respiratory infection. The barking cough tends to occur at night, with symptoms worsening on the second night.

The parents are usually alarmed by the sound of the cough or the child's breathing difficulty. The throat is clear and normal in appearance, and there may be varying degrees of stridor (predominately inspiratory) or retractions of the accessory chest muscles.

What to Do

✅ **Perform a complete examination, with attention directed to the patient's work of breathing, mental status, hydration status, and upper and lower airway exam.** Although now rare in children, acute epiglottitis should be eliminated as a possibility by noting a healthy-appearing supraglottic region with absence of high fever, sudden onset, drooling, and laryngeal tenderness. There should also be no worsening of the child's condition when lying supine. At times, the epiglottis can be seen (Fig. 32.1), but visualization of a normal epiglottis is not necessary to diagnose croup. A thorough vaccination history can help in understanding risk of having *Haemophilus influenzae,* the most common cause of epiglottitis. Consider a foreign body as a possible cause of airway obstruction by obtaining a good history, and during exam ensure no foreign bodies are seen.

✅ **Many clinical scoring tools are available and can be helpful to reference for classifying the severity of the disease and appropriate treatment and disposition algorithms.**

✅ Make the child as comfortable as possible. Avoid agitating the child with unnecessary procedures and examinations because many patients will improve significantly simply with calming techniques.

✅ Humidified air or cool-mist therapy may be used, but neither has been proven to be effective.

✅ Humidified oxygen should be administered to any patient with O_2 saturation less than 92%.

✅ **Treatments are aimed at reducing airway edema. For patients with stridor or significant work of breathing at rest, give a combination of nebulized epinephrine and a corticosteroid.**

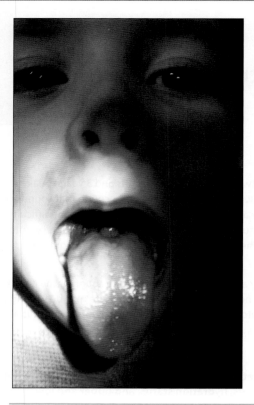

Fig. 32.1 A normal-appearing epiglottis.

For racemic epinephrine, nebulize 0.05 mL/kg/dose (max dose 0.5 mL) of a 2.25% solution diluted in 3 mL of normal saline. (Confirm your dosages with local pharmacists, and review your concentration prior to administration)

⊘ An adjunct to treatment with epinephrine is the use of a continuous 70/30 helium and oxygen mixture (heliox) administered through a facemask, usually reserved for patients with severe respiratory compromise.

⊘ **Give glucocorticoids to patients with all severities of croup. Dexamethasone 0.6 mg/kg once PO (maximum dose 10 mg) is recommended. If the patient is vomiting or unable or unwilling to take dexamethasone PO, it can be given intramuscularly (IM) as an injectable suspension, or even nebulized in 3 mL normal saline. The oral suspension of dexamethasone has a foul taste and requires a higher volume. The intravenous (IV) formulation, which is more concentrated at 4 mg/mL, may be given orally and is often tolerated well in juice or a syrup.**

⊘ Observe the patient for signs of improvement or worsening over a period of 3 to 4 hours.

⊘ **In general, admit all children with a toxic appearance, with inability to maintain oral hydration, without improvement after nebulized epinephrine administration, or with symptoms that recur during the observation period following initial epinephrine administration.**

✓ For the mildest cases of croup, it is reasonable to treat with supportive measures alone, but adding one dose of dexamethasone can decrease duration of croup symptoms and reduce the need for reevaluation. If the symptoms recur and are not severe, parents should be encouraged to try supportive measures such as calming the child and exposing the child to humidified or cold air at home.

What Not to Do

✗ Do not routinely obtain soft tissue neck radiographs. These should be reserved for atypical presentations or when more severe disease (i.e., epiglottitis or abscess) or a foreign body is suspected. In croup, an anteroposterior soft tissue neck radiograph may show subglottic narrowing, which is called the steeple or pencil-point sign.

✗ Do not routinely obtain blood work. The resultant pain and agitation will do more to worsen symptoms than is justified by the small potential for any useful information that might be obtained.

✗ Do not prescribe antibiotics. This is a viral illness, and unless there is an alternative or suspected concurrent source of bacterial infection, antibiotic use will be ineffective and is inappropriate.

✗ Do not discharge the patient prior to an extended period of observation after racemic epinephrine has been administered. Although the theoretical rebound phenomenon has been discredited, patients might return to an unacceptable baseline.

✗ Do not forget to consider alternate diagnoses, including peritonsillar or retropharyngeal abscess, epiglottitis, allergic reaction, airway foreign body, and airway anomalies, especially when the course is atypical or there are any atypical features in the presentation.

Discussion

Laryngotracheitis, or viral croup, is the most common infectious cause of acute upper airway obstruction in children. While it is usually a mild and self-limited disease, significant upper airway obstruction and, rarely, death can occur. Most cases occur in the late fall and early spring. Parainfluenza viruses cause most cases of croup. Other responsible viruses include influenzae A and B, adenovirus, respiratory syncytial virus, measles, and rhinovirus. The viral infection leads to inflammation of the nasopharynx and subglottic area of the upper airway.

Most children with these viral infections will not develop croup. The barking cough and stridor in children with croup occurs from the mucosal and submucosal edema of this subglottic portion of the airway, which is the narrowest portion of a child's upper airway. Redness and swelling just below the vocal cords are seen in children with croup who have video laryngoscopy performed. When croup is severe, the diameter of the airway can become as small as 1 to 2 mm.

Not all children with stridor have croup. Excluding other causes, especially foreign body aspirations or ingestions, is crucial.

In contrast with viral croup, a nonseasonal allergic variant, known as spasmodic croup, may occur. This disorder typically has an abrupt onset, with no preceding upper respiratory infection and no fever. Spasmodic croup usually resolves quickly with exposure to humidified or cold air.

When high fever, toxicity, and worsening respiratory distress develop after several days of crouplike illness, consider the possibility of the more serious but uncommon diagnosis of bacterial tracheitis.

Consider referring patients with recurrent episodes of croup to otolaryngology (ENT) for further evaluation of possible anatomic or other contributing factors.

133

Suggested Readings

Everard, M. (2009). Acute bronchiolitis and croup. *Pediatric Clinics of North America, 56*, 119–133.

Geelhoed, G. C. (1996). Sixteen years of croup in a western Australian teaching hospital: Effects of routine steroid treatment. *Annals of Emergency Medicine, 28*, 621–626.

Geelhoed, G. C., & Macdonald, W. B. G. (1995). Oral dexamethasone in the treatment of croup. *Pediatric Pulmonology, 20*, 362–368.

Johnson, D. W., Jacobson, S., Edney, P. C., et al. (1998). A comparison of nebulized budesonide, intramuscular dexamethasone, and placebo for moderately severe croup. *New England Journal of Medicine, 339*, 498–503.

Klassen, T. P., Craig, W. R., Moher, D., et al. (1998). Nebulized budesonide and oral dexamethasone for treatment of croup. *Journal of the American Medical Association, 279*, 1629–1632.

Klassen, T. P., Watters, L. K., Feldman, M. E., et al. (1996). The efficacy of nebulized budesonide in dexamethasone-treated outpatients with croup. *Pediatrics, 97*, 463–466.

Kunkel, N. C., & Baker, M. D. (1996). Use of racemic epinephrine, dexamethasone, and mist in the outpatient management of croup. *Pediatric Emergency Care, 12*, 156–159.

Luria, J. W., Gonzalez-del Rey, J. A., Digiulio, G. A., et al. Effectiveness of oral or nebulized dexamethasone for children with mild croup. *Archives of Pediatric and Adolescent Medicine, 155,* 1340–1345.

McDonogh, A. J. (1994). The use of steroids and nebulized adrenaline in the treatment of viral croup over a seven-year period at a district hospital. *Anesthesia and Intensive Care Journal, 22*, 175–178.

Neto, G. M., Kentab, O., Klassen, T. P., et al. (2002). A randomized controlled trial of mist in the acute treatment of moderate croup. *Academic Emergency Medicine, 9*, 873–879.

Prendergast, M., Jones, J. S., & Hartman, D. (1994). Racemic epinephrine in the treatment of laryngotracheitis: can we identify children for outpatient therapy? *American Journal of Emergency Medicine, 12*, 613–616.

Rittichier, K. K., & Ledwith, C. A. (2000). Outpatient treatment of moderate croup with dexamethasone: Intramuscular versus oral dosing. *Pediatrics, 106*, 1344–1348.

Rizos, J. D., DiGravio, B. E., Sehl, M. J., et al. (1998). The disposition of children with croup treated with racemic epinephrine and dexamethasone in the emergency department. *Journal of Emergency Medicine, 16*, 535–539.

Rowe, B. H. (2002). Corticosteroid treatment for acute croup. *Annals of Emergency Medicine, 40*, 353–355.

Sobol, S. E., & Zapata, S. (2008). Epiglottitis and croup. *Otolaryngology Clinics of North America, 41*, 551–566.

Weber, J. E., Chudnosfsky, C. R., Younger, J. G., et al. (2001). A randomized comparison of helium-oxygen mixture (heliox) and racemic epinephrine for the treatment of moderate to severe croup. *Pediatrics, 107*, e96.

Mononucleosis

(Glandular Fever)

Presentation

The patient is usually an adolescent or a young adult between the ages of 15 and 25 complaining of several days of fever, malaise, myalgias, and anorexia, culminating in a severe sore throat. The physical examination is remarkable for lymphadenopathy, typically bilateral posterior cervical chains, and enlarged tonsils, at times meeting in the midline and covered with an exudate, which can be white, green, yellow, or necrotic appearing. There may also be palatal petechiae and swelling, periorbital edema, splenomegaly (often not evident clinically), hepatomegaly, and, less commonly, a diffuse maculopapular rash or jaundice (more common in patients who are >40 years of age).

What to Do

✓ **Perform a complete physical examination, including lymph nodes, the entire oropharynx, abdomen, and skin. Look for signs of other ailments and the rare complications of airway obstruction, encephalitis, hemolytic anemia, thrombocytopenic purpura, myocarditis, pericarditis, hepatitis, peritonsillar abscess, and splenic rupture.**

✓ **Send blood samples to be tested. Obtain a differential white cell count (looking for lymphocytosis and atypical lymphocytes), an Epstein-Barr and cytomegalovirus panel, and monospot test.** Each of these tests, along with the lymphadenopathy, will help confirm the diagnosis of mononucleosis.

✓ **Culture the throat.** Patients with mononucleosis often harbor group A *Streptococcus,* and they can concurrently have mononucleosis and a bacterial infection.

✓ **When the diagnosis has been confirmed, warn the patient that the period of convalescence for mononucleosis is longer than that for most other viral illnesses (typically 2–4 weeks, occasionally more), and that they should seek attention if they experience lightheadedness, abdominal or shoulder pain, or any other sign of the rare complications mentioned earlier.**

✓ **Symptomatic treatment is the mainstay of care. This includes adequate hydration, analgesics, antipyretics, and adequate rest. Bed rest should not be enforced, and the patient's energy level should guide activity.**

✓ **These patients should be withdrawn from contact or collision sports or any strenuous athletic activity for at least 4 weeks after the onset of symptoms.**

✓ Patients should be warned that, in a few cases, fatigue, myalgias, and an excessive need for sleep may persist for several months.

✓ Corticosteroids, acyclovir, and antihistamines are not recommended for routine treatment. If there is impending airway obstruction caused by tonsillar swelling, hospitalization may be necessary, along with intravenous (IV) fluids, humidified air, and corticosteroids.

✓ **Dexamethasone, in doses up to 0.6 mg/kg (max of 10 mg), has been used to treat impending airway obstruction caused by markedly enlarged "kissing tonsils."**

What Not to Do

✗ Do not routinely begin therapy with penicillin for the pharyngitis unless there is clinical suspicion for streptococcal pharyngitis. In a patient with mononucleosis, penicillin derivatives can produce an uncomfortable maculopapular rash, which incidentally does not imply that the patient is allergic to the antibiotic.

✗ Do not forget to advise patients of the unlikely complication of splenic rupture. This complication usually occurs within 3 weeks of onset of symptoms. Refer patients with clinically notable splenomegaly to their primary care provider for reevaluation before they resume contact sports.

Discussion

Infectious mononucleosis is caused by Epstein-Barr virus (EBV) in 90% of cases. EBV is a tumorigenic herpes virus so ubiquitous that close to 100% of the adult population worldwide has serologic evidence of prior exposure. EBV establishes a harmless lifelong infection in almost everyone worldwide and rarely causes disease unless the host-virus balance is upset. After an acute infection, a patient can shed and transmit virus through saliva for months, and intermittent shedding can occur for decades. The incubation period for infectious mononucleosis is 4 to 8 weeks. In most cases, primary infection occurs subclinically during childhood, often spread between family members by salivary contact. When the primary infection is delayed until adolescence or beyond, clinical illness is caused by an intense immunopathologic reaction. Similar mononucleosis-like illnesses can be caused by other infectious agents, including cytomegalovirus, streptococcal infection, adenovirus, human immunodeficiency virus (HIV), human herpes virus 6, and *Toxoplasma gondii*. Infectious mononucleosis should be suspected in patients who are 10 to 30 years of age who present with sore throat, fever, and lymphadenopathy. Sore throat may be absent in up to 15% of cases.

Atypical lymphocytosis of at least 10%, total lymphocytosis of 50%, or absolute lymphocyte count above 4500 strongly support the diagnosis. False-negative results of monospot tests are relatively common early in the course of infection. In the first week of symptoms 25% of patients can have a false-negative result, followed by 5% to 10% in the second week and 5% in the third week. Results can remain positive for up to 1 year after initial infection. Patients typically only have mononucleosis once in a lifetime. Patients with negative results for the heterophile test, atypical lymphocytes, and lymphocytosis may have another infection, such as the examples given earlier. Based on the clinical scenario, consider sending EBV-specific antibodies to confirm or retesting later in the course. Consider sending HIV testing in patients with heterophile-negative antibody test or if there are mucocutaneous ulcerations seen. Although reasonably specific, positive tests are also seen in other conditions, including HIV, lymphoma, systemic lupus, rubella, parvovirus, and other viral infections.

Mild thrombocytopenia, elevations of hepatocellular enzymes, microscopic hematuria, and proteinuria are often present but self-limiting abnormalities.

Although there are some cases of prolonged fatigue after infectious mononucleosis, there is no convincing evidence that EBV infection or recurrence of EBV infection is linked to a chronic fatigue syndrome. For previously healthy adolescents and young adults, infectious mononucleosis is a self-limited illness. Many have symptoms for less than 1 week, and most have returned to their usual state of health within 1 month.

Splenic rupture is the most well-known complication. Up to 60% of patients with mononucleosis will have splenomegaly. Rupture is quite rare, but when it occurs, 50% have no known associated trauma.

Suggested Readings

Auwaeter, P. G. (2004). Infectious mononucleosis: Return to play. *Clinics in Sports Medicine, 23*, 485–497.

Bass, M. H. (1954). Periorbital edema as the initial sign of infectious mononucleosis. *Journal of Pediatrics, 45*, 204–205.

Ebell, M. H. (2004). Epstein-Barr virus infectious mononucleosis. *American Family Physician, 70*, 1279–1287.

Ellen Rimsza, M. E., & Kirk, G. M. (2005). Common medical problems of the college student. *Pediatric Clinics of North America, 52*, 9–24.

Macsween, K. F., & Crawford, D. H. (2003). Epstein-Barr virus—recent advances. *Lancet Infectious Diseases, 3*, 131–140.

Mandell, G. L., Bennett, J. E., & Dolin, R. (2011). *Mandell, Douglas, and Bennett's principles and practice of infectious diseases* (7th ed.). Philadelphia: Churchill Livingstone.

Rea, T. D., Russo, J. E., Katon, W., Ashley, R. L., & Buchwald, D. S. (2001). Prospective study of the natural history of infectious mononucleosis caused by Epstein-Barr virus. *Journal of the American Board of Family Practice, 14*(4), 234–242.

Nasal Fracture

(Broken Nose)

Presentation

After a direct blow to the nose, a patient may present with concern that their nose is broken. There is usually minimal bleeding. There may be tender ecchymotic swelling over the nasal bones or the anterior maxillary spine, and inspection and palpation may or may not reveal nasal deformity.

What to Do

✓ **To help determine the nature and extent of the injury, obtain a history of the mechanism of injury. A direct frontal blow can cause fractured bones to telescope posteriorly. A laterally directed injury can cause a depression on the side of the impact, often with a corresponding outward displacement on the opposite side of the nose.**

✓ Additional history should include information regarding previous surgeries and injuries, as well as a subjective assessment of baseline nasal function and appearance.

✓ **Examine the patient for any associated injuries** (e.g., blowout fractures, zygoma fractures, mandible fractures, dental injuries, naso-orbital-ethmoid fracture, concussion, intracranial hemorrhage, and eye injuries). A general screening exam should include special attention to the cervical spine, other facial bones, extraocular movements, and dentition.

✓ **A deformity of the nose usually will be evident when a nasal fracture has occurred.** Edema and ecchymosis of the nose and periorbital structures ordinarily will be present. **Palpation of the nasal structures should be done to elicit crepitus, indentation, or irregularity of the nasal bone. Bony crepitus and nasal segment mobility are both diagnostic for nasal fracture.**

✓ **If another facial or mandibular fracture is suspected, assessment with a computed tomography (CT) scan may be indicated.** Uncommon findings, such as a cerebrospinal fluid leak posing as clear rhinorrhea, subcutaneous emphysema, mental status changes, new malocclusion, or limited extraocular movement, also may require CT evaluation and subspecialty consultation.

✓ **An internal nasal examination should be conducted with good lighting, suction, and vasoconstriction with topical anesthesia. A nasal speculum and a headlamp will improve visualization.** Anxiolysis may be needed. Clots should be removed with Frazier tip suction and cotton-tipped applicators. If swelling or continued bleeding obscure adequate visualization, instill cotton pledgets soaked in vasoconstrictive medication such as 0.25% to 1% phenylephrine or oxymetazoline (Afrin).

✅ After removing the pledgets, **inspect for nasal airway patency, ongoing epistaxis, septal deformities, and, most importantly, septal hematoma, which may appear as slightly white or purple areas of fluctuance lying on one or both sides of the nasal septum.** Bimanual palpation of the septum with cotton-tipped applicators helps to differentiate hematoma, which tends to be more compressible than tissue edema. Areas of increased mobility are suggestive of septal fracture. If bleeding continues, treat this epistaxis as described in Chapter 28.

✅ **When an uncomplicated nasal fracture is suspected, plain radiography is not indicated.** Because of poor sensitivity and specificity, plain radiographs may serve only to confuse the clinical picture.

✅ Explain to the patient that for minor injuries, radiographic examinations are not routinely used. These studies expose the patient to unnecessary radiation and are not helpful. **Therapeutic decisions are made on the basis of the physical examination and patient symptoms.** If there is a fracture but it is stable and in a good position clinically, the nose need not be reset. Conversely, a broken and displaced cartilage may obstruct breathing and require reduction or operation but may not be evident on imaging studies.

✅ **Patients with suspected or possible nondisplaced fractures and no nasal deformity should be sent home with cold packs and instructions to keep the head elevated and avoid contact sports and related activities for 6 weeks.** When nasal deformity cannot be visualized or palpated because of marked swelling, have the patient follow up within 3 to 5 days when the swelling has decreased. Alternatively, recent studies show that, for determining the orientation and location of a displaced/depressed fracture, **nasal sonography** is as accurate as facial CT.

✅ **Patients with suspected displaced fractures, nasal deformity, or both should be referred for otolaryngology (ENT) or plastic surgery consultation to discuss immediate or delayed reduction. Patients can be instructed that reduction is more accurate after the swelling subsides and that there is no greater difficulty if it is done within 2 weeks of the injury.**

✅ **Septal hematomas should be drained immediately. Untreated septal hematomas can lead to pressure-induced avascular necrosis** and subsequent septal perforation, saddle nose deformity, or abscess formation. Due to high rate of complications, ENT consultation is advisable.

✅ **A minor isolated fracture of the anterior nasal spine** (in the columella of the nose) does not necessitate restriction of activities. Such fractures hurt only when the patient smiles and do not require any special treatment.

✅ **A laceration over a nasal fracture should be treated with antibiotic prophylaxis with coverage for gram-positive flora after copious irrigation.**

✅ Physical abuse should be considered in vulnerable populations such as children and women and should be appropriately evaluated and managed.

What Not to Do

❌ Do not focus solely on the traumatized nose. Consider cervical spine injury as well as other facial injuries and other remote trauma.

(X) Do not routinely obtain radiographs of the injured nose. Patients may expect this because it used to be standard practice, but plain films typically do not change management. Radiographs can often be inaccurate in determining the presence and nature of a nasal fracture. Rely on the clinical assessment (or ultrasound when available). When relying on clinical assessment, if there is significant swelling, arrange for reexamination in 3 to 5 days when the swelling has subsided.

(X) Do not pack an injured nose that does not continue to bleed. Packing is generally unnecessary and will only add to the patient's discomfort.

Discussion

The nose is easily exposed to trauma because it is the most prominent and anterior feature of the face. The nose is supported by cartilage, anteriorly and inferiorly, and by bone, posteriorly and superiorly. Although most of the nasal structures are cartilaginous, the nasal bones usually are fractured in an injury.

Fights and sports injuries account for most nasal fractures in adults, followed by falls and vehicle crashes.

The two most common indications for reduction of a nasal fracture are an unacceptable appearance and the patient's inability to breathe through the nose. If neither breathing nor cosmesis is a concern, it is not necessary to reduce the fracture.

Nasal fractures are uncommon in young children because the nose at this age is composed of mostly pliable cartilage. For this reason, radiographic examination has even less accuracy than in an adult.

It should be noted, however, that with significant trauma to the face, children may develop devastating growth retardation of the nose and midface. Refer all young children with posttraumatic nasal asymmetry, bony crepitus, epistaxis, periorbital ecchymosis, significant edema, or overlying skin lacerations to a pediatric ENT for reexamination within 2 to 4 days. Because of faster rates of bone healing, realignment in children should ideally be performed within 4 days of injury.

Suspect septal hematoma when a patient's nasal airway is completely occluded. Within 48 to 72 hours, a hematoma can compromise the blood supply to the cartilage and cause irreversible damage.

Suggested Readings

Alshaikh, N., & Lo, S. (2011). NNasal septal abscess in children: From diagnosis to management and prevention. *International Journal of Pediatric Otorhinolaryngology*, *75*(6), 737–744. https://doi.org/10.1016/j.ijporl.2011.03.010. Epub 2011 Apr 14. PMID: 21492944.

Fattahi, T., Steinberg, B., Fernandes, R., Mohan, M., & Reitter, E. (2006). Repair of nasal complex fractures and the need for secondary septo-rhinoplasty. *Journal of Oral and Maxillofacial Surgery*, *64*(12), 1785–1789. https://doi.org/10.1016/j.joms.2006.03.053. PMID: 17113446.

Kang, W. K., Han, D. G., Kim, S. E., Lee, Y. J., & Shim, J. S. (2020). Bone remodeling after conservative treatment of nasal bone fracture in pediatric patients. *Archives Caniofacial of Surgery*, *21*(3), 166–170. https://doi.org/10.7181/acfs.2020.00192. Epub 2020 Jun 29. PMID: 32630988 Free PMC article.

Kopacheva-Barsova, G., & Arsova, S. (2016). The impact of the nasal trauma in childhood on the development of the nose in future. *Open Access Maced J Med Sci*, *4*(3), 413–419. https://doi.org/10.3889/oamjms.2016.081. Epub 2016 Aug 2. PMID: 27703565 Free PMC article.

Kühnel, T. S., & Reichert, T. E. (2015). Trauma of the midface. *GMS Current Topics in Otorhinolaryngology, Head and Neck Surgery*, *14*, Doc06. https://doi.org/10.3205/cto000121. eCollection 2015.

Mondin, V., Rinaldo, A., & Ferlito, A. (2005). Management of nasal bone fractures. *American Journal of Otolaryngology*, *26*(3), 181.

Olsen, K. D., Carpenter, R. J., 3rd, & Kern, E. B. (1979). Nasal septal trauma in children. *Pediatrics*, *64*(1), 32–35. PMID: 450557.

Otitis Externa (Swimmer's Ear), Acute

Presentation

In acute otitis externa (AOE), the patient complains of ear pain, which is always uncomfortable and sometimes unbearable, often accompanied by drainage and a blocked sensation, decreased hearing, and sometimes fever. When the condition is mild or chronic, there may be itching rather than pain. Pulling on the auricle (Fig. 35.1) or pushing on the tragus of the ear classically causes increased pain. The tissue lining of the canal may be swollen; in severe cases, the swelling can extend into the soft tissue surrounding the ear. Tender erythematous swelling or an underlying furuncle may be present, and it may be pointing or draining.

The canal may be erythematous and dry, or it may be covered with fuzzy cottonlike grayish or black fungal plaques (wet newspaper appearance). Most often, the canal lining is moist and covered with purulent drainage and debris, and cerumen is characteristically absent. The canal may be so swollen that it is difficult or impossible to view the tympanic membrane (TM) (Fig. 35.2), which, when visible, often looks dull.

A pruritic vesiculopapular eruption in the canal is most consistent with an allergic reaction to a topical agent (often neomycin) (see Chapter 162).

What to Do

✅ Determine if the patient has had tympanostomy tubes within the past year or a history of chronic suppurative otitis media with recurrent ear drainage; if so, the patient will probably have an open TM. Those who can taste topical otic medications after placement of the medication in the external auditory canal and those who can expel air from the ear are also indicators of a defect in the TM.

✅ **Meticulous and repeated clearing of the canal is the cornerstone of treatment. Irrigation can be very effective** in cleaning out the canal, using a 1:1 dilution of 3% hydrogen peroxide **(if the TM is intact)** or just plain warm water may be best. Other cleaning methods include suction, cotton swabs, and ear curettes.

✅ **Inspect the ear for the presence of a foreign body.**

✅ **Incise and drain any furuncle that is pointing or fluctuant.**

✅ **If the ear canal is too narrow to allow medication to flow freely, insert a wick. The best wick is the Pope ear wick (Merocel Corporation, Mystic, CT),** which is about 1×10 mm of compressed cellulose; it is thin enough to slip into an occluded canal but expands when wet. If this wick is not available, try using alligator forceps to insert a 1-cm strip of 0.25-inch

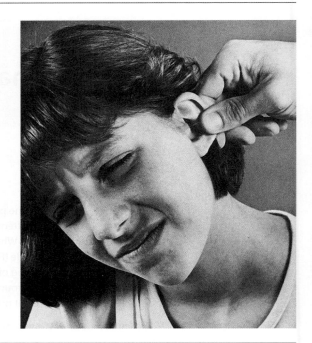

Fig. 35.1 Pulling on the ear causes increased pain.

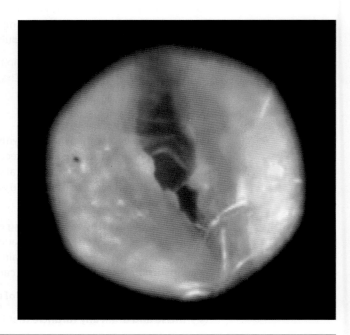

Fig. 35.2 Otoscopic view of otitis externa. Edema of the ear canal obscures the tympanic membrane. (With permission from Point of Care. [2019]. *Otitis externa*. Amsterdam, Netherlands: Elsevier BV.)

plain gauze or a twisted wisp of cotton that may be obtained from a cotton ball or the end of a cotton-tipped applicator. (This method is more painful.) Advance the wick cautiously to avoid damaging the middle-ear structures or puncturing the TM. **After the wick is inserted, instill the otic drops noted below. Water must then be kept out of the ear, and the patient must be instructed to use soft wax earplugs while showering or, alternatively, a cotton ball covered with petroleum jelly.** Wicks may be replaced every 1 to 3 days if the symptoms persist.

✓ **Studies have shown no difference in cure rate between topical antibiotics, topical antiseptics, and topical antibiotic/steroid preparations but that these agents are significantly superior to placebo.**

✓ **Acidifying solutions**, such as acetic acid, work by lowering canal pH, thus inhibiting fungal and bacterial growth. **The addition of a steroid to the antimicrobial or acidifying solution has been shown to decrease time to symptom relief.** A typical acidifying solution is 2% acetic acid. (Add two parts of 5% acetic acid [or household vinegar] to three parts water and you will render 2% acetic acid.) *Pseudomonas aeruginosa* and *Staphylococcus* are the most common bacteria responsible for AOE.

✓ **There are several antibiotic choices, but ciprofloxacin and ofloxacin have the advantage of good bacterial coverage, bid dosing, and ability to use if the TM is perforated, but unfortunately these topical medications can be very expensive. Suggestions are ciprofloxacin-hydrocortisone (Cipro HC Otic) otic suspension, 10 mL, 3 drops in ear(s) twice daily for 7 days, or ofloxacin (Floxin Otic), 10 mL, 0.3%, 5 drops in ear(s) twice daily for 7 days.**

✓ **If the TM is intact, other choices are gentamycin (Garamycin) or tobramycin (Tobrex) ophthalmic solution 0.3%, 5 mL, 4 to 6 drops in ear(s) four times a day for 7 days. (Yes, this eye medication can be placed in the ear canal.)**

✓ **Fungal infections cause about 2% to 10% of AOE. Patients usually complain more of itching than pain,** and edema of the canal is often milder than in bacterial infection. Fungal filaments can sometimes be seen, and *Candida* typically reveals sebaceous-like material in the canal. **Topical antifungals**, such as acetic acid and aluminum acetate (Domeboro Otic), 60 mL, 4 to 6 drops in ear(s) every 2 to 3 hours for 7 days; acetic acid (VoSol Otic) 15%, 30 mL, 5 drops in ear(s) three to four times a day (VoSol HC Otic adds hydrocortisone 1% [only generic is available]); or clotrimazole (Lotrimin) 10 mL, 1% solution, 4 to 6 drops in ear(s) twice daily for 7 days, may be prescribed. VoSol Otic (or 2% acetic acid) can be used **to prevent recurrent AOM** if used two to four times a day for 4 to 5 days after water exposure. **Acetic acid preparations should not be used if an open TM is known or suspected to be present because of theoretic ototoxicity.**

✓ **For moderate to severe pain and soft tissue swelling or other signs of cellulitis, prescribe an appropriate analgesic.**

✓ **Systemic antibiotics are indicated in patients with diabetes mellitus, immunodeficiency, history of radiation to the ear, or when infection has spread beyond the external ear canal, or if the canal cannot be adequately cleared to allow the topical agent to work. Systemic antibiotics include levofloxacin (Levaquin), 500 mg once daily for 10 days, or ciprofloxacin (Cipro), 500 mg twice daily 10 days.**

✓ Provide follow-up in 2 to 3 days to remove a wick and any remaining debris from the ear canal.

✓ **In general, prognosis is excellent with adequate treatment. Full recovery is expected within 1 week, and patients often experience marked improvement after 1 day.**

✓ **Patients should be instructed** to avoid using cotton-tipped swabs and other devices to clean wax out of the ear canals. These techniques are usually counterproductive and often increase their risk for AOM. Also have them thoroughly dry the external auditory canal after exposure to moisture or swimming.

✓ When administering eardrops without a wick in the ear canal, instruct the patient to lie on that side for 20 minutes after instilling, to maximize medication exposure.

What Not to Do

✗ Do not routinely culture ear drainage. This should be reserved for severe cases or where there is persistent or refractory infection.

✗ Do not use oral antibiotics to treat simple otitis externa without evidence of cellulitis or concurrent otitis media.

✗ Do not use topical antibiotics for prophylaxis. Long-term use of any topical antibiotic can lead to a fungal superinfection.

✗ Do not instill medication without first cleansing the ear canal, unless restricted because of pain and/or swelling.

✗ Do not expect medicine to enter a canal that is swollen shut without using a wick.

✗ Do not use eardrops containing neomycin, which sometimes causes severe allergic contact dermatitis.

✗ Do not miss the case of malignant (necrotizing) external otitis in the elderly diabetic patient who presents with exquisitely painful otorrhea. These patients require otolaryngologic consultation, special diagnostic evaluation, and prolonged administration of an oral quinolone.

Discussion

Common predisposing factors to the development of otitis externa are excessive moisture in the external auditory canal, obstruction of canal, disrupted epithelial integrity, and disrupted protective cerumen layer in the canal.

Acute otitis externa has a seasonal occurrence, being more frequently encountered in the summer months, when the climate and contaminated swimming water will most likely precipitate a fungal or *Pseudomonas aeruginosa* bacterial infection. *P. aeruginosa* is the most common bacterium involved in this infection, with *Staphylococcus* species being the next most common pathogen. Fungi are only responsible for approximately 2% of cases but may well be more prominent in cases of persistent or chronic infection. Various dermatoses (eczema, psoriasis, seborrhea), diabetes, aggressive ear cleaning with cotton-tipped swabs, previous external ear infections, and furunculosis also predispose patients to developing otitis externa.

The healthy ear canal is coated with cerumen and sloughed epithelium. Cerumen is water repellent and acidic and contains a number of antimicrobial substances. Repeated washing or cleaning can remove this defensive coating. Moisture retained in the ear canal is readily absorbed by the stratum corneum. The skin becomes macerated and edematous, and the accumulation of debris may block gland ducts, preventing further production of the protective cerumen. Finally, endogenous or exogenous organisms invade the damaged canal epithelium and cause the infection.

In most cases of uncomplicated acute otitis externa, topical antibiotics are the first-line treatment choice. There is no evidence that systemic antibiotics alone or combined with topical preparations improve treatment outcome compared with topical antibiotics alone, and they may contribute to the development of bacterial resistance. **When a perforation exists or a patent**

Discussion continued

tympanostomy tube is present, quinolone drops offer superior safety and efficacy. It should be realized, however, that the risk for ototoxicity is negligible when using aminoglycoside combination drops or acetic acid drops when the TM is intact, and that these preparations are consistently effective and less expensive first-line treatments. Clearly, systemic antibiotics are indicated to treat the more serious manifestations of the disease, such as periauricular cellulitis or necrotizing otitis externa.

Malignant or necrotizing external otitis

is a potentially life-threatening condition that occurs primarily in elderly diabetic patients and immunocompromised individuals. *P. aeruginosa* is isolated from the aural drainage in more than 90% of cases. The pathophysiology is incompletely understood, although irrigation for cerumen impaction has been reported as a potential iatrogenic factor.

The typical patient presents with severe headache or ear pain, swelling, and drainage. Granulation tissue on the floor of the ear canal may be present. The TM is almost always intact. Disease progression is associated with osteomyelitis of the skull base and temporomandibular joint. Cranial nerve palsies generally indicate advancing infection. Paralysis of the facial nerve is most common. Patients are usually afebrile with normal white blood cell (WBC) and differential counts. The erythrocyte sedimentation rate (ESR) is usually markedly increased. CT scans are ideal to assess for bone erosion. In a prospective study, presence of bone erosion and soft tissue abnormalities in the infratemporal fossa were most helpful in making the diagnosis of malignant external otitis. There is no role for topical antibiotics, even

quinolones, in the treatment of this disease. Instillation of antipseudomonal topical agents only increases the difficulty of isolating the pathogenic organism from the ear canal. Systemic antipseudomonal antibiotics are the primary therapy for malignant external otitis. The availability of oral agents has eliminated the need for hospitalization in all but the most recalcitrant cases. Ciprofloxacin (Cipro), 750 mg orally bid, seems to be the antibiotic of choice. Despite the rapid relief of symptoms (pain and otorrhea), prolonged treatment for 6 to 8 weeks is still recommended, as indicated for osteomyelitis. Early consultation should be obtained if there is any suspicion of this condition in a susceptible patient with a draining ear.

The ear is innervated by the fifth, seventh, ninth, and tenth cranial nerves and the second and third cervical nerves. Because of this rich nerve supply, the skin is extremely sensitive. Otalgia may arise directly from the seventh cranial nerve (geniculate ganglion), ninth cranial nerve (tympanic branch), external ear, mastoid air cells, mouth, teeth, or esophagus. **Ear pain can result from sinusitis, trigeminal neuralgia, and temporomandibular joint dysfunction or may be referred from disorders of the pharynx and larynx.** A mild pain referred to the ear may be felt as itching, may cause the patient to scratch the ear canal, and may present as external otitis.

It is important to consider the possibility of malignancy in the evaluation of a patient with otalgia and apparently refractory otitis externa. When the source of ear pain is not readily apparent, the patient should be referred for a more complete otolaryngologic investigation.

Suggested Readings

Cummings, C. (Ed.). (2004). *Otolaryngology: Head and neck surgery* (4th ed.). St. Louis, MO: Mosby.

Hannley, M. T., Denneny, J. C., & Holzer, S. S. (2000). Use of ototopical antibiotics in treating 3 common ear diseases. *Otolaryngology-Head and Neck Surgery, 122,* 934–940.

Kaushik, V., Malik, T., & Saeed, S. R. (2010). Interventions for acute otitis externa. *Cochrane Database of Systematic Reviews, 1,* CD004740.

Point of Care. (2019). *Otitis externa.* Amsterdam, Netherlands: Elsevier BV.

Rosenfeld, R. M., Brown, L., Cannon, C. R., et al. (2006). Clinical practice guideline: Acute otitis externa. *Otolaryngology-Head and Neck Surgery, 134*(Suppl. 4), S4–S23.

Rosenfeld, R. M., Singer, M., Wasserman, J. M., & Stinnett, S. S. (2006). Systematic review of topical antimicrobial therapy for acute otitis externa. *Otolaryngology-Head and Neck Surgery, 134*(Suppl. 4), S24–S48.

Ruben, R. J. (2001). Efficacy of ofloxacin and other otic preparations for otitis externa. *The Pediatric Infectious Disease Journal, 20,* 108–110.

Rubin Grandis, J. R., Branstetter, I. V. B. F., & Yu, V. L. (2004). The changing face of malignant (necrotizing) external otitis: Clinical, radiological, and anatomic correlations. *The Lancet Infectious Diseases, 4*, 34–39.

van Balen, F. A., Smit, W. M., Zuithoff, N. P., & Verheij, T. J. (2003). Clinical efficacy of three common treatments in acute otitis externa in primary care: Randomised controlled trial. *BMJ, 327*, 1201–1205.

van Balen, F. A., Zuithoff, B. P., & Verheij, T. J. (2003). Clinical efficacy of three common treatments in acute otitis externa in primary care: Randomized controlled trial. *BMJ, 327*, 1201–1205.

Wong, D. L. H., & Rutka, J. A. (1994). Do aminoglycoside otic preparations cause ototoxicity in the presence of tympanic membrane perforations? *Otolaryngology-Head and Neck Surgery, 116*, 404–410.

Wooltorton, E. (2002). Ototoxic effects from gentamicin ear drops. *Canadian Medical Association Journal, 167*, 56.

CHAPTER 36

Otitis Media, Acute

Presentation

In acute otitis media (AOM), adults and older children will complain of ear pain (and/or fever) that is usually rapid in onset. There may or may not be accompanying symptoms of upper respiratory tract infection. In the younger child or infant, parents may report irritability, decreased appetite, and sleeplessness, with or without fever or pulling at the ears. The real diagnosis comes not from symptoms or history but from tympanic membrane (TM) findings (Figs. 36.1 and 36.2). The TM may show marked redness, but contrary to what many clinicians were taught during training, erythema of the TM is the least specific finding for AOM.

Expanding middle-ear effusion volume and intense inflammation produce the key TM findings that are essential for an AOM diagnosis. These findings point to fullness or a bulging TM, with decreased clarity of the bony landmarks and decreased mobility on pneumatic otoscopy. A normal TM snaps briskly like a sail filling with air from a sudden breeze. With fluid behind the TM, there will be either sluggish or no movement at all. A diagnosis of AOM also can be established if the TM has perforated and acute purulent otorrhea is present that is not attributable to otitis externa (see Chapter 35).

Note that increased vascularity or erythema is not sufficient to diagnose AOM but does strengthen the diagnosis by providing the identification of possible TM inflammation. Keep in mind that a child's vigorous crying is a common cause of an erythematous TM that otherwise has normal findings. Therefore, under these circumstances, avoid diagnosing AOM if erythema of the TM is the only finding suggesting AOM.

What to Do

✅ Investigate for any other underlying illness. When clinical evidence of AOM is obscure or absent, consider other sources of ear pain such as dental or oral disease, temporomandibular joint dysfunction, or disorders of the mastoid, pharynx, or larynx.

✅ There are many antibiotics available for the treatment of AOM. **Amoxicillin remains the treatment of choice** according to the guidelines of the American Academy of Pediatrics, based on efficacy, palatability, side-effect profile, and cost. **High-dose amoxicillin at 80 mg/kg/day twice daily provides better coverage of resistant organisms than standard 40 mg/kg/day dosing.**

✅ **Amoxicillin should not be used if** there has been a treatment failure with amoxicillin in the past 30 days, concurrent purulent conjunctivitis is present (usually caused by *Haemophilus influenzae*), or the patient is already on chronic suppressive therapy with amoxicillin.

✅ **For those patients in whom an alternative to amoxicillin is needed and there is no penicillin allergy, choices include amoxicillin-clavulanate (Augmentin), 90 mg/kg/day**

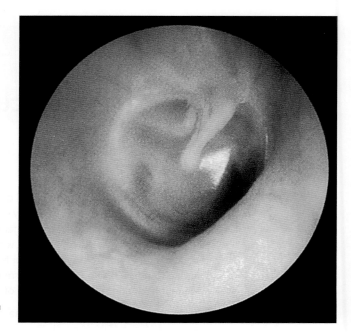

Fig. 36.1 Normal right tympanic membrane and middle ear. (From Meniscus Educational Institute. [1998]. *Otitis media: Management strategies for the 21st century*. Bala Cynwyd, PA: Meniscus.)

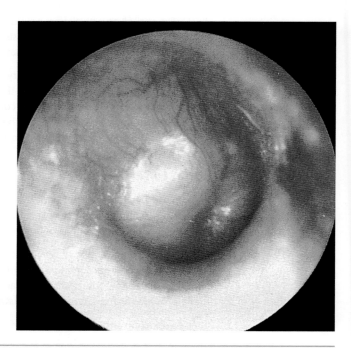

Fig. 36.2 Bulging right tympanic membrane in acute otitis media. (From Meniscus Educational Institute. [1998]. *Otitis media: Management strategies for the 21st century*. Bala Cynwyd, PA: Meniscus.)

twice daily (maximum dose 3 g/day); cefpodoxime, 10 mg/kg once daily (maximum dose 800 mg/day); or cefuroxime, 30 mg/kg/day twice daily (maximum dose 1 g/day).

✓ **For patients allergic to penicillin, the best choice is erythromycin plus sulfisoxazole (Pediazole), 75 mg/kg/day of the erythromycin component divided either three or four times a day (maximum dose 2 g erythromycin component) × 10 days.** Azithromycin and trimethoprim-sulfamethoxazole have significant problems with resistance.

✓ **Studies suggest that 10 days of oral therapy for AOM is more effective than shorter courses in children less than 2 years of age. After 2 years of age, consideration may be given to shorter courses of 5 to 7 days.**

✓ **Ceftriaxone (Rocephin) can be used in a dose of 50 mg/kg IM once daily for 1 to 3 days when compliance problems are anticipated.** A three-dose regimen of IM ceftriaxone may be more efficacious than a single dose for patients with nonresponsive AOM.

✓ **When there is reliable follow-up and the parents are responsible, mild cases of AOM may be treated initially with analgesics alone, adding antimicrobials as an option if symptoms persist or worsen.**

✓ **All children younger than 6 months and all those with moderate to severe ear pain and fever greater than 39 °C in the past 24 hours, bilateral disease, or otorrhea should be treated immediately.**

✓ **Parents can be very satisfied with a wait-and-see approach, in which an antibiotic is prescribed, but the parents are asked to wait 72 hours before filling it.** They are to have the prescription filled only if the child still has substantial ear pain or fever at that point or if the child is not starting to get better. **Most viral and certain bacterial infections (most commonly those infections caused by Haemophilus influenzae) will resolve spontaneously without antibiotic treatment.** Overall, up to 80% of symptoms of acute otitis media resolve spontaneously within 3 days. Provide follow-up by telephone or office visit within 3 days to reassess.

✓ **Acute draining OM** (by either spontaneous perforation or tympanostomy tube) usually is caused by standard AOM pathogens. The usual systemic antibiotics are, in most cases, successful at curing the otitis and stopping the drainage. **In children with no symptoms other than the drainage, ofloxacin (Floxin Otic), 5 mL 0.3%, 5 drops in ear(s) twice daily for 7 to 10 days, has been shown to produce clinical success in more than 75% of cases, although it can be very expensive.** Topical agents alone, however, are not recommended for children whose draining AOM is accompanied by fever or otalgia. Aminoglycoside topical agents should not be used with an open TM because of the potential for ototoxicity.

✓ **Provide pain and fever control with acetaminophen or ibuprofen elixir. Additional pain relief may be obtained using antipyrine, benzocaine, oxyquinoline, and glycerin (Auralgan Otic) drops if perforation or tympanostomy tubes are not present.**

✓ **Advise parents** that pacifier use, exposure to tobacco smoke, and bottle feeding an infant in a reclining rather than an upright position all increase the risk for AOM. Daycare with more than five attendees has been shown to be the most powerful risk factor for frequent AOM. Children who have one or more parents or siblings who experienced frequent AOM or who had pressure-equalizing tubes also will often have frequent AOM or need pressure-equalizing tubes.

✅ **Recommend a 10-day follow-up examination for all patients younger than 2 years of age, in those cases in which the parents do not believe that the infection has resolved or the child's symptoms persist, and when there is a family history of recurrent otitis or the accuracy of the parental observations may be in doubt.**

✅ **Persistent, severe symptoms and unimproved otologic findings after 48 to 72 hours in patients treated with antibiotics** indicate the need to consider changing to second-line antibiotic.

✅ **Because otitis media is much less common in adults**, these patients should also have follow-up in 2 weeks, with possible otolaryngologic consultation.

✅ **Middle-ear effusion will often persist after resolution of acute infection.** Otitis media with effusion (nonacute; also called serous otitis media) represents a noninfected middle ear effusion. Clinically this effusion lacks signs and symptoms of acute middle ear inflammation indicative of acute otitis media. **Persistence of this effusion without symptoms does not indicate a need for further antibiotics.**

What Not to Do

❌ Do not overlook a serious underlying illnesses such as meningitis or mastoiditis.

❌ Do not prescribe antihistamines or decongestants. These drugs do not decrease the incidence or hasten the resolution of AOM in children of any age. The American Academy of Pediatrics recommends that over-the-counter cough and cold medications should not be given to children younger than 2 years of age because of the risk of life-threatening side effects.

❌ Do not overdiagnose AOM. It is critical to avoid inappropriate use of antibiotics.

❌ Do not continue the initial treatment for a persistent effusion. Otitis media with effusion (nonacute persistent effusion) can take up to months to resolve following an acute infection; do not treat with antibiotics unless new symptoms or signs of middle ear inflammation appear.

Discussion

AOM is primarily a disease of children younger than 3 years of age, although AOM is not totally unexpected up to age 5. Age-related factors that directly cause AOM are the result of immature anatomy and immature immune systems coupled with excessive exposure to pathogens. The main reasons for AOM are not bacterial, although bacteria are the final precipitating factor leading to infection. Bacterial AOM pathogens merely take advantage of the main cause of AOM (i.e., dysfunction of the middle ear–flushing mechanism, the eustachian tube). Eustachian tubes are dysfunctional to some degree in every young child but gradually become fully functional by age 5.

Most AOM is caused by a viral infection, and most patients do well regardless of the antibiotic chosen. **Some 50% to 80% of cases of AOM will spontaneously clear without antibiotics.** (Older children with infrequent AOM are more

likely to experience spontaneous clearing, whereas more severe AOM or AOM occurring soon after a previous episode is less likely to clear spontaneously.) Because AOM usually occurs secondary to acute viral infections (respiratory syncytial virus, influenza, and rhinovirus), rapid initiation of antibiotic treatment may result in eradication or reduction of the susceptible organisms in both the middle-ear fluid and the nasopharynx, permitting the overgrowth of the nasopharyngeal flora organisms that are not susceptible to the drug. Because the predisposing condition (the viral infection causing ciliary and mucosal damage, plus overproduction of secretions) may still be present, a new infection of the middle ear may then take place with the newly selected resistant pathogen. Despite the increase in antimicrobial resistance of community-acquired *Streptococcus pneumoniae, Haemophilus influenzae,* and *Moraxella catarrhalis* and the plethora of alternative antibiotics

Discussion continued

available, amoxicillin remains the drug of choice in the treatment of uncomplicated AOM.

Bullous myringitis is the result of acute bacterial infection of the tympanic membrane, producing intraepithelial fluid collections. These patients present with bullae on the TM and can have severe pain. They respond well to anesthetic otic drops (Auralgan), oral antibiotics, corticosteroids, and analgesia.

Suggested Readings

American Academy of Pediatrics. (1997). Use of codeine- and dextromethorphan-containing cough remedies in children. (A statement of reaffirmation for this policy was published on February 1, 2007). Committee on Drugs. *Pediatrics, 99*, 918–920.

American Academy of Pediatrics Subcommittee on the Management of Otitis Media. (2004). Diagnosis and management of acute otitis media. *Pediatrics, 113*, 1451–1465.

Arguedas, A., Emparanza, P., Schwartz, R. H., et al. (2005). A randomized, multicenter, double blind, double dummy trial of single dose azithromycin versus high dose amoxicillin for treatment of uncomplicated acute otitis media. *The Pediatric Infectious Disease Journal, 24*, 153–161.

Bell, L. M. (2005). The new clinical practice guidelines for acute otitis media: An editorial. *Annals of Emergency Medicine, 45*, 514–516.

Cohen, R., Levy, C., Boucherat, M., et al. (2000). Five vs. ten days of antibiotic therapy for acute otitis media in young children. *The Pediatric Infectious Disease Journal, 19*, 458–463.

Culpepper, L., & Froom, J. (1997). Routine antimicrobial treatment of acute otitis media: Is it necessary? *Journal of the American Medical Association, 278*, 1643–1645 [editorial].

Del Mar, C., Glaszion, P., & Hayem, M. (1997). Are antimicrobials indicated as initial treatment for children with acute otitis media? A meta-analysis. *BMJ, 314*, 1526–1529.

Eskin, B. (2004). Evidence-based emergency medicine/systemic review abstract. Should children with otitis media be treated with antibiotics? *Annals of Emergency Medicine, 44*, 537–539.

Froom, J., Culpepper, L., Jacobs, M., et al. (1997). Antimicrobials for acute otitis media? A review for the international primary care network. *BMJ, 315*, 98–102.

Garbutt, J., St Geme, J. W., May, A., et al. (2004). Developing community-specific recommendations for first-line treatment of acute otitis media: Is high-dose amoxicillin necessary? *Pediatrics, 114*, 342–347.

Klein, J., & Pelton, S. (n.d.). Acute otitis media in children: Treatment. UpToDate. http://www.uptodate.com.

Kozyrskyj, A. L., Hildes-Ripstein, E., Longstaffe, S., et al. (1998). Treatment of acute otitis media with a shortened course of antibiotics. *Journal of the American Medical Association, 279*, 1736–1742.

Le Saux, N., Gaboury, I., Baird, M., et al. (2005). A randomized, double-blind, placebo-controlled noninferiority trial of amoxicillin for clinically diagnosed acute otitis media in children 6 months to 5 years of age. *Canadian Medical Association Journal, 172*, 335–341.

Marchetti, F., Ranfani, L., Nibali, S. C., et al. (2005). Delayed prescription may reduce the use of antibiotics for acute otitis media. *Archives in Pediatric and Adolescent Medicine, 159*, 679–684.

McCormick, D. P., Chonmaitree, T., Pittman, C., et al. (2005). Nonsevere acute otitis media: A clinical trial comparing outcomes of watchful waiting versus immediate antibiotic treatment. *Pediatrics, 115*, 1455–1465.

Niemela, M., Uhari, M., Jounio-Ervasti, K., et al. (1994). Lack of specific symptomatology in children with acute otitis media. *The Pediatric Infectious Disease Journal, 13*, 765–768.

Paradise, J. L. (1995). Managing otitis media: A time for change. *Pediatrics, 96*, 712–715 [editorial].

Pelton, S. I. (1998). Otoscopy for the diagnosis of otitis media. *The Pediatric Infectious Disease Journal, 17*, 540–543.

Point of Care. (2019). *Acute otitis media*. Amsterdam, Netherlands: Elsevier BV.

Rosenfeld, R. M., Vertrees, J. E., Carr, J., et al. (1994). Clinical efficacy of antimicrobial drugs for acute otitis media: Meta-analysis of 5400 children from thirty-three randomized trials. *The Journal of Pediatrics, 124*, 355–367.

Otitis Media With Effusion; Serous (Secretory) Otitis Media (Glue Ear)

Presentation

After an upper respiratory tract infection, an episode of acute otitis media (AOM), an airplane flight, or during a bout of allergies, an adult may complain of a feeling of fullness in the ears, an inability to equalize middle ear pressure, decreased hearing, and a clicking, popping, or crackling sound, especially when moving the head. There is little or no pain or tenderness. Otitis media with effusion (OME) is usually asymptomatic in children, except for tugging at the ears or signs of decreased hearing (lack of attention, talking too loudly, sitting nearer to the television set). When viewed through the otoscope, the tympanic membrane (TM) appears retracted, with bony landmarks that are clearly visible and associated with a dull to normal light reflex with minimal if any injection. The best test to diagnose OME is pneumatic otoscopy, showing poor motion of the TM on insufflation. An air-fluid level or bubbles through the eardrum may be visible (Fig. 37.1). There may be a lack of translucency, with a yellow or grayish effusion (Fig. 37.2). Hearing may be decreased, and the Rinne test may show decreased air conduction (i.e., a tuning fork is heard no better through air than through bone).

It should be emphasized that there is no pain, fever, inflammation, or bulging of the TM, as one might expect to see in AOM (see Chapter 36).

What to Do

✓ **In children without underlying developmental delay, preexisting hearing or vision problems, or other prior speech or language issues, OME can be observed for 3 months from the time of symptom onset or diagnosis without specific workup or treatment.** If the OME lasts longer than 3 months or the child has preexisting problems, as outlined earlier, a hearing evaluation should be obtained.

✓ **Adults with OME may request symptomatic relief of the nasal congestion or middle ear symptoms. Over-the-counter vasoconstrictor nose sprays, such as phenylephrine (Neo-Synephrine) or oxymetazoline 0.05% (Afrin), may be recommended but not for more than a 72-hour period.**

✓ **Also, fluticasone (Flonase) topical corticosteroid spray may be prescribed (two sprays per nostril daily).** However, in studies of children, neither vasoconstrictor sprays nor corticosteroids have been shown to lead to long-term resolution of OME.

✓ **Autoinflation has been shown to afford some improvement without side effects in audiometry at 1 month.** To perform this, instruct the patient to insufflate the middle ear through the eustachian tube by closing the mouth, pinching the nose shut, and blowing until the ears "pop."

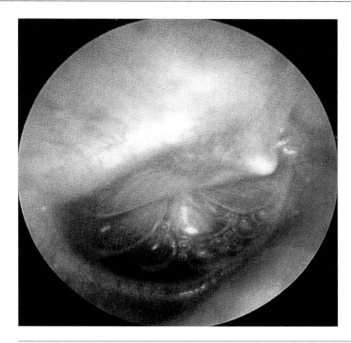

Fig. 37.1 Air-fluid level and bubbles visible through right retracted, translucent tympanic membrane in otitis media with effusion. (From Meniscus Educational Institute. [1998]. *Otitis media: Management strategies for the 21st century*. Bala Cynwyd, PA: Meniscus.)

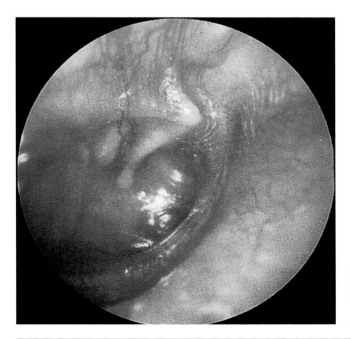

Fig. 37.2 Severely retracted, opaque right tympanic membrane in otitis media with effusion. (From Meniscus Educational Institute. [1998]. *Otitis media: Management strategies for the 21st century*. Bala Cynwyd, PA: Meniscus.)

✓ **A course of antibiotics may improve clearance of OME. Use the same antibiotics as for AOM. Do not prescribe more than one course.**

✓ Instruct the patient to seek follow-up with a primary care doctor or ear-nose-throat (ENT) specialist if the condition does not improve within 1 week.

✓ Parents of children should be informed that bottle feeding, feeding a supine child, attending daycare, and living in a home in which people smoke increases the prevalence of OME.

What Not to Do

✗ Do not allow the patient to become habituated to vasoconstrictor sprays. After a few days of use, the sprays become ineffective, and the nasal mucosa develops a rebound swelling known as rhinitis medicamentosa, when the medicine is withdrawn.

✗ Do not use oral antihistamines or decongestants. They have been shown to be ineffective in the treatment of OME.

✗ Do not use oral or topical corticosteroids for the treatment of children with OME. There may be significant side effects with use of these medications in children. The American Academy of Pediatrics guidelines recommend against their use.

✗ Do not miss a nasopharyngeal mass, which should be considered in all patients with unilateral OME.

Discussion

Among children who have had an episode of AOM, as many as 45% have persistent effusion after 1 month. OME is defined as fluid in the middle ear without signs or symptoms of ear infection. Approximately 90% of cases of OME resolve spontaneously within 6 months. There is significant controversy regarding the routine treatment of this condition.

Most episodes resolve spontaneously within 1 to 2 months. The treatments described here are directed mainly at reestablishing normal function of the eustachian tube. It is unclear if any of these recommended treatments alter the natural course of this disease; therefore **symptomatic relief should guide the clinician toward the most effective management for each individual patient.**

Fluid in the middle ear is more common in children because of frequent viral upper respiratory tract infections and an underdeveloped eustachian tube. The highest incidence of OME occurs in children younger than 2 years, and the incidence decreases dramatically in those older than 6 years. Children are also more prone to bacterial superinfection of the fluid in the middle ear. When accompanied by fever and pain with inflammation and/or purulence, this condition merits treatment with analgesics and antibiotics.

When the diagnosis of OME is uncertain, the patient should be referred for tympanometry or acoustic reflectometry. Children with persistent OME who do not have the aforementioned risk factors should be examined at intervals of 3 to 6 months until the effusion clears or hearing abnormalities are discovered. Tympanostomy tube insertion is now recommended if there is hearing loss of 40 dB or greater persisting for 4 to 6 months and/or speech and language delay or learning difficulties.

Repeated bouts of OME in an adult, especially if unilateral, should raise suspicion regarding a tumor obstructing the eustachian tube.

Suggested Readings

American Academy of Family Physicians. (2004). American Academy of Otolaryngology—head and neck surgery; American Academy of Pediatrics subcommittee on otitis media with effusion. Otitis media with effusion. *Pediatrics*, *113*, 1412–1429.

Csortan, E., Jones, J., Haan, M., et al. (1994). Efficacy of pseudoephedrine for the prevention of barotrauma during air travel. *Annals of Emergency Medicine*, *23*, 1324–1327.

Griffin, G. H., Flynn, C., Bailey, R. E., & Schultz, J. K. (2006). Antihistamines and/or decongestants for otitis media with effusion (OME) in children. *Cochrane Database of Systematic Reviews*, *4*, CD003423.

Harrison, C. J. (2003). The laws of acute otitis media. *Primary Care*, *30*, 109–135.

Jones, J. S., Sheffield, W., White, L. J., et al. (1998). A double-blind comparison between oral pseudoephedrine and topical oxymetazoline in the prevention of barotraumas during air travel. *American Journal of Emergency Medicine*, *16*, 262–264.

Klein, J., & Pelton, S. (2010). *Otitis media with effusion (serious otitis media) in children*. UpToDate. http://www.uptodate.com.

McCracken, G. H. (2002). Diagnosis and management of acute otitis media in the urgent care setting. *Annals of Emergency Medicine*, *39*, 413–421.

Onusko, E. (2004). Tympanometry. *American Family Physician*, *70*, 1713–1720.

Reidpath, D. D., Glasziou, P. P., & Del Mar, C. (1999). Systematic review of autoinflation for treatment of glue ear in children. *BMJ*, *318*, 1177.

Rosenfeld, R. M., & Post, J. C. (1992). Meta-analysis of antibiotics for the treatment of otitis media with effusion. *Otolaryngology-Head and Neck Surgery*, *106*, 378–386.

Williams, R. L., Chalmers, T. C., Strange, K. C., et al. (1993). Use of antibiotics in preventing recurrent acute otitis media and in treating otitis media with effusion. A meta-analytic attempt to resolve the brouhaha. *Journal of the American Medical Association*, *270*, 1344–1351.

CHAPTER

Perforated Tympanic Membrane

(Ruptured Eardrum)

38

Presentation

The patient experiences ear pain after barotrauma, such as a blow or slap on the ear, an exploding firecracker, a fall while water skiing or during a deep-water dive, or after direct trauma inflicted with a sharp object, such as an open paper clip, cerumen curette, or sharp plant part. Hemorrhage is often noticed within the external canal, and the patient will experience the acute onset of pain (which tends to subside quickly) and some partial hearing loss. Tinnitus or transient vertigo may also be present. Otoscopic examination reveals a defect in the tympanic membrane (TM) that may or may not be accompanied by disruption of the ossicles (Fig. 38.1). The presence of blood may make assessment difficult.

What to Do

✓ When necessary, clear any debris from the canal, using gentle suction.

✓ **Determine if this is just an abrasion of the wall of the ear canal or if an actual TM perforation is present. If so, note its size and location.**

✓ Test for nystagmus and gross hearing loss.

✓ **With a true TM perforation, place a protective cotton plug inside the ear canal and instruct the patient to keep the canal dry by using soft wax earplugs while showering (petroleum jelly–covered cotton can be used as a substitute when soft wax earplugs are unavailable). The patient should also avoid submerging the head under water until the perforation is completely healed.**

✓ **Prescribe an appropriate analgesic,** such as ibuprofen (Motrin), naproxen (Anaprox), or acetaminophen (Tylenol). Opioids, such as hydrocodone or oxycodone, should be reserved for patients with severe pain and limited to a supply of 1 to 2 days.

✓ **Prescribe the ototopic antibiotic ofloxacin (Floxin Otic), 5 mL, two to three drops in the effected ear twice daily for 3 to 5 days, only if the lacerated TM and middle ear were contaminated with lake water, seawater, or a dirty object such as a tree branch.** Systemic antibiotics may be added in cases when contamination is severe or substituted for in cases when the patient cannot afford this expensive ototopic.

✓ **Some authors recommend water precautions alone,** with an overall success rate of spontaneous healing (without surgical intervention) of up to 95%, depending on the size of the perforation.

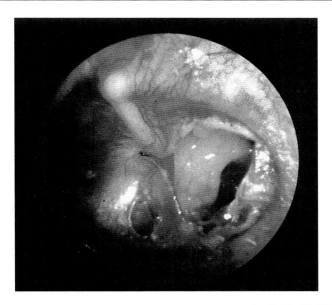

Fig. 38.1 Small traumatic perforation of the tympanic membrane.

✅ **Ensure that the patient gets early follow-up with an otolaryngologist for a thorough assessment of the injury and to test for any hearing loss. This is especially important with sharp, penetrating trauma in the posterior superior quadrant of the TM, where disruption of the ossicles is most likely to occur.**

✅ **Persistent vertigo suggests inner ear involvement (perilymphatic fistula), requiring urgent Otolaryngologist (ENT) consultation.**

✅ In all cases, the patient should be seen regularly until the TM is well healed.

What Not to Do

❌ Do not suction or attempt to clear blood or debris close to the TM if the canal is filled with clotted blood or if damage to the ossicles has occurred; vigorous suctioning may further traumatize these structures.

❌ Do not attempt to remove a foreign body you feel may have penetrated the middle ear space. Consult an ENT specialist (otolaryngologist) in these cases.

❌ Do not instill any fluid other than Floxin Otic into the external canal or allow the patient to get water into the ear. Water in the middle ear is painful and irritating and may introduce bacteria. Wax earplugs or a cotton plug covered with petroleum jelly will allow the patient to shower more safely.

Discussion

Small, uncomplicated perforations usually heal without sequelae over a period of days to weeks. Small defects (<2 mm) will heal spontaneously almost 100% of the time, but larger defects or marginal defects may not heal and would then require either myringoplasty or tympanoplastic procedures. When there is nystagmus, vertigo, profound hearing loss, or disruption of the ossicles, early otolaryngologic consultation is advisable.

If healing has not taken place after 8 weeks or if there is persistent hearing loss after healing, then surgical repair may be indicated.

Suggested Readings

Amadasun, J. E. O. (2002). An observational study of the management of traumatic tympanic membrane perforations. *Journal of Laryngology & Otology, 116*, 181–184.

Evans, A. K., & Handler, S. D. (2010). *Evaluation and management of middle ear trauma*. UpToDate. http://www.uptodate.com.

Fagan, P., & Patel, N. (2002). A hole in the drum. An overview of tympanic membrane perforations. *Australian Family Physician, 31*, 707–710.

Isaacson, J. E., & Vora, N. M. (2003). Differential diagnosis and treatment of hearing loss. *American Family Physician, 68*, 1125–1132.

Sagiv, D., Migirov, L., Glikson, E., Mansour, J., Yousovich, R., Wolf, M., et al. (2018). Traumatic perforation of the tympanic membrane: A review of 80 cases. *Journal of Emergency Medicine, 54*(2), 186–190.

Segal, S. (2003). Inner ear damage in children due to noise exposure from toy cap pistols and firecrackers: A retrospective review of 53 cases. *Noise and Health, 5*, 13–18.

Pharyngitis

(Sore Throat)

Presentation

The patient with **bacterial pharyngitis** complains of a rapid onset of throat pain worsened by swallowing. There is usually sudden onset of the following: fever; pharyngeal erythema; edematous uvula; palatine petechiae (Fig. 39.1); purulent, patchy yellow, gray, or white exudate; tender anterior cervical adenopathy; headache; and absence of a cough. Children who are younger than 3 years of age more often have coryza and are less likely to present with exudative pharyngitis.

Viral infections are typically accompanied by conjunctivitis, nasal congestion, hoarseness, cough, aphthous ulcers on the soft palate, and myalgias. There are circumstances where the appearance of the pharynx may be seen in either bacterial or viral infections (Fig. 39.2). Children with viral pharyngitis can present with mouth breathing, vomiting, abdominal pain, and diarrhea.

It is helpful to differentiate pain on swallowing (odynophagia) from difficulty swallowing (dysphagia); the latter is more likely to be caused by obstruction or abnormal muscular movement.

What to Do

✅ Obtain important historical information, including onset, exposure history, duration, and progression of symptoms as well as the presence of associated fever, cough, respiratory difficulty, or tender swollen lymph nodes.

✅ First, examine the ears, nose, and mouth, which are, after all, connected to the pharynx and often contain clues to the diagnosis. The pharynx should be evaluated for erythema, hypertrophy, foreign body, exudates, and petechiae (using a tongue blade). It is also important to assess the patient for fever, rash, cervical adenopathy, and coryza. Also, listen for the presence of a heart murmur and evaluate the patient for hepatosplenomegaly.

✅ Patients usually fall into three clinical categories: those who appear to have *Streptococcus* pharyngitis, those who clearly have a viral illness, and those with symptoms of both. **Scoring systems have been developed that can aid in decision making.**

✅ There are other uncommon causes of pharyngitis that should be kept in mind, such as primary human immunodeficiency virus (HIV) infection, diphtheria, and noninfectious causes such as gastroesophageal reflux, postnasal drip, thyroiditis, allergies, and foreign bodies.

✅ **The Centor scoring system has been validated for adults and places people into high-, moderate-, and low-risk groups (for Streptococcus pharyngitis), based on four criteria: tonsillar exudates, tender anterior cervical lymphadenopathy, absence of a cough, and history of fever. High-risk patients have three or four positive criteria. Low-risk patients have zero or one positive criterion.**

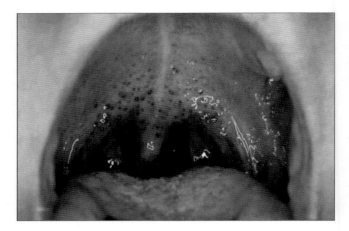

Fig. 39.1 Palatal petechiae in a child with *Streptococcus pyogenes* pharyngitis. (With permission from Asher, M. I., et al. [2008]. Infections of the upper respiratory tract. In L. M. Taussig, et al. (Eds.), *Pediatric respiratory medicine* [2nd ed., pp. 453–480]. Philadelphia, PA: Mosby.)

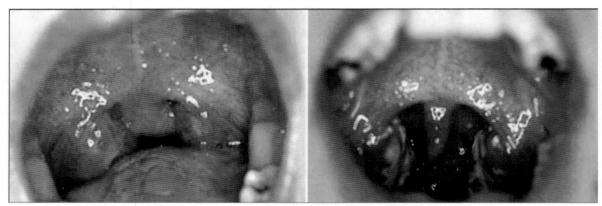

Fig. 39.2 Pharyngotonsillitis. *(Left)* The diffuse tonsillar and pharyngeal erythema seen here is a nonspecific finding that can be produced by a variety of pathogens. *(Right)* This photograph of exudative tonsillitis is most commonly seen in either group A streptococcal or Epstein-Barr virus infection. (With permission from Wetmore, R. F. [2016]. Tonsils and adenoids. In R. M. Kliegman, et al. (Eds.), *Nelson textbook of pediatrics* (20th ed., pp. 2023–2026,e1]. Philadelphia, PA: Elsevier.)

✅ **The McIsaac scoring system** has been validated in both children and adults and uses the following factors: fever, absence of a cough, tender anterior cervical adenopathy, tonsillar swelling or exudates, age younger than 15 years, each of which scores 1 point. Age 15 to 45 years scores 0 points. Age over 45 scores −1 point. High-risk patients have a score of 4 or 5 points. Low-risk patients have a score of 0 or −1 point.

✅ **Patients in the low-risk category**, in either scoring system, should be neither treated nor tested for group A Strep.

✅ **Patients in the high-risk category** may be treated empirically with antibiotics or tested and then treated if positive.

✅ **Patients with moderate risk** should be tested and only treated if positive for group A *Streptococcus* (GAS) infection.

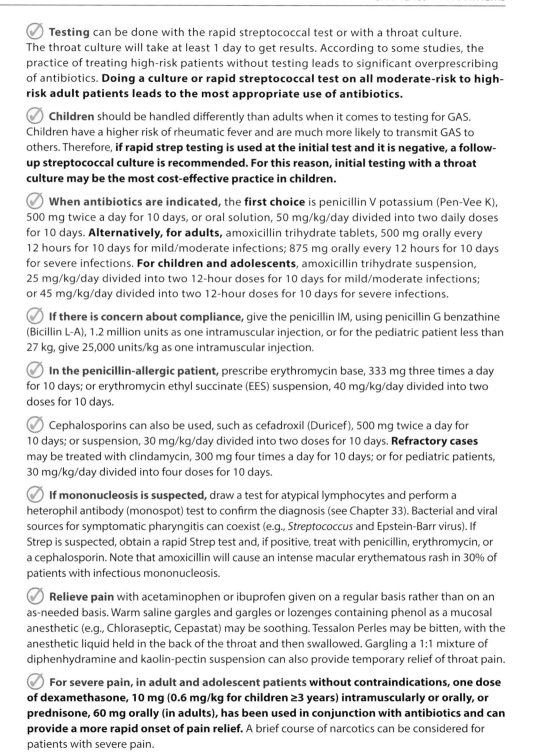

✅ **Testing** can be done with the rapid streptococcal test or with a throat culture. The throat culture will take at least 1 day to get results. According to some studies, the practice of treating high-risk patients without testing leads to significant overprescribing of antibiotics. **Doing a culture or rapid streptococcal test on all moderate-risk to high-risk adult patients leads to the most appropriate use of antibiotics.**

✅ **Children** should be handled differently than adults when it comes to testing for GAS. Children have a higher risk of rheumatic fever and are much more likely to transmit GAS to others. Therefore, **if rapid strep testing is used at the initial test and it is negative, a follow-up streptococcal culture is recommended. For this reason, initial testing with a throat culture may be the most cost-effective practice in children.**

✅ **When antibiotics are indicated,** the **first choice** is penicillin V potassium (Pen-Vee K), 500 mg twice a day for 10 days, or oral solution, 50 mg/kg/day divided into two daily doses for 10 days. **Alternatively, for adults,** amoxicillin trihydrate tablets, 500 mg orally every 12 hours for 10 days for mild/moderate infections; 875 mg orally every 12 hours for 10 days for severe infections. **For children and adolescents**, amoxicillin trihydrate suspension, 25 mg/kg/day divided into two 12-hour doses for 10 days for mild/moderate infections; or 45 mg/kg/day divided into two 12-hour doses for 10 days for severe infections.

✅ **If there is concern about compliance,** give the penicillin IM, using penicillin G benzathine (Bicillin L-A), 1.2 million units as one intramuscular injection, or for the pediatric patient less than 27 kg, give 25,000 units/kg as one intramuscular injection.

✅ **In the penicillin-allergic patient,** prescribe erythromycin base, 333 mg three times a day for 10 days; or erythromycin ethyl succinate (EES) suspension, 40 mg/kg/day divided into two doses for 10 days.

✅ Cephalosporins can also be used, such as cefadroxil (Duricef), 500 mg twice a day for 10 days; or suspension, 30 mg/kg/day divided into two doses for 10 days. **Refractory cases** may be treated with clindamycin, 300 mg four times a day for 10 days; or for pediatric patients, 30 mg/kg/day divided into four doses for 10 days.

✅ **If mononucleosis is suspected,** draw a test for atypical lymphocytes and perform a heterophil antibody (monospot) test to confirm the diagnosis (see Chapter 33). Bacterial and viral sources for symptomatic pharyngitis can coexist (e.g., *Streptococcus* and Epstein-Barr virus). If Strep is suspected, obtain a rapid Strep test and, if positive, treat with penicillin, erythromycin, or a cephalosporin. Note that amoxicillin will cause an intense macular erythematous rash in 30% of patients with infectious mononucleosis.

✅ **Relieve pain** with acetaminophen or ibuprofen given on a regular basis rather than on an as-needed basis. Warm saline gargles and gargles or lozenges containing phenol as a mucosal anesthetic (e.g., Chloraseptic, Cepastat) may be soothing. Tessalon Perles may be bitten, with the anesthetic liquid held in the back of the throat and then swallowed. Gargling a 1:1 mixture of diphenhydramine and kaolin-pectin suspension can also provide temporary relief of throat pain.

✅ **For severe pain, in adult and adolescent patients without contraindications, one dose of dexamethasone, 10 mg (0.6 mg/kg for children ≥3 years) intramuscularly or orally, or prednisone, 60 mg orally (in adults), has been used in conjunction with antibiotics and can provide a more rapid onset of pain relief.** A brief course of narcotics can be considered for patients with severe pain.

✅ Instruct the parents of a child being treated for *Streptococcus* pharyngitis that their child should not return to school or daycare until after a 24-hour course of antibiotics has been completed and symptoms have improved.

What Not to Do

❌ Do not prescribe an antibiotic to patients with a clear viral infection (low-risk Centor or McIsaac scores). Treatment of viral pharyngitis with antibiotics is a major source of antibiotic resistance.

❌ Do not miss scarlet fever, which is associated with group A beta-hemolytic *Streptococcus* (GABHS) pharyngitis and usually presents as a punctate, erythematous, blanchable, sandpaper-like exanthema. The rash is found in the neck, groin, and axilla and is accentuated in body folds and creases (the Pastia lines). The tongue may be bright red with a white coating (strawberry tongue).

❌ Do not overlook acute epiglottic or supraglottic inflammation. In children, this presents as a sudden, severe pharyngitis, with a guttural rather than hoarse voice (because it hurts to speak), drooling (because it hurts to swallow), and respiratory distress (because swelling narrows the airway). Adults usually have a more gradual onset over several days and are not as prone to a sudden airway occlusion, unless they present later in the progression of the swelling and are already experiencing some respiratory distress.

❌ Do not prescribe ciprofloxacin, tetracycline, doxycycline, and sulfamethoxazole/trimethoprim for acute pharyngitis. These drugs are considered to be ineffective.

❌ Do not give ampicillin to a patient with mononucleosis. Although the resulting rash helps make the diagnosis, it does not imply ampicillin allergy and can be uncomfortable.

❌ Do not overlook peritonsillar abscesses, which often require hospitalization and IV penicillin, incision and drainage, or needle aspiration. Peritonsillar abscesses or cellulitis causes the tonsillar pillar to bulge toward the midline. Patients typically have a toxic appearance and may present with a "hot potato voice." With an abscess, there is a very tender, fluctuant, peritonsillar mass and asymmetric deviation of the uvula. Intraoral ultrasound examination or computed tomography (CT) examination are diagnostic tests that can provide an accurate diagnosis if the clinical picture is unclear.

❌ Do not overlook gonococcal pharyngitis in sexually active patients at risk. This can produce a clinical syndrome with fever, severe sore throat, dysuria, and characteristic greenish exudates that require special culture on Thayer-Martin medium or testing with a nucleic acid probe. This requires special treatment (see Chapter 83).

❌ Do not overlook Kawasaki disease. A malady that most often affects children younger than 5 years of age, it has characteristic signs and symptoms that include sore throat, fever, bilateral nonpurulent conjunctivitis, anterior cervical node enlargement, erythematous oral mucosa, and an inflamed pharynx with a strawberry tongue. Within 3 days of the onset of fever, the patient will develop cracked red lips, a generalized erythematous rash with edema and erythema of the hands and feet, and periungual desquamation followed by peeling of the palms.

❌ Do not overlook diphtheria. This acute upper respiratory tract infection is characterized by a sore throat, low-grade fever, and an adherent grayish membrane with surrounding inflammation of the tonsils, pharynx, and nasal passages with a serosanguineous nasal discharge.

⊗ Do not overlook retropharyngeal abscess, which may cause more pain with neck extension and requires more advanced imaging.

Discussion

Pharyngitis is an inflammation of the pharynx or tonsils. Most cases of pharyngitis are caused by viruses; up to 10% of adult and 30% of childhood pharyngitis are caused by group A *Streptococcus*. Almost all people with viral and streptococcal pharyngitis recover completely without complications.

Members of the general public know to see a doctor for a sore throat, but the actual benefit of this visit is unclear. Rheumatic fever is exceedingly rare in the United States and other developed countries (annual incidence less than one case per 100,000). Only 15% to 30% of cases in children and 5% to 15% of cases in adults are culture-positive GABHS pharyngitis. Poststreptococcal glomerulonephritis is usually a self-limiting illness and is not prevented with antibiotic treatment.

On the other hand, penicillin and other antibiotic therapies do prevent the rare development of acute rheumatic fever and may sometimes reduce symptoms or shorten the course of a sore throat. Antibiotics probably inhibit the infection from progressing into tonsillitis, peritonsillar and retropharyngeal abscesses, adenitis, and pneumonia.

Group A streptococcal infection cannot be diagnosed reliably based on clinical signs and symptoms. Typically, 25% of throat cultures grow group A *Streptococcus*, and 50% of those represent carriers who do not raise antistreptococcal antibodies and risk rheumatic fever.

Rapid streptococcal screens are less sensitive than cultures, but because of improvements in rapid streptococcal antigen tests, throat culture can be reserved for patients whose symptoms do not improve over time or who do not respond to antibiotics.

Clinical prediction rules have been developed that use several key elements of the history and physical examination to predict the probability of strep throat. Using a clinical prediction rule gives the clinician a rational basis for assigning a patient to a low-risk category (requires neither testing nor treatment), a high-risk category (empiric antibiotic may be indicated), or a moderate-risk category (may require further diagnostic testing). One of the best validated scoring systems is a simple four-item clinical prediction rule developed by Centor. The Centor score has been validated in three distinct adult populations. McIsaac modified the Centor score and validated it prospectively in a mixed population of adults and children. There is controversy surrounding these and other similar clinical prediction rules. Therefore clinical judgment and monitoring of the most recent literature on the subject are still advised when deciding whether to test or treat with antibiotics.

Suggested Readings

Adam, D., Scholz, H., & Helmerking, M. (2000). Short-course antibiotic treatment of 4782 culture-proven cases of group A streptococcal tonsillopharyngitis and incidence of poststreptococcal sequelae. *Journal of Infectious Diseases*, *182*, 509–516.

Bisno, A., & Lichtenberger, P. (2010). *Evaluation of acute pharyngitis in adults*. UpToDate. http://www.uptodate.com.

Bisno, A. L., Garnet, S. P., & Kaplan, E. L. (2002). Diagnosis of strep throat in adults: Are clinical criteria really good enough? *Clinics in Infectious Disease*, *35*, 126–129.

Bisno, A. L., Gerber, M. A., Gwaltney, J. M., et al. (1997). Diagnosis and management of group A streptococcal pharyngitis: A practice guideline. *Clinics in Infectious Disease*, *25*, 574–583.

Bulloch, B., Kabani, A., & Tenenbein, M. (2003). Oral dexamethasone for the treatment of pain in children with acute pharyngitis: A randomized, double-blind, placebo-controlled trial. *Annals of Emergency Medicine*, *41*, 601–608.

Casey, J. R., & Pichichero, M. E. (2004). Meta-analysis of cephalosporins versus penicillin for treatment for group A streptococcal tonsillopharyngitis in adults. *Clinics in Infectious Disease*, *38*, 1526–1534.

Cohen, R., Reinert, P., de la Rocque, F., et al. (2002). Comparison of two dosages of azithromycin for three days versus penicillin V for ten days in acute group A streptococcal tonsillopharyngitis. *The Pediatric Infectious Disease Journal, 21,* 297–303.

Coonan, K. M., & Kaplan, E. L. (1994). In vitro susceptibility of recent North American group A streptococcal isolates to eleven oral antibiotics. *The Pediatric Infectious Disease Journal, 13,* 630–635.

Cooper, R. J., Hoffman, J. R., Bartlett, J. G., et al. (2001). Principles of appropriate antibiotic use for acute pharyngitis in adults: Background. *Annals of Emergency Medicine, 37,* 711–719.

DiMatteo, L. A., Lowenstein, S. R., & Brinhall, B. (2001). The relationship between the clinical features of pharyngitis and the sensitivity of a rapid antigen test: Evidence of spectrum bias. *Annals of Emergency Medicine, 38,* 648–652.

Ebell, M. H., Smith, M. A., Barry, H. C., et al. (2000). Does this patient have strep throat? *Journal of the American Medical Association, 284,* 2912–2918.

Hall, M. C., Kieke, B., Gonzales, R., et al. (2004). Spectrum bias of a rapid antigen detection test for group A beta-hemolytic streptococcal pharyngitis in a pediatric population. *Pediatrics, 114,* 182–186.

Huovinen, P., Lahhtonen, R., Ziegler, T., et al. (1989). Pharyngitis in adults: The presence and coexistence of viruses and bacterial organisms. *Annals of Internal Medicine, 110,* 612–616.

Marvez-Valls, E. G., Stuckey, A., & Ernst, A. A. (2002). A randomized clinical trial of oral versus intramuscular delivery of steroids in acute exudative pharyngitis. *Academy of Emergency Medicine, 9,* 9–14.

Mayes, T., & Pichichero, M. E. (2001). Are follow-up throat cultures necessary when rapid antigen detection tests are negative for group A streptococcus? *Clinics in Pediatrics, 40,* 191–195.

McIsaac, W. J. (2000). The validity of a sore throat score in family practice. *Canadian Medical Association Journal, 163,* 811–815.

McIsaac, W. J., Kellner, J. D., Aufricht, P., et al. (2004). Empirical validation of guidelines for the management of pharyngitis in children and adults. *Journal of the American Medical Association, 291,* 1587–1595.

Neuner, J. M., Hamel, M. B., Phillips, R. S., et al. (2003). Diagnosis and management of adults with pharyngitis. *Annals of Internal Medicine, 139,* 113–122.

O'Brien, J. F., Meade, J. L., & Falk, J. L. (1993). Dexamethasone as adjuvant therapy for severe acute pharyngitis. *Annals of Emergency Medicine, 22,* 212–214.

Pichichero, M. E. (1995). Group A streptococcal tonsillopharyngitis: Cost-effective diagnosis and treatment. *Annals of Emergency Medicine, 25,* 390–403 [editorial, 404–406].

Point of Care. (2020). *Pharyngitis.* Amsterdam, Netherlands: Elsevier BV.

Vincent, M. T., Celestin, N., & Hussain, N. (2004). Pharyngitis. *American Family Physician, 69,* 1465–1470.

Webb, K. H., Needham, C. A., & Kurtz, S. R. (2000). Use of a high-sensitivity rapid strep test without culture confirmation of negative results. *Journal of Family Practice, 49,* 34–38.

Yeh, B., & Eskin, B. (2005). Evidence-based emergency medicine/systematic review abstract. Should sore throats be treated with antibiotics? *Annals of Emergency Medicine, 45,* 82–84.

CHAPTER 40

Rhinitis, Acute
(Runny Nose)

Presentation

In **allergic rhinitis**, patients typically complain of rhinorrhea ("runny nose"), nasal congestion, sneezing, nasal itching, and "itchy eyes." There may be a problem with sleep disturbance (from nasal congestion), malaise, fatigue, irritability, and neurocognitive deficits.

Typically patients with allergic rhinitis have clear discharge, swollen turbinates, and bluish or pale mucosa. There may be "allergic shiners"—infraorbital darkening thought to be caused by chronic venous pooling—or an "allergic salute" in children who rub their noses upward because of nasal discomfort, sometimes producing a persistent horizontal crease across the nose. Mild bilateral conjunctivitis with nonpurulent discharge is strongly suggestive of an allergic cause when it is accompanied by pruritus. The patient with a "summer cold" lasting a full month is likely to have allergic rhinitis.

Precipitating factors may be known or may be elicited from the patient. Common allergens include airborne dust-mite fecal particles, cockroach residues, animal danders (especially cats and dogs), molds, and pollens (hence the origin of the term *hay fever*).

Vasomotor (idiopathic) rhinitis may occur in response to environmental conditions such as changes in temperature or relative humidity, odors (e.g., perfume or cleaning materials), passive tobacco smoke, alcohol, sexual arousal, or emotional factors.

Drug-induced rhinitis may be caused by oral medications, including angiotensin-converting enzyme (ACE) inhibitors, beta-blockers, various antihypertensive agents, chlorpromazine, aspirin, other nonsteroidal anti-inflammatory drugs (NSAIDs), and oral contraceptives as well as topical α-adrenergic decongestant sprays that have been used for more than 5 to 7 days (rhinitis medicamentosa). Repeated use of intranasal cocaine and methamphetamines may also result in rebound congestion and, on occasion, nasal septal erosion and perforation.

In **viral rhinitis (the common cold)**, patients generally complain of an annoying, persistent mucoid nasal discharge accompanied by nasal and facial congestion, along with a constellation of viral symptoms, including low-grade fever, myalgias, and sore throat. These patients generally seek care because they feel miserable, cannot sleep, and want relief. They often believe that antibiotics are needed to cure their problem.

On physical examination, there is only nasal mucous membrane congestion, which may appear erythematous, along with cloudy nasal secretions, which may become somewhat yellow and thick after several days. Resolution occurs within 10 days to 2 weeks.

Always keep in mind that young children may place intranasal foreign bodies (e.g., beads or beans) in the nose, leading to foul-smelling, purulent, unilateral nasal discharge (see Chapter 30).

What to Do

Allergic Rhinitis

✅ **Determine which specific symptoms are most bothersome to the patient** (e.g., nasal congestion, pruritus, rhinorrhea, sneezing), the pattern of the symptoms (e.g., intermittent, seasonal, perennial), any precipitating factors in the home or occupational environment, the response to previous medications, and any coexisting conditions.

✅ **Use a handheld otoscope or headlamp with nasal speculum to view the anterior nasal airway.** (A topical decongestant improves visualization of the nasal cavity.)

✅ **Educate the patient** about avoidance of any known inciting factors. In particular, patients who are allergic to house dust mites should use allergen-impermeable encasings on the bed and pillows. For patients with seasonal allergies, pollen exposure can be reduced by having them keep windows closed, using an air conditioner, and limiting the amount of time spent outdoors.

✅ **Intranasal corticosteroids are the most effective medication class for treatment of allergic rhinitis and should be used as a single first-line agent,** although it should be kept in mind that these are generally expensive items. These preparations are generally not associated with significant systemic side effects in adults. Prescribe fluticasone (Flonase) nasal spray (which has been shown to be beneficial even when used on an as-needed basis) for adults and children older than 12 years of age, two sprays (50 µg/spray) in each nostril once daily or one spray in each nostril twice daily. Other options include flunisolide (Nasalide) nasal spray, two sprays in each nostril twice daily (may increase to three or four times a day), or, for children 6 to 14 years old, one spray in each nostril three times a day or two sprays in each nostril twice daily; mometasone furoate (Nasonex) for adults and children older than 12 years of age, two sprays in each nostril once daily; and budesonide (Rhinocort Aqua) nasal spray for adults and children older than 6 years of age, one spray in each nostril every morning. **It is generally accepted that these sprays are most effective if taken daily compared with as-needed use.**

✅ Patients should be instructed to direct sprays away from the nasal septum to avoid irritation and not to tilt the head back when spraying, to avoid having the drug run out of the nasal cavity and into the throat.

✅ **Antihistamines are a second-line agent in allergic rhinitis treatment** but have less effect on nasal congestion. Recommend an over-the-counter (OTC) nonsedating second-generation antihistamine, such as fexofenadine (Allegra), 180 mg once daily (for children 6–11 years old, 30 mg twice daily); loratadine (Claritin), 10 mg once daily, or syrup, 10 mg/10 mL (for children 2–5 years old, 5 mg once daily; for children 6–11 years old, 10 mg once daily); cetirizine (Zyrtec), 5 to 10 mg once daily, or syrup, 5 mg/5 mL (for children 2–5 years old, 0.5–1 tsp [2–2.5 mg] once daily; for children 6–11 years old, 1–2 tsp [5–10 mg] once daily).

✅ At this time, desloratadine (Clarinex), 5 mg once daily, can be offered by prescription only.

✅ **An alternative to oral antihistamines is the intranasal antihistamine azelastine (Astelin Nasal Spray) for adults and children older than 12 years of age,** two sprays per nostril twice a day. This medication is by prescription only and its side effects may include a bitter taste in the mouth and sedation. Combination therapy with intranasal azelastine and fluticasone is more effective than either monotherapy alone and is approved for moderate to severe allergic rhinitis.

✓ **Topical decongestant nasal sprays and oral decongestants can effectively reduce nasal congestion for both allergic and nonallergic forms of rhinitis, but they can cause side effects** (especially the oral forms) of insomnia, nervousness, loss of appetite, and urinary retention in males. They should be used with caution or not at all in patients with arrhythmias, hypertension, or hyperthyroidism. Recommend behind-the-counter (BTC) pseudoephedrine (Sudafed), 60 mg every 6 hours; time-released version, 120 mg twice daily; or syrup, 3 mg/mL (for children 2–5 years old, 5–30 mg every 4–6 hours; for children 6–12 years old, 30 mg every 4–6 hours or 4 mg/kg/day divided into equal doses every 6 hours [1 mg/kg/dose]).

✓ **Two effective OTC nasal decongestant sprays** are oxymetazoline (Afrin) 0.05%, two sprays per nostril twice daily (or, for pediatric patients, 0.025%, one to two sprays per nostril twice daily), and phenylephrine (Neo-Synephrine Nasal) 0.025%, 0.05%, or 1%, one to two sprays per nostril every 3–4 hours (or, for pediatric patients >2 years, 0.125% or 0.25%). **Use must be limited to 3 to 5 days to avoid rebound nasal congestion (rhinitis medicamentosa). However,** studies indicate that they can be safely used longer term in conjunction with an intranasal corticosteroid (INCS) for adult and adolescent patients with nasal congestion not responsive to steroid sprays alone or in combination with an intranasal antihistamine. The longest double-blind randomized trial evaluating an intranasal decongestant in combination with an INCS was 6 weeks and found this combination to be effective and safe without evidence of rhinitis medicamentosa.

✓ **The same cautions and contraindications exist for nasal decongestants as for the oral medications.** Because of the use of pseudoephedrine in the illegal manufacture of amphetamine drugs, it now must be purchased behind the counter.

✓ **Other products that have some efficacy in allergic rhinitis are cromolyn sodium, a mast cell stabilizer, and montelukast (Singulair), a leukotriene receptor antagonist,** for adults, 10 mg every night at bedtime (for children 2–5 years old, 4 mg chewable tab every night at bedtime; for children 6–14 years old, 5 mg chewable tab every night at bedtime).

✓ **In addition, ipratropium bromide (Atrovent Nasal Spray) 0.06%, two sprays per nostril three to four times a day, have been shown to help but works best in vasomotor (idiopathic) rhinitis.**

Viral Rhinitis

✓ **Determine which specific symptoms are most bothersome to the patient** (e.g., nasal congestion, rhinorrhea, scratchy throat, general aches, fever, or cough).

✓ **Perform a general examination,** including a careful nasal examination, to exclude any associated diseases, such as rhinosinusitis, otitis media, bacterial pharyngitis, and asthmatic bronchitis.

✓ **For nasal congestion, prescribe oral or topical decongestants, as you would for allergic rhinitis (described earlier). For rhinorrhea, you can prescribe ipratropium bromide (Atrovent Nasal Spray) 0.06%, two sprays per nostril three to four times a day.**

✓ Although **antihistamines** are effective for treatment of rhinitis related to allergy, they are much less effective for rhinitis related to the common cold. The side effects often outweigh the benefit and thus are **not recommended**.

✓ **Nasal saline irrigation** has been shown to have some efficacy in the relief of viral rhinitis. This can easily be accomplished with a commercially available neti pot or other nasal irrigation products.

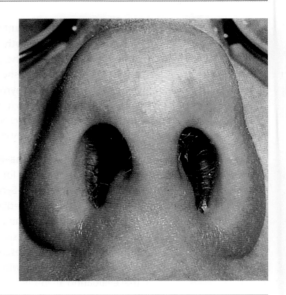

Fig. 40.1 Example of nasal vestibulitis. (Adapted from Park, Y. W., Littlejohn, R., & Eley, J. [2002]. Diagnosis at a glance. *Emergency Medicine, 5,* 9.)

✓ Provide symptomatic relief for associated symptoms (e.g., acetaminophen [Tylenol] or ibuprofen [Motrin] for fever, general aches, and scratchy throat; or, with signs and symptoms consistent with asthma, albuterol [Ventolin] metered-dose inhaler for cough). For an uncomplicated nonproductive cough, the adult patient may get some relief from a prescription for Tessalon Perles 100 to 200 mg three times a day as needed.

✓ Warm facial compresses, steam inhalation, warm tea, and chicken soup are all comforting, and chicken soup may possibly be therapeutic.

✓ **When pain, redness, and tender swelling around the nostrils occur** because of nose picking or excessive rubbing or blowing of the nose **(nasal vestibulitis)** (Fig. 40.1), treat with an antistaphylococcal antibiotic ointment—mupirocin (Bactroban) 2%, apply three times a day for 2 weeks—and recommend warm compresses. Patients with diabetes, immune deficiency, or progressive infection should be placed on a systemic antistaphylococcal antibiotic to avoid potential spread to the cavernous sinus.

What Not to Do

✗ Do not prescribe sedating antihistamines for symptoms of hay fever.

✗ Do not prescribe antihistamines or nasal steroids for the common cold.

✗ Do not obtain imaging studies of the sinuses unless the criteria for bacterial rhinosinusitis are met (symptoms lasting >7 days and including facial or dental pain or tenderness along with purulent nasal drainage).

✗ Do not prescribe antibiotics for cold symptoms. Antibiotics should only be considered if symptoms persist for >7 days and are accompanied by signs of rhinosinusitis (see Chapter 41).

✗ Do not bother recommending the use of zinc lozenges. Despite numerous randomized trials, the evidence for their effectiveness in reducing the duration of common cold symptoms is still lacking.

Discussion

Rhinitis is an inflammation of the nasal mucous membranes. Allergic rhinitis triggers a systemic increase in inflammation. Within minutes of allergen exposure, immune cells release histamine, proteases, cysteinyl leukotrienes, prostaglandins, and cytokines. Systemic circulation of inflammatory cells permits their infiltration into other tissues where chemoattractant and adhesion molecules already exist. Consequently, allergic rhinitis is linked to comorbid conditions: asthma, chronic hyperplastic eosinophilic sinusitis, nasal polyposis, and serous otitis media. Effective therapy should ideally be directed at the underlying inflammation and its systemic manifestations. It should improve the rhinitis and the comorbid conditions.

Antihistamines relieve early symptoms, but they do not significantly influence the proinflammatory loop. Oral corticosteroids provide the systemic anti-inflammatory effect needed, but their toxicity precludes extended routine use. Intranasal corticosteroids effectively target the local inflammatory processes of rhinitis, but they only reduce the local inflammatory cells within the nares. Leukotriene modifiers have both systemic anti-inflammatory effects and an acceptable safety profile.

Immunotherapy (allergy shots) is the only treatment that produces long-term relief of symptoms. Patients should be considered candidates for these treatments, based on the severity of their symptoms and the failure or unacceptability of the other treatment modalities.

Nasal polyps are benign inflammatory growths that arise from the inflamed mucosa lining the paranasal sinuses. They are frequently associated with sinus disease. Unilateral nasal polyps should raise consideration of a possible neoplasm.

Suggested Readings

Borish, L. (2003). Allergic rhinitis: Systemic inflammation and implications for management. *The Journal of Allergy and Clinical Immunology, 112*, 1021–1031.

Diamond, L., Dockhorn, R. J., Grossman, J., et al. (1995). A dose-response study of the efficacy and safety of ipratropium bromide nasal spray in the treatment of the common cold. *The Journal of Allergy and Clinical Immunology, 95*, 1139–1146.

Dykewicz, M. S. (2003). Rhinitis and sinusitis. *The Journal of Allergy and Clinical Immunology, 111*, S520–S529.

Fletcher, R. (2010). *An overview of rhinitis.* UpToDate. http://www.uptodate.com.

Friedman, N., & Sexton, D. (2910). *The common cold in adults: Treatment and prevention.* UpToDate. http://www.uptodate.com.

Jackson, J. L., Peterson, C., & Lesho, E. (1997). A meta-analysis of zinc salts lozenges and the common cold. *Archives of Internal Medicine, 157*, 2373–2376.

Linder, J. A., & Singer, D. E. (2003). Desire for antibiotics and antibiotic prescribing for adults with upper respiratory tract infections. *Journal of General Internal Medicine, 18*, 795–801.

Macknin, M. L., Piedmonte, M., Calendine, C., et al. (1998). Zinc gluconate lozenges for treating the common cold in children. *Journal of the American Medical Association, 279*, 1962–1967.

Mainous, A. G., Hueston, W. J., & Clark, J. R. (1996). Antibiotics and upper respiratory infection: Do some folks think there is a cure for the common cold? *Journal of Family Practice, 42*, 357–361.

Patel, G. B., Kern, R. C., Bernstein, J. A., Hae-Sim, P., & Peters, A. T. (2020). Current and future treatments of rhinitis and sinusitis. *The Journal of Allergy and Clinical Immunology: In Practice, 8*(5), 1522–1531.

Prasad, A. S., Fitzgerald, J. T., Bao, B., et al. (2001). Duration of symptoms and plasma cytokine levels in patients with the common cold treated with zinc acetate: A randomized double-blind, placebo-controlled trial. *Annals of Emergency Medicine, 38*, 245–252.

Rosenwasser, L. J. (2002). Treatment of allergic rhinitis. *The American Journal of Medicine, 113*(Suppl. 9A), S17–S24.

Rhinosinusitis

(Sinusitis)

Presentation

After a viral infection or with chronic allergies, the patient may complain of a dull facial pain, which is usually unilateral, gradually increases over a couple of days, is exacerbated by sudden motion of the head or bending over with the head dependent, may radiate to the upper molar teeth (through the maxillary antrum), and may increase with eye movement (through the ethmoid sinuses). Often there is a sensation of facial congestion and stuffiness. The child with sinusitis often has a cough, rhinorrhea, and fetid breath. The patient's voice may have a resonance similar to that of an individual with a "stopped up" nose and may complain of a foul taste in the mouth or reduced sense of smell. Stuffy ears and impaired hearing are common because of associated otitis media with effusion and eustachian tube dysfunction. A colored nasal discharge is a particularly sensitive finding. Fever is present in only half of all patients with acute infection and is usually low grade. A high fever and severe headache usually indicate a serious complication, such as meningitis or another diagnosis altogether. Transillumination of sinuses in the acute care setting is usually unrewarding, but tenderness may be elicited on gentle percussion or firm palpation over the maxillary or frontal sinuses or between the eyes (ethmoid sinuses). Swelling and erythema may exist. Pus may be visible draining below the nasal turbinates (most often in the middle meatus) with a purulent yellow-green appearance, sometimes with a foul-smelling discharge from the nose or running down the posterior pharynx.

What to Do

✅ **Rule out other possible causes of facial pain or headache through the patient's history and physical examination** (palpate the scalp muscles, temporal arteries, temporomandibular joints, eyes, and teeth). Consider the diagnosis of viral or allergic rhinitis (see Chapter 40).

✅ **Shrink swollen nasal mucosa (and thereby provide symptomatic relief of nasal obstruction) with 1% phenylephrine (Neo-Synephrine) or 0.05% oxymetazoline (Afrin) nose drops.** Instill two drops in each nostril, allow the patient to lie supine for 2 minutes, and then repeat the process. (Repeating the process allows the first applications to open the anterior nose so that the second dose gets farther back.) Have the patient repeat this process every 4 hours but for no more than 3 to 5 days (to avoid rhinitis medicamentosa).

✅ **Examine the nose for purulent drainage** before and, when practical, after shrinking the nasal mucosa with a topical vasoconstrictor.

✓ **Unless contraindicated by age, hypertension, benign prostatic hypertrophy, or underlying cardiac disease, prescribe systemic sympathomimetic decongestants such as pseudoephedrine (Sudafed), 60 mg every 6 hours.**

✓ **Antibiotics should be limited to patients who have symptoms lasting 7 or more days, with unilateral maxillary pain or tenderness of the face or teeth accompanied by purulent nasal secretions or to those patients who present initially with more severe symptoms.**

✓ **Prescribe amoxicillin (Amoxil),** 500 mg every 12 hours or 250 mg every 8 hours for mild to moderate symptoms, 875 mg every 12 hours or 500 mg every 8 hours for severe symptoms. Studies have shown that the newer broad-spectrum antibiotics are no better than the older, less expensive narrow-spectrum ones.

✓ **If the patient has taken antibiotics within the past month or the prevalence of drug-resistant Streptococcus pneumoniae is greater than approximately 30% in the community,** prescribe amoxicillin clavulanate (Augmentin XR), 875 mg every 12 hours for 5 to 7 days, or extra-strength pediatric suspension, 90 mg amoxicillin component/kg/day divided into two daily doses for 10 days.

✓ **The best choice in penicillin-allergic patients** is either trimethoprim-sulfamethoxazole (Bactrim) 1 by mouth twice a day for 7 days or azithromycin (Zithromax) 500 mg orally on day 1 then 250 mg orally once daily days 2 to 5.

✓ The more expensive respiratory fluoroquinolones should be considered in adults only if penicillin-resistant *S. pneumoniae* is a major concern or for treatment failures.

✓ **Most cases of acute rhinosinusitis are viral in origin,** and the clinical differentiation of viral from bacterial causes is difficult. Therefore, when a patient presents early in the course of the illness, unnecessary treatment with antibiotics can often be avoided by not starting a patient on antibiotics initially, but instead writing a **backup prescription** that can be filled if symptoms persist for a total of 7 days.

✓ **Provide pain relief** (e.g., ibuprofen, naproxen, acetaminophen, oxycodone, hydrocodone) when necessary.

✓ If allergic rhinitis is suspected (see Chapter 40), a second-generation antihistamine is a logical addition to therapy, or an intranasal steroid may be helpful but it may be difficult to distinguish viral from allergic sinus symptoms.

✓ **For symptomatic relief,** recommend that the patient try hot facial compresses and hot water vapor inhalation using a simple teakettle, a hot shower, a steam vaporizer, or a home facial sauna device. Hot soups or teas can also be comforting. Plain saline nasal sprays and irrigations have been shown to lessen symptoms as well. Have the patient sleep with their head elevated and avoid cigarette smoke.

✓ **Arrange for follow-up within 1 to 7 days,** depending on the severity of the initial findings. Specialist evaluation is appropriate when sinusitis is refractory to treatment or is recurrent.

✓ Give the patient an explanation of the rationale for management and inform about the signs and symptoms of worsening that should prompt the patient to seek immediate medical attention.

What Not to Do

(X) Do not ignore signs of orbital cellulitis (swelling, erythema, decreased extraocular movements, and possible proptosis). These patients require consultation and hospital admission for IV antibiotic therapy.

(X) Do not ignore the toxic patient who has marked swelling, high fever, severe pain, profuse drainage, or other signs and symptoms of a serious infection. (See the potential complications described later.) These patients require immediate consultation and intervention.

(X) Do not order routine radiograph or computed tomography (CT) examinations. Reserve them for difficult diagnoses and treatment failures.

(X) Do not prescribe first-generation antihistamines, which are sedating and can make mucous secretions dry and thick and can interfere with necessary drainage.

(X) Do not allow the patient to use decongestant nose drops for more than 3 to 5 days; this will prevent the nasal mucosa from becoming habituated to topical sympathomimetic medication. If using the drops for more than 5 days, the patient may suffer rebound nasal congestion (rhinitis medicamentosa) when use of the drops is discontinued; resolution of this condition requires time, topical steroids, and reeducation.

(X) Do not prescribe long-term topical or systemic sympathomimetic decongestants to a patient who suffers from increased intraocular pressure, hypertension, ischemic heart disease, tachycardia, or difficulty initiating urination, all of which may be exacerbated.

(X) Do not prescribe antibiotics to patients with mild symptoms who do not have persistent maxillary facial or dental pain or tenderness or who do not have purulent nasal drainage. These patients are unlikely to have bacterial rhinosinusitis, regardless of duration of illness.

Discussion

The term *rhinosinusitis* is considered to be more accurate than sinusitis because sinusitis is, in most instances, a continuum and eventual consequence of rhinitis (see Chapter 40). Acute sinusitis is defined as inflammation of the sinuses for less than 4 weeks.

Sinusitis is the most common health care complaint in the United States. The paranasal sinuses drain through tiny ostia under the nasal turbinates. Occlusion of these ostia allows secretions and pressure differences to build up, resulting in the pressure and pain of acute sinusitis and the air-fluid levels sometimes visible on radiographs. Early mild cases do not require treatment with antibiotics. However, congested sinuses can become a site for bacterial superinfection.

Most cases of rhinosinusitis begin with ostial obstruction caused by mucosal swelling associated with viral upper respiratory tract infection. Other causes include allergic rhinitis; barotraumas caused by flying, swimming, or diving; nasal polyps and tumors; and foreign bodies, including nasogastric and endotracheal tubes placed in hospitalized patients. Abscessed teeth can also be the source of maxillary sinusitis. If there is tenderness on percussion of the bicuspids or molars, arrange for dental consultation.

A CT scan of the sinuses is the study of choice for evaluating sinusitis but is needed urgently only with complicated cases or treatment failures. Radiologic studies performed within days of the onset of symptoms may lead to an incorrect conclusion that bacterial infection is present. Up to 40% of sinus radiographs and more than 80% of CT scans may be abnormal in viral sinusitis if obtained within 7 days of the onset of illness.

Most patients can receive initial treatment on the basis of the history and physical examination alone. **Anyone who has moderate to severe unilateral facial or dental pain or purulent nasal discharge persisting for more than 7 days, with**

(continued)

Discussion continued

or without fever, should probably be treated empirically for acute bacterial rhinosinusitis. Be aware that most cases of milder acute bacterial rhinosinusitis will resolve without the need to prescribe antibiotics, and complications of untreated bacterial disease are rare.

Many patients have been conditioned by the advertising of over-the-counter antihistamines for "sinus" problems (usually meaning "allergic rhinitis") and may relate a history of "sinuses," which on closer questioning turns out to be uncomplicated rhinitis.

Suggested Readings

Clement, P. A. R., Bluestone, C. D., Gordts, F., et al. (1998). Management of rhinosinusitis in children. *Archives of Otolaryngology - Head and Neck Surgery*, *124*, 31–124.

Dykewicz, M. S. (2003). Rhinitis and sinusitis. *The Journal of Allergy and Clinical Immunology*, *111*, S520–S529.

Garbutt, J. M., Goldstein, M., Gellman, E., et al. (2001). A randomized, placebo-controlled trial of antimicrobial treatment for children with clinically diagnosed acute sinusitis. *Pediatrics*, *107*, 619–625.

Gwaltney, J. (1996). Acute community-acquired sinusitis. *Clinics in Infectious Disease*, *23*, 1209–1223.

Hickner, J. M., Bartlett, J. G., & Besser, R. E. (2001). Principles of appropriate antibiotic use for acute rhinosinusitis in adults: Background. *Annals of Emergency Medicine*, *37*, 703–710.

Hwang, P., & Getz, A. (2010). *Acute rhinosinusitis*. UptoDate. http://www.uptodate.com.

Low, D. E., Desrosiers, M., McSherry, J., et al. (1997). A practical guide for the diagnosis and treatment of acute sinusitis. *Canadian Medical Association Journal*, *156*(Suppl. 6), S1–S14.

Piccirillo, J. F., Mager, D. E., Frisse, M. E., et al. (2001). Impact of first-line vs second-line antibiotics for the treatment of acute uncomplicated sinusitis. *Journal of the American Medical Association*, *286*, 1849–1856.

Rosenfeld, R. M., Andes, D., Bhattacharyya, N., et al. (2007). Clinical practice guidelines: Adult sinusitis. *Otolaryngology-Head and Neck Surgery*, *137*, S1–S31.

Slavin, R. G. (1997). Nasal polyps and sinusitis. *Journal of the American Medical Association*, *278*, 1849–1854.

Tang, A., & Frazee, B. Antibiotic treatment for acute maxillary sinusitis. *Annals of Emergency Medicine, 42*, 705–708.

Van Buchem, F. L., Knottnerus, J. A., & Schrijnemaekers, V. J. (1997). Primary-care-based randomized placebo-controlled trial of antibiotic treatment in acute maxillary sinusitis. *Lancet*, *349*, 683–687.

Williams, J. W., & Simel, D. L. (1993). Does this patient have sinusitis? Diagnosing acute sinusitis by history and physical examination. *Journal of the American Medical Association*, *270*, 1242–1246.

PART 4

Oral and Dental Emergencies

■ Daniel Wolfson   ■ Nathaniel Moore

CHAPTER

42

Aphthous Ulcer, Acute

Presentation

Patients present with a painful lesion in their mouth, often worried about having herpes. Lesions may interfere with eating, speaking, or swallowing. Minor oral trauma from dental appliances, dentures, and orthodontic hardware may be causative, or patients may inadvertently produce traumatic ulcers through biting of their oral mucosa.

Simple aphthosis (apthous ulcers), episodic lesions that are few in number, healing within 1 to 2 weeks, and recurring infrequently, is the more common scenario. Conversely, **complex aphthosis** presents with numerous severe lesions, which are persistent and associated with marked pain or disability.

Aphthous ulcers, also known as **canker sores**, are the most common oral ulcer and are characterized by a painful prodrome lasting 2 to 48 hours followed by the appearance of shallow, erythematous ulcers with a gray base. They can present as one or more flat, even-bordered, round or oval ulcers with a central friable pseudomembranous base surrounded by a bright red halo. They may be seen on nonkeratinized unattached mucosa, such as the buccal or labial mucosa, lingual sulci, soft palate, pharynx, lateral and ventral tongue, or gingiva. Lesions are usually solitary but can be multiple and recurrent without antecedent vesicles or bulla. The pain is usually greater than the size of the lesions would suggest.

Minor aphthae (<10 mm in circumference) comprise 80% of all aphthae, are usually located on the buccal or labial mucosa, and heal spontaneously in 7 to 10 days without scarring (Fig. 42.1). Ten percent of all lesions are **major aphthae**, which are larger than 10 mm in circumference and deeper. They may heal over weeks to months and often result in scarring. Major aphthae may also be located posteriorly on the soft palate, tonsils, and pharynx (Fig. 42.2). Major aphthae that last for months and are slow to heal may be associated with human immunodeficiency virus (HIV) infection. The remaining 10% of aphthae are **herpetiform aphthae**, which are smaller (1–3 mm), grouped, or coalescent ulcers that may be present on keratinized mucosa of the dorsal tongue and palate and heal spontaneously over 1 to 4 weeks (Fig. 42.3). Herpes simplex virus is not, by definition, found in these lesions.

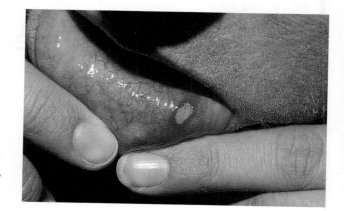

Fig. 42.1 Aphthous ulcers. A gray-white oval ulcer with a bright red margin is typical. These lesions are usually quite painful. (From White, G., & Cox, N. [2006]. *Diseases of the skin* [2nd ed.]. St. Louis, MO: Mosby.)

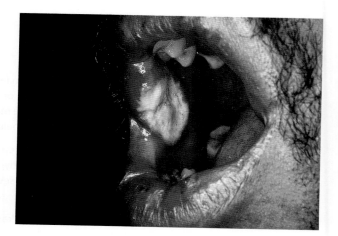

Fig. 42.2 Aphthae major in a patient with AIDS. (From Bolognia, J., Jorizzo, J., & Rapini, R. [2003]. *Dermatology*. St. Louis, MO: Mosby.)

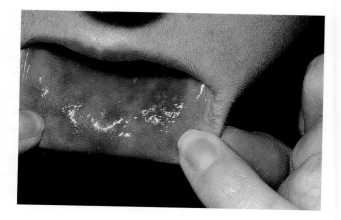

Fig. 42.3 Herpetiform mouth ulcers. (From White, G., & Cox, N. [2006]. *Diseases of the skin* [2nd ed.]. St. Louis, MO: Mosby.)

What to Do

☑ Through a careful history and physical examination, decide whether the patient is troubled with simple aphthosis or is more likely to have the potentially more serious complex aphthosis.

☑ Attempt to differentiate between the patient's mucosal sores and lesions of herpes simplex, which more commonly appear on the lips and skin outside the mouth (see Chapter 54).

☑ **For simple aphthosis with minor aphthae, inform the patient that these lesions are benign and usually last 1 to 2 weeks. They should avoid heavily spiced, acidic, or other irritating food and drink, such as pretzels and citrus fruit, and avoid any precipitating factors, such as ill-fitting dentures, a hard-bristled toothbrush, or habitual biting.** Sodium lauryl sulfate–containing mouthwash and dentifrices (used for its foaming action) are irritative to the skin and may increase the risk and incidence of aphthous ulcers. Switching to toothpaste, mouthwash, and other personal care products marked "SLS free" may help reduce this risk.

☑ **If food allergens such as cereal, fruit, chocolate, nuts, and tomatoes can be identified as triggering recurrent canker sores, their elimination will reduce or completely relieve symptoms in approximately 90% of cases.**

☑ **Treatments include topical anesthetics for pain control and topical or systemic corticosteroids to reduce inflammation.**

☑ Recommend acetaminophen (Tylenol) as an analgesic.

☑ **Prescribe triamcinolone 0.1% in Orabase. Apply a thin film to dried ulcers two to four times daily until healed.**

☑ **Prescribe amlexanox 5%, 5-g tube. Apply about 0.5 cm to affected area in mouth after brushing teeth four times daily.** This medication may increase initial discomfort, but it is the first drug to be approved by the US Food and Drug Administration (FDA) for aphthous ulcers in healthy people. This treatment may help canker sores heal only a little faster and could be **reserved for those cases in which pain is severe and sores recur frequently.**

☑ **An alternative treatment that can be used for transient pain relief is a tablet of sucralfate crushed in a small amount of warm water and swirled in the mouth or gargled. Another alternative is tetracycline elixir (or a capsule dissolved in water), not swallowed but applied to the lesions to cauterize them or used as a mouthwash.**

☑ **Diphenhydramine (Benadryl) elixir mixed 1:1 with kaolin-pectin, lidocaine (2% viscous solution), and hydrocortisone applied topically with a cotton-tipped swab can also provide symptomatic relief.** Bioadhesive 2-octyl cyanoacrylate (Dermabond) has been recommended as a topical nonprescription treatment for pain reduction, but cost is prohibitive if applied repeatedly.

☑ **For more severe cases prescribe dexamethasone elixir 0.5 mg/5 mL, swish/spit 5 mL four times a day and take nothing by mouth for 30 min. Alternatively, prescribe the topical steroid clobetasol propionate gel 0.05%. Apply a thin film after drying the area four times per day until healed. The gel may be mixed with Orabase (over the counter [OTC]) mucosal adherent, although the dilution may affect the strength. Not recommended for patients under 12 years of age.**

☑ **In very severe cases**, try a burst dose of prednisone, 40 to 60 mg daily by mouth for 5 days (no tapering required).

✅ A recent study showed that use of barrier-forming hyaluronic acid containing mouth rinse (GUM® AftaClear® rinse) or the topical gel formulation (GUM® AftaClear® gel) is effective in the treatment of minor recurrent aphthous ulcers. Patients using the GUM® AftaClear® mouth rinse formulation rinsed for 60 seconds three times per day, after meals, repeating as necessary. Patients using the gel formulation applied around 1 cm of the oral gel to each ulcer three times per day, after meals, repeating as necessary.

✅ Patients with complex aphthosis or with major aphthae can be treated with the same measures as outlined earlier. Approximately 15% of these patients have a systemic disorder in which the oral ulcers are a mucocutaneous marker of the systemic disease. These patients should also be referred for further evaluation of these possible associated systemic diseases, which may require management with systemic agents to control the aphthae (e.g., colchicines, thalidomide, dapsone, and cyclosporine). You may also consider vitamin supplementation: zinc lozenges, vitamin C, and vitamin B complex.

What Not to Do

❌ Do not give steroids to a patient in whom you suspect there may be an underlying herpes infection.

❌ Do not forget to consider hematologic etiologies if recurrent or slow-healing ulcers are associated with fevers. Check a complete blood count (CBC) with differential to rule out neutropenia or leukemias.

Discussion

Aphthae is a term of ancient origin referring to ulceration of any mucosal surface.

Aphthous stomatitis has been studied for many years by numerous investigators. Although many exacerbating factors have been identified, the cause as yet remains unknown. Lesions can be precipitated by minor trauma (often from a hard-bristled toothbrush), food allergy, stress, genetic predisposition, allergy, medications, nutritional hematinic deficiencies (e.g., iron, folic acid, vitamin B_{12}), systemic illnesses (e.g., inflammatory bowel disease or gluten-sensitive enteropathy [celiac sprue]), or HIV-associated immunosuppression. Recurrent aphthous ulcers may also accompany malignancy or autoimmune disease.

- Periodic fever with pharyngitis, aphthous stomatitis, and cervical adenitis (PFAPA syndrome) is characterized by periodic fever accompanied by pharyngitis, aphthous stomatitis, and cervical adenitis. In children the fever may occur with clockwork periodicity, while recurrences may be more variable in adults. The condition is associated with elevated inflammatory markers (CBC, C-reactive protein [CRP]) during flares, and the mainstay of treatment is oral steroids.

Behçet syndrome is a multisystem inflammatory disorder characterized by recurrent oral ulcers that are clinically indistinguishable from aphthae but are accompanied by genital ulcers, conjunctivitis, retinitis, iritis, leukocytosis, eosinophilia, and increased erythrocyte sedimentation rate. Patients with posterior uveitis (i.e., retinal vasculitis) are at risk for blindness. Patients with Behçet disease usually present with oral aphthae (minor, major, and herpetiform), which may be the only manifestation of disease for an average of 6 to 7 years before the second major manifestation is apparent.

Herpangina and hand-foot-and-mouth disease can produce ulcers resembling aphthous ulcers, but these ulcers are instead part of Coxsackie viral exanthems, usually occurring with fever and in clusters among children.

At present, the treatment for both simple and complex aphthosis is only supportive and may not alter the course of the syndrome. Aphthous ulcers may be an immune reaction to damaged mucosa or altered oral bacteria.

Although the lesions are painful, patients with simple aphthosis and minor aphthae can be reassured that they do not have a serious problem and that they are not contagious.

Suggested Readings

Bruce, A. J., & Rogers, R. S. (2003). Acute oral ulcers. *Dermatology Clinics*, *21*, 1–15.

Dalessandri, D., Zotti, F., Laffranchi, L., Migliorati, M., Isola, G., Bonetti, S., et al. (2019). Treatment of recurrent aphthous stomatitis (RAS; aphthae; canker sores) with a barrier forming mouth rinse or topical gel formulation containing hyaluronic acid: A retrospective clinical study. *BMC Oral Health*, *19*(1), 153, PMID: 31311529.

Diebold, S., & Overbeck, M. (2019). Soft tissue disorders of the mouth. *Emergency Medicine Clinics of North America*, *37*(1), 55–68, PMID: 30454780.

Letsinger, J. A., McCarty, M. A., & Jorizzo, J. L. (2005). Complex aphthosis: A large case series with evaluation algorithm and therapeutic ladder from topicals to thalidomide. *Journal of the American Academy of Dermatology*, *52*, 500–508.

Marques, D. P., Rocha, S., Manso, M., & Domingos, R. (2019). Periodic fever with pharyngitis, aphthous stomatitis and cervical adenitis syndrome: A rare cause of fever in adults. *European Journal of Case Reports in Internal Medicine*, *6*(3), 001041, PMID: 30931275.

Ship, J. A. (1996). Recurrent aphthous stomatitis: An update. *Oral Surgery, Oral Medicine, Oral Pathology*, *81*, 141–147.

Vincent, S. D., & Lilly, G. E. (1992). Clinical, historic and therapeutic features of aphthous stomatitis. *Oral Surgery, Oral Medicine, Oral Pathology*, *74*, 79–86.

Zunt, S. L. (2003). Recurrent aphthous stomatitis. *Dermatology Clinics*, *21*, 33–39.

Avulsed Tooth, Dental Subluxation, and Dental Luxation

43

Presentation

After a direct blow to the mouth, the patient, usually a child 7 to 9 years old, may have a permanent tooth that has been completely knocked out of its socket (avulsion) (Fig. 43.1). The tooth is intact down to its root, from which hangs the delicate periodontal ligament that used to be attached to alveolar bone. Alternatively, the tooth may have only become loosened within its normal anatomic position (subluxation) or partially displaced laterally, partially extruded from the socket, or intruded into the alveolar ridge (luxation) (Fig. 43.2). These disfiguring, hemorrhagic injuries are often dramatic and a frightening experience for the patient, the parents, and other bystanders.

What to Do

✅ Reassure everyone that you will be doing everything that can be done to save the patient's tooth (or teeth) and provide comfort.

✅ Obtain a detailed history that includes the mechanism of injury, conditions that may have led to dental contamination, the length of time that any avulsed tooth has been out of its socket, and how that tooth was stored and handled. **Determine whether there are any missing teeth that cannot be accounted for, and determine if the injured teeth were primary or permanent.** This is a key question, as while permanent (adult) teeth should be reimplanted, primary (baby) teeth should not. By age 6 to 8 years it is common for the primary (baby) tooth to have fallen out and have been replaced by the permanent (adult) tooth.

✅ **Check to see whether prophylaxis against bacterial endocarditis is required** because of an implanted heart valve, abnormal native valve (leakage/blockage), congenital heart defect (ventricular septal defect [VSD], atrial septal defect [ASD], patent ductus arteriosus [PDA], complex anomaly), significant mitral valve prolapse, pacemaker, or Dacron or Teflon vascular graft or patch over cardiac defect.

✅ Examination should include evaluation of surrounding soft tissue for lacerations (see Chapter 52), with special attention to possible embedded foreign bodies (e.g., chipped teeth). Grasp the injured teeth between your gloved fingers to see if a tooth or an entire segment of teeth (e.g., alveolar ridge fractures) is mobile.

✅ Check for malocclusion and other signs of mandibular fracture as well as any other associated injuries that might be overlooked with the distracting oral trauma.

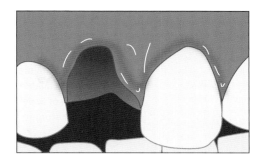

Fig. 43.1 The site of an avulsed tooth. (Adapted from Honsik, K. A. [2004]. Emergency treatment of dentoalveolar trauma. *Physician and Sports Medicine, 32*, 23–29.)

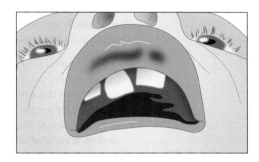

Fig. 43.2 A partially extruded and laterally displaced tooth (luxation). (Adapted from Honsik, K. A. [2004]. Emergency treatment of dentoalveolar trauma. *Physician and Sports Medicine, 32*, 23–29.)

⊘ **Radiographs need only be obtained if a mandibular or alveolar fracture is suspected, if a dental fragment is missing in the soft tissues of the mouth, or if a tooth may have been intruded down into its socket, is no longer visible, and appears to be missing.**

⊘ **If a tooth is lost and cannot be accounted for,** order a chest radiograph to rule out bronchial aspiration.

⊘ **The best way to preserve a tooth that has been knocked out (avulsed) is to put it back in its socket as quickly as possible.** Do not delay replanting a tooth because you are waiting for radiograph results unless you suspect an alveolar ridge fracture. Keep in mind that more accurate dental films can be done at the time of dental follow-up.

⊘ **A primary tooth that has been avulsed should not be reimplanted. The risk of injury to the developing permanent tooth is high.**

⊘ **If the permanent tooth is only partially avulsed and is just protruding farther out of its socket than normal or is angulated, simply push it back in, using firm pressure until it sits in its proper position.** If the tooth is very sensitive and painful to touch, first provide analgesia, using an appropriate oral nerve block (see Appendix D). To ensure that the tooth is firmly reseated, have the patient bite down hard on a piece of gauze.

⊘ **In the field, fully extruded permanent teeth may be stored under the tongue or in the buccal vestibule between the gums and the cheek. If the patient is unconscious, the tooth can be stored in cold milk or saline solution—or, if nothing else is available, water—until**

a better preservation solution is available. A child's permanent tooth might be preserved, if necessary, in the parent's mouth.

✅ **Place the tooth in protective solution as soon as possible after patient arrival,** even before obtaining additional history. Milk is an ideal storage medium that is inexpensive and readily available. Commercially available protective solutions, such as Hank balanced salt solution or Save-A-Tooth kit, may also be utilized. *Note:* Contact-lens solution is not an appropriate storage medium.

✅ **If the tooth is contaminated,** *hold it by the crown only* **and irrigate it with normal saline.** *Do not rub or scrub the root surface.*

✅ **Replacing a tooth into its socket can be facilitated by first anesthetizing the tooth socket with a dental block (see Appendix D). After the socket is numb, irrigate the socket and gently suction out any remaining debris or blood. Once the socket is prepared in this manner, replace the tooth back into the socket.**

✅ **If the permanent tooth has been out of its socket for less than 15 minutes, take it by the crown, drop it in a tooth-preservation solution (see earlier), and gently flush the socket with the same solution or normal saline. Then reimplant the tooth firmly, first checking its proper orientation. Instruct the patient to bite down hard on a piece of gauze to help stabilize the tooth. While most of the time the tooth will remain stable in the socket, if instead, after reimplantation the tooth is assumed to still be unstable, it should be secured with wax or dental cement (Coe-Pak) to the two adjacent teeth.** Wire or arch bars can also be utilized if available (see EM-RAP videos if available). If there is significant resistance when reimplanting a tooth, there may be hematoma or clot in the socket. Pad the tooth with gauze and ask the patient to bite down gently avoiding too much pressure that could cause a fracture at the root or the socket. Teeth that are unable to be reimplanted will have to be referred to a dentist or oral surgeon.

✅ **Zinc oxide periodontal pack (Coe-Pack)** is a dressing that comes in the form of a base and a catalyst. Mix together the two parts and mold the resulting paste, which will eventually set semihard, over the gingival line and between the dried teeth on both the buccal and lingual sides but not over the occlusive surface of the teeth. For a video describing how to use a Coe-Pak dressing to stabilize a tooth, see the following link: https://youtu.be/REKJuYm5OpM. Another useful video is available at Thedentalbox.com: https://youtu.be/2GNAQwOid1l.

✅ **If a temporary zinc oxide periodontal splint (Coe-Pak) or wire is not available** to stabilize loose teeth, spread soft wax over palatal and labial tooth surfaces and neighboring teeth as a temporary splint. If this item is not available, there is a case report showing the use of a pliable metal nasal bridge from a respirator mask to stabilize the replanted tooth. This splint is molded to the outer surface of the teeth and then glued to the reimplanted tooth and the stabilizing adjacent teeth using 2-octyl cyanoacrylate (2-OCA; Dermabond and others) (Fig. 43.3).

✅ **Put the patient on a soft diet, prescribe doxycycline 100 mg twice a day for 7 days. Other alternatives include penicillin, amoxicillin, clindamycin, or erythromycin. In children under age 12, prescribe amoxicillin 12.5 mg/kg twice a day or penicillin V potassium 12.5 mg/kg four times a day for 7 days** and schedule a dental appointment as soon as possible. Instruct the patient to brush all but the splinted teeth. Some endorse chlorhexidine mouth rinse in addition to brushing.

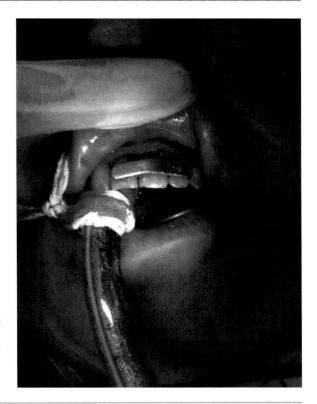

Fig. 43.3 Pliable metal nasal bridge of respirator mask bonded to teeth using 2-OCA for reimplantation and stabilization of avulsed left upper central incisor (tooth 9). (Adapted from Rosenberg, H., Rosenberg, H., & Hickey, M. [2011]. Emergency management of a traumatic tooth avulsion. *Annals of Emergency Medicine, 57,* 375–377.)

✅ **If the permanent tooth has been out of its socket for 15 minutes to 2 hours, first soak it in the previously mentioned protective solution for 30 minutes to replenish nutrients before reimplanting. Local anesthesia will probably be needed before the tooth can be reimplanted as described earlier (see Appendix D).**

✅ **If the permanent tooth has been out of its socket for longer than 2 hours, the periodontal ligament is dead and should be removed, along with the pulp.** Soak the tooth in 2% sodium fluoride solution for 20 minutes before reimplanting. Another option is to soak the tooth for 30 minutes in 5% sodium hypochlorite (Clorox) and 5 minutes each in saturated citric acid, 1% stannous fluoride, and 5% doxycycline. The dead tooth should ankylose into the alveolar bone of the socket as with a dental implant.

✅ **Even when the tooth has been out less than 2 hours, if the patient is between 6 and 10 years of age, soak the tooth for 5 minutes in 5% doxycycline to kill bacteria that could enter the immature apex and form an abscess.**

✅ **If all this cannot be done right away, simply keep the tooth soaking in the preservation solution until a dentist can get to it. The solution should preserve the tooth safely for up to 4 days.**

✅ **After the tooth has been reimplanted, suture gingival lacerations if present.**

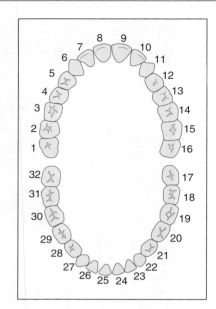

Fig. 43.4 Dental map.

✅ **When consulting a dentist or an oral surgeon, the use of a dental map will help in communicating the exact tooth/teeth involved** (Fig. 43.4).

✅ **Provide antibiotic prophylaxis to all patients, with even minor dental trauma (e.g., subluxation), if they are at risk for bacterial endocarditis.**

✅ **Consider the possibility of domestic or child abuse** as the source of the trauma; if suspected, notify the appropriate authorities.

✅ Add tetanus prophylaxis to the treatment protocol if required (see Appendix G).

✅ Inform the patient or the parents that any trauma to the teeth can lead to the death of a tooth or infection or root absorption and the eventual loss of the tooth. Also advise that the patient will require dental referral for possible repositioning, more durable splinting, possible root canal therapy, and long-term follow-up. **Root canal therapy will definitely be required on all permanent teeth that have been completely avulsed.**

✅ **Prescribe appropriate pain medication, such as ibuprofen and acetaminophen. Adults may use 600 mg of ibuprofen every 6 hours and 1000 mg of acetaminophen every 6 hours. Tell the patient to alternate by taking one and then the other every 3 hours. Children can follow the same timing of doses using 10 mg/kg of ibuprofen and 15 mg/kg of acetaminophen.** For uncontrolled pain, you may use oxycodone oral solution 5 mg/5 mL concentration. Give 0.05 to 0.15 mg/kg PO q4-6h prn for 1-2 days.

What Not to Do

❌ Do not allow an avulsed tooth to dry out. The total length of dry storage time has the greatest negative impact on the success or failure of dental reimplantation.

ⓧ Do not touch a viable root with fingers, forceps, gauze, or anything else, and do not try to scrub or clean it. The periodontal ligament will be injured and unable to revascularize the reimplanted tooth. Only hold an avulsed tooth by its crown.

ⓧ Do not overlook fractures of teeth and alveolar ridges.

ⓧ Do not substitute the calcium hydroxide composition (Dycal) used for covering fractured teeth for the temporary periodontal pack (Coe-Pak) used to stabilize luxated teeth. They are different products.

ⓧ Do not reimplant an avulsed tooth if there is a complicated crown fracture, a fractured root, or an alveolar ridge fracture. An avulsed tooth with a simple fracture but an intact root may still be reimplanted.

ⓧ Do not replace primary deciduous or baby teeth, although this has been done under very special circumstances. Reimplanted primary teeth heal by ankylosis; they literally fuse to the bone, which can lead to cosmetic deformity because the area of ankylosis will not grow at the same rate as the rest of the dentofacial complex. Ankylosis can also interfere with eruption of the permanent tooth.

ⓧ Do not confuse an avulsed adult tooth with a child's deciduous tooth, which would fall out soon anyway. Normal developmental shedding of primary decidual teeth is preceded by absorption of the root. If such a tooth is brought in by mistake, there is no root to reimplant and little or no empty socket; instead, a new permanent tooth may be visible or palpable underneath.

ⓧ Do not release a patient with an unsplinted tooth that is so loose that it is in danger of falling out and being aspirated.

Discussion

Accidents at home, at school, or in a motor vehicle, as well as altercations and contact sports, lead to injuries of the teeth. The maxillary central incisors are the teeth most commonly affected. When teeth are avulsed, the prognosis is best when teeth are reimplanted within 5 minutes of avulsion; yet, such optimal treatment is not always possible.

Before commercially available reconstitution solutions (e.g., Hank balanced salt solution, 320 mOsm, pH 7.2), the best treatment that could be offered the avulsed tooth was rapid reimplantation. Without a preservation solution, the chances of successful reimplantation decline approximately one percentage point every minute the tooth is absent from the oral cavity. Remember that milk is also an ideal storage medium.

In mature teeth (those >10 years old), the pulp will not survive avulsion, even if the periodontal ligament does. At the 1-week follow-up visit with the dentist, the necrotic pulp will be removed (root canal) to prevent a chronic inflammatory reaction from interfering with the healing of the periodontal ligament.

The primary goal of rapid reimplantation is to preserve the periodontal ligament, not the tooth. With survival of the periodontal ligament, the tooth is more likely to function for a longer period of time, with less resorption of the root and reduced ankylosis.

Almost half of teeth with luxation injuries become necrotic after 3 years (Fig. 43.5). The correct and timely management of these cases can increase the success of treatment.

Successful reimplantation of avulsed anterior permanent teeth can delay or negate the need for prosthetic or complex and expensive restorative procedures. Several studies have shown that teeth can function for 20 years or more after reimplantation. A number of cases have been reported in which reimplanted teeth have been functional for 20 to 40 years with a normal periodontium.

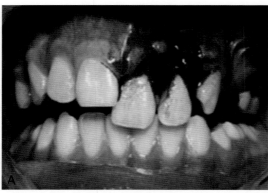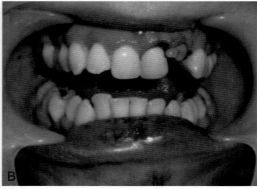

Fig. 43.5 Tooth luxation: (A) extrusive luxation, (B) intrusive luxation. (With permission from Piccininni P, Clough A, Padilla R, et al. Dental and orofacial injuries. *Clin Sports Med* 2017;36:369–405.

Suggested Readings

Cho, S., & Cheng, A. C. (2002). Replantation of an avulsed incisor after prolonged dry storage: A case report. *Journal of the Canadian Dental Association, 68,* 297–300.

Douglass, A. B. (2003). Common dental emergencies. *American Family Physician, 67,* 511–516.

Hammel, J. M., & Fischel, J. (2019). Dental emergencies. *Emergency Medicine Clinics of North America, 37*(1), 81–93.

Krasner, P. (1994). Modern treatment of avulsed teeth by emergency physicians. *American Journal of Emergency Medicine, 12,* 241–246.

Martins, W. D., Westphalen, V. P. D., & Westphalen, F. H. (2004). Tooth replantation after traumatic avulsion: A 27-year follow up. *Dental Traumatology, 20,* 101–105.

Moran, I., James, M., Cook, W., & Perry, M. (2016). Tooth avulsion. *British Medical Journal, 25*(4), 353–i1394.

Rosenberg, H., Rosenberg, H., & Hickey, M. (2011). Emergency management of a traumatic tooth avulsion. *Annals of Emergency Medicine, 57,* 375–377.

Zamon, E. L., & Kenny, D. J. (2001). Replantation of avulsed primary incisors: A risk–benefit assessment. *Journal of the Canadian Dental Association, 67,* 386.

Bleeding After Dental Surgery

Presentation

The patient may have had an extraction or other dental surgery performed earlier in the day and now has excessive bleeding at the site and is unable to visit the dentist. The patient may also be using aspirin, warfarin, or direct-acting oral anticoagulants (DOACs) such as apixaban, dabigatran, or rivaroxaban. In addition, patients may be taking aspirin in combination with one of the newer dual antiplatelet therapy (DAPT) medications: clopidogrel, prasugrel, or ticagrelor.

What to Do

✓ Ask the patient what procedure was done and estimate how much bleeding has occurred. Inquire about medications such as antiplatelet drugs (aspirin, warfarin, clopidogrel, DOACs, or DAPT medications), underlying coagulopathies, and previous experiences with unusual bleeding.

✓ **Using suction and saline irrigation, clear any packing and blood from the bleeding site.**

✓ **Roll a 2 × 2–inch gauze pad, insert it over the bleeding site, and have the patient apply constant pressure on it (biting down usually suffices) for 30 to 45 minutes.**

✓ **If the site is still bleeding after 30 to 45 minutes of gauze pressure,** infiltrate the extraction area and inject a local anesthetic and vasoconstrictor, such as 2% lidocaine with 1:100,000 or 1:200,000 epinephrine, into the socket and surrounding gingiva until the tissue blanches. Again, have the patient bite on a gauze pad for 45 minutes. The anesthetic allows the patient to bite down harder, and the epinephrine helps decrease the bleeding.

✓ **If this injection does not stop the bleeding, pack the bleeding site with Gelfoam, Surgicel, or gauze soaked in topical thrombin. Then place the gauze pad on top and reapply pressure. Alternatively, HemCon dental gauze can be applied. Place the HemCon dental dressing into the extraction wound. The dressing is most effective when in contact with blood from the wound, which wets the dressing. The top of the dressing should be flush with the gingival margin. Place sterile gauze over the HemCon dental dressing, and have the patient bite down, applying gentle pressure for 1 to 2 minutes. Visualize the site to confirm proper placement of the dressing, and replace the gauze on top. The HemCon dressing dissolves in 48 hours to 7 days and does not need to be removed. The patient may irrigate the wound site at 7 days to ensure removal of any residual material.**

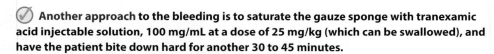 **Another approach** to the bleeding is to saturate the gauze sponge with tranexamic acid injectable solution, 100 mg/mL at a dose of 25 mg/kg (which can be swallowed), and have the patient bite down hard for another 30 to 45 minutes.

✅ An arterial bleeder resistant to all the aforementioned treatments may require ligation with a figure-eight stitch to achieve hemostasis.

✅ If bleeding cannot be controlled with the abovementioned measures, consider reversal of any anticoagulation or coagulopathy.

✅ Bleeding that cannot otherwise be controlled may involve injury to an artery, vein, or arteriovenous malformation and require consult with an oral surgeon or interventional radiology to consider surgical management or embolization.

✅ Assess any possible significant blood loss by obtaining orthostatic vital signs.

✅ **When the bleeding stops,** remove the overlying gauze and instruct the patient to leave the site alone for a day and see the dentist for follow-up.

What Not to Do

❌ Do not routinely obtain laboratory clotting studies or hematocrit levels unless there is reason to suspect a bleeding disorder such as hemophilia A or von Willebrand disease, the patient is taking warfarin, or there is suspected severe blood loss.

❌ Do not allow a patient to intermittently remove the gauze. It is the constant, prolonged pressure that is most likely to provide successful hemostasis.

Discussion

Serious hemorrhage is rare even in the presence of a bleeding diathesis or anticoagulant therapy. Most patients are merely annoyed by the continued bleeding and often only need to stop dabbing the area and apply constant pressure to get the bleeding to stop.

Occasionally this problem can be handled with telephone consultation alone. Some say a moistened tea bag, which contains the hemostatic effects of tannic acid, works better than a gauze pad when constant pressure is applied.

Suggested Readings

Engelen, E. T., Schutgens, R. E., Mauser-Bunschoten, E. P., van Es, R. J., & van Galen, K. P. (2018). Antifibrinolytic therapy for preventing oral bleeding in people on anticoagulants undergoing minor oral surgery or dental extractions. *Cochrane Database of Systematic Reviews, 2*(7), 7. CD012293 PMID: 29963686.

Federici, A. B. (2004). Clinical diagnosis of von Willebrand disease. *Haemophilia, 10,* 169–176.

Gazda, H., & Grabowska, A. (1993). Topical treatment of oral bleeding in children with clotting disturbances [in Polish]. *Wiadomosci Lekarskie, 46,* 111–115.

Hammel, J. M., & Fischel, J. (2019). Dental emergencies. *Emergency Medicine Clinics of North America*, *37*(1), 81–93. PMID: 30454782.

Ockerman, A., Bornstein, M. M., Leung, Y. Y., Li, S. K. Y., Politis, C., & Jacobs, R. (2019). Incidence of bleeding after minor oral surgery in patients on dual antiplatelet therapy: A systematic review and meta-analysis. *International Journal of Oral and Maxillofacial Surgery*, *24*, PMID: 31248706.

Petersen, J. K., Krogsgaard, J., Nielsen, K. M., et al. (1984). A comparison between 2 absorbable hemostatic agents: Gelatin sponge (Spongostan) and oxidized regenerated cellulose (Surgicel). *International Journal of Oral Surgery*, *13*, 406–410.

Senghore, N., & Harris, M. (1999). The effect of tranexamic acid (Cyclokapron) on blood loss after third molar extraction under a day case general anaesthetic. *British Dental Journal*, *186*, 634–636.

Songra, A. K., & Darbar, U. R. (1998). Post-extraction bleeding—an aid to diagnosis? *Australian Dental Journal*, *43*, 242–243.

Waly, N. G. (1995). Local antifibrinolytic treatment with tranexamic acid in hemophilic children undergoing dental extractions. *Egyptian Dental Journal*, *41*, 961–968.

Zanon, E., Martinelli, F., Bacci, C., et al. (2003). Safety of dental extraction among consecutive patients on oral anticoagulant treatment managed using a specific dental management protocol. *Blood Coagulation and Fibrinolysis*, *14*, 27–30.

Burning Mouth Syndrome, Burning Tongue

(Glossodynia)

Presentation

Patients present with a painful sensation of the tongue or mouth. The pain is variably described as a burning, tingling, hot, scalded, or numb sensation, the magnitude of which is similar to a toothache. The sensation occurs most commonly on the anterior two-thirds and tip of the tongue but may include the upper alveolar region, palate, lips, and lower alveolar region. Burning mouth syndrome (BMS) affects women seven times more frequently than men. It particularly affects the middle-aged and elderly population (mean age 60 years) and has not been reported in children.

There may be xerostomia (dry mouth) (Fig. 45.1), dental disease or dentures, geographic tongue (Fig. 45.2), smooth tongue (Fig. 45.3), candidiasis (see Chapter 53), or no visible explanation for the pain. True BMS is characterized by oral pain and discomfort in a patient with normal-appearing mucosa and no local or systemic condition typically associated with stomatodynia.

What to Do

⊘ **First, attempt to classify the patient with BMS into either primary BMS, which does not have an association with any other evident disease, or secondary BMS, which is oral burning from other clinical abnormalities. In the case of secondary BMS, once other conditions are treated, the oral burning symptoms should improve or resolve. The diagnosis of primary BMS is clinical and consists of the classic burning pain in the absence of any physical findings.**

⊘ **Determine the type of primary BMS the patient has by the character of the symptoms.**

⊘ **In type 1 (35%), the patient has daily pain that is not present on awakening but progresses throughout the day and is most severe during the evening hours.** This type of pain is usually not associated with psychiatric disorders.

⊘ **In type 2 (55%), the patient awakens with a constant daily pain. This type of pain is associated with psychiatric conditions, especially chronic anxiety.**

⊘ **In type 3 (10%), the patient has intermittent pain with symptom-free intervals. The pain occurs in unusual sites, such as the buccal mucosa, floor of the mouth, and throat. This type of pain is associated with allergies to food additives or flavorings.**

⊘ Try to determine if the patient's pain is associated with systemic, local, psychiatric, psychological, or idiopathic factors.

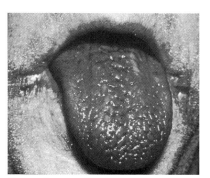

Fig. 45.1 Xerostomia. (From Drage, L. A., & Rogers, R. S. [2003]. Burning mouth syndrome. *Dermatology Clinics, 21,* 135–145.)

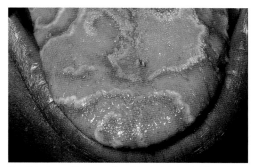

Fig. 45.2 Geographic tongue. (From Bolognia, J., Jorizzo, J., & Rapini, R. [2003]. *Dermatology.* St. Louis, MO: Mosby.)

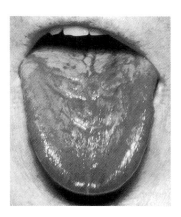

Fig. 45.3 Smooth tongue. (From Drage, L. A., & Rogers, R. S. [2003]. Burning mouth syndrome. *Dermatology Clinics, 21,* 135–145.)

⊘ **The most common associations include psychiatric or psychological disorders, xerostomia, nutritional deficiencies, allergic contact stomatitis, denture-related factors, parafunctional behavior (e.g., bruxism and tongue thrusting), candidiasis, diabetes mellitus, and drug-related BMS. There may be more than one cause.**

⊘ A history should include the duration, character, pattern, and site of pain. Ask about depression, anxiety, and fear of specific conditions. Are there any exacerbating factors such as food, mouthwash, mints, lip cosmetics, or smoking? Is there a relationship of the pain to denture use, dental work, tongue thrusting, bruxism, or jaw clenching? Look into medication use that has xerostomic potential.

⊘ A general physical examination should be performed with emphasis on a thorough oral evaluation. Look for erythema, ulcers, glossitis, atrophy, candidiasis, dentures, geographic tongue, lichen planus, and xerostomia.

⊘ **When a psychiatric disorder is suspected**, referral for psychiatric evaluation or psychotherapy evaluation may play a role in alleviating the symptoms. Antidepressants and anxiolytics with less anticholinergic impact (therefore less xerostomia) are preferred. Selective serotonin reuptake inhibitors (SSRIs) may be a good choice in this setting (paroxetine 10–20 mg/day with dose increase to a maximum 30 mg/day). Medical management may also include tricyclic antidepressants (amitriptyline 10–25 mg once a day at night and can be titrated up by the provider in follow-up), benzodiazepines (clonazepam starting at 0.25 mg once a day at night), or anticonvulsants (gabapentin starting at 100 mg three times a day).

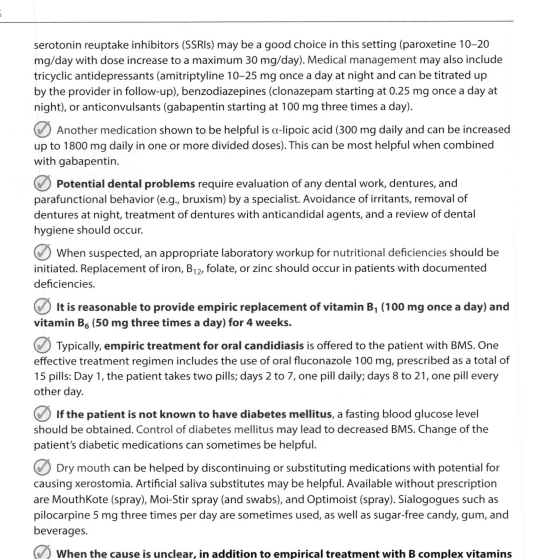 Another medication shown to be helpful is α-lipoic acid (300 mg daily and can be increased up to 1800 mg daily in one or more divided doses). This can be most helpful when combined with gabapentin.

Potential dental problems require evaluation of any dental work, dentures, and parafunctional behavior (e.g., bruxism) by a specialist. Avoidance of irritants, removal of dentures at night, treatment of dentures with anticandidal agents, and a review of dental hygiene should occur.

When suspected, an appropriate laboratory workup for nutritional deficiencies should be initiated. Replacement of iron, B_{12}, folate, or zinc should occur in patients with documented deficiencies.

It is reasonable to provide empiric replacement of vitamin B_1 (100 mg once a day) and vitamin B_6 (50 mg three times a day) for 4 weeks.

Typically, **empiric treatment for oral candidiasis** is offered to the patient with BMS. One effective treatment regimen includes the use of oral fluconazole 100 mg, prescribed as a total of 15 pills: Day 1, the patient takes two pills; days 2 to 7, one pill daily; days 8 to 21, one pill every other day.

If the patient is not known to have diabetes mellitus, a fasting blood glucose level should be obtained. Control of diabetes mellitus may lead to decreased BMS. Change of the patient's diabetic medications can sometimes be helpful.

Dry mouth can be helped by discontinuing or substituting medications with potential for causing xerostomia. Artificial saliva substitutes may be helpful. Available without prescription are MouthKote (spray), Moi-Stir spray (and swabs), and Optimoist (spray). Sialogogues such as pilocarpine 5 mg three times per day are sometimes used, as well as sugar-free candy, gum, and beverages.

When the cause is unclear, in addition to empirical treatment with B complex vitamins and anticandidal agents, patients should be instructed to discontinue all potentially irritating substances, such as alcohol-based mouthwashes, cinnamon, mint products, and smoking.

You can provide symptomatic relief with a 1:1 mixture of diphenhydramine elixir and kaolin-pectin or prescribe viscous lidocaine 15 to 20 mL, swish and spit every 3 hours.

If the onset is recent, an alternative approach is to have the patient rinse with a topical anesthetic mouth rinse for 3 minutes and then apply capsaicin gel (0.025%) for 3 minutes. This is repeated morning and evening for 6 weeks. (This works best in neuropathic pain of recent onset.) The patient should be informed that using oral capsaicin may cause gastrointestinal discomfort.

If the cause is uncertain and persists, refer the patient for a comprehensive medical evaluation.

What Not to Do

Ⓧ Do not assume that the patient has a purely psychiatric cause for the pain until all other potential causes have been considered and appropriate consultations have been made.

Discussion

Burning mouth syndrome is a chronic condition characterized by a burning pain sensation of the oral mucosa in a patient with a normal oral mucosal examination and for which no cause can be identified. Etiologies are multifactorial, and the biggest barrier to identifying a core pathophysiology is the heterogeneity of the syndrome.

Psychiatric disease is a common underlying factor in patients with BMS. At least one-third of patients may have an underlying psychiatric diagnosis, most commonly depression or anxiety disorders. A phobic concern regarding cancer is also prominent in 20% of patients. Remember that depression and psychological disturbance are common in chronic pain populations and may be secondary to the chronic pain, rather than the cause of BMS. In addition, many of the medications that are used to treat psychiatric disease can cause xerostomia and exacerbate BMS.

Dry mouth is a frequent complaint among BMS patients. Drug-related xerostomia is common and can occur with many medications, including tricyclic antidepressants, benzodiazepines, monoamine oxidase inhibitors, antihypertensives, and antihistamines. Connective tissue diseases, such as Sjögren syndrome or sicca syndrome, can cause xerostomia, as can a history of local irradiation or diabetes mellitus. Even stress and anxiety can lead to a dry mouth.

Because of rapid cell turnover and trauma, the oral cavity is especially sensitive to nutritional deficiencies and may be the first indicator of such a problem. Iron-deficiency anemia, pernicious anemia (an autoimmune B_{12} deficiency), zinc deficiency, and B complex vitamin deficiency have all been reported to cause BMS.

Flavoring or food additives have been implicated as possible allergens in BMS. Cinnamon aldehyde (cinnamon), sorbic acid, tartrazine, benzoic acid, propylene glycol, menthol, and peppermint have all been identified as potential causes of mouth pain.

Denture-related pain is usually caused by faulty design, irritation, or parafunctional behavior. Candidiasis can also contribute to denture-related pain. Most BMS patients with dentures or significant dental work benefit from referral for a formal dental consultation to assess dental work, dentures, occlusion, and the need for modification or replacement.

Candidiasis is reported as a causative factor in 6% to 30% of patients with BMS. The mucosal alterations typically seen with candidiasis (thrush) may be minimal or absent. Candidal overgrowth occurs with xerostomia, corticosteroid treatment, antibiotic treatment, denture use, and diabetes mellitus. Empiric treatment for oral candidiasis is often prescribed to patients with BMS.

Approximately 5% of BMS patients have diabetes mellitus. BMS is the second most common oral complaint after xerostomia in a study of diabetic patients. Improved control of the diabetes mellitus may lead to improvement or cure of BMS.

The angiotensin-converting enzyme inhibitors enalapril, captopril, and lisinopril can cause scalded mouth or BMS. There is often improvement with reduction or discontinuation of the medication.

Although they are often regarded as asymptomatic variants of normal, multiple studies have shown geographic, fissured, or scalloped tongues more frequently in patients with tongue pain. When these patients complain of pain, they do not by definition fall under the rubric of BMS but can be treated as such and should be assessed for fear of cancer.

Identification of correctable causes of BMS should be emphasized, and psychiatric causes should not be invoked without thorough evaluation of the patient. A thoughtful and structured evaluation has been associated with improvement in approximately 70% of these patients.

Suggested Readings

Drage, L. A., & Rogers, R. S. (2003). Burning mouth syndrome. *Dermatology Clinics, 21*, 135–145.

Grushka, M., Epstein, J., & Gorsky, M. (2002). Burning mouth syndrome. *American Family Physician, 65*, 615–621.

Klasser, G. D., Grushka, M., & Su, N. (2016). Burning mouth syndrome. *Oral and Maxillofacial Surgery Clinics of North America, 28*(3), 381–396.

Moghadam-Kia, S., & Fazel, N. (2017). A diagnostic and therapeutic approach to primary burning mouth syndrome. *Clinics in Dermatology, 35*(5), 453–460.

Tu, T. T. H., Takenoshita, M., Matsuoka, H., Watanabe, T., Suga, T., Aota, Y., et al. (2019). Current management strategies for the pain of elderly patients with burning mouth syndrome: A critical review. *BioPsychoSocial Medicine, 13*, 1.

Vickers, R. (n.d.). Burning mouth/tongue syndrome (glossodynia/glossopyrosis). www.painmanagement.usyd.edu.au/html/orofacial_burning_mouth.htm.

Dental Pain, Periapical Abscess

(Tooth Abscess)

Presentation

The patient complains of severe, constant facial or dental pain, often associated with facial swelling, regional lymphadenopathy, and cellulitis, and may exhibit signs of systemic toxicity. The pain may be gnawing, throbbing, or sharp and shooting. Dental caries may or may not be apparent. Percussion of the offending tooth causes increased pain (Fig. 46.1). The severe toothache may be exacerbated by thermal changes, especially cold drinks. On the other hand, hot and cold sensitivity may no longer be present because of necrosis of the pulp. A fluctuant abscess may be palpated in the buccal or palatal gingiva, but usually extends toward the buccal side and to the gingival-buccal reflection.

See normal anatomy (Fig. 46.2) with subsequent development of periapical abscess and cellulitis (Fig. 46.3).

What to Do

✓ **The quickest way to control dental pain is with a dental block. See Appendix D for inferior alveolar, infraorbital, mental, or apical nerve block.** See instructional videos at https://www.thedentalbox.smartpractice.com/shop/wa/category?cn=How-To-Videos&id=3&m=SPDB&mc=true. Use of bupivacaine (Marcaine) as the anesthetic agent will give prolonged pain relief. For instructional videos on how to perform dental blocks, see the following links at www.thedentalbox.com:

Infraorbital Nerve Block: https://www.youtube.com/watch?v=QWOt3kkvw90
Mental Nerve Block: https://youtu.be/hPALXAq9pTo
Inferior Aveolar Nerve Block: https://youtu.be/58CY6-5uyYI

✓ **Adequate pain medication should be administered and prescribed for continued pain relief until dental follow-up can be arranged.** Nonsteroidal anti-inflammatory drugs (NSAIDs) are excellent for dental pain and often suffice or can be administered in combination with acetaminophen. Have the patient use ibuprofen 600 mg (10 mg/kg, child max dose 600 mg) and acetaminophen 1000 mg (15 mg/kg, child max dose 1000 mg) every 6 hours. Alternate so the patient is taking one and then the other every 3 hours. Narcotic pain medications are generally not needed for dental pain but can be prescribed for synergistic analgesia if absolutely necessary. Provide a small prescription for five tabs of hydrocodone or oxycodone to help manage the patient's pain until they can follow up with a dentist.

✓ Antibiotics are not necessary to treat apical abscesses unless there is concurrent cellulitis, systemic involvement such as fever or lymphadenopathy or malaise, progressive swelling, and/

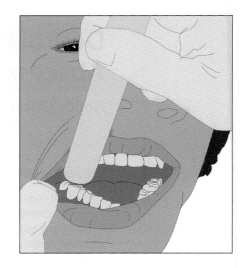

Fig. 46.1 Percussion of tooth with tongue blade.

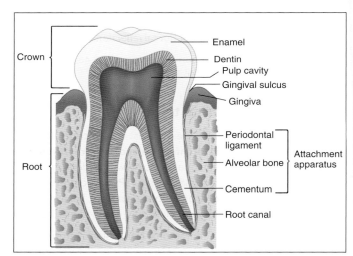

Fig. 46.2 Normal tooth anatomy.
(From Marx, J. A., Hockberger, R. S., Walls, R. M., et al. [2010]. *Rosen's emergency medicine concepts and clinical practice* [7th ed.]. Philadelphia, PA: Mosby.)

or trismus. Immunocompromised patients should also be considered for treatment even in the absence of other findings.

✓ **When cellulitis and facial swelling are present, depending on the level of toxicity, the patient initially should be treated with either parenteral or oral antibiotics. A course (7–10 days) of penicillin VK, 500 mg four times per day, may be prescribed in adults (50 mg/kg/day divided into three doses in children). Amoxicillin 500 mg every 8 to 12 hours (25 mg/kg/day divided every 12 hours in children) may provide more rapid improvement in pain or swelling due to its broader spectrum of antimicrobial activity and easier dosing schedule. For more severe infections use amoxicillin/clavulanate (Augmentin) 875 mg/125 mg orally every 12 hours (30 mg/kg/day divided every 12 hours in children). Erythromycin or clindamycin may be substituted if the patient is allergic to penicillin.**

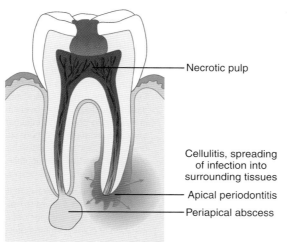

Necrotic pulp

Cellulitis, spreading
of infection into
surrounding tissues

Apical periodontitis

Periapical abscess

Fig. 46.3 Apical periodontitis, periapical abscess, and cellulitis.

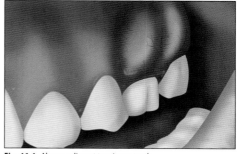

Fig. 46.4 Abscess adjacent to primary tooth.

✅ **If a fluctuant gingival abscess cavity is present** (Fig. 46.4), **perform incision and drainage at the most dependent location.** Provide local anesthesia with 1% lidocaine (Xylocaine) with epinephrine. With gingival swelling and fluctuance, incision and drainage can often be accomplished by sliding a No. 15 scalpel blade between the tooth and gingiva.

✅ **Instruct the patient to apply warm compresses to the affected area and seek follow-up care from a dentist within 24 hours. Definitive therapy is root canal treatment or extraction.**

What Not to Do

❌ Do not obtain radiographs for an uncomplicated abscess.

❌ Do not insert an obstructing pack into a tooth cavity when an abscess or cellulitis is present.

❌ Do not prescribe aspirin if it is possible that a tooth will need to be extracted.

Discussion

A periapical abscess originates in the dental pulp, usually secondary to dental caries that erodes the protective layers of the tooth (enamel, dentin) and allows bacteria to invade the pulp, producing a pulpitis. A severely inflamed pulp (pulpitis) will eventually necrose, causing apical periodontitis, which is inflammation around the apex of the tooth. Apical abscess is a localized, purulent form of apical periodontitis. Cellulitis may follow apical periodontitis or abscess if the infection spreads into the surrounding tissues (see Fig. 46.4). This is the most common dental abscess in children.

Dental pain may be referred to the ear, temple, eye, neck, or other teeth. Conversely, what appears to be dental pain may in fact be caused by overlying maxillary sinusitis or otitis.

(continued)

Discussion continued

Diabetes, immune deficiency diseases, and valvular heart disease increase the risk for complications from bacteremia. Local extension of infection can lead to retropharyngeal abscess, Ludwig cellulitis, cavernous sinus thrombosis, osteomyelitis, mediastinitis, and pulmonary abscess, which are all serious complications requiring immediate consultation with an appropriate specialist.

An acute periodontal (as opposed to periapical) abscess involves the supporting structures of the teeth (periodontal ligaments, alveolar bone) and causes localized, painful, fluctuant swelling of the gingiva, either between the teeth or laterally, and is associated with vital teeth that are not usually sensitive to percussion. This condition is found in patients with chronic periodontal disease and is the most common dental abscess in adults. It may also occur in patients (including children) who have a foreign object lodged in the gingiva. The involved tooth may be tender to percussion and show increased mobility. Treatment consists of local infiltrative anesthesia and drainage by subgingival curettage. In severe cases or cases in which there is fever, prescribe doxycycline, 100 mg twice per day for 10 days. Also instruct the patient to rinse the mouth with warm salt water and consult a dentist for further treatment. Severe periodontitis in a young patient should raise the possibility of an underlying immune disorder. Dental infections may be associated with complications such as endocarditis, brain abscesses, and mediastinitis. Fever may be the only symptom. Consider dental infections when evaluating patients with unexplained fever.

The opioid crisis necessitates that health care providers seek alternatives to opioid (ALTO) pain management strategies, including avoidance of initiation of opioids, limiting prescription amounts, and using a state prescription-monitoring database to inform prescribing practices. Most dental pain can be managed by use of NSAIDs. Ibuprofen can be combined with acetaminophen for a synergistic effect. Dental nerve blocks provide effective long-lasting pain management without the use of opioid pain medications.

Suggested Readings

Arslan, F., Karagöz, E., Arslan, B. Y., & Mert, A. (2016). An unnoticed origin of fever: Periapical tooth abscess. Three case reports and literature review. *Le Infezioni in Medicina, 24*(1), 67–70.

Douglass, A. B. (2003). Common dental emergencies. *American Family Physician, 67*, 511–516.

May, E., & Wilbeck, J. (2019). Dental pain relief in the age of ALTO. *Advanced Emergency Nursing Journal, 41*(3), 229–233.

Siqueira, J. F., & Rôças, I. N. (2013). Microbiology and treatment of acute apical abscesses. *Clinical Microbiology Reviews, 26*(2), 255–273.

Dental Pain, Pericoronitis

Presentation

Patients, typically between the ages of 17 and 29, seek help because of painful swelling and signs of infection around a partially erupted or impacted third molar (wisdom tooth). There may be a bad taste caused by pus oozing from the area. The pain is usually quite intense and may radiate to the external neck, throat, ear, or oral floor. Occasionally there is trismus (the inability to open the jaws more than a few millimeters) or pain on biting. The site appears red and swollen, with a flap that may reveal a partial tooth eruption beneath it (Fig. 47.1). There may be purulent drainage when the flap is pulled open. There should be no pain on percussion of the tooth.

Even with relatively minor enlargement of the operculum (flap), the third molar region of the mandible can be very painful. Cervical lymphadenopathy, fever, and malaise may be present in advanced cases. In severe cases there can be compromise of the airway.

What to Do

☑ **Irrigate with a weak (2%) hydrogen peroxide solution. Purulent material can be released by placing the catheter tip of the irrigating syringe under the tissue flap overlying the impacted molar.** A syringe with an Angiocath catheter will work well to accomplish this. The patient should not swallow the solution.

☑ **Prescribe oral analgesics for comfort.**

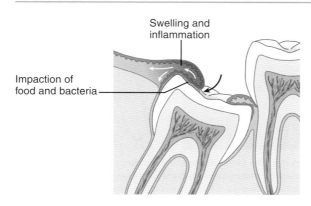

Swelling and inflammation

Impaction of food and bacteria

Fig. 47.1 Mild pericoronitis.

✅ **If the problem is not localized and there is evidence of cellulitis, prescribe amoxicillin 500 mg every 8 hours or penicillin V potassium, 500 mg four times per day.** In penicillin-allergic individuals use erythromycin, azithromycin, or clindamycin. Cefuroxime is also effective in the treatment of acute dental infections.

✅ **Patients with signs of systemic infection, including fever, trismus, lymphadenopathy, deep tissue space infections of the face, difficulty swallowing, or airway compromise, need parenteral antibiotics and immediate consultation with an oral surgeon for extraction of the tooth and drainage of infection** (Figs. 47.2, 47.3, and 47.4).

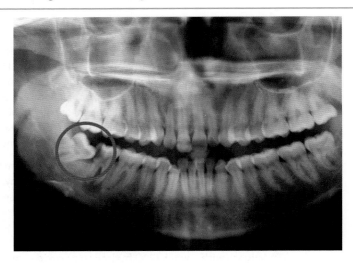

Fig. 47.2 Radiograph showing a full set of 32 permanent teeth. In three quadrants, the third permanent molars (M3s) have erupted into a normal position. The lower right M3 *(circled)* became impacted into the adjacent second permanent molar, which as a consequence has suffered extensive dental caries *(the radiolucent area in the crown of the tooth)* resulting in a dental abscess *(the radiolucent area around the apices of the roots of the tooth).* (With permission from Renton, T., & Wilson, N. H. [2016]. Problems with erupting wisdom teeth: Signs, symptoms, and management. *British Journal of General Practice, 66*[649], e606–e608.)

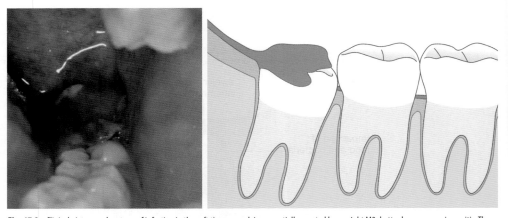

Fig. 47.3 Clinical picture and cartoon of infection in the soft tissues overlying a partially erupted lower right M3, better known as pericoronitis. The white patches in the clinical picture are scarring caused by trauma from the opposing, fully erupted upper left M3. (With permission from Renton, T., & Wilson, N. H. [2016]. Problems with erupting wisdom teeth: Signs, symptoms, and management. *British Journal of General Practice*, 66[649], e606–e608.)

✅ Instruct the patient regarding the importance of cleansing away any food particles that collect beneath the gingival flap. This can be accomplished simply by using a soft toothbrush or by using water-jet irrigation. Have the patient rinse and swish with a hot, salty mouthwash after meals and at least four times per day. A chlorhexidine-containing mouthwash can also be used.

✅ **A follow-up visit with a dentist should be arranged** so that the resolution of the acute infection can be observed. In addition, the patient can be evaluated to see if symptomatic treatment can suffice until eruption is complete or if surgical therapy to remove the overlapping gingival tissue (operculectomy) is necessary. Extraction of the underlying wisdom tooth will be considered if it is poorly positioned and does not erupt completely. This method eliminates any future occurrences of a wisdom tooth infection.

What Not to Do

❌ Do not undertake any major blunt dissection while draining pus. This could spread a superficial infection into the deep spaces of the head and neck or follow a deep abscess posteriorly into the carotid sheath.

❌ Do not place analgesic tablets adjacent to the area of inflamed pericoronitis. Analgesic tablets should always be swallowed.

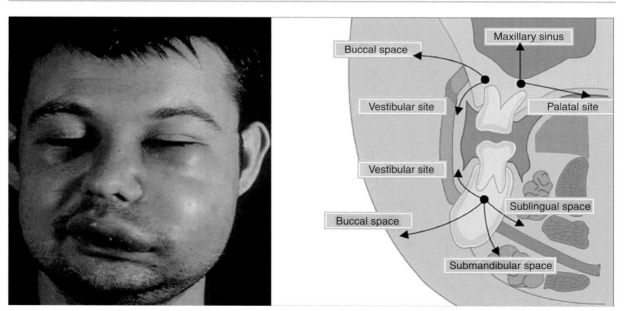

Fig. 47.4   *(Left)* Clinical picture of a patient presenting with acute spreading infection, stemming from a right mandibular M3 pericoronitis. Given the risk of significant morbidity, this patient requires referral to an oral-maxillofacial surgeon for urgent care. *(Right)* Illustration of potential tissue spaces where infection can spread from an M3 pericoronitis. (With permission from Renton, T., & Wilson, N. H. [2016]. Problems with erupting wisdom teeth: Signs, symptoms, and management. *British Journal of General Practice, 66*[649], e606–e608.)

Discussion

Pericoronitis is a special type of acute periodontal abscess that occurs when gingival tissue (gum flap, or operculum) that overlies a partially erupted or impacted tooth (usually a third molar, also known as a wisdom tooth) becomes inflamed. Recurring acute symptoms are usually initiated by trauma inflicted by the opposing tooth or by impaction of food or debris under the flap of tissue that partially covers the erupting tooth.

When dental referral is not readily available, one procedure that can relieve the pain is **surgical removal of the operculum. Inject local anesthetic, such as lidocaine (Xylocaine) 1% with epinephrine, directly into the overlying tissue and then cut it away using the outline of the tooth as a guide for the incision.** Sutures are not required.

There is evidence that periodontal treatment of mandibular third molar teeth may effectively reduce symptoms, whereas tooth extraction seems to be more effective in eliminating recurrences.

Suggested Reading

Douglass, A. B., & Douglass, J. M. (2003). Common dental emergencies. *American Family Physician*, *67*(3), 511–516.

Renton, T., & Wilson, N. H. (2016). Problems with erupting wisdom teeth: Signs, symptoms, and management. *British Journal of General Practice*, *66*(649), e606–e608.

Sasaki, I., Morihana, T., Kaneko, A., et al. (1990). Clinical evaluation of cefuroxime axetil in acute dental infections [in Japanese]. *Japanese Journal of Antibiotics*, *43*, 2035–2068.

Stephens, M. B., Wiedemer, J. P., & Kushner, G. M. (2018). Dental problems in primary care. *American Family Physician*, *98*(11), 654–660.

Yurttutan, M. E., Karaahmetoğlu, Ö., Üçok, C., & Bağış, N. (2020). Comparison of the quality of life of patients with mandibular third molars and mild pericoronitis treated by extraction or by a periodontal approach. *British Journal of Oral and Maxillofacial Surgery*, *58*(2), 179–184.

Dental Pain, Postextraction Alveolar Osteitis

(Dry Socket, Septic Socket, Necrotic Socket, Localized Osteitis)

Presentation

Patients present with severe, dull, throbbing pain 2 to 4 days after a tooth extraction, usually a wisdom tooth in the lower jaw. The pain is often excruciating and continuous; may radiate to the ear, temple, or neck; and is not relieved by oral analgesics. There may be associated foul taste and odor (halitosis). There may also be localized swelling and lymph node involvement. The extraction blood clot is absent from the tooth socket, the bony walls of which are denuded and exquisitely sensitive to even gentle probing.

If untreated, the pain may last weeks to more than 1 month.

What to Do

✓ **Treatment is optimized by first administering an anesthetic nerve block with a long-acting local anesthetic, such as bupivacaine 0.5% or ropivacaine 0.5% (see Appendix D).**

✓ **Irrigate the socket with warm normal saline solution or with 0.12% warmed chlorhexidine and remove all retained debris.**

✓ Pack the socket with 0.25-inch iodoform gauze (soaked in oil of cloves if available).

✓ **An alternative to packing with iodoform gauze is to fill the socket with zinc oxide or dry socket dressing material or other commercially available dry socket paste.** Immediate pain relief can be obtained by mixing this paste with one crushed aspirin and 2 drops of eugenol. This mixture can be inserted with the wooden end of a cotton-tipped applicator. Placing a moistened, folded gauze pad over the site will prevent this material from coming out. Have the patient keep it covered for a few hours.

✓ **One study suggests that 4000 mg per day of vitamin C may be associated with rapid recovery from dry socket.**

✓ **Adequate pain medication should be administered and prescribed for continued pain relief until dental follow-up can be arranged.** Nonsteroidal anti-inflammatory drugs (NSAIDs) are excellent for dental pain and often suffice or can be administered in combination with acetaminophen. Have the patient use ibuprofen, 600 mg (10 mg/kg child max dose 600 mg), and acetaminophen, 1000 mg (15 mg/kg child max dose 1000 mg), every 6 hours. Alternate so the patient is taking one and then the other every 3 hours. Narcotic pain medications are generally not needed for dental pain but can be prescribed for synergistic analgesia if absolutely necessary. Provide a small prescription for five tabs of hydrocodone or oxycodone if necessary to help manage the patient's pain until the follow-up appointment with a dentist.

⊘ Refer the patient back to the dentist for follow-up. The gauze packing should be removed and replaced every 24 hours until symptoms subside. Advise the patient that the dry socket paste will dissolve over the next few days and likely need to be replaced by the dentist at least one more time in most cases.

What Not to Do

⊗ Do not try to create a new clot by creating bleeding. Scraping the socket can implant bacteria in the alveolar bone, setting the stage for osteomyelitis.

⊗ Do not routinely prescribe antibiotics. Despite the lack of evidence to support the use of antibiotics, these are still commonly prescribed for prophylaxis and postoperative purposes despite the potential for negative side effects.

Discussion

Dry socket results from a pathologic process combining loss of the healing blood clot with a localized inflammation (alveolar osteitis). Fibrinolysis produced by bacterial activity may contribute to production of the dry socket.

The condition most commonly occurs with difficult extractions of the mandibular molars, especially third retained molars. This condition may be promoted by smoking, spitting, or drinking through a straw—activities that create negative pressure in the oral cavity. The vasoconstrictive effect of nicotine, poor oral hygiene, and the use of oral contraceptives are also considered significant risk factors.

Topical application of chlorhexidine gel to the surgical wound during the postoperative week may decrease the incidence of aveolar osteitis (AO). Another alternative is perioperative rinsing with 0.12% chlorhexidine. A randomized controlled trial showed that prophylactic

0.2% chlorhexidine gluconate and amoxicillin plus clavulanic acid, when compared with chlorhexidine gluconate alone, demonstrated a significant reduction in AO in patients given combination therapy. In the same trial there was minimal difference between control (saline) and chlorhexidine mouthwash–only groups. Other studies suggest that there is no current evidence base for the administration of prophylactic antibiotics to prevent AO.

The primary aim of dry socket management is pain control until commencement of normal healing. This is facilitated by the use of intraalveolar dressing materials such as iodoform gauze with zinc oxide or commercial dry socket paste. Alvogyl contains butamben (anesthetic), eugenol (analgesic), and iodoform (antimicrobial). Intractable pain usually responds to a nerve block with long-acting local anesthetics.

Suggested Readings

Carvalho, P., Mariano, R., & Okamoto, T. (1997). Treatment of fibrinolytic alveolitis with rifamycin B diethylamide associated with Gelfoam: A histological study. *Brazilian Dental Journal, 8*, 3–8.

Chow, O., Wang, R., Ku, D., & Huang, W. (2020). Alveolar osteitis: A review of current concepts. *Journal of Oral and Maxillofacial Surgery, 78*(8), 1288–1296.

Daly, B., Sharif, M. O., Newton, T., Jones, K., & Worthington, H. V. (2012). Local interventions for the management of alveolar osteitis (dry socket). *Cochrane Database of Systematic Reviews, 12*, CD006968.

Dodson, T. (2013). Prevention and treatment of dry socket. *Evidence Based Dental Practice, 14*(1), 13–14.

Halberstein, R. A., & Abrahnsohn, G. M. (2003). Clinical management and control of alveolalgia ("dry socket") with vitamin C. *American Journal of Dentistry, 16,* 152–154.

Hita-Iglesias, P., Torres-Lagares, D., Flores-Ruiz, R., Magallanes-Abad, N., Basallote-Gonzalez, M., & Gutierrez-Perez, J. L. (2008). Effectiveness of chlorhexidine gel versus chlorhexidine rinse in reducing alveolar osteitis in mandibular third molar surgery. *Journal of Oral and Maxillofacial Surgery, 66*(3), 441–445.

Jesudasan, J. S., Wahab, P. U., & Sekhar, M. R. (2015). Effectiveness of 0.2% chlorhexidine gel and a eugenol-based paste on postoperative alveolar osteitis in patients having third molars extracted: A randomised controlled clinical trial. *British Journal of Oral and Maxillofacial Surgery, 53*(9), 826–830.

Kolokythas, A., Olech, E., & Miloro, M. (2010). Alveolar osteitis: A comprehensive review of concepts and controversies. *International Journal of Dentistry,* 249073 2010.

Supe, N. B., Choudhary, S. H., Yamyar, S. M., Patil, K. S., Choudhary, A. K., & Kadam, V. D. Efficacy of alvogyl (combination of iodoform + butylparaminobenzoate) and zinc oxide eugenol for dry socket. *Annals of Maxillofacial Surgery,* 8(2), 193–199.

Torres-Lagares, D., Serrera-Figallo, M. A., Romero-Ruíz, M. M., et al. (2005). Update on dry socket: A review of the literature (in Spanish). *Medicina Oral, Patología Oral y Cirugía Bucal, 10,* 77–85.

Turner, P. S. (1982). A clinical study of "dry socket. *International Journal of Oral Surgery, 11,* 226–231.

Dental Pain, Pulpitis

Presentation

The patient presents with a sharp, throbbing pain in a tooth. This pain is often worse when the patient is in a recumbent position. This individual may or may not be aware of a cavity in the affected tooth. Initially, the pain is decreased by heat application and increased by cold application, but as the condition progresses, heat application worsens the pain, whereas application of ice dramatically relieves it. (The patient may arrive with their own cup of ice and may not allow examination unless ice can be kept on the tooth.) Oral examination may reveal dental cavities (caries) or an extensive tooth restoration, without facial or gingival swelling.

What to Do

✅ **Reach the appropriate diagnosis by clinical exam:** Obtain a thorough dental history, including location of the offending tooth, when the pain started, intensity and duration of pain, aggravating or alleviating factors (including heat or cold application), and pain description (dull, sharp, throbbing). Look for dental caries, exposed dentin, a deep or defective restoration, or trauma. Confirm there is no cellulitis or facial swelling.

✅ **Adequate pain medication should be administered and prescribed for continued pain relief until dental follow-up can be arranged.** Nonsteroidal anti-inflammatory drugs (NSAIDs) are excellent for dental pain and often suffice or can be administered in combination with acetaminophen. Have the patient use ibuprofen, 600 mg (10 mg/kg child max dose 600 mg), and acetaminophen, 1000 mg (15 mg/kg child max dose 1000 mg) every 6 hours. Alternate so the patient is taking one and then the other every 3 hours. Narcotic pain medications are generally not needed for dental pain but can be prescribed for synergistic analgesia if absolutely necessary. Provide a small prescription for five tabs of hydrocodone or oxycodone if necessary to help manage the patient's pain until the follow-up appointment with a dentist.

✅ **Severe pain may necessitate a nerve block with a long-acting local anesthetic, such as bupivacaine 0.5% or ropivacaine 0.5% (see Appendix D).**

✅ If a cavity is present, insert a small cotton pledget soaked in oil of cloves (eugenol). The cotton should fill the cavity loosely without rising above the opening (where it would strike the opposing tooth). An alternative to eugenol is a perle of benzonatate (Tessalon) opened so that the contents can soak the small cotton pledget. Alternatively, benzonatate perles can be prescribed, and the patient can bite them for repeated topical anesthesia.

✅ **Refer the patient to a dentist for urgent definitive therapy (removal of caries, removal of pulp, or removal of the tooth).**

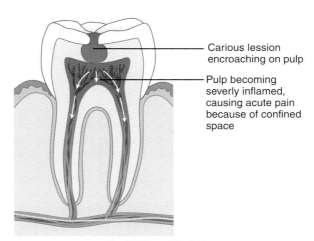

Carious lesion encroaching on pulp

Pulp becoming severly inflamed, causing acute pain because of confined space

Fig. 49.1 Irreversible pulpitis.

What Not to Do

(X) Do not prescribe antibiotics if there are no signs of cellulitis or visible abscess formation.

(X) Do not pack a tooth cavity tightly with eugenol-soaked cotton. If an abscess develops, this cavity may serve as a route for drainage.

Discussion

Pulpitis can be classified as reversible (pain resolves after etiology is removed) or irreversible (pain will not resolve until definitive treatment with root canal, tooth extraction, or pulpotomy). Dental decay presents visually as opaque white areas of enamel with gray undertones or, in more advanced cases, as brownish, discolored cavitations. Caries is initially asymptomatic. Pain does not occur until the decay impinges on the pulp and an inflammatory process develops. Reversible pulpitis is mild inflammation of the tooth pulp caused by caries or defective restorations encroaching on the pulp. Pain is triggered by hot, cold, and sweet stimuli; it lasts for a few seconds; and it resolves spontaneously. Treatment involves removal of the carious tissue and replacement with a dental restoration or filling. Pain should resolve once the etiology is removed.

As the condition progresses from reversible pulpitis to irreversible pulpitis (Fig. 49.1), the patient experiences excruciating pain due to ongoing inflammation causing rapid buildup of fluid and gaseous pressure within the pulp chamber, occlusion of blood vessels at the apical foramen,

ischemia, and ultimately necrosis of the pulp tissue. Heat increases the pressure and pain, whereas cold reduces it. The pain is persistent and is often poorly localized.

Intractable pain usually responds to nerve block techniques with injection of long-acting local anesthetics.

The opioid crisis necessitates that health care providers seek alternatives to opioid (ALTO) pain management strategies, including avoidance of initiation of opioids, limiting prescription amounts, and using a state prescription-monitoring database to inform prescribing practices. Most dental pain can be managed by use of NSAIDs. Ibuprofen can be combined with acetaminophen for a synergistic effect. Dental nerve blocks provide effective long-lasting pain management without the use of opioid pain medications.

The only way to definitively treat the discomfort of irreversible pulpitis is root canal treatment (removal of the pulp and filling of the empty pulp chamber and canal), extraction of the tooth, or pulpotomy.

Discussion continued

Pulpotomy is a minimally invasive procedure whereby the inflamed/diseased pulp tissue is removed from the coronal pulp chamber of the tooth leaving healthy pulp tissue, which is then dressed with a dental biomaterial that maintains pulpal vitality and promotes repair. The procedure can either be partial (whereby 2–3 mm of the coronal pulp is removed) or complete pulpotomy (in which the entire coronal pulp is removed).

Antibiotics are often overprescribed for irreversible pulpitis despite research clearly indicating that antibiotics are not effective for treating the condition or reducing pain. The urgency of referral to a dentist should be determined by the patient's level of discomfort, but examination should not be delayed for more than a few days. **Patients should be warned to return if they develop signs of cellulitis, such as facial swelling, fever, and/or malaise.**

Suggested Readings

Agnihotry, A., Gill, K. S., Stevenson, R. G., Fedorowicz, Z., Kumar, V., Sprakel, J., et al. (2019). Irreversible pulpitis—a source of antibiotic over-prescription? *Brazilian Dental Journal, 30*(4), 374–379.

Cushley, S., Duncan, H. F., Lappin, M. J., Tomson, P. L., Lundy, F. T., Cooper, P., ... El Karim, I. A. Pulpotomy for mature carious teeth with symptoms of irreversible pulpitis: A systematic review. *Journal of Dentistry*, 88, 103158.

Dabuleanu, M. (2013). Pulpitis (reversible/irreversible). *Journal of the Canadian Dental Association, 79*, d90.

Douglass, A. B., & Douglas, J. M. (2003). Common dental emergencies. *American Family Physician, 67*, 511–516.

May, E., & Wilbeck, J. (2019). Dental pain relief in the age of ALTO. *Advanced Emergency Nursing Journal, 41*(3), 229–233.

Nagle, D., Reader, A., Beck, M., & Weaver, J. (2000). Effect of systemic penicillin on pain in untreated irreversible pulpitis. *Oral Surgery, Oral Medicine, Oral Pathology, Oral Radiology & Endodontics, 90*(5), 636–640.

Dental Trauma

(Fracture, Subluxation, and Displacement)

Presentation

After a direct blow to the mouth, a portion of a patient's tooth (most often one of the maxillary incisors) may be broken off, or a tooth may be loosened to a variable degree.

Ellis class I dental fractures (Fig. 50.1) involve only the enamel and are problematic only if a sharp edge remains, which can be filed down with an emery board. These fractures are painless, do not bleed, and can be referred to a dentist for cosmetic repairs. Athletes with only this type of injury may return to play. Ellis class II fractures (Fig. 50.2) expose yellow dentin, which is sensitive to temperature, percussion, and forced air. This type of fracture can become infected and may bleed slightly. Ellis class III fractures (Fig. 50.3) expose pulp that is pink, typically bleed, and are usually painful. Ellis II and III fractures should be covered to help control pain and prevent pulp infection.

A tooth that is either impacted inward or partially avulsed outward is recognizable because its occlusal surface is out of alignment compared with adjacent teeth. There is also usually some hemorrhaging at the gingival margin. If several teeth move together, suspect a fracture of the alveolar ridge. Fig. 50.4 shows normal dental anatomy.

What to Do

⊘ Assess the patient for any associated injuries, such as facial or mandibular fractures. Pay special attention to the temporomandibular joints. Clean and irrigate the mouth to expose all injuries. Touch injured teeth with a tongue depressor or grasp them between gloved fingers to see if they are loose, sensitive, painful, or bleeding.

⊘ **Consider possible locations of any tooth fragments.** Broken tooth fragments may be embedded in the soft tissue, swallowed, or aspirated. Intraoral wounds should be explored for retained dental fragments. **Ultrasonography can be used to detect foreign bodies that may be deeply imbedded and difficult to palpate. A chest radiograph examination can disclose tooth fragments that have been aspirated into the bronchial tree.**

⊘ When there is an open wound, provide tetanus prophylaxis as indicated.

⊘ For uncomplicated **Ellis class I fractures**, the patient can be instructed to file the rough edges with an emery board and to see a dentist for reshaping and polishing the broken tooth or, for larger fractures, providing composite fillings to replace the broken portion.

⊘ **For sensitive Ellis class II fractures with exposed dentin, cover the surface with a calcium hydroxide composition, zinc oxide, tooth varnish (copal ether varnish),**

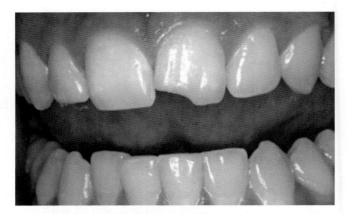

Fig. 50.1 Ellis class I dental fracture. (From Benko, K. [2014]. Dental procedures. In: J. R. Roberts, C. B. Custalow, T. W. Thomson, et al. [Eds.], *Roberts and Hedges' clinical procedures in emergency medicine*. Philadelphia, PA: Elsevier.)

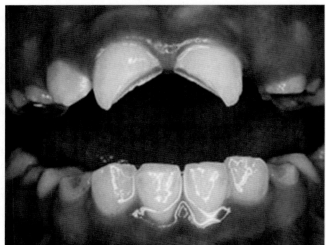

Fig. 50.2 Ellis class II dental fracture. (From Zitelli BJ, McIntire SC, Nowalk AJ, editors: Zitelli and Davis' atlas of pediatric physical diagnosis, ed 6, St. Louis, 2012, Saunders.)

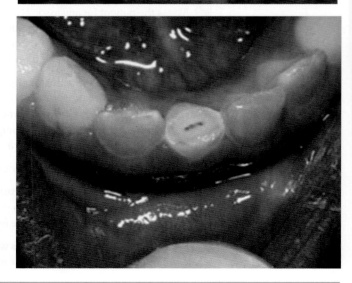

Fig. 50.3 Ellis class III dental fracture. (From Zitelli BJ, McIntire SC, Nowalk AJ, editors: Zitelli and Davis' atlas of pediatric physical diagnosis, ed 6, St. Louis, 2012, Saunders.)

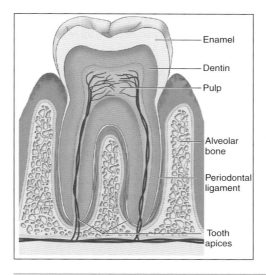

Fig. 50.4 Anatomy of the tooth.

cyanoacrylate (Dermabond), a strip of Stomahesive, or clear nail polish to decrease sensitivity. Younger patients have less dentin; therefore the pulp is closer to the enamel and is at greater risk for injury and infection. Treat these patients aggressively. **Provide nonsteroidal pain medications and acetaminophen,** instruct the patient to avoid hot and cold food or drink, and arrange for follow-up with a dentist the following day. Children should be referred the same day if possible. For a video explaining how to care for dental fractures and apply calcium hydroxide paste, see the following link: https://youtu.be/6iwhdkbNcZM. Another useful video is available at thedentalbox.com: https://youtu.be/m91RDKY4nyE.

⊘ Patients with **Ellis class III fractures exposing pulp should be seen by a dentist immediately (ideally the same day or within 24 hours). The tooth should be cleaned, then calcium hydroxide or moist cotton covered with foil be used as a temporary covering. Alternatively, medical-grade cyanoacrylate (Dermabond) can be placed on the exposed pulp to decrease the risk for infection and reduce the pain of an exposed nerve.**

⊘ **For Ellis II and III fractures, prescribe penicillin V, 500 mg four times a day for 10 days, or amoxicillin, 500 mg three times a day for 7 days. Use clindamycin or erythromycin in penicillin-allergic individuals.**

⊘ Root canal will have to be performed to avoid dental extraction.

⊘ **Bleeding must be controlled and teeth dried prior to application of calcium hydroxide dental cement.** Bleeding can be controlled with the application of pressure with sterile gauze. If simple pressure does not suffice, apply topical tranexamic-soaked gauze (500 mg in 10 mL) to the bleeding site and hold pressure or ask the patient to gently bite down on the gauze.

⊘ **Minimally subluxed (loosened) teeth** may require no emergency treatment other than a soft diet for 1 to 2 weeks and dental follow-up. **Very loose teeth** should be pressed back into their sockets (see Chapter 43) and wired or covered with a temporary periodontal splint (Coe-Pak) for stability for up to 48 hours. The patient should be scheduled for dental follow-up, definitive fixation, and a possible root canal. These patients should be placed on a soft food or liquid diet to prevent further tooth motion. Antibiotic prophylaxis with penicillin should be provided 500 mg four times a day, amoxicillin, 500 mg three times a day, or doxycycline, 100 mg twice a day 1 week.

✅ **Intruded primary teeth and permanent teeth of young patients** can be left alone and allowed to reerupt. Intruded teeth of adolescents and older patients are usually repositioned by an oral surgeon.

✅ **An extruded primary or permanent tooth** can be readily returned to its original position by applying firm pressure with the fingers. Both intrusive and extrusive injuries require early dental follow-up and antibiotic prophylaxis as discussed (see Chapter 43).

✅ **Inform patients that any trauma to teeth can disrupt the blood supply to a tooth and lead to the eventual need for root canal. Recommend a soft diet, no biting on the side of the injured tooth, and urgent follow-up with a dentist.**

What Not to Do

❌ Do not fail to consider or recognize domestic abuse and/or child abuse.

❌ Do not overlook associated injuries of the alveolar ridge, mandible, facial bones, or neck.

❌ Do not use bone wax on complicated crown fractures with exposure of the pulp. It can cause inflammatory reactions.

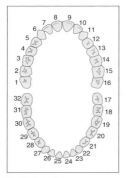

Fig. 50.5 Dental map.

Discussion

Accurately describing the dental anatomy can be very helpful when communicating with a dental consultant. The adult mouth consists of 32 teeth, named from midline to lateral. There is a set of central incisors and lateral incisors, a set of canines (or cuspids), two sets of premolars (or bicuspids), and three sets of permanent molars (first, second, and third molars). The third molars are referred to as wisdom teeth.

Each tooth is assigned a number starting with the right maxillary third molar as number 1, ending with the left maxillary third molar as number 16. The number 17 is assigned to the left mandibular third molar and the number 32 to the right mandibular third molar (Fig. 50.5).

Dentists generally no longer use the Ellis system for classifying dental fractures. These fractures can simply be described as being an uncomplicated enamel fracture, a fracture with exposed dentin, or a complicated crown fracture that involves the pulp of the tooth. Exposure of dentin leads to variable sequelae, depending on the age of the patient. Because it is composed of microtubules, dentin can serve as a conduit for pathogenic microorganisms.

In children, the exposed dentin in an Ellis class II fracture lies nearer the neurovascular pulp and is more likely to lead to a pulp infection. Therefore, in patients younger than 12 years of age, this injury requires a dressing such as a calcium hydroxide composition. Mix a drop of resin and catalyst over the fracture, and consider covering it with dry aluminum foil. When in doubt, consult a dentist. If these fractures are covered quickly, pulpal contamination can be prevented, and subsequent root canal may be avoided.

In older patients with Ellis class II fractures, the previously mentioned treatment may be applied; however, avoidance of hot and cold foods and follow-up with a dentist within 24 hours are usually adequate.

If a temporary periodontal splint or wire is not available to stabilize loose teeth, spread soft wax over palatal and labial tooth surfaces and neighboring teeth as a temporary splint (see Chapter 43 for additional techniques).

Root fractures are clinically difficult to diagnose; patients may notice abnormal mobility and sensitivity to percussion of the tooth.

Suggested Readings

Hammel, J. M., & Fischel, J. (2019). Dental emergencies. *Emergency Medicine Clinics of North America*, *37*(1), 81–93.

Hile, L. M., & Linklater, D. R. (2006). Use of 2-octyl cyanoacrylate for the repair of a fractured molar tooth. *Annals of Emergency Medicine*, *47*, 424–426.

Piccininni, P., Clough, A., Padilla, R., & Piccininni, G. (2017). Dental and orofacial injuries. *Clinics in Sports Medicine*, *36*(2), 369–405.

Gingivitis and Acute Necrotizing Ulcerative Gingivitis

(Trench Mouth)

Presentation

With mild gingivitis, the patient's gums bleed easily and become red and swollen with increased sensitivity. As symptoms worsen, the gums begin to recede and take on a beefy red, inflamed color.

Further progression leads to the most severe periodontal infection, trench mouth, or acute necrotizing ulcerative gingivitis (ANUG).

The patient complains of generalized severe pain of the gums, often with a foul taste or fetid odor (halitosis). The gingiva will appear edematous and red, with a grayish necrotic membrane between the teeth. The gums bleed spontaneously or on gentle touch, and there is loss of gingival tissue, especially the interdental papillae. The teeth will eventually become loose, and the patient may become febrile and show signs of systemic infection with generalized weakness.

What to Do

✅ **For extensive gingival involvement, lymphadenopathy, or systemic signs, prescribe a course of 7 to 10 days of either metronidazole, 500 mg every 8 hours, amoxicillin-clavulanate, 875 mg every 12 hours, or clindamycin, 450 mg orally every 8 hours.**

✅ **For milder cases, instruct the patient to rinse with warm saline every 1–2 hours, floss, and gently brush with sodium bicarbonate toothpaste and an ultrasoft brush.**

✅ **In all cases, have the patient rinse the mouth with an antiseptic solution: Use chlorhexidine 0.12% oral rinse (1 Tbsp), swish and spit four times a day. Half-strength hydrogen peroxide may also be used as a mouth rinse, but caution the patient not to swallow.**

✅ **Have patients avoid tobacco, alcohol, and condiments.**

✅ For comfort, prescribe topical viscous lidocaine 2%. Rinse and spit 1 Tbsp up to four times per day.

✅ **Nonsteroidal anti-inflammatory drugs (NSAIDs) have been shown to speed the resolution of inflammation** when teeth are being cleaned and scaled to remove plaque. With appropriate treatment, patients usually respond dramatically in 48 to 72 hours. Use ibuprofen, 600 mg, up to four times per day if there are no contraindications.

⊘ **For definitive care and the prevention of periodontal disease, refer the patient for dental follow-up. The dentist will remove any dead gum tissue to promote healing and help reduce pain. In severe cases, periodontal surgery may be required to restore gum tissue.**

What Not to Do

⊗ Do not obtain radiographs or diagnostic blood work. Gingivitis is a clinical diagnosis, and special testing is required only if the patient is very ill or not responding to initial therapy or when a more serious underlying disease is suspected.

Discussion

Gingivitis and trench mouth are infections of the gum tissue. The most common type of gingivitis involves the marginal gingiva and is brought on by the accumulation of microbial plaques in persons with inadequate oral hygiene. Eventually, the gingiva separates from the tooth, pockets develop, the periodontal ligaments break down, and, along with alveolar bone destruction, the teeth loosen and eventually fall out. In advanced stages, pseudomembrane slough may occur along the gingiva (Fig. 51.1).

Acute necrotizing ulcerative gingivitis is also known as trench mouth or Vincent angina. This condition is usually seen in those patients who practice very poor oral hygiene, those who are under stress, smokers, malnourished, and the immunocompromised, especially human immunodeficiency virus (HIV)/acquired immunodeficiency syndrome (AIDS). ANUG may be the first clinical sign of HIV infection. The term *trench mouth* was coined in World War I, when ANUG was common among trench-bound soldiers.

ANUG is different from simple gingivitis in that it is an acute infection of the gingiva,

with organisms such as *Prevotella intermedia*, α-hemolytic streptococci, *Actinomyces* species, or any number of different oral spirochetes. Diagnosis is based on the acute clinical presentation with three distinctive characteristics: rapid onset of gingival pain, interdental gingival necrosis, and bleeding, together with the risk factors of poor oral hygiene, malnutrition, and/or immunocompromise. Systemic diseases that may simulate the appearance of ANUG include infectious mononucleosis, leukemia, aplastic anemia, and agranulocytosis. ANUG may be confused with other periodontal infectious disease such as herpetic gingivostomatitis or gonococcal or streptococcal gingivitis.

Treatment of the acute phase of ANUG is focused on stopping the disease process and tissue destruction. Once the acute phase is under control, treatment should focus on any preexisting conditions. Treatment of trench mouth is generally highly effective, and complete healing often occurs in a few weeks. Healing may take longer if the patient's immune system is compromised.

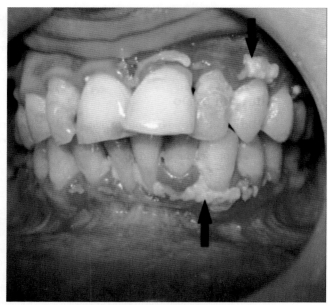

Fig. 51.1 Maxillary and mandibular gingiva showing pseudomembrane slough (black arrows). (With permission from Tanay Chaubal and Ranjeet Bapat; *American Journal of Medicine,* The, 2017-11-01, Volume 130, Issue 11, Pages e493-e494, Copyright © 2017 Elsevier Inc.)

Suggested Readings

Chaubal, T., & Bapat, R. (2017). Trench mouth. *The American Journal of Medicine, 130*(11), e493–e494.

Herrera, D., Alonso, B., de Arriba, L., Santa Cruz, I., Serrano, C., & Sanz, M. (2014). Acute periodontal lesions. *Periodontology 2000, 65*(1), 149–177.

Malek, R., Gharibi, A., Khlil, N., & Kissa, J. (2017). Necrotizing ulcerative gingivitis. *Contemporary Clinical Dentistry, 8*(3), 496–500.

Martos, J., Ahn Pinto, K. V., Feijó Miguelis, T. M., Cavalcanti, M. C., & César Neto, J. B. (2019). Clinical treatment of necrotizing ulcerative gingivitis: A case report with 10-year follow-up. *General Dentistry, 67*(3), 62–65.

Lacerations of the Mouth

Presentation

Because of the rich vascularity of the soft tissues of the mouth, impact injuries often lead to dramatic hemorrhages that bring patients with relatively trivial lacerations to the emergency department (ED) and other health care facilities. Blunt trauma to the face can cause secondary lacerations of the lips, frenulum, buccal mucosa, gingiva, and tongue. Active bleeding has often stopped by the time a patient with a minor laceration has reached the clinic or ED.

What to Do

Provide appropriate tetanus prophylaxis (see Appendix G), and check for associated injuries, such as loose teeth and mandibular or facial fractures. Crushed ice wrapped in clean gauze and held inside the cheek may help limit swelling, bleeding, and discomfort.

If dental fractures or avulsions are present, explore wounds thoroughly with a gloved finger, looking for a dental fragment within the wound. **In deep wounds or whenever there is the question of a retained foreign body, obtain radiographs or perform ultrasonography.** Ideally, all missing teeth or dental fragments should be accounted for (see Chapter 50).

When only small lacerations (<2 cm) are present or only minimal gaping of the wound occurs, only reassurance and simple aftercare are required. Inform the patient that the wound will become somewhat uncomfortable over the next 48 hours, and **instruct the patient to rinse with lukewarm water or half-strength hydrogen peroxide for several days after meals and every 1 to 2 hours while awake. Have them follow a bland diet. Patients may rinse with chlorhexidine 0.12% oral rinse, swished in mouth for 30 seconds and spit out four times daily.**

If there is continued bleeding, **if the wound edges fall between chewing surfaces, if the wound edges gape significantly (especially on the edge of the tongue), or if there is a flap or deformity when the underlying musculature contracts, the wound should be anesthetized using lidocaine with epinephrine, cleansed thoroughly with saline, and loosely approximated using a 5-0 or 6-0 absorbable suture.**

Most tongue lacerations heal well without suturing. The decision of whether to repair tongue lacerations depends on the estimated risk of compromised function after healing. Lacerations that should be considered for repair include large lacerations (>1 cm in length) that extend into or pass through the muscular layers of the tongue, deep lacerations on the lateral border of the tongue, gaping lacerations or those with large flaps, or lacerations that may cause dysfunction if healed improperly (anterior split tongue). Tongue lacerations that do not need repair include those less than 2 cm in length, nongaping lacerations, or lacerations assessed to be clinically minor.

✓ Consider using procedural sedation and analgesia when suturing children who cannot cooperate (see Appendix E).

✓ A traction stitch or special rubber-tipped clamp can be very helpful when attempting to suture the tongue of a small child or an intoxicated adult (Fig. 52.1). The same aftercare as described earlier applies here as well.

✓ **When the exterior surface of the lip is lacerated, any separation of the underlying musculature must be repaired with buried absorbable sutures.**

✓ **To avoid an unsightly scar when the lip heals, precise skin approximation is very important. First, approximate the vermilion border, making this the key suture** (Fig. 52.2). (See Video 52.1) Fine, nonabsorbable suture material (e.g., 6-0 nylon or Prolene) is most appropriate for the skin surfaces of the lip, whereas a fine absorbable suture (e.g., 6-0 Dexon or Vicryl) is acceptable for use on the mucosa and vermilion.

✓ Although in most cases of minor lacerations antibiotics are not indicated, **for deep lacerations of the mucosa or lip or for any sutured laceration in the mouth, prescribe prophylactic penicillin (penicillin V potassium, 500 mg three times per day for 3–4 days) to help prevent deep tissue infections. (Erythromycin or clindamycin may be substituted in penicillin-allergic individuals.)**

✓ Recommend acetaminophen or ibuprofen for pain.

✓ **Instruct patient to be reevaluated in 48 hours.**

✓ Recommend that the patient consume only cool liquids and soft foods beginning 4 hours after the repair.

What Not to Do

✗ Do not repair a simple laceration or avulsion of the frenulum of the upper lip. It will heal quite nicely on its own (Fig. 52.3).

✗ Do not use nonabsorbable suture material on the tongue, gingiva, or buccal mucosa. There is no advantage, and suture removal on a small child will be an unpleasant struggle.

✗ Do not overlook domestic abuse or child abuse.

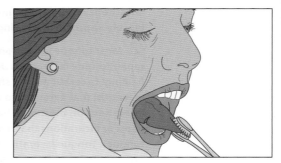

Fig. 52.1 Proper use of a rubber-tipped clamp.

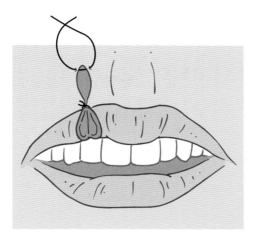

Fig. 52.2 In the repair of lip lacerations, the first stitch should be placed at the vermilion-cutaneous border to obtain proper alignment. (From Grabb, W. C., & Kleinert, H. E. [1980]. *Techniques in surgery: Facial and hand injuries.* Somerville, NJ: Ethicon, Inc.)

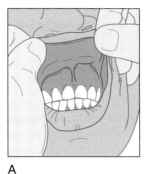

A

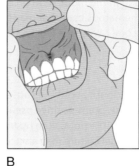

B

Fig. 52.3 Simple laceration or avulsion of the frenulum of the upper lip. (A) Normal frenulum. (B) Lacerated frenulum.

Discussion

Imprecise repair of the vermilion border will lead to a step-off or puckering that is unsightly and difficult to repair later.

Fortunately, the tongue and oral mucosa usually heal with few complicating infections, and there is a low risk for subsequent tissue necrosis.

Suggested Readings

Armstrong, B. D. (2000). Lacerations of the mouth. *Emergency Medicine Clinics of North America, 18*(3), 471–480. https://doi.org/10.1016/S0733-8627(05)70139-5

Grabb, W. C., & Kleinert, H. E. (1980). *Techniques in surgery: Facial and hand injuries.* Somerville, NJ: Ethicon, Inc.

Seiler, M., Massaro, S. L., Staubli, G., & Schiestl, C. (2018). Tongue lacerations in children: To suture or not? *Swiss Medical Weekly, 148.* https://doi.org/10.4414/smw.2018.14683

Oral Candidiasis

(Thrush or Yeast Infection)

Presentation

A parent may present with an infant with white patches in the mouth, or an older patient—classically with either poor oral hygiene, diabetes, a hematologic malignancy, an immunodeficiency, or on antibiotic, cytotoxic, or steroid therapy—may complain of a sore mouth and sensitivity to foods that are spicy or acidic. On physical examination, painless white patches are found in the mouth and on the tongue. The patches wipe off easily with a swab, leaving an erythematous base that may bleed. There also may be intense, dark red inflammation throughout the oral cavity (see Fig. 53.1).

What to Do

✓ If there is any doubt about the cause, confirm the diagnosis by smearing, Gram stain, or microscopy for large, gram-positive pseudohyphae and spores. Mycologic confirmation can be achieved rapidly by 10% potassium hydroxide (KOH preparation) or normal saline microscopic examination. A fungal culture may also confirm the diagnosis but is usually unnecessary and does not distinguish between colonization and true infection.

✓ **Mild cases in infants may be watched without treatment. For topical treatment, prescribe an oral suspension of nystatin 100,000 U/mL; place 1 mL in each cheek for infants and 4 to 6 mL in each cheek for children and adults.** Instruct the patient to gargle and swish the liquid in the mouth as long as possible before swallowing, four times a day, for at least 2 days beyond resolution of symptoms. Nystatin is also available in lozenges of 200,000 U; one or two lozenges can be dissolved in the mouth four to five times daily. Alternatively, for children 3 years and older, prescribe clotrimazole in 10-mg troches to be dissolved slowly in the mouth five times a day for 7 to 14 days. The best time to administer medication is between meals because this allows longer contact time. Nystatin suspension is the least expensive option, more palatable, and possibly more effective. When treating patients with diabetes, remember that nystatin suspension has a high sugar content.

✓ **For adults who do not have immunodeficiency, fluconazole 100 mg per day for 14 days may be a better regimen. A single 200-mg oral dose is effective, but the longer course decreases the risk for recurrence. An acceptable compromise is to give 200 mg on day 1, followed by 100 mg per day for 4 more days.** Itraconazole (Sporanox) suspension (10 mg/mL), 100 to 200 mg daily for 7 days, is as effective as fluconazole.

✓ For immunocompromised patients, prescribe fluconazole, 200 mg on day 1, then 100 mg per day for 14 days.

⊘ **Have patients with removable dental appliances or dentures soak them overnight in any of the commercial denture soaking solutions, or in mouthwashes such as Listerine, or chlorhexidine gluconate (Peridex).** Alternatively, have patients soak them overnight in a nystatin suspension to prevent reinfection with these contaminated objects.

⊘ **Look elsewhere for *Candida* infection** (e.g., esophagitis, intertrigo, vaginitis, diaper rash, angular cheilitis), and treat these conditions appropriately.

⊘ For healthy newborns or infants, reassure the parents about the benign origin and course of this minor superficial yeast infection.

What Not to Do

⊗ Do not overlook diarrhea, rashes (other than diaper rash), failure to thrive, hepatosplenomegaly, or repeated infections that may suggest an underlying immunodeficiency. Beyond infancy, be especially vigilant with patients who have no apparent underlying cause for thrush (e.g., antibiotics, steroids).

Discussion

Oropharyngeal candidiasis or thrush is a local infection commonly found in infants, older individuals with poor oral hygiene or dentures, diabetics, or patients treated with antibiotics, steroids, chemotherapy, or radiation therapy. Thrush can also be found in those with a hematologic malignancy or immunodeficiency, such as human immunodeficiency virus (HIV)/acquired immunodeficiency syndrome (AIDS).

In the healthy newborn, thrush is a self-limited infection, but it usually should be treated to avoid feeding problems. The neonate acquires the yeast from the mother at the time of delivery. Most often, thrush will appear at about 1 week of age; the incidence peaks around the fourth week of life. In infants who fail to respond to treatment with nystatin, oral fluconazole (in age 6 months or older) 6 mg/kg on day 1, followed by 3 mg/kg daily for at least 14 days (may cause nausea/vomiting).

In adults, oral candidiasis can be acute or chronic. The pseudomembranous form is the most common and appears as white plaques on the buccal mucosa, palate, tongue, or the oropharynx. The atrophic form does not have plaques, is more common in adults with dentures, and is known as denture stomatitis. This form of oral candidiasis presents with localized erythema and erosions with minimal white exudate, which may be caused by candidal colonies beneath dentures. Thrush may also present simply as a beefy red tongue.

Thrush may be the first sign of HIV infection (see Fig. 53.1). Maintenance prophylaxis may be required in patients with AIDS who have several recurrences of symptomatic oral candidiasis. After an initial 200-mg dose, fluconazole can be continued at 100 mg per day or given intermittently (200 mg weekly). A recurrence rate of 10% to 20% can be anticipated with intermittent prophylaxis.

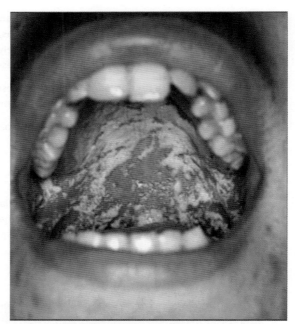

Fig. 53.1 White plaques of oral candidiasis (which can be scraped off to reveal an erythematous base) in an HIV-positive patient. (Reprinted from Peters, J., Green, J., & Hijazi, L. [2018]. Urogenital system. In M. Glynn & W. Drake (Eds.), *Hutchison's clinical methods: An integrated approach to clinical practice* (24th ed., pp. 355–377). Amsterdam, The Netherlands: Elsevier.)

Suggested Readings

Baumgardner, D. J. (2019). Oral fungal microbiota: To thrush and beyond. *Journal of Patient Centered Research and Reviews, 6(4)*, 252–261.

Millsop, J. W., & Fazel, N. (2016). Oral candidiasis. *Clinics in Dermatology, 34*(4), 487–494. ISSN0738-081X. https://doi.org/10.1016/j.clindermatol.2016.02.022.

Vazquez, J. A., & Sobel, J. D. (2002). Mucosal candidiasis. *Infectious Disease Clinics of North America, 16*, 793–820.

Oral Herpes Simplex

(Cold Sore, Fever Blister)

Presentation

Patients present with swelling, burning, or soreness at the vermilion border of the lips followed by the appearance of clusters of small painful vesicles on an erythematous base (Fig. 54.1). The vesicles can rupture to produce red, irregular ulcerations with swollen borders and crusting, which eventually heal without leaving a scar. These lesions can also occur on the hard palate or gingiva. Episodes may recur after exposure to sunlight or emotional or physical stress. The initial episode is usually the worst, with generalized malaise, low-grade fever, tender cervical adenopathy, and occasional exudative pharyngitis lasting 2 to 3 weeks. Recurrences are milder and shorter, with a prodrome of itching or burning at the lesion site. The painful ulcers that eventually form last 7 to 10 days.

What to Do

✓ **If the diagnosis is not clinically apparent,** scrape the base of a vesicle, stain a prepped slide with Wright or Giemsa solution, and examine it for multinucleate giant cells (look for nuclear molding). This is called a Tzanck preparation, and it establishes the diagnosis of herpes. Alternatively, a swab can be sent for viral cultures. When performing a culture, the ulcer base should be swabbed vigorously, because herpes simplex virus (HSV) is an intracellular infection, and adequate cell sampling is required.

✓ **For minor symptoms, docosanol, a topical cream available without a prescription,** started within 12 hours of prodromal symptoms, decreases time to healing by about half a day.

✓ **For moderate-to-severe symptoms, prescribe penciclovir (Denavir) 0.1% cream. Have the patient apply it every 2 waking hours for 4 days.** This treatment has been shown to hasten the resolution of lesions and pain in immunocompetent adults who have recurrent herpes simplex labialis, regardless of whether it is applied early or late in the course of the eruption. Started within 1 hour of papule appearance and applied every 2 hours while awake, it will decrease healing time by approximately 1 day.

✓ **An alternative treatment is oral acyclovir (Zovirax) 400 mg five times per day for 7 days.** This therapy reduces viral shedding, appearance of new lesions, and severity of pain and has been shown to decrease time to healing by 1 day. **A much more convenient regimen with the same efficacy is a single-day course of valacyclovir** (Valtrex) to begin with the first symptoms of herpes labialis (1 g twice on the day of therapy).

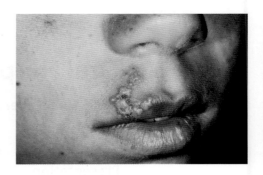

Fig. 54.1 Herpes simplex labialis. (From Bolognia, J., Jorizzo, J., & Rapini, R. [2003]. *Dermatology.* St. Louis, MO: Mosby.)

Treat recurrences early, if possible during the prodrome or at the first sign of the first skin lesion.

For comforting topical treatment, an equal mixture of kaolin-pectin and diphenhydramine elixir can coat and dry the area and reduce pain. By adding an equal part of lidocaine 2% viscous solution, a mouthwash is created that can be swished in the mouth and then expectorated (do every 3–4 hours). **Topical lip salves and application of cold compresses will also relieve the pain.**

Prescribe nonsteroidal anti-inflammatory drugs (NSAIDs) for discomfort if there are no contraindications.

Instruct the patient to keep lesions clean and to avoid touching them, which will prevent spreading the virus to the eyes, unaffected skin, and other people. Instruct the patient about the benefits of thorough hand washing. **The patient should avoid oral and other close contact while lesions are apparent.**

Inform the patient that oral herpes need not be related to genital herpes and that the vesicles and pain should resolve over about 2 weeks. Advise the patient about being infectious during this period (and perhaps at other times as well), and that the HSV, residing in sensory ganglia, can be expected to cause recurrences from time to time, especially during periods of illness or stress. If more than six outbreaks occur a year, the patient should discuss prophylaxis with a primary care provider.

What Not to Do

Do not prescribe topical acyclovir or corticosteroids, as they are ineffective.

Do not use topical anesthetics on keratinized skin. They are effective only on oral mucosa and lip vermilion.

Discussion

In most cases, herpes labialis is caused by herpes simplex virus type 1 (HSV-1). Primary herpes usually appears as gingivostomatitis (Fig. 54.2), pharyngitis, or a combination of the two, whereas recurrent infections usually occur as intraoral or labial ulcers.

Primary infection is acquired mainly by direct person-to-person contact. Health care workers are at particular risk for finger or hand infections (whitlows). Primary infection tends to be a disease of childhood or young adulthood; is more severe than recurring episodes; is preceded by a temperature of up to 105° F, sore throat, and headache; and is followed by red, swollen gums that bleed easily.

This gingivostomatitis may need to be differentiated from herpangina, acute necrotizing ulcerative gingivitis, Stevens-Johnson syndrome, Behçet syndrome, and hand-foot-and-mouth disease. Herpangina is caused by Coxsackievirus group A and involves the posterior pharynx. The intraoral vesicles are 1 to 4 mm and do not extend beyond the soft palate and tonsillar pillars. Acute necrotizing ulcerative gingivitis, also known as Vincent angina or trench mouth, is bacterial in origin, causes characteristic blunting of the interdental gingival papillae, and responds rapidly to treatment with penicillin. Stevens-Johnson syndrome is a severe form of erythema multiforme. In this syndrome, there are characteristic lip lesions, the gingiva is only rarely affected, and there may be bull's-eye skin lesions on the hands and feet. Behçet syndrome is thought to be an autoimmune response and is associated with genital ulcers and inflammatory ocular lesions. Hand-foot-and-mouth disease is also caused by Coxsackievirus group A and is associated with concurrent lesions of the palms and soles. Fifteen percent of these cases present with oral ulceration only, making differentiation from herpes difficult, but tender cervical adenopathy is uncommon in hand-foot-and-mouth disease. Recurrent aphthous stomatitis (RAS) (see Chapter 42) is usually located on the loose mucosal surfaces of lips or buccal mucosa of the cheeks.

Recurrent HSV infection most commonly occurs on the cutaneous lip and vermilion (herpes simplex labialis). Primary infection, unlike recurrent HSV, affects both the keratinized surfaces of the oral mucosa (such as the hard palate and gingiva, where the mucosa is tightly adherent to underlying bone) and the nonkeratinized mucosal surfaces.

Secondary recurrences of cold sores are due to reactivation of latent infection in the trigeminal ganglion. Possible causes of HSV-1 reactivation include stress, fever, infection, fatigue, and exposure to cold or sunlight.

Among immunocompetent patients, HSV infections are usually self-limiting, and reactivation is rapidly controlled by the host's immune system. In the immunocompromised person, however, the reactivated virus might continue to replicate, forming large, slowly expanding, long-lasting ulcerative lesions.

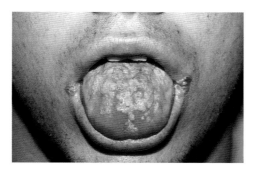

Fig. 54.2 Acute herpes simplex gingivostomatitis in a young adult. (From White, G., & Cox, N. [2006]. *Diseases of the skin* [2nd ed.]. St. Louis, MO: Mosby.)

Suggested Readings

Balasubramaniam, R., Kuperstein, A. S., & Stoopler, E. T. (2014). Update on oral herpes virus infections. *Dental Clinics of North America, 58*(2), 265–280. ISSN0011-8532. https://doi.org/10.1016/j.cden.2013.12.001.

Bruce, A. J., & Rogers, R. S. (2003). Acute oral ulcers. *Dermatology Clinics, 21,* 1–15.

Spruance, S. L., Rea, T. L., Thoming, C., et al. (1997). Penciclovir cream for the treatment of herpes simplex labialis: A randomized, multicenter, double-blind, placebo-controlled trial. *Journal of the American Medical Association, 277,* 1374–1379.

Orthodontic Complications

Presentation

Patients with orthodontic appliances may present after traumatic injury or discomfort in the absence of distinct trauma. There may be bleeding, lacerations, or patient anxiety. Other problems include impacted food, candy, or chewing gum causing gingival infection.

What to Do

✅ Irrigate and cleanse the mouth so that the nature of the problem can be clearly visualized.

✅ **Inject local anesthetic (e.g., lidocaine 1% with epinephrine) into entrapped or punctured mucosa to ease discomfort and allow treatment.**

✅ **Release mucosa from mechanical attachments** by pushing the lip against the teeth and moving it (usually upward) to unhook it. You may have to use a closed hemostat to manipulate the mucosa off of the bent wire or hooked piece of metal.

✅ **Bend any exposed sharp wire end so that it points toward the teeth rather than toward sensitive lips and gums.** Use a hemostat to grasp the wire. If a brace wire has popped out of the bands around the molars, and the grooves (that the wire fits in) are visible, just slide the wire back in place.

✅ **When a sharp wire cannot be moved, cover the point with any soft wax, orthodontic wax, cotton, or sugarless chewing gum.**

✅ A loose band or bracket can generally be left in place until the patient is seen by the orthodontist. If a bracket or wire becomes excessively loose, it can usually be removed with judicious tinkering. If a wire must be cut and small wire cutters are unavailable, try repeatedly bending the appliance until the metal fatigues and breaks.

✅ Treat gingival infections with frequent warm saline rinses and, if severe, with penicillin or erythromycin (see Chapter 51).

✅ For any continued discomfort, recommend over-the-counter (OTC) analgesics.

✅ **Arrange for early orthodontic follow-up and definitive repair. Dental fractures or loosened or avulsed teeth require follow-up by a general dentist** (see Chapters 43 and 50).

What Not to Do

(X) If at all possible, do not cut a protruding wire. This will only create another sharp edge.

(X) Do not administer antibiotics for minor oral abrasions, punctures, or small lacerations.

Discussion

Broken or disturbed appliances are likely to occur from time to time during orthodontic treatment. Fortunately, after orthodontic trauma, the tongue and oral mucosa usually heal with few complicating infections and little tissue necrosis.

Suggested Reading

Thilander BL. Complications of orthodontic treatment. *Curr Opin Dent*. 1992; 2: 28–37. PMID: 1298455.

Perlèche
(Angular Cheilitis)

Presentation

Patients present with inflammation and soreness of the skin and contiguous labial mucous membranes at the angles of the mouth (Fig. 56.1). On examination, there is erythema, fissuring, and maceration of the oral commissures. In severe cases, bleeding can occur when the mouth is opened, and shallow ulcers or a crust may form.

What to Do

✓ Attempt to identify a precipitating cause, and advise corrective action when possible.

✓ **Prescribe topical antifungal cream, such as ketoconazole (Ketozole; Nizoral) 2%, econazole (Ecoza; Spectazole) 1%, or ciclopirox olamine (Loprox; Penlac) 0.77% applied twice per day, followed by a corticosteroid such as triamcinolone (Aristocort; Kenalog) 0.1% cream 15 g.**

✓ Keep the oral commissure dry to decrease the chances of reinfection. Continue the antifungal cream for a few weeks for greatest efficacy.

✓ Treat any associated oral candidiasis with an appropriate oral antimycotic (see Chapter 53).

What Not to Do

✗ Do not use ointments or creams containing neomycin. They are unlikely to be effective and may cause unnecessary contact dermatitis.

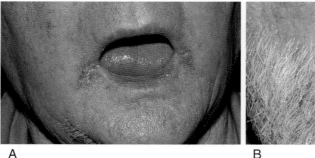
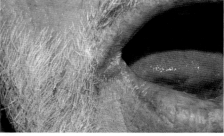

A   B

Fig. 56.1 (A, B) Perlèche. (From White, G., & Cox, N. [2006]. *Diseases of the skin*. St. Louis, MO: Mosby.)

Discussion

Perlèche is associated with the collection of moisture at the corners of the mouth, which encourages invasion by *Candida albicans*, staphylococci, streptococci, and other organisms. The differential diagnosis includes impetigo (see Chapter 174) and herpes simplex (see Chapter 54) infections. Vitamin B2 or zinc deficiency or iron-deficiency anemia can cause perlèche, but this is rare and should not be treated presumptively. Angular cheilitis can also be a sign of anorexia or bulimia secondary to the associated malnutrition and frequent vomiting. Potassium hydroxide (KOH) preparation will confirm a yeast infection. Cheilosis may also be part of a group of symptoms (dysphagia resulting from upper esophageal webs, iron-deficiency anemia, burning mouth syndrome with a shiny red tongue resulting from glossitis) defining the condition called Plummer-Vinson syndrome.

Suggested Readings

Loo, D. S. (2004). Cutaneous fungal infections in the elderly. *Dermatology Clinics*, *22*, 33–50.

Mancini, A. J., & Krowchuk, D. P. (Eds.). (2019). Chéilite angulaire/perlèche. In *Dermatologie de L'enfant* (pp. 220–222, chap. 35A). Issy les Moulineaux Cedex, France: Elsevier Masson. https://doi.org/10.1016/B978-2-294-75852-2.00118-8.

Martin, E. S., & Elewski, B. E. (2002). Cutaneous fungal infections in the elderly. *Clinics in Geriatric Medicine*, *18*, 59–75.

Sialolithiasis

(Salivary Duct Stones)

Presentation

Although most common in men of age 30 to 60 years, patients of any demographic may develop salivary duct stones. Most salivary stones occur in the Wharton duct from the submandibular gland. **The patient typically presents after rapid swelling that suddenly appears beneath the jaw while eating.** The swelling may be painful but is not inflamed and usually subsides within hours. This swelling may be intermittent and may not occur with every meal. Infection can occur, accompanied by increased pain, exquisite tenderness, erythema, and fever. Under these circumstances, pus can sometimes be expressed from the opening of the duct when the gland is pressed (Fig. 57.1).

What to Do

✅ Conservative care is the mainstay of treatment for salivary duct stones. Patients should be advised to stay well hydrated and to apply warm compresses frequently while gently massaging the gland or "milking" the duct. Lemon drops or other hard tart candy (sialogogues, which promote ductal secretions) may help express the stone.

✅ If possible, discontinue anticholinergic medications that may inhibit ductal secretions, such as diphenhydramine or amitriptyline.

✅ Control pain with nonsteroidal anti-inflammatory drugs (NSAIDs) if there are no contraindications.

✅ **Bimanually palpate the course of the salivary duct, feeling for stones.** For the submandibular gland, palpate the floor of the mouth anteriorly to find a stone in the Wharton duct. For the parotid gland, palpate the buccal mucosa around the orifice to the Stensen duct and along the line from the earlobe to the jawline (see Fig. 57.1).

✅ **When a small superficial stone can be felt, anesthetize the tissue beneath the duct and its orifice with a small amount of lidocaine 1% with epinephrine. If available, a punctum dilator can be used to widen the orifice of the blocked duct. Milk the gland and duct with the fingers to express the stone(s).**

✅ **If the stone cannot be palpated, refer the patient to an otolaryngologist for further workup, which may include ultrasonography, sialoendoscopy, computed tomography (CT) imaging, magnetic resonance (MR) sialography, or operative intervention.**

✅ If the patient has pain, swelling, erythema, and purulent discharge expressed from the gland or systemic infectious symptoms, suspect an associated infection (sialadenitis). Initiate

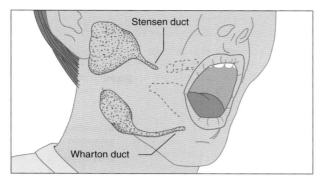

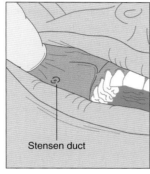

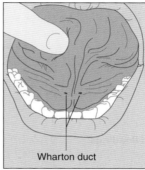

Fig. 57.1 Most salivary duct stones occur in the Wharton duct.

treatment with amoxicillin/clavulanate (Augmentin) 875/125 mg twice per day or clindamycin (Cleocin) 300 mg every 6 hours for 10 days. For the more severe infections (e.g., when there is fever, tachycardia, severe swelling, and pain), consider hospitalization for administration of intravenous (IV) antibiotics.

What Not to Do

Ⓧ Do not attempt to dilate a salivary duct if the patient has a suspected case of mumps. Acute, persistent pain and swelling of the parotid gland along with inflammation of the papilla of the Stensen duct, fever, lymphocytosis, hyperamylasemia, and malaise should raise suspicion for mumps or other viruses that may cause sialadenitis.

Ⓧ Do not obtain sialography with acute infection. Injection of dye into an acutely inflamed gland may push the infection outside the gland capsule and into the surrounding soft tissues.

Discussion

Sialolithiasis is the most common disorder of the salivary glands and may range from tiny particles to stones that are several centimeters in length. Salivary duct stones are generally composed of calcium phosphate and hydroxyapatite. Uric acid stones may form in patients with gout. Although the majority (approximately 92%) form in the Wharton duct arising from the medial surface of the submandibular glands in the floor of the mouth, others occur in the Stensen duct (which arises from the anterior border of the parotid gland) in the cheek, and 1% to 2% occur in the sublingual ducts. The exact cause of stone formation is unclear. Secretion of saliva rich in calcium in the setting of partial obstruction of the duct caused by local inflammation, foreign body, or ductal injury may promote stone formation. Dehydration, anticholinergic medications, and trauma may also contribute to salivary duct stones. Depending on the location and the size of the stone, the presenting symptoms vary. Although most salivary stones are asymptomatic or cause minimal discomfort, larger stones may interfere with the flow of saliva and may cause pain and swelling. **As a rule, the onset of swelling is sudden and associated with salivation during a meal.**

The differential diagnosis for sialolithiasis includes other disease processes that may affect the salivary gland: infections, inflammatory conditions, and neoplastic and nonneoplastic masses.

If left untreated, salivary stones can result in chronic sialadenitis and glandular atrophy. Conservative treatment may consist of oral analgesics and antibiotics. Surgical management may include salivary lithotripsy, basket retrieval, and sialoendoscopy.

Suggested Readings

Iwai, T., Sugiyama, S., Hayashi, Y., Oguri, S., Hirota, M., Mitsudo, K., et al. (2017). Sialendoscopic removal of fish bone-induced sialoliths in the duct of the submandibular gland. *Auris Nasus Larynx*, *45*(2), 343–345.

Knight, J. (2004). Diagnosis and treatment of sialolithiasis. *Irish Medical Journal*, *97*, 314–315.

Saliva: Secretion and functions. A. J. M. Ligtenberg, & E. C. I. Veerman (Eds.). (2014). *Monographs in Oral Science*, *24*, 135–148. https://doi.org/10.1159/000358794

Temporomandibular Disorder

Presentation

Patients usually complain of poorly localized facial pain or headache that does not appear to conform to a strict anatomic distribution. The pain is generally dull and unilateral, centered in the temple above and behind the eye, and in and around the ear. The pain may be associated with mastication and passive movement of the mandible, instability of the temporomandibular joint (TMJ), crepitus, or clicking with movement of the jaw. It is often described as an earache.

Other, less obvious symptoms include radiation of pain down the carotid sheath, tinnitus, dizziness, decreased hearing, itching, sinus symptoms, a foreign-body sensation in the external ear canal, and trigeminal, occipital, and glossopharyngeal neuralgias.

Patients may have been previously diagnosed with migraine headaches, sinusitis, or recurrent external otitis. Predisposing factors include malocclusion, trauma, recent extensive dental work, or a habit of grinding the teeth (bruxism), all of which put unusual stress on the TMJ.

Clinical signs include tenderness of the chewing muscles, the ear canal, or the joint itself; restricted opening of the jaw or lateral deviation on opening; and a normal neurologic examination.

What to Do

✅ The patient should be asked about TMJ pain with jaw motion, such as chewing or yawning. Determine if there is a history of jaw trauma or involvement of other joints (which may be indicative of an underlying rheumatologic disorder).

✅ Examine the head thoroughly for other causes of the pain, including assessment of visual acuity, examination of the cranial nerves, and palpation of the scalp muscles and the temporal arteries.

✅ The TMJ examination should focus on the joint and the muscles of mastication, with careful attention to whether palpation can reproduce the patient's pain. While firmly palpating the preauricular area, ask the patient to repeatedly open and close the mouth. This maneuver will be painful if the TMJ is the source of the pain. Intraoral palpation of the pterygoid muscles allows evaluation of spasm and tenderness of the muscle. The mandible can be distracted laterally by the patient to assess for pain during range of motion of the TMJ. Crepitus or a "click" may be heard or palpated with movement of the mandible. One should note, however, that given the prevalence of TMJ crepitus, the presence of these findings does not necessarily implicate the TMJ as the cause of the patient's symptoms.

✅ Muscular trigger points that reproduce or intensify the patient's pain on firm palpation indicate a myofascial origin. Look for signs of bruxism, such as ground-down teeth, and percuss the teeth to possibly elicit dental pain as the source of the patient's discomfort.

✅ If the patient has a headache, perform a complete neurologic examination, including fundoscopy. If the temporal artery is tender, swollen, or inflamed, send bloodwork for an erythrocyte sedimentation rate (see Chapters 6 and 9).

✅ Complete evaluation of TMJ disorders, in addition to a thorough physical examination, includes panoramic or plain radiographs and can include magnetic resonance imaging (MRI) studies. These **imaging studies can be deferred until it is clear that symptoms are not resolving after 3 to 4 weeks of conservative therapy.**

✅ **If the pain is severe and clearly isolated to the joint, try an injection into the TMJ, just anterior to the tragus** (Fig. 58.1)**, with 1 to 2 mL of plain lidocaine 1% (Xylocaine) or bupivacaine 0.5%. If symptoms have been prolonged, add 10 mg of methylprednisolone (Depo-Medrol).**

✅ Explain to the patient the pathophysiology of the syndrome, including how many different symptoms may be produced by inflammation at one joint and how TMJ pain is not necessarily related to arthritis at other joints.

✅ **Prescribe anti-inflammatory analgesics (e.g., ibuprofen, naproxen), a soft diet, and application of heat or ice.**

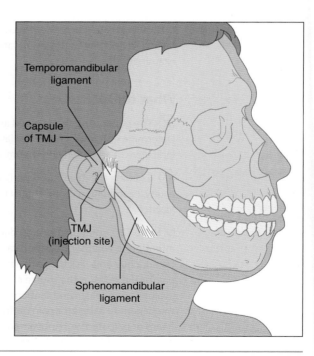

Fig. 58.1 Proper temporomandibular joint *(TMJ)* injection site.

Have the patient avoid extreme jaw movements as well as chewing unnecessarily.

✓ If the symptoms do not clear after 2 to 4 weeks, the patient should follow up with a dentist for possible correction of dental malocclusion or an otolaryngologist. Long-term treatments include orthodontic correction, physical therapy, and (sometimes) psychotherapy and treatment with antidepressants. Surgical intervention should be a last resort. Earlier follow-up should be provided if symptoms dramatically worsen or change.

What Not to Do

✗ Do not rule out TMJ arthritis simply because the joint is not tender on examination. This syndrome typically fluctuates, and the diagnosis is often made based on the history alone.

✗ Do not omit examining the TMJ in the workup of any headache or earache.

✗ Do not administer narcotics.

Discussion

Painful disorders of the TMJ involve the trigeminal nerve. Other areas innervated by the trigeminal nerve help explain referred pain from the TMJ. Included are the dura mater, orbit, paranasal sinuses, tympanic membrane, and oral cavity and teeth, which help explain headaches, eye pain, sinus pressure, otalgia, and dental pain, respectively.

The muscles of mastication are abductors (jaw-opening muscles) and adductors (jaw-closing muscles). The temporalis, masseter, and medial pterygoids are adductors; the lateral pterygoids are the primary abductors of the jaw.

The relative causative roles of abnormal joint anatomy, poor dentition, unsatisfactory occlusion, bruxism, dysfunction of the masticatory muscles, and emotional disorders remain controversial. To stress the role played by muscles, it has been suggested that the term *myofascial pain dysfunction syndrome* is more accurate than the term *TMJ arthritis*. Both these terms, as well as TMJ syndrome, are now considered to be outdated. The term *temporomandibular joint disorder* (TMD)

is an umbrella term that combines a true disorder of the TMJ with involvement of the muscles of mastication. There is also much debate as to the indications for and the efficacy of treatment modalities aimed at these presumed causes. At the least, irreversible treatments such as surgery should be replaced by more conservative therapy.

In the emergency department or urgent care clinic, the diagnosis of TMJ pain is often suspected but seldom made definitively. It can be gratifying, however, to see patients with a myriad of seemingly unrelated symptoms respond dramatically after only conservative measures and advice are offered.

It is worth noting that a study of approximately 450 patients with TMJ pain demonstrated otalgia to be the presenting complaint in 48%. In this study, the TMD (and hence otalgia) was successfully managed with conservative therapies such as heat, massage, patient education, occlusal splints, and pain control.

Suggested Readings

Guralnick, W., Kaban, L. B., & Merrill, R. G. (1978). Temporomandibular joint afflictions. *New England Journal of Medicine*, *299*, 123–128.

Seedorf, H., & Jüde, H. D. (2006). Otalgia as a result of certain temporomandibular joint disorders [article in German]. *Laryngo-Rhino-Otologie*, *85*, 327–332.

Shah, R. K., & Blevins, N. H. (2003). Otalgia. *Otolaryngology Clinics of North America*, *36*, 1137–1151.

Stepan, C. L., & Shaw, S. (2017). Temporomandibular disorder in otolaryngology: Systematic review. *Journal of Laryngology & Otology*, *131*(Suppl. 1), S50–S56. https://doi.org/10.1017/S0022215116009191

Temporomandibular Joint Dislocation

(Jaw Dislocation)

Presentation

Patients present with the inability to close the jaw, usually after yawning, laughing, taking a large bite of food, suffering a traumatic jaw injury, or having a dystonic drug reaction. Such patients have difficulty enunciating clearly. Although they usually have only mild to moderate discomfort, they may have severe pain anterior to the ear. A depression can be seen or felt in the preauricular area, and the jaw may appear to be protruding forward (underbite). If only one side is dislocated, the mandible appears tilted and lies lower on the affected side.

What to Do

✓ If there was no trauma (and especially if the patient's jaw is dislocated often), attempt reduction immediately before muscle spasm around the joint makes the reduction more difficult. If there is any possibility of an associated fracture, obtain radiographs first. A history of trauma and/or excessive pain and tenderness are suggestive of an underlying fracture.

✓ **When the possibility of a fracture has been ruled out, first try two simple reduction techniques:**

   ○ **The gag reflex method: Stimulate the back of the tongue with a tongue blade to cause a gag reflex; muscle relaxation occurs, and the mandible descends caudally so that the condyle moves inferiorly and relocates back into place.**

   ○ **The syringe technique: With the patient seated, depending on how wide the patient can open the mouth, place a 5-mL or 10-mL syringe between the posterior upper and lower molars on the dislocated side. Instruct the patient to then bite down on the syringe and role the syringe back and forth between the teeth. The gliding action moves the mandible posteriorly and the displaced condyle is allowed to slide back into its normal position. In bilateral dislocations, reducing one side will spontaneously reduce the other.**

✓ If these techniques are unsuccessful, **have the patient sit on a low stool, with back and head braced against something firm, either against the wall (facing you) or, as most clinicians prefer, against your body (facing away from you).**

✓ **With gloved hands, wrap your thumbs in gauze, place them on the lower molars, grasp both sides of the mandible, lock your elbows, and, bending from the waist, exert slow, steady pressure downward and posteriorly. The mandible should be at or below the level of your forearm** (Fig. 59.1).

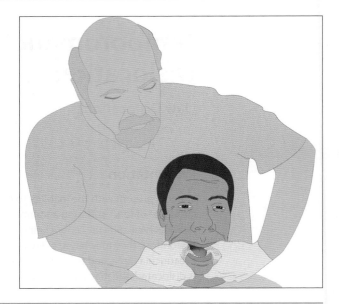

Fig. 59.1 Dislocation reduction of the jaw.

✅ **In a bilateral dislocation, attempt to reduce one side at a time. This helps to reduce the risk for an inadvertent bite to your thumbs. Use of a bite block may also help to prevent being bitten.**

✅ **Successful reduction is usually evident with the sensation of a palpable "clunk." The teeth will again be able to close easily without malocclusion.**

✅ If the jaw does not relocate easily or convincingly, it may be necessary to reassess the dislocation with radiographs and to reattempt relocation using intravenous (IV) midazolam to overcome the muscle spasm and 1 to 2 mL of intraarticular 1% lidocaine to overcome the pain. Inject the lidocaine directly into the palpable depression left by the displaced condyle. If you are still unsuccessful, consider using procedural sedation and analgesia, using your institution's standard protocols (see Appendix E).

✅ **A wrist pivot method for temporomandibular joint (TMJ) reduction has been described and may be more effective than the traditional techniques described earlier.** While the examiner is facing the patient, who is sitting on a high surface, the mandible is grasped with the clinician's thumbs at the apex of the mentum and fingers on the occlusal surface of the inferior molars (Fig. 59.2). Cephalad force is then applied with the thumbs and caudad pressure with the fingers while pivoting at the wrists until the mandible is reduced.

✅ Recommend a soft food diet for several days, and instruct the patient to refrain from opening the mouth widely over the next 24 hours.

✅ All patients should be referred for follow-up by an appropriate specialist (i.e., oral and maxillofacial surgeon).

✅ If reduction cannot be accomplished using the aforementioned techniques, consult oral-maxillofacial or otolaryngology.

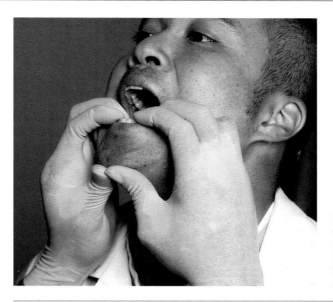

Fig. 59.2 The wrist pivot method for temporomandibular joint dislocation reduction. (From Lowery, L. E., Beeson, M. S., & Lurn, K. K. [2004]. The wrist pivot method, a novel technique for temporomandibular joint reduction. *Journal of Emergency Medicine, 27*, 167–170.)

What Not to Do

⊗ Be careful to not be bitten when the jaw snaps back into position. Maintain firm, steady traction, protect the thumbs with gauze, and consider using a bite block.

⊗ Do not apply pressure to oral prostheses, which could cause them to break.

⊗ Do not overlook associated injuries if trauma is involved.

⊗ Do not try to force the patient's jaw shut.

Discussion

Certain patients with a congenitally shallow mandibular fossa or underdeveloped condyle are predisposed to mandibular dislocation. Most cases of dislocation occur spontaneously without direct trauma.

The mandible usually dislocates anteriorly and subluxes when the jaw is opened wide. Dislocation is often a recurring problem (avoided by limiting motion) and is associated with TMJ dysfunction. If dislocation is not obvious, consider other possible conditions such as fracture, hemarthrosis, closed lock of the joint meniscus, and myofascial pain.

Suggested Readings

Gorchynski, J., Karabidian, E., & Sanchez, M. (2014). The "syringe" technique: A hands-free approach for the reduction of acute nontraumatic temporomandibular dislocations in the emergency department. *Journal of Emergency Medicine, 47*(6), 676–681.

Liddell, A., & Perez, D. E. (2015). Temporomandibular joint dislocation. *Oral and Maxillofacial Surgery Clinics of North America, 27*(1), 125–136. ISSN1042-3699. https://doi.org/10.1016/j.coms.2014.09.009.

Lowery, L. E., Beeson, M. S., & Lurn, K. K. (2004). The wrist pivot method: A novel technique for temporomandibular joint reduction. *Journal of Emergency Medicine, 27*, 167–170.

Luyk, N. H., & Larsen, P. E. (1989). The diagnosis and treatment of the dislocated mandible. *American Journal of Emergency Medicine, 7*, 329–335.

Uvular Edema, Acute

Presentation

The patient presents with a foreign-body sensation or a fullness or lump in the throat, possibly associated with a slightly muffled voice and gagging. Often patients have seen their swollen uvula after looking in a mirror. On examination of the throat, the uvula is boggy, swollen, pale, and somewhat translucent and gelatinous appearing (uvular hydrops). If greatly enlarged, the uvula might rest on the tongue and move in and out with respiration. There should be no associated rash or pruritus, soreness, fever, dyspnea, or other areas of edematous involvement, such as the tongue, sublingual region, soft palate, and tonsils.

What to Do

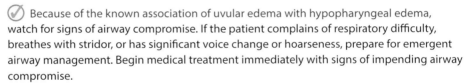 Because of the known association of uvular edema with hypopharyngeal edema, watch for signs of airway compromise. If the patient complains of respiratory difficulty, breathes with stridor, or has significant voice change or hoarseness, prepare for emergent airway management. Begin medical treatment immediately with signs of impending airway compromise.

✓ If there is no acute respiratory difficulty, ask the patient about precipitating events. **Consider foods, medications, physical agents, trauma, inhalants, insect bites, and hereditary angioneurotic edema,** although most of the time the cause remains unidentified.

✓ **When fever, sore throat, and pharyngeal injection are present,** test the throat for streptococcus.

✓ **If there is general pruritus, urticaria, flushing, or facial edema, and an allergic reaction is suspected, the patient should receive parenteral antihistamines, such as diphenhydramine (Benadryl) 50 mg intravenously (IV). H_2 blockers such as famotidine (Pepcid) 20 mg IV over 2 minutes can also be given.**

✓ **For more severe cases, give epinephrine, 0.3 mL of 1:1000 subcutaneously (SC) every 20 minutes for up to three doses. Nebulized isomeric or racemic epinephrine is also effective. Topical application of a vasoconstrictor, such as cocaine gel, works very well.**

✓ **Parenteral corticosteroids, such as methylprednisolone 125 mg IV, are also typically used.**

✅ When symptoms are mild and there is no clear cause (**idiopathic isolated uvular edema**), it is reasonable to provide the same treatment as one would give for an allergic reaction, although it is unclear whether this will bring about any diminution of the patient's uvular swelling.

✅ **If the patient is on an angiotensin-converting enzyme (ACE) inhibitor, use of that medication should be discontinued, and therapy with an alternative antihypertensive should begin.** The patient will more likely have swelling of the tongue or lips and should be held for several hours of observation. Hospital admission should be considered if the swelling worsens. **Airway compromise can occur rapidly and unpredictably when it is secondary to ACE inhibitor administration, and standard treatments are usually ineffective.** Pronounced edema of the tongue and floor of the mouth are predictors of a need for airway intervention.

✅ Eight patients with acute ACE inhibitor–induced angioedema, in a case series, were successfully treated with a single SC injection of icatibant (Firazyr) 30mg SC. This small series showed complete relief of symptoms at 4.4 hours (standard deviation [SD] 0.8 hour), with the first symptom improvement occurring at a mean time of 50.6 minutes (SD 21 min). There were no adverse effects, except erythema occurring at the injection site. The external validity of these impressive results still needs to be confirmed in a prospective, randomized, controlled clinical trial.

✅ If the patient has a history of recurrent episodes of edema, and there is a family history of the same, consider ordering tests to determine the C4 complement level or the C1 esterase inhibitor level to screen for hereditary angioedema. In this condition, the edema often involves the uvula and soft palate together. This is a rare condition that also does not respond to standard therapy but can be treated with C1 esterase inhibitor administered IV or with icatibant as noted above.

✅ **All patients should be observed for an adequate period of time to ensure that there is either improvement or no further increase in the swelling before being sent home.** When discharged, the patient with an allergic or idiopathic cause for the edema should be given a supply (4–5 days) of H_1 and H_2 blockers and steroids if required.

What Not to Do

❌ Do not perform a comprehensive laboratory evaluation on every patient. Order only those specific tests that are clearly indicated and will provide results that can be followed up.

❌ Do not obtain lateral soft tissue neck radiographs on patients with acute spontaneous uvular edema who are asymptomatic other than for the sensation of a lump in the throat.

Discussion

The uvula (Latin for "little grape") is a small, conical, peduncular process hanging from the middle of the lower border of the soft palate. The soft palate is composed of muscle, connective tissue, and mucous membrane, and the bulk of the uvula consists of glandular tissue with diffuse muscle fibers interspersed throughout. During the acts of deglutition and phonation, the uvula and soft palate are directed upward, thereby walling off the nasal cavity from the pharynx. During swallowing, this prevents ingested substances from entering the nasal cavity.

(continued)

Discussion continued

Most patients who present acutely with isolated angioedema of the uvula have mild symptoms and a benign clinical course with an obscure cause. This idiopathic form of spontaneous swelling of the uvula may or may not be related to other forms of angioedema.

Angioedema, also known as angioneurotic edema or Quincke disease, is defined as a well-localized edematous condition that may variably involve the deeper skin layers, subcutaneous tissues, and mucosal surfaces of the upper respiratory and gastrointestinal tracts.

Immediate hypersensitivity type I reactions, seen with atopic states and specific allergen sensitivities, are the most common causes of angioedema. These reactions involve the interaction of an allergen with IgE antibodies bound to the surface of basophils or mastocytes. Physical agents, including cold, pressure, light, and vibration, or other processes that increase core temperature may also cause edema through the IgE pathway.

Hereditary angioedema, a genetic disorder of the complement system, is characterized by either an absence or a functional deficiency of C1 esterase inhibitor. This absence or deficiency allows unopposed activation of the first component of complement, with subsequent breakdown of its two substrates, the second (C2) and fourth (C4) components of the complement cascade. This process, in the presence of plasmin, generates a vasoactive kinin-like molecule that causes angioedema. Acquired C1 esterase inhibitor deficiency and other complement consumption states have been described in patients with malignancies and immune complex disorders, including serum sickness and vasculitides.

Other causes of angioedema include certain medications and diagnostic agents (e.g., opiates, d-tubocurarine, curare, radiocontrast materials) that have a direct degranulation effect on mast cells and basophils; substances such as aspirin, nonsteroidal anti-inflammatory drugs (NSAIDs), azo dyes, and benzoates that alter the metabolism of arachidonic acid, thus increasing vascular permeability; and ACE inhibitors, implicated presumably by promoting the production of bradykinin.

The known infectious causes of uvulitis include group A streptococci, *Haemophilus influenzae,* and *Streptococcus pneumoniae.* An associated cellulitis may contiguously involve the uvula and the tonsils, posterior pharynx, or epiglottis.

Suggested Readings

Bas, M., Greve, J., Stelter, K., et al. (2010). Therapeutic efficacy of icatibant in angioedema induced by angiotensin-converting enzyme inhibitors: A case series. *Annals of Emergency Medicine, 56,* 278–282.

Chiu, A. G., Newkirk, K. A., Davidson, B. J., et al. (2001). Angiotensin-converting enzyme inhibitor-induced angioedema: A multicenter review and an algorithm for airway management. *Annals of Otology, Rhinology & Laryngology, 110,* 834–840.

Goldberg, R., Lawton, R., Newton, E., et al. (1993). Evaluation and management of acute uvular edema. *Annals of Emergency Medicine, 22,* 251–255.

Gurmen, E. S., Dogan, S., Sert, E., Dikmetas, C., & Hussein, S. (2017). Effect of C1 esterase inhibitor in hereditary angioedema treatment. *American Journal of Emergency Medicine, 35*(6), 942 e5–e6.

Ishoo, E., Shah, U. K., Grillone, G. A., et al. (1999). Predicting airway risk in angioedema: Staging system based on presentation. *Otolaryngology - Head and Neck Surgery, 121,* 263–268.

Kestler, A., & Keyes, L. (2003). Images in clinical medicine. Uvular angioedema (Quincke's disease). *New England Journal of Medicine, 349,* 867.

Neustein, S. M. (2006). Acute uvular edema after regional anesthesia. *Journal of Clinical Anesthesia, 19*(5), 365–366. ISSN0952-8180. https://doi.org/10.1016/j.jclinane.2006.06.009.

Riviello, R. J. (DATE). Otolaryngologic procedures. In *Roberts and Hedges' clinical procedures in emergency medicine and acute care* (pp. 1338–1383, chap. 63). Philadelphia, PA: Elsevier.

PART 5

Pulmonary and Thoracic Emergencies

■ Alison Sullivan ■ Katherine A. Walsh

Bronchitis (Chest Cold), Acute

Presentation

The patient's symptoms generally begin with 1 to 5 days of fever, malaise, and myalgias that are often indistinguishable from other acute upper respiratory tract infections (URIs). With acute bronchitis, the acute phase is followed by a second phase characterized by persistent cough, often accompanied by phlegm production or wheezing. This second phase usually lasts 1 to 3 weeks but may last as long as 2 months in some patients. The cough may produce hoarseness or may be accompanied by difficulty breathing and chest tightness. The patient may be fearful about developing pneumonia, is seeking relief from the symptoms, and is frequently seeking antibiotics that are errantly believed to improve the condition.

The patient's vital signs are within normal limits and they do not appear toxic. They commonly produce sputum, which may be clear, white, yellow, brown, or green, and lung sounds may be clear or reveal rhonchi or wheezes. The presence or absence of purulent sputum is a poor predictor of bacterial infections.

What to Do

⊘ Perform a complete history and physical examination. Document which of the aforementioned signs and symptoms are present, rule out other underlying ailments, and note any sign of bacterial superinfection of the ears, sinuses, pharynx, tonsils, epiglottis, bronchi, or lungs, which might require antibiotics or other therapy. In the absence of significant comorbid conditions or asthma, **the primary objective when evaluating patients who have acute cough illness is to exclude pneumonia.**

⊘ The absence of abnormal vital signs (heart rate >100 beats/min, respiratory rate >24 breaths/min, oral temperature >100.4° F [38° C], hypoxemia), along with the absence of abnormalities on chest examination (focal consolidation [e.g., rales, egophony, fremitus, increased work of breathing]), reduces the likelihood of pneumonia.

⊘ **We recommend against routine antibiotic treatment for acute bronchitis. This practice has no benefit and is potentially harmful.** On the other hand, a Cochrane review concluded that antibiotics may be of some value in subpopulations (e.g., frail elderly patients with other significant medical comorbidities). In addition, the European Respiratory Society/European Society of Clinical Microbiology and Infectious Diseases suggests antibiotics be considered for patients with serious comorbidities (e.g., chronic obstructive pulmonary disease (COPD), cardiac failure, insulin-dependent diabetes). For such patients, amoxicillin or doxycycline is recommended as a first-line agent. If there is a contraindication to first-line agents, a macrolide (e.g., erythromycin, clarithromycin, azithromycin) may be substituted. (See treatment of patients with COPD later.)

✅ **Fever, tachycardia, tachypnea, focal chest pain, or focal abnormalities on chest examination should prompt the ordering of a chest radiograph or performance of bedside thoracic ultrasound.** Consider chest imaging with radiography or ultrasound in all elderly patients, as they may present with atypical manifestations of pneumonia (and without vital sign or examination abnormalities).

✅ **In settings where chest radiography or ultrasound is not readily available, elderly patients with clinical findings consistent with pneumonia may be prescribed antibiotics.**

✅ **Patients who have a cough accompanied by the sudden onset of high fever (>101° F), headache, moderate to severe myalgias, and fatigue with normal chest imaging should be considered to have influenza (or coronavirus, given the local disease incidence).** Laboratory testing to make the diagnosis of influenza in patients not requiring hospital admission is not necessary during an outbreak. Treatment of influenza with antiviral agents has the limited efficacy of reducing duration of illness by 1 day. This effect is only significant if initiated within the first 48 hours. **If symptoms have been present less than 48 hours, consider treating with oseltamivir (Tamiflu) 75 mg twice daily × 5 days (varies by weight in children. For children less than 1 year, 3 mg/kg twice daily, If 1 yr or older, dose varies by child's weight: 15 kg or less, the dose is 30 mg twice a day >15 to 23 kg, the dose is 45 mg twice a day >23 to 40 kg, the dose is 60 mg twice a day >40 kg, the dose is 75 mg twice a day).** In patients younger than 65 years, who are otherwise healthy and not pregnant, treatment is not necessary but may shorten the duration of illness if initiated promptly. For unvaccinated or high-risk vaccinated patients (elderly, children <2 years old, pregnant women, immunosuppressed patients, or those with underlying lung disease), evidence is lacking, but the Centers for Disease Control and Prevention (CDC) advises treatment regardless of time from onset of symptoms.

✅ **Explain the course of the viral illness and the inadvisability of indiscriminate use of antibiotics.** Provide the patient with realistic expectations for the duration of the cough (typically 1–3 weeks) and the ineffectiveness and potential adverse side effects of antibiotics. In addition, inform the patient that the condition could worsen because resistant bacteria may be produced.

✅ Tailor drug treatment to the patient's specific complaint as follows:

○ **For fever, headache, and myalgia in adults, suggest acetaminophen 1 g up to four times per day and ibuprofen 600 mg up to four times per day.**

○ **For bronchitis with suspected bronchospasm (wheeze), treat the cough using inhaled bronchodilators, such as albuterol, two puffs every 4 hours as needed.** A Cochrane review suggested that β_2-agonists may improve symptoms of acute cough in subpopulations of children and adults with airflow restriction (asthma) but found no evidence for benefit otherwise (i.e., in a general population).

✅ **Recommend comforting regimens, such as using a vaporizer in a dry environment and staying hydrated.** Zinc and vitamin C have been shown to be beneficial in reducing the duration and severity of the common cold when taken within 24 hours of onset of symptoms. Hot tea and honey as well as chicken soup can also be recommended as comforting agents.

✓ Parents of children with an acute cough resulting from URI should be advised that there is no meaningful evidence regarding the effectiveness of over-the-counter (OTC) cough preparations, and that the available evidence does not support such treatment. European Respiratory Society/European Society of Clinical Microbiology and Infectious Diseases guidelines recommend against cough suppressants, mucolytics, expectorants, antihistamines, inhaled corticosteroids, and bronchodilators.

✓ Patients with COPD who have an acute bacterial exacerbation of chronic bronchitis (increased sputum volume or purulence and difficulty breathing) are more likely than patients without underlying lung disease to benefit from antibiotic therapy. For mild to moderate disease, either no treatment or doxycycline or trimethoprim/sulfamethoxazole (TMP/SMX) can be prescribed. For severe disease, amoxicillin/clavulanate, azithromycin, or a respiratory quinolone may be given for a period of 3 to 7 days. If the patient is at risk for Pseudomonas (i.e., severe COPD, recent hospitalization, or requiring antibiotics frequently), consider treatment with levofloxacin.

✓ Consider gastroesophageal reflux disease as a possible etiology of new cough, and treat accordingly.

✓ **Arrange for follow-up if symptoms persist for a prolonged period of time or worsen or if new problems such as fever or wheeze develop.**

✓ **Inform patients that a simple cough may persist for as long as 3 weeks.**

What Not to Do

✗ Do not prescribe antibiotics inappropriately. Antibiotics cause frequent side effects, especially of the gastrointestinal tract.

✗ Do not obtain sputum for Gram stains and cultures. These have no clinical usefulness in patients with acute bronchitis.

Discussion

Data from the National Health Interview Survey suggest that 4% to 5% of all adults experience one or more episodes of acute bronchitis each year. More than 90% of acute bronchitis episodes will come to medical attention.

Acute bronchitis is a clinical diagnosis applied to otherwise healthy adults with acute respiratory illness lasting 1 to 3 weeks, with cough as the predominant feature. A **cough lasting longer than 3 weeks** should be considered a persistent or chronic cough, with diagnostic considerations different than those addressed in this chapter.

The underlying pathophysiology of acute bronchitis is hypersensitivity of the tracheobronchial epithelium and airway receptors (reactive airway disease). **Recurrent episodes of acute bronchitis** may suggest underlying asthma, but a workup for asthma should be reserved for patients with a cough that lasts longer than 3 weeks.

In epidemiologic studies, respiratory viruses cause most cases of acute bronchitis. *Mycoplasma pneumoniae* and *Chlamydia pneumoniae* have been recognized as possible bacterial causes of acute bronchitis. In several studies in which these

(continued)

Discussion continued

pathogens were present (as determined by antibody titer or gene amplification), however, treatment with antibiotics appropriate to these pathogens did not change the outcome.

Adults with pertussis generally present with a persistent cough, with a mean duration of 36 to 48 days. The cough is mostly paroxysmal and often disturbs sleep. Choking or vomiting and whooping can be present, more often in children or previously unimmunized adults. The diagnosis is made by swabbing the posterior nasopharynx and sending the specimen for polymerase chain reaction (PCR) testing. Antibiotic therapy does not seem to decrease duration of symptoms for pertussis unless it is initiated within 7 to 10 days of the onset of illness. Macrolide prophylaxis during outbreaks and after intrafamilial contact seems effective, however, and decreases spread of disease.

The societal cost of inappropriate antibiotic use includes the rapid emergence of antibiotic resistance among bacterial pathogens and unnecessary prescription expenditures. On an individual level, a person's risk for carriage and invasive infection with antibiotic-resistant bacteria is associated strongly with previous antibiotic use. There is ongoing research on using serum levels of **procalcitonin** as a surrogate biomarker of bacterial infection to help guide the need for antibiotic therapy in acute bronchitis. Further research is needed before this is incorporated into standard clinical practice.

Evidence suggests that physicians and patients are more likely to believe that antibiotics are appropriate if purulent secretions are present or if the patient is a smoker, despite significant evidence to the contrary. Patients frequently expect to receive antibiotics for uncomplicated acute bronchitis, and patients or parents who expect antibiotics are more likely to receive them. Despite physician concerns about patient expectations, most studies find that satisfaction with care for acute respiratory infections is tied more closely to how much time the physician spent explaining the illness rather than receipt of antibiotics.

Influenza is the most common cause of acute bronchitis, and influenza vaccination is the most effective strategy for preventing influenza illness. Prophylactic treatment for high-risk exposed individuals is indicated. Antiviral agents have limited efficacy in the treatment of influenza, however. Oseltamivir decreases illness duration by approximately 1 day and led to a half-day quicker return to normal activities. The relative proportion of cases caused by each type of influenza virus varies from year to year and is determined best through consultation with local public health agencies. Because each of these therapies is effective only if initiated within the first 48 hours (preferably the first 30 hours) of symptom onset, rapid diagnosis is key. During documented influenza outbreaks, the positive predictive value of clinical diagnosis based on clinical judgment is good (correct approximately 70% of the time) and compares favorably with rapid diagnostic tests for influenza (sensitivities of 63–81%). Diagnosis of influenza in a non-outbreak period is more difficult, and diagnostic testing should be considered.

The effectiveness of **antitussive therapy** seems to depend on the cause of a cough illness. An acute or early cough caused by colds and other URIs does not seem to respond to dextromethorphan. Codeine has a significant side effect profile and should be avoided.

For patients who present with a cough persisting longer than 1 week, pertussis should be considered, as well as bronchial hyperresponsiveness.

Suggested Readings

Aagaard, E., & Gonzales, R. (2004). Management of acute bronchitis in healthy adults. *Infectious Disease Clinics of North America*, *18*, 919–937.

American Lung Association. (2019). *Diagnosing and treating acute bronchitis*. American Lung Association. https://www.lung.org/lung-health-diseases/lung-disease-lookup/bronchitis/symptoms-diagnosis-treatment.

Becker, L. A., Hom, J., Villasis-Keever, M., & van der Wouden, J. C. (2015). Beta2-agonists for acute cough or a clinical diagnosis of acute bronchitis. *Cochrane Database of Systematic Reviews*, *9*, CD001726.

Brent, S., Saint, S., Vittinghoff, E., et al. (1999). Antibiotics in acute bronchitis: A meta-analysis. *The American Journal of Medicine*, *107*, 62–67.

Chavez, M. A., Shams, M., Ellington, L. E., et al. (2014). Lung ultrasound for the diagnosis of pneumonia in adults: A systematic review and meta-analysis. *Respiratory Research*, *15*(1), 50.

Edmonds, M. L. (2002). Antibiotic treatment for acute bronchitis. *Annals of Emergency Medicine*, *40*, 110–112.

Glezen, W. P. (2008). Clinical practice. Prevention and treatment of seasonal influenza. *New England Journal of Medicine*, *359*, 2579–2585.

Gonzales, R., Bartlett, J. G., Besser, R. E., et al. (2001). Principles of appropriate antibiotic use for treatment of uncomplicated acute bronchitis: Background. *Annals of Internal Medicine*, *134*, 521–529.

Hamm, R. M., Hicks, R. J., & Bemben, D. A. (1996). Antibiotics and respiratory infections: Are patients more satisfied when expectations are met? *Journal of Family Practice*, *43*, 56–62.

Kaiser, L., Wat, C., Mills, T., et al. (2003). Impact of oseltamivir treatment on influenza-related lower respiratory tract complications and hospitalizations. *Archives of Internal Medicine*, *163*, 1667–1672.

Knutson, D., & Braun, C. (2002). Diagnosis and management of acute bronchitis. *American Family Physician*, *65*, 2039–2044.

Linder, J. A., & Sim, I. (2002). Antibiotic treatment of acute bronchitis in smokers. *Journal of General Internal Medicine*, *17*, 230–234.

Linder, J. A., & Singer, D. E. (2003). Desire for antibiotics and antibiotic prescribing for adults with upper respiratory tract infections. *Journal of General Internal Medicine*, *18*, 795–801.

Macfarlane, J., Holmes, W., Gard, P., et al. (2002). Providing patient information reduces antibiotic use in acute bronchitis. *BMJ*, *324*, 1–6.

Paul, I. M., Yoder, K. E., Crowell, K. R., et al. (2004). Effect of dextromethorphan, diphenhydramine, and placebo on nocturnal cough and sleep quality for coughing children and their parents. *Pediatrics*, *114*, e85–e90.

Rothberg, M. B., Bellantonio, S., & Rose, D. N. (2003). Management of influenza in adults older than 65 years of age: Cost-effectiveness of rapid testing and antiviral therapy. *Annals of Internal Medicine*, *139*, 321–329.

Singh, M., & Das, R. (2011). Zinc for the common cold. *Cochrane Database of Systematic Reviews*, *2*, CD001364.

Smith, S. M., Schroeder, K., & Fahey, T. (2014). Over-the-counter (OTC) medications for acute cough in children and adults in community settings. *Cochrane Database of Systematic Reviews*, *11*(11), CD001831.

Smucny, J., Becker, L. A., & Glazier, R. (2006). Beta2-agonists for acute bronchitis. *Cochrane Database of Systematic Reviews*, *4*, CD001726.

Snow, V., Mottur-Pilson, C., & Gonzales, R. (2001). Principles of appropriate antibiotic use for treatment of acute bronchitis in adults. *Annals of Internal Medicine*, *134*, 518–520.

Treanor, J. J., Hayden, F. G., Vrooman, P. S., et al. (2000). Efficacy and safety of the oral neuraminidase inhibitor oseltamivir in treating acute influenza. *Journal of the American Medical Association*, *283*, 1016–1024.

Wark, P. (2015). Bronchitis (acute). *BMJ Clinical Evidence*, *1508*. PMID: 26186368.

Wilson, A. A., Crane, L. A., Barrett, P. H., et al. (1999). Public beliefs and use of antibiotics for acute respiratory illness. *Journal of General Internal Medicine*, *14*, 658–662.

Zambon, M., Hays, J., Webster, A., et al. (2001). Diagnosis of influenza in the community: Relationship of clinical diagnosis to confirmed virological, serologic, or molecular detection of influenza. *Archives of Internal Medicine*, *161*, 2116–2122.

Costochondritis and Musculoskeletal Chest Pain

Presentation

Patients, typically younger than age 40, present with a day or more of steady aching with intermittent stabbing chest pain. The pain may follow an episode of minor trauma, a period of frequent coughing, or unusual physical activity or overuse. The symptoms may be localized to the left or right of the sternum and may worsen when the patient takes a deep breath, changes position, twists at the torso, pushes or pulls against resistance, or reaches overhead. There may be associated anxiety about the etiology of the pain, but there is no associated nausea, vomiting, diaphoresis, or dyspnea, and most patients do not have significant cardiac risk factors. The middle anterior costal cartilages (connecting the ribs to the sternum) may be diffusely tender to firm palpation, without swelling or erythema, and exactly matching the patient's complaint. There may be sites other than the sternal borders, such as the anterior ribs, xiphoid process, or thoracic spine that are the source of the patient's pain. The rest of the physical examination is normal, along with normal vital signs that include pulse oximetry.

What to Do

✅ Obtain a thorough history and perform a complete physical examination. Pay special attention to the specific location and character of the pain (e.g., onset, severity, quality, radiation, duration, and whether it is related to strenuous activity, movement, deep breathing, and cough) and associated symptoms (e.g., sensation of a racing heart, palpitations, pallor, syncope or near-syncope, shortness of breath, nausea, vomiting, fever, weight loss, fatigue, diaphoresis, cough, or wheezing). Inquire about any risk factors for pulmonary embolism (PE; e.g., estrogen use, recent surgery, immobilization, malignancy, personal or family history of thromboembolic disease) or about a history of preexisting cardiac risk factors (e.g., family history of early-onset coronary artery disease, smoking, hypertension, diabetes mellitus, obesity, elevated cholesterol levels, or stimulant abuse).

✅ Be attentive to abnormal vital signs, pleural or pericardial rubs, new murmurs and dysrhythmias, single or paradoxic splitting of the second heart sound, new gallops, unilateral leg swelling, asymmetric pulses, and signs of congestive heart failure, which include rales, peripheral edema, and jugular venous distention. Carefully examine the abdomen using deep palpation under the costal margins, looking for signs of intraabdominal tenderness.

✅ **At a minimum, obtain an electrocardiogram (ECG) and have a low threshold for chest radiograph or sonography.** If there is concern for PE, but the patient is low risk, consider applying the PE rule-out criteria (PERC rule: age <50 years, pulse <100, SaO_2 ≥95%, no hemoptysis, no estrogen use, no surgery/trauma requiring hospitalization within 4 weeks, no prior venous thromboembolism [VTE], no unilateral leg swelling) to determine need for D-dimer testing to exclude PE.

✅ If any abnormalities are discovered and there is any suspicion of a pulmonary, cardiac, vascular, or gastrointestinal disorder, begin the appropriate treatment and clinical investigation. **The presence of costochondritis does not exclude the possibility of aortic dissection, myocardial infarction, pericarditis, esophageal or peptic ulcer perforation, PE, pneumomediastinum, pneumothorax, pneumonia, mediastinitis, or pleural effusion. When there is a reasonable possibility of one of these more serious clinical entities to be present, a more complete medical workup is required.**

✅ If there is any suggestion of cardiac, aortic, or serious gastrointestinal or pulmonary disease; if there are complaints of chest tightness or pressure; or if there are significant cardiac risk factors or risk factors for PE, obtain appropriate consultation and strongly consider admission.

✅ **If the ECG and chest radiograph are normal and there is no evidence of other disease (the symptoms are purely musculoskeletal, there are no associated symptoms or significant risk factors, vital signs are normal, and the abnormal physical findings are limited to the chest wall tenderness that mimics their pain), prescribe anti-inflammatory analgesics, have the patient apply heat to ease discomfort, explain the pathophysiology, and reassure the patient that this discomfort usually subsides within 3 weeks. Direct the patient to seek follow-up with a primary care practitioner.**

✅ Exquisite tenderness localized over the xiphoid cartilage may represent the rare condition of xiphoidalgia, which may be treated with a course of nonsteroidal anti-inflammatory drugs (NSAIDs) as described earlier.

✅ Instruct all of these patients to return if they experience any fever, palpitations, lightheadedness, shortness of breath, diaphoresis, change in the character of their pain, or radiation of pain to their arm, shoulder, or jaw.

What Not to Do:

❌ Do not rule out myocardial infarction or acute coronary syndrome, especially in the middle-aged or elderly patient, simply because there is tenderness over the costal cartilage.

Discussion

This local inflammatory process is often related to minor trauma and would not be brought to medical attention so often in the absence of patient anxiety about cardiac disease. Reassuring the patient is important when the diagnosis of costochondritis is evident. This disorder is self-limited, usually resolving within 3 weeks. There may be a low rate of remissions and exacerbations.

Tietze syndrome is a rare variant that is generally less diffuse and is associated with characteristic nonsuppurative painful swelling over the rib cartilages.

Precordial catch syndrome is described as a sharp, needlelike pain that is well localized. The pain usually occurs at rest and has a split-second onset, taking the patient by surprise. Typically, the pain lasts only seconds to minutes, with deep breathing making the pain worse. Patients may sit straight up to help relieve the pain. Physical examination is normal, without reproducible pain. These patients are usually young, of light or medium build, and apparently healthy. It can occur once or twice in some people or several times a day for a number of weeks in others. Patients with these symptoms require only reassurance and a chest x-ray with expiratory view to rule out a spontaneous pneumothorax.

(continued)

Discussion continued

Slipping rib syndrome may cause lower chest and upper abdominal pain because of hypermobility at the anterior ends of lower costal cartilages. The diagnosis is made by eliciting tenderness over the costal margin, as well as by performing the hooking maneuver, which is done by curving the fingers under the costal margin and pulling the ribs forward, thereby eliciting a click that reproduces the patient's pain. Treat with rest and physical therapy.

Chest pain in the pediatric population is most commonly benign, but a careful history and physical examination are critical. If there are any concerning elements in the history (e.g., syncope, dyspnea or pain with exertion, shortness of breath, family history of sudden death), or abnormalities on examination, a workup is indicated. When the history and physical examination reveal a healthy child, routine testing has not been shown to be helpful. An ECG may be useful for providing reassurance, which is the mainstay of therapy in this situation.

In adults, one study showed that almost 3% of patients thought to have noncardiac chest pain had an adverse cardiac event (myocardial infarction, coronary artery bypass graft, death) within 30 days. **It is always the medical practitioner's primary responsibility to consider the most serious etiology of symptoms. Even when the initial impression is that of noncardiac chest pain, if the patient has known coronary artery disease or a history of congestive heart failure, coronary risk factors, weakness, diaphoresis, or chest pain similar to what they may have experienced in a previous acute coronary syndrome event, it may be prudent to pursue a more extensive workup.**

Suggested Readings

Ayloo, A., et al. (2013). Evaluation and treatment of musculoskeletal chest pain. *Primary Care, 40*(4), 863–887.

Boran, M., & Boran, E. (2018). Idiopathic costochondritis and Tietze syndrome: Atypical chest pain syndromes—recurrence rates, treatment modalities, seasonality. *The American Journal of Cardiology, 121*(8), e40.

Fanaroff, A. C., & Rymer, J. A. (2015). Does this patient with chest pain have acute coronary syndrome? The rational clinical examination systematic review. *Journal of the American Medical Association, 314*(18), 1955–1965.

Kline, J. A., & Kabrhel, C. (2015). Emergency evaluation for pulmonary embolism, part 1: Clinical factors that increase risk. *Journal of Emergency Medicine, 48*(6), 771–780.

Miller, C. D., Lindsell, C. J., & Khandelwal, S. (2004). Is the initial diagnostic impression of "noncardiac chest pain" adequate to exclude cardiac disease? *Annals of Emergency Medicine, 44*, 565–574.

Perron, A. D. (2003). Chest pain in athletes. *Clinics in Sports Medicine, 22*, 37–50.

Proulx, A., & Zyrd, T. Costochondritis: Diagnosis and treatment. *American Family Physician, 80*, 617–620.

Thull-Freedman, J. (2010). Evaluation of chest pain in the pediatric patient. *Medical Clinics of North America, 94*(2), 327–347.

Inhalation Injury

(Smoke Inhalation)

Presentation

The patient was trapped in an enclosed space with toxic gases or fumes (e.g., produced by a fire, a leak, evaporation of a solvent, a chemical reaction, or fermentation of silage) and comes to the emergency department or acute care center complaining of coughing, wheezing, shortness of breath, irritated or runny eyes or nose, or skin irritation. More severe symptoms include confusion and narcosis, dizziness, headache, chest pain, nausea, vomiting, and rapidly evolving upper airway obstruction.

Symptoms may develop immediately or after a lag of as much as 1 day. On physical examination, the victim may smell of the agent or be covered with soot or burns. Inflammation of the eyes, nose, mouth, or upper airway may be visible, and pulmonary irritation may be evident in the form of coughing, rhonchi, rales, or wheezing, although these signs may also take up to 1 day to develop.

What to Do

✓ Separate the victim from the toxic agent by removing clothing or washing with soap and water.

✓ **Make sure the victim is breathing adequately, and then add oxygen at 15 L/min through a nonrebreather mask with humidification. Oxygen helps treat most inhalation injuries and is essential in treating carbon monoxide (CO) poisoning.**

✓ **Have a low threshold to check a carboxyhemoglobin (HbCO) level. Carbon monoxide poisoning should be suspected in any patient with smoke inhalation.** Patients present with headache, nausea, vomiting, dizziness, and confusion. Levels above 3% in nonsmokers and 10% in smokers should be treated with 90% to 100% oxygen. This reduces the half-life of HbCO from 4 to 6 hours to 60 to 90 minutes. Otherwise asymptomatic patients can be discharged once their CO levels are less than 5%. For severe disease (neurologic compromise, metabolic acidosis, electrocardiogram [ECG] evidence of myocardial ischemia or dysrhythmias, HbCO >40%, pregnancy with HbCO >15%, or history of coronary artery disease with HbCO >20%), hyperbaric oxygen (HBO) should be considered after consultation with a toxicologist and a hyperbaric center. HBO can reduce the HbCO half-life to 20 to 30 minutes.

✓ **Bronchodilators should be administered by aerosol inhalation when there is any evidence of bronchospasm.**

✅ The clinical course of inhalation injury is dependent on the agent inhaled and the intensity and duration of exposure. Obtain a detailed history to clarify the nature of the exposure: Was there a fire? What was burning? What was the estimated duration of exposure? Was the patient in an open or a closed space? Was the patient disoriented or unconscious at the scene? What is the status of any other victims? Was there an associated blast?

✅ Determine whether there are significant preexisting conditions, such as smoking, underlying allergies, cardiac or cerebrovascular disease, chronic obstructive pulmonary disease (COPD), asthma, or other chronic illness. Patients with underlying pulmonary disease are less able to compensate for inhalation injuries.

✅ Perform a thorough exam of the patient. What material is on the victim? What do they smell of? What are their current signs and symptoms? Is there soot in the posterior pharynx, singed nasal hair, hoarseness, confusion, tachycardia, tachypnea, use of accessory respiratory muscles, wheezing, rales and rhonchi, or stridor to indicate significant injury to the respiratory tract? Note that the lack of physical findings does not reliably exclude airway injury. If airway injury is suspected, bronchoscopy may be necessary to assess extent.

✅ There may be evidence of exposure to a specific toxin that calls for a specific antidote (e.g., muscle fasciculations, small pupils, and wet lungs may imply inhalation of organophosphates, which should be treated with atropine. Cyanide toxicity should be suspected in critically ill smoke inhalation patients with lactic acidosis).

✅ **Unless the exposure is insignificant, obtain a chest radiograph, pulse oximetry, and arterial or venous blood gases.** Record the percentage of oxygen being inhaled (Fio_2 approximately 90% at 15 L/min). An increased alveolar-arterial partial pressure of oxygen (Po_2) difference (A-a O_2 gradient) may be the earliest sign of pulmonary injury, but even if the chest radiograph film and arterial blood gases are normal (as they often are), they can serve as a baseline for evaluation of possible later pulmonary problems. An abnormal initial chest radiograph is a poor prognostic factor.

✅ **With significant smoke inhalation, obtain a HbCO level, complete blood count (CBC) and electrolytes, and serial peak flow measurements, if available. With carbon monoxide poisoning, pulse oximetry (Spo_2) is unreliable because of similar light absorption by carboxyhemoglobin and oxyhemoglobin. HbCO saturation can be directly measured by co-oximetry.** Blood and urine toxicology studies may be obtained to identify coexisting toxicity that may have contributed to the cause of the inhalation injury and complicate its course.

✅ **Obtain an ECG if there is loss of consciousness, a history of coronary artery disease, or complaint of chest pain or palpitations.** Inhalation injuries result in decreased oxygen delivery to the tissues, increasing the risk of cardiac ischemia.

✅ **Consider cyanide toxicity in any patient with smoke inhalation.** Some burning plastics give off cyanide. An anion gap acidosis may be the result of elevated lactate levels secondary to cyanide, carbon monoxide, or hypoxia. A lactate level greater than 8 mmol/L is considered a surrogate marker of elevated cyanide levels and requires treatment. Treatment consists of hydroxocobalamin and/or sodium thiosulfate.

✓ If the patient has difficulty breathing, hoarseness, change in voice, or throat pain—or if he has any abnormality evidenced by the radiography examination, arterial blood gas levels, or physical examination, suggesting acute pulmonary injury—administration of oxygen should be continued to maintain saturation above 90%, and the patient should be admitted to the hospital or transferred to an appropriate tertiary center. Consider early, elective endotracheal intubation in patients at risk for developing airway compromise, particularly those with hoarseness, difficulty breathing, throat pain, drooling, or difficulty swallowing.

✓ **If stridor or other physical evidence of upper airway edema is present or if there is impending respiratory failure, endotracheal intubation should be performed as soon as possible.** Bronchoscopy may be useful in evaluating the extent of injury.

✓ Wheezing and bronchospasm may be allergic reactions and may respond to conventional doses of aerosolized bronchodilators but, if not promptly reversible, are probably signs of pulmonary injury. The elderly (>64 years), the young (<5 years), and persons under the influence of alcohol or other drugs require a lower threshold for admission or transfer.

✓ **After minimal exposure, if no signs or symptoms of inhalation injury develop or if all have resolved in 3 to 4 hours, it may be safe to send the patient home with instructions to return for reevaluation the next day or sooner if any pulmonary signs or symptoms (e.g., stridor, coughing, wheezing, shortness of breath) occur.**

✓ **With minimal to moderate exposure, the patient should be more closely observed for a period of at least 24 hours. Serial arterial blood gas levels, chest radiography, peak expiratory flow rate, airway and lung examination, and bedside spirometry, where available, help detect the evolution of delayed-onset distal airway and pulmonary parenchymal injury.**

What Not to Do

✗ Do not assume that the patient has not suffered any inhalation injury simply because there are no symptoms or abnormalities evidenced by chest radiography or arterial blood gases in the first few hours after exposure. Some agents produce pulmonary inflammation that develops over 12 to 24 hours.

✗ Do not wait until carboxyhemoglobin levels have been determined before giving 100% oxygen to treat suspected carbon monoxide poisoning. Begin oxygen administration as soon as possible.

✗ Do not insist that the patient breathe room air for a long period before obtaining arterial blood gases.

✗ Do not prescribe corticosteroids unless there is a history of asthma or allergy. Evidence of reduced clearance of lung bacteria and of increased incidence of bacterial pneumonia as a late complication of inhalation injury outweighs any potential anti-inflammatory effects.

✗ Do not prescribe antibiotics unless there is a proven infection.

Discussion

Inhalation injury can be caused by several different mechanisms. One type of inhalation injury is caused by relatively inert gases, such as carbon dioxide and fuel gases (e.g., methane, ethane, propane, acetylene), which displace air and oxygen, producing asphyxia. Treatment consists of removing the victim from the gas, allowing them to breathe fresh air or oxygen, and attending to any damage (e.g., myocardial infarction, cerebral injury) caused by the period of hypoxia.

A second category of inhalation injury is caused by irritant gases, including ammonia (NH_3), formaldehyde (HCHO), chloramine (NH_2Cl), chlorine (Cl_2), nitrogen dioxide (NO_2), and phosgene ($COCl_2$). When dissolved in the water lining the respiratory mucosa, irritant gases produce a chemical burn and an inflammatory response. The first three gases listed, which are more soluble in water, tend to produce more upper airway burns, irritating the eyes, nose, and mouth, whereas the latter two gases, being less water soluble, produce more pulmonary injury and respiratory distress. Phosgene can be found in household solvents and can cause delayed severe pulmonary edema, mandating prolonged observation if this agent is suspected. Chlorine is a gas of intermediate solubility and may exert irritant effects widely throughout the respiratory tract. Household bleach contains hypochlorite. Mixing hypochlorite bleach or cleaners with acids, such as hydrochloric acid, sulfuric acid, or phosphoric acid, generates chlorine. Mixing hypochlorite solutions with ammonium hydroxide–containing cleaners generates chloramine.

A third type of inhalation injury is caused by gases that are systemic toxins, such as carbon monoxide, hydrogen cyanide (HCN), and hydrogen sulfide (H_2S). All interfere with the delivery of oxygen for use in cellular energy production and with aromatic and halogenated hydrocarbons, which can result in later liver, kidney, brain, lung, and other organ damage.

A fourth cause of inhalation injury is allergic; inhaled gases, particles, or aerosols produce bronchospasm and edema similar to that caused by asthma or spasmodic croup.

A fifth cause of inhalation injury is direct thermal burns. They are usually limited to the upper airway and produce varying degrees of local edema. Inhalation of steam is far more injurious than heated air. (Steam has approximately 4000 times the heat-carrying capacity of heated air.) Consequently, steam can result in rapidly fatal obstructive glottic edema and lower airway destruction.

The diagnosis of inhalation injury is largely clinical, based on history (disorientation or unconsciousness at the scene, closed space exposure) and physical examination (singed nasal hairs and carbonaceous endobronchial secretions).

In general, treatment of inhalation injury is supportive. There has been no demonstrated value to prophylactic steroids or antibiotics, but in cases when the patient is experiencing an exacerbation of underlying COPD or asthma, routine use of steroids is appropriate. Inhaled β-adrenergics can be added if there is bronchospasm. There is promising research being conducted that is evaluating nebulized anticoagulants and N-acetylcysteine for treating inhalation injury.

Because symptoms of acute inhalation injury can be delayed in onset, a key decision that has to be made during the acute evaluation concerns how long to observe a patient for development of more severe respiratory involvement, and whether to admit the patient for hospital treatment. **Current diagnostic tools cannot stratify inhalation injury by severity or accurately predict subsequent clinical course. Again, knowledge of the agent involved and the intensity/duration of exposure is critical.**

Indicators of poor prognosis include a history of altered mental status at the scene, progressive respiratory difficulty, sputum production, rales, burns to the face, hypoxemia, and altered mental status at time of presentation.

- Although inhalation injuries are often self-limited events, **even mild exposures require early follow-up with clear instructions to the patient** to seek medical care immediately if symptoms worsen.

Suggested Readings

Hall, A. H., Saiers, J., & Baud, F. (2009). Which cyanide antidote? *Critical Reviews in Toxicology, 39,* 541–552.

Miller, K., & Chang, A. (2003). Acute inhalation injury. *Emergency Medicine Clinics of North America, 21,* 533–557.

Rabinowitz, P. M., & Siegel, M. D. (2002). Acute inhalation injury. *Clinics in Chest Medicine, 23,* 707–715.

Sheridan, R. (2002). Specific therapies for inhalation injury. *Critical Care Medicine, 30*(3), 718–719.

Walker, P. F., et al. (2015). Diagnosis and management of inhalation injury: An updated review. *Critical Care, 19*(1), 351.

Woodson, L. C. (2009). Diagnosis and grading of inhalation injury. *Journal of Burn Care and Research, 30,* 143–145.

You, K., Yang, H. T., Kym, D., Yoon, J., Haejun, Y., & Cho, Y. S. (2014). Inhalation injury in burn patients: Establishing the link between diagnosis and prognosis. *Burns, 40,* 1470–1475.

Irritant Incapacitant Exposure

(Lacrimators, Riot Control Agents, Tear Gas)

Presentation

The patient may have been sprayed with tear gas (e.g., Mace) during a riot being dispersed by the police or may have accidentally sprayed oneself. The patient might complain of burning of the eyes, nose, mouth, and skin, as well as tearing and inability to open the eyes because of the severe stinging. There may be sneezing, coughing, runny nose, and perhaps a metallic taste with a burning sensation of the tongue possibly accompanied by nausea, vomiting, and abdominal pain. These signs and symptoms last 15 to 30 minutes after exposure. Redness and edema may be noted for 1 to 2 days after exposure to these aerosol agents.

What to Do

✅ **Segregate victims so that others are not contaminated.** Ideally this should be done outdoors in the fresh air. Secondary contamination can cause adverse symptoms and injuries in emergency medical personnel, can further contaminate your medical facility, and can potentially lead to costly medical facility closures and evacuations. Medical personnel should don gowns, gloves, and masks before helping victims. (Level C protection with an appropriate air-filtering gas mask approved for riot control agents is adequate.)

✅ **Remove contaminated clothing in a predesignated decontamination area, place the clothing in sealed plastic bags, and then shower with soap and water to remove the irritant incapacitants from the skin.**

✅ **Exposed eyes should be irrigated with copious amounts of tepid water or saline for at least 15 minutes, and contact lenses should be removed. If available, use a Morgan Lens (MorTan, Missoula, MT).** Washing the skin with water will remove the residue but will not inactivate it. Removal of contaminated clothing will aid in preventing reexposure. Effects on the eyes and respiratory system generally dissipate within 15 to 30 minutes of cessation of exposure.

✅ **If pepper spray (oleoresin capsicum) was the offending agent, some studies suggest that magnesium-aluminum hydroxide suspension (MgAl) (Mylanta), applied to the affected area of skin during the initial 30 minutes, can provide prompt and dramatic relief.** Because MgAl is cheap and readily available and has minimal side effects, it is considered an appropriate early treatment for such dermal exposure. If MgAl is not available, milk has anecdotally been found to be helpful, as its hydrophobic protein casein displaces capsaicin, relieving pain.

✅ **If eye pain lasts longer than 15 to 20 minutes, examine the eyes with fluorescein dye, looking for corneal erosions, which may be produced by tear gas or capsicum** (see Chapter 16). **Eye pain from pepper spray is largely dissipated within 1 hour. Short-term use of topical ophthalmic anesthetics will alleviate the pain, but topical nonsteroidal**

anti-inflammatory drugs (NSAIDs) will not. Patients should be cautioned against rubbing the eyes to prevent inflicting further damage.

✓ Look for signs of, and warn the patient about, allergic reactions to tear gas, including bronchospasm and contact dermatitis. Minor prolonged skin irritation can be treated with hydrocortisone cream 2.5% (1 tube, 30 g), applied two to four times a day, or lotion 2.5% (1 bottle, 59 mL), applied two to four times a day.

What Not to Do

✗ Do not rush or allow others to rush to the aid of the patient who has been exposed to tear gas; rushing heedlessly can result in contamination and incapacitation of those attempting to help the patient.

✗ Do not allow the patient to rub the eyes. This may cause mechanical corneal abrasions in addition to the chemical irritation.

Discussion

Irritant incapacitants, also called riot control agents, lacrimators, and tear gases, are currently used by law enforcement agencies and are available to the public for personal protection. These relatively nontoxic agents cause temporary incapacitation by inducing eye pain, lacrimation, and uncontrollable blepharospasm. Exposure to these agents may also result in irritation in the nose and mouth, throat, and airways, causing difficulty breathing and burning sensations in the chest, abdominal pain, vomiting, and skin irritation (particularly in moist and warm areas).

Two of the most common riot control agents include chlorobenzylidene malononitrile (CS) (named after its creators, Ben Corson and Roger Stoughton) and oleoresin capsicum (OC), also known as pepper spray.

CS is a white crystalline powder with a pungent pepperlike odor that is immediately detectable. It is used extensively in tear gas.

OC is a mixture of compounds obtained by extracting dried ripe fruit of cayenne peppers. Capsaicin is the principal constituent that works through direct irritation and neurogenic inflammation.

There is no antidote for OC. Treatment consists of thorough early decontamination and symptom-directed supportive measures. Decontamination should be carefully carried out to avoid contamination of the surrounding skin and clothing.

Although most exposures do not result in life-threatening emergencies, bronchospasm and noncardiogenic pulmonary edema have been seen. Those exposures resulting in respiratory distress should be treated with supplemental oxygen and inhaled bronchodilators. Standard asthma treatment should be initiated in patients with an exacerbation of underlying disease triggered by exposure.

Suggested Readings

Blain, P. G. (2003). Tear gases and irritant incapacitants. *Toxicology Review*, *22*, 103–110.

Bozeman, W. P., Dilbero, D., & Schauben, J. L. (2002). Biologic and chemical weapons of mass destruction. *Emergency Medicine Clinics of North America*, *20*, 975–993.

Horton, D. K., Burgess, P., Rossiter, S., et al. (2002). Secondary contamination of emergency department personnel from o-chlorobenzylidene malononitrile exposure, 2002. *Annals of Emergency Medicine*, *45*, 655–658.

Lee, D. C., & Ryan, J. R. (2003). Magnesium-aluminum hydroxide suspension for the treatment of dermal capsaicin exposures. *Academic Emergency Medicine*, *10*, 688–690.

Miller, K., & Chang, A. (2003). Acute inhalation injury. *Emergency Medicine Clinics in North America*, *21*, 533–557.

Schep, L. J., Slaughter, R. J., & McBride, D. I. (2015). Riot control agents: The tear gases CN, CS and OC-a medical review. *Journal of the Royal Army Medical Corps*, *161*(2), 94–99.

Sivathasan, N. (2010). Educating on CS or 'tear gas. *Emergency Medicine Journal*, *27*(11), 881–882.

Yenigun, O. M., & Thanassi, M. (2019). Capsaicin: An uncommon exposure and unusual treatment. *Clinical Practice and Cases in Emergency Medicine*, *3*(3), 219–221.

Zollman, T. M., Bragg, R. M., & Harrison, D. A. (2000). Clinical effects of oleoresin capsicum (pepper spray) on the human cornea and conjunctiva. *Ophthalmology*, *107*, 2186–2189.

Rib Fracture and Costochondral Separation

(Broken Rib)

Presentation

A patient with an isolated rib fracture or a minor costochondral separation usually has recently fallen, injuring the side of the chest; been struck by a blunt object; coughed violently; or leaned over a rigid edge. The initial chest pain may subside, but over the next few hours or days the pain increases with movement, interferes with sleep and activity, and becomes severe when the patient coughs or breathes deeply. The patient is often worried about having a broken rib and may have a sensation of bony crepitus or abnormal rib movement. Breath sounds bilaterally should be normal unless there is substantial splinting or a pneumothorax or hemothorax is present. There is point tenderness over the site of the injury, and occasionally bony crepitus can be felt.

What to Do

⊘ Examine the patient for possible associated injuries, and palpate the abdomen for any signs of a splenic or hepatic injury. What appear to be insignificant mechanisms of injury, such as falling over a chair, hitting the edge of a table, or colliding into a strong ocean wave, all have resulted in splenic injury. **Maintain a high index of suspicion of severe underlying injuries. Consider intraabdominal injuries in all patients with lower rib fractures, and mediastinal injury in those with fractures of the first three ribs. Keep a low threshold for ordering computed tomography (CT) scans, especially in the patient with altered mental status or other distracting injuries, as well as those who are anticoagulated.**

⊘ **When there is a history of minor trauma and no suspicion of an intraabdominal or intrathoracic injury, check for rib pain and clinical evidence of fracture by applying indirect stress to the suspected fracture site.** Compress the rib anteroposteriorly if a fracture is suspected at a lateral location. Compress the rib medially if a posterior or anterior fracture is suspected (Fig. 65.1) (See Video 65.1). **Pain occurring at the suspected fracture site during application of indirect stress is clinical evidence of a fracture or cartilage separation and should be documented on the chart as "a clinical or occult rib fracture."** If there is pain with deep inspiration, or cough and point tenderness at any position along the rib contours that reproduces this pain, a diagnosis of a clinical rib fracture can also be made. If subcutaneous emphysema is appreciated on examination, the patient is at risk for delayed pneumothorax and should be admitted for observation.

⊘ Obtain any history of chronic pulmonary problems or heavy smoking because these patients are at greater risk for developing pulmonary infections.

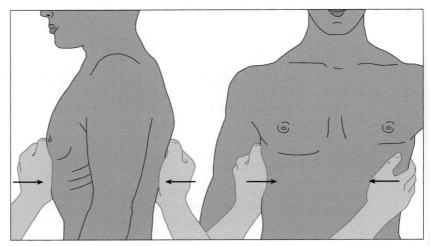

Fig. 65.1 Indirect stress test with anteroposterior compression to reveal a lateral rib fracture and lateral-medial compression to reveal an anterior or posterior fracture.

✓ **Send the patient for posteroanterior and lateral chest radiographs to evaluate for pneumothorax, hemothorax, and pulmonary contusion. Additional oblique rib films for radiologic documentation of a fracture are generally not recommended and rarely add clinical or therapeutic benefit. These films may be indicated to document the extent of injury when there is a suspicion of multiple rib fractures and CT is not available. Ultrasound is a useful modality to evaluate for rib fracture as well as associated complications such as pneumothorax (Fig. 65.3).**

✓ Elderly patients with multiple rib fractures have an increased incidence of pneumonia and overall increased mortality and usually require hospital admission with aggressive analgesic management and respiratory care.

✓ **If there is no suspicion of a more serious underlying injury, and there is clinical or radiologic evidence of a rib fracture or chondral separation, provide as potent an oral analgesic as needed to control pain.** Adequate pain control has been shown to improve pulmonary function and reduce complications. Ibuprofen and acetaminophen are excellent first-line agents, although initially, opioid analgesia may be necessary.

✓ While generally not recommended, **if the patient is young and healthy**, you can place a rib belt on the patient to see if this provides comfort. If there is significant pain relief, you can instruct the patient regarding the intermittent use of this elastic and Velcro belt. Place the bottom of the belt at the inferior tip of the xiphoid process, tightening it around the chest enough to obtain maximum pain relief (Fig. 65.2). The rib belt may be worn almost continuously for the first 1 to 4 days, removing it intermittently to cough and deep breath, but it should thereafter be removed as comfort allows.

✓ **Instruct the patient regarding the importance of deep breathing and coughing (using a pillow held against the painful rib as a splint) to help prevent pneumonia. Tell**

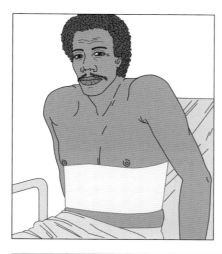

Fig. 65.2 Proper placement of elastic and Velcro rib belt.

the patient to take enough pain medicine to allow coughing and deep breathing. When available, provide incentive spirometry.

✓ **Provide the patient with appropriate documentation for missing work, and refer for follow-up care in 48 hours.** Tell the patient to expect gradually decreasing discomfort for about 2 to 4 weeks but to be prepared for an extended period of disability (it will take several weeks to heal and become pain free). **Forbid strenuous activity for approximately 8 weeks.** One study showed that patients with isolated rib fractures returned to work or their usual activities at a mean of 51 days (±39 days).

✓ Severe worsening of chest pain, shortness of breath, fever, or purulent sputum may signal pulmonary complications and should prompt a return visit. A greater incidence of complications can be expected in patients with displaced rib fractures.

✓ **When there is no clinical or radiologic evidence of a fracture, treat the pain as any other contusion would be treated, using an appropriate analgesic.**

What Not to Do

✗ Do not confuse simple rib fractures with massive blunt trauma to the chest. The evaluation and management are quite different.

✗ Do not overlook child or elder abuse. Rib fractures are uncommon in younger children and are found in 5% to 27% of documented cases of child abuse. Child abuse should be considered in the absence of a plausible history of trauma or conditions of bony fragility, such as osteogenesis imperfecta or rickets.

✗ Do not tape ribs or, in the elderly, use rib belts. This will lead to hypoventilation and an atelectatic lung that is prone to developing pneumonia.

✗ Do not assume that there is no fracture just because the radiographs are normal. Rib fractures are often not apparent on radiographs, especially when they occur in the cartilaginous portion of the rib. The patient deserves the disability period and analgesics commensurate with the real injury.

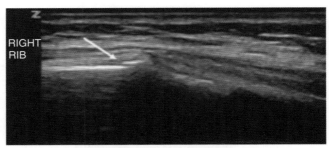

Fig. 65.3 Point-of-care ultrasound (POCUS) image of rib fracture *(arrow)*. (From Simard, R. [2020]. Ultrasound imaging of orthopedic injuries. *Emergency Medicine Clinics of North America, 38*[1], 243–265.)

Discussion

Rib fracture pain can be significant, and is usually reported by patients to be exacerbated by any movement of the chest wall (e.g., with respiration and most certainly with deep breathing and coughing). Although most commonly secondary to trauma, rib fractures may also occur because of repetitive stressors, such as that experienced with coughing or in athletes such as golfers and rowers.

Most isolated fractures and separations cause minimal morbidity or mortality and are treated with immobilization, but ribs are a special problem because patients have to continue breathing. Pain management is crucial. Patients with pain often splint, hypoventilate, and avoid coughing; thus they are predisposing themselves to pneumonia. With this in mind, outpatient management of isolated single rib fractures with oral pain medication is generally adequate for most healthy patients.

Rib and sternal fractures are notoriously difficult to see on plain films in the acute setting. **Point-of-care ultrasound (POCUS)** can be used over a patient's area of maximal pain to identify rib fractures (Fig. 65.3). A systematic review revealed that US for diagnosing rib fractures was superior to plain films. In another study, US for sternal fractures also was considered superior to plain films. Both rib and sternal fractures seem to have a high specificity (98% and 97%, respectively) and only moderate sensitivity (67% and 83%, respectively).

In the presence of severe pain or multiple rib fractures, consider the use of an intercostal nerve block with 0.5% bupivacaine (Marcaine). Because of the risk for pneumothorax or hemothorax, in most cases, this procedure should be reserved for secondary management when initial treatment has proven inadequate.

Although rib belts are no longer commonly used and their use is discouraged, they can sometimes provide significant pain relief for young, active patients who are at low risk for pulmonary complications. If used, it may be worn almost continuously for the first 1 to 4 days, but it should be removed as comfort allows thereafter.

Suggested Readings

Bansidhar, B., Lagares-Garcia, J. A., & Miller, S. L. (2002). Clinical rib fractures: Are follow-up chest x-rays a waste of resources? *The American Journal of Surgery, 68,* 449–453.

Bhavnagri, S. J., & Mohammed, T. L. (2009). When and how to image a suspected broken rib. *Cleveland Clinic Journal of Medicine, 76,* 309–314.

Bliss, D., & Silen, M. (2002). Pediatric thoracic trauma. *Critical Care Medicine, 30*(Suppl. 11), S409–S415.

Bulger, E. M., Arneson, M. A., Mock, C. N., & Jurkovich, G. H. (2002). Rib fractures in the elderly. *Annals of Emergency Medicine, 39,* 1040–1046.

Fabricant, L., Ham, B., et al. (2013). Prolonged pain and disability are common after rib fractures. *The American Journal of Surgery, 205*(5), 511–515.

Holcomb, J. B., McMullin, N. R., Kozar, R. A., et al. (2003). Morbidity from rib fractures increases after age 45. *Journal of the American College of Medicine*, *196*, 549–555.

Holmes, J. F., Nguyen, H., Jacoby, R. C., et al. (2005). Do all patients with left costal margin injuries require radiographic evaluation for intraabdominal injury? *Annals of Emergency Medicine*, *46*, 232–236.

Kerr-Valentic, M. A., Arthur, M., Mullins, R. J., et al. (2003). Rib fracture pain and disability: Can we do better? *The Journal of Trauma*, *54*, 1058–1064.

Kieninger, A. N. (2005). Epidural versus intravenous pain control in elderly patients with rib fractures. *The American Journal of Surgery*, *189*, 327–330.

Lazcano, A., Dougherty, J., & Kruger, M. (1989). Use of rib belts in acute rib fractures. *American Journal of Emergency Medicine*, *7*, 97–100.

Lu, M. S., Huang, Y. K., Liu, Y. H., et al. (2008). Delayed pneumothorax complicating minor rib fracture after chest trauma. *American Journal of Emergency Medicine*, *26*, 551–554.

Quick, G. (1990). A randomized clinical trial of rib belts for simple fractures. *American Journal of Emergency Medicine*, *8*, 277–281.

Sikka, R. (2004). Unsuspected internal organ traumatic injuries. *Emergency Medicine Clinics of North America*, *22*, 1067–1080.

Simard, R. (2019). Ultrasound imaging of orthopedic injuries. *Emergency Medicine Clinics of North America*, *38*(1), 243–265.

Ullman, E. A., Donley, L. P., & Brady, W. J. (2003). Pulmonary trauma. *Emergency Medicine Clinics of North America*, *21*, 291–313.

PART 6

Gastrointestinal Emergencies

■ Daniel Ackil ■ Nicholas J. Koch

Anal Fissure

Presentation

In most patients, the symptoms are so characteristic that they are nearly diagnostic. Initial onset of pain often occurs during or after defecation, usually after passing a large, hard bowel movement or following an explosive bout of diarrhea. Later, patients complain of severe intense pain with subsequent defecation. It can be described as knifelike, cutting, or tearing in character. This pain can persist for a few minutes to hours, with a tight, throbbing quality followed by relative comfort prior to the next bowel movement. Often patients will complain of constipation that predates their anal symptoms. Occasionally patients have diarrhea or an alternating pattern of constipation and diarrhea.

Bright red bleeding with defecation may occur but is usually slight, only staining the toilet tissue. Mucous discharge may increase perineal moisture and cause itching. Examination of the anus reveals a radial tear or ulceration of the posterior midline 95% of the time (the fissure is anterior in 10% of women but only 1% of men) (Fig. 66.1). If the condition becomes chronic (>8 weeks), the skin distal to the fissure becomes edematous and enlarged and may form a fibrous skin tag called a sentinel pile.

What to Do

✔ Most patients with an anal fissure cannot tolerate a digital rectal examination or anoscopy without general anesthesia. Parenteral analgesia may be necessary prior to attempting any examination.

✔ To examine, place the patient in the left lateral decubitus position with knees bent toward the chest. (Use proper draping to maintain the patient's dignity and to minimize any embarrassment.) Good lighting is essential.

✔ **Gentle retraction of the perianal skin usually allows one to visualize the fissure directly, even in patients with significant spasm.**

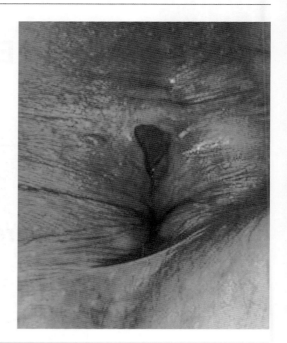

Fig. 66.1 With the patient in prone jackknife position, a posterior acute anal fissure is visible once the buttocks are separated. (Courtesy Richard P. Billingham, MD, Seattle, WA.)

✅ **When you are confident in the diagnosis, the mainstay of medical treatment for both acute and chronic anal fissures is the avoidance of hard stools.** This can be accomplished with fiber supplementation and stool softeners. **Advise the patient to take methylcellulose (Citrucel), 1 heaping tablespoon (2 g) in 8 oz of water three to four times a day, along with docusate sodium (Colace), 50 to 200 mg/day orally, divided in one to four doses (50-, 100-, 250-mg capsules). Lubricating glycerin suppositories used twice a day can also be helpful. All of these products may be purchased over the counter.**

✅ **To break the cycle of sphincter spasm and tearing of anal mucosa**, and thereby promote subsequent healing of the fissure, medical therapy is often necessary. **Prescribe topical nifedipine 0.2%, twice a day for 3 weeks, or diltiazem gel 2%** (these prescriptions often need to be filled at a compounding pharmacy) **with lidocaine HCl 2% gel, maximum dose 4.5 mg/kg, not to exceed 300 mg, to be applied once every 12 hours for 8 weeks.**

✅ Topical glyceryl trinitrate 0.2% or nitroglycerin ointment 0.2% (these prescriptions also may need to be filled at a compounding pharmacy) can be substituted for the topical diltiazem and nifedipine, but many patients are unable to tolerate the headaches that frequently occur. Avoid nitroglycerin therapy in patients taking sildenafil (Viagra) or other erectile dysfunction medications.

✅ **Instruct the patient to use warm, soothing sitz baths after each painful bowel movement.**

✅ Prescribe analgesics if needed but remember that narcotics are constipating.

✅ **When the condition becomes chronic**, Botox injection into the sphincter may be considered if the abovementioned therapies fail; however, flatus or fecal incontinence is a potential side effect of this. Lateral sphincterotomy is usually 95% successful when medical therapies fail, although complications such as fecal incontinence may occur.

(✓) Inform the patient that an acute superficial fissure will take about 4 to 6 weeks to heal. He or she should follow up if symptoms continue. At that point, or whenever there is uncertainty as to the diagnosis, gastrointestinal (GI) consultation and endoscopy to assess for possible Crohn disease and other diagnoses, including malignancy, should be considered.

What Not to Do

(X) Do not attempt a digital rectal exam when there is a high likelihood of an anal fissure because such an exam would be expected to cause intolerable pain.

(X) Do not confuse this condition with a thrombosed hemorrhoid (see Chapter 74), because the management is very different.

(X) Do not assume that a lesion located outside the anteroposterior midline sagittal plane of the anus is an uncomplicated anal fissure. Lateral location, extension onto the anal verge or above the dentate line, and extension of the base of the ulcer through the internal sphincter are all atypical features that warrant further investigation. Other possibilities include ulcerative colitis, squamous cell carcinoma, leukemia, tuberculosis, syphilis, herpes, Crohn disease, sexually transmitted diseases, and trauma from instrumentation and anal intercourse. Appropriate follow-up should be arranged.

(X) Do not confuse a sentinel pile with a hemorrhoidal vein.

(X) Do not prescribe 0.2% nitroglycerin ointment for use in patients taking sildenafil (Viagra) and other phosphodiesterase inhibitors.

(X) Do not fail to refer a patient for GI consultation and possible endoscopy when the diagnosis of anal fissure is in doubt or when there is rectal bleeding.

Discussion

Anal fissures probably begin by the tearing of the mucosa during defecation. Hard stools are most commonly implicated, but explosive liquid stools can produce the same results. This starts a vicious cycle of pain, causing spasm in the anal sphincter, which results in increased friction during defecation and leads to further tearing and pain.

Currently, ischemia is considered the most likely cause for development of an anal fissure. There is a paucity of anal blood vessels, especially in the posterior midline, and it is thought that anal spasm further reduces blood flow.

After a period of about 4 to 8 weeks, a fissure can be considered chronic. The cycle can be broken with analgesia, stool softening, lubrication, relaxation of spasm, or all four.

Although many acute anal fissures with a fresh skin tear heal spontaneously, some do not. With those that do not, secondary changes develop, with raised edges exposing the white, horizontally oriented fibers of the internal sphincter (chronic fissure). Botulinum toxin, which is a potent inhibitor of acetylcholine release from nerve endings, can be injected into the anal sphincter and can improve healing in patients with chronic fissures. One uncommon adverse effect associated with the drug is flatus incontinence. If the fissure is large, it may become ulcerated and infected, not heal spontaneously, and require surgical excision.

Pruritus ani has multiple causes, although most cases are idiopathic. Infections such as pinworms, *Candida albicans, Tinea cruris,* and erythrasma can

Discussion continued

cause anal itching. Mechanical trauma from overly vigorous cleansing of the perianal area may also cause pruritus. The latter may be aggravated by diarrhea and the presence of external or prolapsed hemorrhoids or multiple skin tags, which make cleansing more difficult. Another cause of pruritus ani is allergic or contact dermatitis from agents such as soaps, perfumes in toilet tissue, and feminine hygiene sprays, as well as spicy foods, tomatoes, citrus fruits, colas, coffee, and chocolate. Psoriasis, seborrheic dermatitis, atopic eczema, and lichen planus are additional dermatologic sources of itching. Other causes of pruritus ani include chronic anorectal disease, human immunodeficiency virus (HIV)–related infections, diabetes, cancer, and illnesses that produce hyperbilirubinemia. If a specific cause of anal pruritus can be determined, treat it accordingly. If the cause is obscure, the patient can be treated with hydrocortisone cream to reduce itching, scratching, and inflammation, followed by zinc oxide as a barrier cream.

In general, any medications such as antibiotics and laxatives should be discontinued, and the diet should be adjusted as necessary. A bulk-forming agent can be administered to allow for complete and predictable bowel evacuation, followed by bathing appropriately with warm water and little soap (to reduce chemical irritation). Using a hair dryer will provide gentle drying without further irritation. Moistened rectal wipes can be a reasonable alternative, but wipes containing chemicals such as perfumes, alcohol, or witch hazel should be avoided to reduce any effect of chemical contact dermatitis. Irritation from vigorous cleansing may actually worsen the itch. A systemic antipruritic agent, such as hydroxyzine (Vistaril), 25 mg orally three to four times a day, may be prescribed. Follow-up is required.

Proctalgia fugax is a unique entity found mostly in males, causing severe, brief, lancinating episodes of rectal pain lasting seconds to minutes. The pain is excruciating but is spontaneous and unrelated to defecation. The physical examination is completely normal, and treatment primarily consists of reassurance with an explanation of this benign disorder.

Suggested Readings

American Gastroenterological Association. (2003). American gastroenterological association medical position statement: Diagnosis and care of patients with anal fissure. *Gastroenterology, 124*, 233–234. http://www.gastro.org/practice/medical-position-statements.

Brenner, B. E., & Simon, R. R. (1983). Anorectal emergencies. *Annals of Emergency Medicine, 12*, 367–376.

Brisinda, G., Cadeddu, F., Brandara, F., et al. (2007). Randomized clinical trial comparing botulinum toxin injections with 0.2 percent nitroglycerin ointment for chronic anal fissure. *British Journal of Surgery, 94*, 162–167.

Clinical key. (2019). Clinical overview: Anal fissure. © 2019.

Ezri, T., & Susmallian, S. (2003). Topical nifedipine vs. topical glyceryl trinitrate for treatment of chronic anal fissure. *Diseases of the Colon & Rectum, 46*, 805–808.

Gopal, D. V. (2002). Diseases of the rectum and anus: A clinical approach to common disorders. *Clinical Cornerstone, 4*, 34–48.

Herzig, D. O., & Lu, K. C. (2010). Anal fissure. *Surgery Clinics of North America, 90*, 33–44.

Lieberman, D. A. (1984). Common anorectal disorders. *Annals of Internal Medicine, 101*, 837–846.

Lund, J. N., & Scholefield, J. H. (1997). A randomized, prospective, double-blind, placebo-controlled trial of glyceryl trinitrate ointment in treatment of anal fissure. *Lancet, 349*, 11–14.

Madoff, R. D., & Dykes, S. L. (2004). What's new in colon and rectal surgery. *Journal of the American College of Surgeons, 198*, 98–104.

Metcalf, A. M. (2002). Anal fissure. *Surgery Clinics of North America, 82*, 1291–1297.

Parellada, C. (2004). Randomized, prospective trial comparing 0.2 percent isorbide dinitrate ointment with sphincterotomy in treatment of chronic anal fissure: A two year follow-up. *Diseases of the Colon & Rectum*, *47*, 437–443.

Poritz, L. S., Geibel, J., et al. (2020). *Anal fissure guidelines. Medscape clinical guidelines*. https://emedicine.medscape.com/article/196297-guidelines.

Samim, M., Twigt, B., Stoker, L., & Pronk, A. (2012). Topical diltiazem cream versus botulinum toxin a for the treatment of chronic anal fissure: A double-blind randomized clinical trial. *Annals of Surgery*, *255*(1), 18–22.

Slawson, D. (2003). Topical nifedipine plus lidocaine gel effective for anal fissures. *American Family Physician*, *67*, 1781.

Wald, A., Bharucha, A., Cosman, B., & Whitehead, W. (2014). American college of gastroenterology clinical guideline on the management of benign anorectal disorders. *American Journal of Gastroenterology*, *109*(8), 1141–1157. https://doi.org/10.1038/ajg.2014.190.

Zhao, X., & Pasricha, P. J. (2003). Botulinum toxin for spastic GI disorders: A systematic review. *Gastrointestinal Endoscopy*, *57*, 219–235.

Blocked Tubes

(G-Tube, J-Tube)

67

Presentation

The patient presents complaining of a gastrostomy tube (G-tube) or jejunostomy tube (J-tube) that is not functioning properly. The most common complaints are that the tube is obstructed, leaking, displaced, or that there is pain and/or redness surrounding the stoma. Depending on how long the complication has persisted and how dependent on the tube the patient is, the presentation can range from otherwise well-appearing patients to severely dehydrated or malnourished patients. Patients may also have missed several doses of their medications if they are usually given through the tube.

What to Do

✅ **Perform a thorough history, including how long the tube has been in place, how long it has been malfunctioning, and what exactly is not working.** Perform a physical exam, including a thorough exam of the tube site. In addition to your normal abdominal exam, look for evidence of infection or skin changes at the gastrostomy site and leakage from the gastrostomy site.

✅ **If the patient presents with a clogged tube, first attempt to aspirate the clogging material using a catheter tip syringe.** Use a smaller syringe to allow you to exert a larger amount of force. If this is not successful, try gently flushing with saline. **You may need to gently and alternately flush and aspirate small amounts repeatedly.** Be patient because this can take several minutes and may be successful even if you don't feel anything moving initially.

✅ **If this is not successful, you can attempt to use a guidewire, small stylet, or Fogarty catheter to clear the exterior part of the tube of debris (the visualized portion of the tube before it enters the stoma). Do not attempt to clear the subcutaneous portion (proximal to the stoma), as this creates a perforation risk. Confirm tube integrity and positioning with a contrast radiograph once it is flushing normally.**

✅ **Pharmacologic adjuncts may be helpful.** Use of cola, cranberry juice, and meat tenderizer have been described; however, these have not been shown to be effective. **There are commercially available decloggers that are effective, such as Clog Zapper or Bionix. Instilled pancreatic enzymes have also been shown to be effective. Crush one tablet of pancreatin or pancrelipase and one 324-mg tablet of nonenteric sodium bicarbonate to a fine powder and dissolve in 5 mL of warm water.** Instill the mixture into the tube and let it sit for 30 to 60 minutes, then flush with water. **Confirm tube integrity and positioning with a contrast radiograph once it is flushing normally.**

✅ **Patients often present complaining of moisture coming from the gastrostomy tube site.** This is often just due to secretions related to a foreign-body reaction of the skin to the silicone tube, especially in recently placed tubes. **These reactions can generally be managed with local skin care, including cleaning with warm water and hydrogen peroxide. If there appears to be leakage of gastric contents through the gastrostomy, this may indicate that the percutaneous tract is too large for the tube.** The service that placed the tube should be consulted regarding management decisions. Sometimes this can be managed by removing the tube for a period of time to allow for shrinking of the tract.

✅ **If the patient has a dislodged jejunostomy tube, the provider or service that placed the tube should be consulted. If a gastrostomy tube is displaced, be sure to determine when the original tube was placed at that site. The percutaneous tract takes at least 2 to 3 weeks to mature.** If the tube has been in place for a shorter period, consult the service or physician that placed the tube. If the timing is unclear, consult gastroenterology or general surgery. Note that if the patient has a skin-level tube, as opposed to a tube that protrudes a distance out of the skin, this is likely a mature tract as skin-level tubes are generally not used in the initial tube placement.

✅ **If it can be determined that the G-tube has been in place long enough for the tract to mature, the tube should be replaced as soon as possible because the tract can become stenotic within hours.** Sometimes patients will arrive with replacement tubes or Foley catheters because a family member or caretaker had been instructed to do so if the tube becomes dislodged. Before attempting reinsertion of a tube, make sure to perform an abdominal exam and examine the stoma for signs of infection. **Gather your supplies, including a G-tube (ideally the same size as the patient had before, but if the tube has been out a few hours, it may be helpful to use a smaller tube), lubricant, saline, and a syringe to inflate the balloon.** Put on clean gloves (this is not a sterile procedure). Determine from the box or package insert how much saline to use to inflate the balloon. Check the balloon. Clean the skin. Lubricate the tube and stoma and push the end of the tube into the stoma using gentle pressure until the external bumper is at the level of the skin. Inflate the balloon with saline and pull back on the tube to ensure the balloon is up against the gastric wall, then slide the bumper down the tube until it is flush against the skin. **Confirm tube positioning with a contrast radiograph.**

✅ **When infection is suspected,** it is necessary to take the patient's whole clinical picture into consideration. **Local erythema at the feeding tube site is a common reason for patients to seek medical care.** When considering if surrounding erythema is a true infection or just skin inflammation, important questions to ask are: Has the patient had fevers, chills, or sweats? Has the redness come on abruptly or with streaking? Has the tube site also had purulent or malodorous discharge? Some skin changes and erythema can be due to irritation from a leaking tube or from tape or bandage sensitivity. **In a toxic-appearing patient with fevers, tachycardia, and concern for sepsis, usual care should be undertaken, including appropriate lab work (complete blood count [CBC], erythrocyte sedimentation rate [ESR], C-reactive protein [CRP], blood or wound cultures), and imaging should be obtained. If there is concern for a localized abscess, ultrasonography may be obtained. If there is concern for possible intraabdominal infection or peritonitis, advanced imaging such as computed tomography (CT) scan with contrast should be considered to evaluate for gastric leaking/perforation. If there is local tenderness, warmth, and swelling consistent with a superficial skin infection or cellulitis, and antibiotics are to be given, consider coverage for the usual skin flora (staph and strep) and consider patient risk factors for methicillin-resistant *Staphylococcus aureus* (MRSA).** Obtain wound cultures when possible to guide treatment if first-line agents fail to adequately clear the infection. Adding coverage against gram negatives and anaerobes is not routinely necessary.

What Not to Do

(X) Do not remove a recently placed (less than 2–3 weeks) tube without consulting the surgery, gastroenterology, or interventional-radiology teams to confirm a new tube can be placed in a timely manner.

(X) Do not routinely prescribe antibiotics for mildly inflamed skin around a G or J tube.

(X) Do not remove, attempt to unclog, or flush a tube without performing a thorough history and physical examination. More serious etiologies, such as bowel obstruction or perforation, must be considered whenever a G or J tube is not functioning properly.

Discussion

Once a feeding tube is placed, the percutaneous tract begins to mature in 2 weeks but is typically not well formed until 4 to 6 weeks. Patients who are immunocompromised, have large ascites, or have severe malnutrition may take even longer than 6 weeks for their tubes to form a matured tract. Children may take even longer to have their tube tract mature, and some institutions recommend 8 weeks before changing a newly placed tube.

Do not remove a recently placed feeding tube unless in consultation with the gastroenterology service or surgical service that will manage this patient's feeding tube long term.

Clogged tubes are a very common issue. Use of warm water and pressure flushing with a syringe (20–30 cc) is usually enough to declog most tubes. If a clogged tube is still not flushing properly after flushing with warm water, consider using one of the methods noted earlier, including sodium bicarbonate or pancrelipase. Never advance a wire or other instrument in an attempt to declog a tube unless supervised by a gastroenterologist or surgeon.

In a toxic-appearing patient with pain and erythema at the feeding tube site, necrotizing fasciitis must be considered.

Suggested Readings

Blumenstein, I. (2014). Gastroenteric tube feeding: Techniques, problems and solutions. *World Journal of Gastroenterology*, *20*(26), 8505.

DeLegge, M. (2019a). *Gastrostomy tubes: Complications and their management*. UptoDate. https://www.uptodate.com/contents/gastrostomy-tubes-complications-and-their-management.

DeLegge, M. (2019b). *Gastrostomy tubes: Placement and routine care*. UptoDate. https://www.uptodate.com/contents/gastrostomy-tubes-uses-patient-selection-and-efficacy-in-adults.

Fisher, C., & Blalock, B. (2014). Clogged feeding tubes: A clinician's thorn. *Practical Gastroenterology*, 16–22.

MacLean, A. A., Miller, G., Bamboat, Z. M., & Hiotis, K. (2004). Abdominal wall necrotizing fasciitis from dislodged percutaneous endoscopic gastrostomy tubes: A case series. *The American Journal of Surgery*, *70*(9), 827–831.

Shah, R., & Shah, M. (2019). *Gastrostomy tube replacement*. Treasure Island, FL: StatPearls Publishing.

Showalter, C. D., Kerrey, B., Spellman-Kennebeck, S., & Timm, N. (2012). Gastrostomy tube replacement in a pediatric ED: Frequency of complications and impact of confirmatory imaging. *American Journal of Emergency Medicine*, *30*(8), 1501–1506.

Soscia, J., & Friedman, J. N. (2011). A guide to the management of common gastrostomy and gastrojejunostomy tube problems. *Paediatric Child Health*, *16*(5), 281–287.

Constipation, Irritable Bowel Syndrome, and Colic

(Stomach Cramps)

Presentation

Patients with functional constipation will often come in with the complaint of abdominal pain or bloating. Often it is not until they are asked that they will describe infrequent bowel movements, straining at stooling, incomplete evacuation, hard or small stools, a blockage in the anal region, or the need for digital manipulation to enable defecation.

Patients with irritable bowel syndrome (IBS) will complain of abdominal pain or discomfort, with a change in the form or frequency of defecation. They will have constipation (fewer than three bowel movements per week), diarrhea (more than three bowel movements per day), or alternating constipation and diarrhea. Their pain is often but not always relieved by defecation.

At the age of 6 weeks, infants with colic will begin having episodes of inconsolable crying that last more than 3 hours per day for more than 3 days per week and that continue longer than 3 weeks. These infants are well fed and otherwise healthy.

In all of these cases, the patient's discomfort is rarely accompanied by nausea or vomiting. In addition, signs and symptoms should not include fever, anorexia, or weight loss, and rarely are patients awakened with nocturnal symptoms.

The physical examination is generally benign, with normal vital signs and no jaundice, tenderness, masses, organomegaly, rectal bleeding, or other abnormalities, and the patient does not appear ill between the episodes of abdominal pain. Some patients may exhibit vital sign abnormalities such as low-grade tachycardia or tachypnea when in pain and may have minimal tenderness on exam; however, they should not exhibit any rebound or guarding.

What to Do

✓ **Take a thorough history** and try to determine the time of onset of symptoms and whether their severity is increasing or decreasing. Ask if there was a similar episode in the past. A careful medication history should be obtained because many commonly used drugs may cause constipation. It is often helpful to specifically ask the patient about patterns of bowel movements, including frequency and consistency as well as need to strain with bowel movements, as this is information that is crucial in making a diagnosis but not necessarily readily volunteered by the patient.

✓ **Perform a complete physical examination,** including rectal and/or pelvic examination, and a repeat abdominal examination after an interval. The patient's skin is checked for pallor and signs of hypothyroidism (e.g., reduced body hair, skin dryness, fixed edema), and the abdomen is examined for masses, distention, tenderness, and high-pitched bowel sounds. The rectal examination includes careful inspection and palpation for masses, anal fissures, inflammation, and hard stool in the ampulla.

✅ **For patients with symptomatic constipation, it may be appropriate (but not always necessary) to obtain a complete blood count, biochemical profile, serum calcium, glucose levels, and thyroid-stimulating hormone.**

✅ If the presentation is not clear or there is any concern about significant underlying disease, consider using diagnostic tests, such as a urinalysis (to help rule out renal colic or urinary tract infection), abdominal radiographs (to show free peritoneal air or fecal impaction), and ultrasonography (for pyloric stenosis, malrotation and intussusception in children, or gallbladder and pelvic disorders in adults). Computed tomography (CT) imaging should be used if there is suspicion for acute intraabdominal or retroperitoneal infectious or surgical pathology. Adult patients with a change in bowel habits or hemoccult positive stool should be referred for colonoscopy to assess for malignancy.

✅ **If simple constipation is the problem and there is obstructing stool on rectal examination, disimpact the rectum by pulling out hard stool *(scybala)* and follow with one oil retention enema. This may be very painful and require parenteral analgesia. For dry, obstipated feces, repeated tapwater enemas or phosphate enemas should be administered once or twice daily until clear.**

✅ **Disimpaction by the oral route,** using medication, is noninvasive and more easily accepted by adolescents, who will often be reluctant to receive enemas. If there is no mechanically obstructing fecal impaction, this can also be done for adults. **Magnesium citrate (Citro-Mag), 150 to 300 mL, is given once or in divided doses for those 7 to 12 years old. For pediatric patients younger than 6 years, 2 to 4 mL/kg is given once or in divided doses.**

✅ **Disimpaction by means of a combination of the rectal route and the oral route has been shown to be effective.**

✅ Instruct the patient to return if symptoms do not improve over the next 12 to 24 hours or to return immediately if the pain worsens.

✅ **Instruct the patient to drink plenty of fluids.**

✅ **Instruct the patient that the recommended amount of dietary fiber is 20 to 35 g per day.**

✅ **Suggest adding bulk fiber, 20 to 35 g total fiber intake per day, in the form of bran, psyllium (Metamucil), methylcellulose (Citrucel), or calcium polycarbophil (FiberCon tablets) for prophylaxis.** The last two products are made from synthetic fiber and produce less gas. A high-fiber diet, however, does not benefit all patients with constipation. In general, patients with inadequate fiber intake should be advised (with the help of a dietitian) to increase their intake of natural fiber with fruit and vegetable servings.

✅ **When possible, medications that may be constipating should be discontinued or replaced.** These medications include narcotic analgesics, antacids containing aluminum and calcium, antidepressants, diuretics, nutritional supplements such as iron and calcium, anticonvulsants, antispasmodics, antiparkinsonian drugs, antihypertensive agents such as calcium channel blockers, sedatives, first-generation antihistamines, and other anticholinergic agents.

✓ **Laxatives remain the mainstay of treatment for constipation.**

✓ **Osmotic agents with laxative effects include sorbitol solution 70%, 30 to 150 mL or 1 to 2 mL/kg as single adult dose, or lactulose (Cephulac, Chronulac), 30 to 150 mL daily. In recent years, the use of over-the-counter (OTC) polyethylene glycol 3350 without electrolytes (MiraLax), 17 g (1 heaping tablespoonful) of powder dissolved in 8 oz of water, juice, soda, coffee, or tea once daily, titrated to effect with a maximum of 34 g/day, has become increasingly popular.** It is relatively expensive but generally has fewer side effects. Because it is virtually tasteless, it has led to better compliance with treatment. Polyethylene glycol (e.g., GoLYTELY) is another option, and is supplied in 14-oz and 26-oz containers as a powder to be administered after dissolution of **1 heaping tablespoon daily in 4 to 8 oz of water, juice, soda, coffee, or tea.**

✓ **Additionally, bisacodyl (Dulcolax), 5 to 15 mg as single adult dose, or senna (Senokot), 15 mg once daily, are stimulant laxatives that can be given at bedtime and are available OTC.** Both sorbitol and senna are less costly than lactulose and have been shown to be at least as efficacious, if not better.

✓ Functional constipation in infants and toddlers is defined as at least 2 weeks of scybalous, pebblelike, hard stools—or firm stools two or fewer times per week—in the absence of structural, endocrine, or metabolic disease.

✓ Constipation in infants and preschool children is usually treated first with sorbitol-containing juices, such as prune, pear, and apple juice; the addition of pureed fruits and vegetables; formula changes; or treatment with a food product with a high sugar content, such as barley malt extract or corn syrup. If, despite these dietary changes, the stool is still hard and painful to evacuate, osmotic laxatives, such as Milk of Magnesia, 0.5 to 1 mL/kg body weight/day, or polyethylene glycol 3350 without electrolytes (MiraLax), 1 to 1.5 g/kg body weight/day, are easily administered by parents and well accepted by children. They have a 92% success rate. Glycerin suppositories can also be effective. Avoid mineral oil in infants, those with neurologic difficulties, and those with gastroesophageal reflux disease (GERD) because of the risk of aspiration pneumonitis. In addition, avoid enemas and stimulant laxatives, such as senna or bisacodyl, in infants.

✓ **If the problem is chronic or recurrent or associated with alternating constipation and diarrhea, consider irritable bowel syndrome. IBS is characterized by chronic abdominal pain, altered bowel habits, and no organic cause; thus it is a diagnosis of exclusion. The most distinguishing trait of IBS is the presence of discomfort or pain associated with defecation.** The Rome IV criteria of 2016 include the following for IBS: recurrent abdominal pain on average at least once a week over the past 3 months associated with two or more of the following:

  ○ Related to defecation (may be increased, decreased, or unchanged by defecation)
  ○ Associated with change in frequency of stool
  ○ Associated with a change in appearance or form of stool

✓ Warning signs of more serious disease include the following: unintentional or unexpected weight loss; nocturnal symptoms (more common in inflammatory bowel disease, celiac sprue, infection, or cancer); fever, weight loss, and bleeding, which suggest ulcerative colitis infection or cancer; abdominal pain with anorexia, rectal abscess, and constipation, which could signal Crohn disease; abdominal pain with iron deficiency and stress fractures, which could be celiac disease or another small-bowel disorder causing malabsorption; and gastrointestinal blood loss (gross or occult), which could be the result of cancer.

✓ If the patient meets the Rome IV criteria, if routine testing shows no abnormalities, and if the patient has no warning signs of more serious disease, then it is reasonable to initiate treatment for IBS and provide follow-up in 3 to 6 weeks (sooner if symptoms change dramatically or the patient's condition deteriorates).

✓ IBS is a chronic condition without known cure. A meticulous dietary history, as it relates to symptoms, can be helpful. Dietary interventions such as a lactose-free diet, restriction of carbohydrates, avoidance of gluten, and avoidance of foods that produce gas may be undertaken.

✓ **For constipation-predominant IBS, you can give synthetic bulk fiber as described earlier.**

✓ **Antidepressants such as tricyclic antidepressants (TCAs) and selective serotonin reuptake inhibitors (SSRIs) have been found to have some efficacy in IBS symptom reduction, as noted in the 2018 American College of Gastroenterology Monograph on Management of Irritable Bowel Syndrome, which also provides further guidelines for management of this disorder.**

✓ The use of psychological therapies may also be considered; however, evidence of efficacy of psychological therapies is limited.

✓ **Antispasmodic drugs, such as dicyclomine (20 mg PO, four times a day as needed for nongeriatric adult) and hyoscyamine (0.125–0.25 mg orally or sublingual three times a day as needed for adult, maximum 1.5 mg/24 h) may provide short-term relief.** 5-Hydroxytryptamine (serotonin)-3 (5-HT3) receptor antagonists such as alosetron (Lotronex), for female patients with diarrhea-predominant IBS, were removed from the market because of problems with ischemic colitis and severe constipation but are now available with tight restrictions. Tegaserod (Zelnorm), a partial 5-HT4 receptor agonist approved for constipation-variant IBS (IBS-C), was removed from the market in 2007 due to concerns about increased risk of cardiovascular disease and subsequently reintroduced in 2019 for use in IBS-C in women under age 65 years. Lubiprostone for patients with IBS-C has been approved, but there is a lack of controlled studies or long-term safety data and it remains expensive.

✓ Rifaximin is a nonabsorbable antibiotic that has shown modest benefit in studies with relatively short-term follow-up for those with IBS and bloating; however, evidence of efficacy is limited.

✓ **If there is weight loss, anemia, occult blood in the stool, abdominal distension or mass, or a family history of colon cancer, refer the patient for colonoscopy and gastroenterology consultation.**

✓ **For infant colic** (defined as crying for a minimum of 3 hours daily 3 days per week for the previous 3 weeks, without weight loss, vomiting, or diarrhea), **there is no "magic bullet." Use of whey hydrolysate milk is considered likely to be beneficial. Other therapies are**

of uncertain effectiveness. You may instruct the parents to administer for infants, 2 mL of 24% solution of sucrose in distilled water and for neonates, 0.2 mL of 24% solution, with each episode for a trial of 1 to 2 days. If this is not successful, a higher concentration of sucrose may be more effective. Probiotics *(Lactobacillus reuteri)* have been shown to be beneficial in two randomized trials, with no ill effects observed. However, these are not regulated by the Food and Drug Administration. Homeopathic remedies, simethicone, and lactase have no proven benefits.

✓ A product called gripe water, which may include any variety of herbs and herbal oils (such as cardamom, chamomile, cinnamon, clove, dill, fennel, ginger, lemon balm, licorice, peppermint, and yarrow), is available online and in health food stores. It is not entirely without risk. Contaminants and alcohol have been found in some preparations. Parents who choose to use this product should avoid versions made with sugar or alcohol and look for products that were manufactured in the United States.

✓ **With breastfeeding mothers,** there is a possible therapeutic benefit from eliminating milk products, eggs, wheat, and nuts from the mother's diet.

✓ Some studies suggest that casein hydrolysate formulas (considered hypoallergenic) or replacement of cow's milk formula with a soy-based formula may be beneficial; a trial period of formula substitution can be recommended.

✓ Above all, parents need reassurance that their baby is healthy, and that colic is self-limited (80–90% of infants have symptom resolution by 4 months of age). There are no long-term adverse effects.

✓ **The potential for child abuse is a real one;** parents with crying infants have been known to hurt their babies. Parents should be given reassurance and empathy and have their coping mechanisms addressed; they should be counseled to take breaks from the colicky infant and employ actions to relieve stress. One study concluded that a home-based nursing intervention program reduced both parental stress and overall infant crying time.

What Not to Do

Ⓧ Do not discharge the patient with significant abdominal pain without a period of observation and serial abdominal examinations. Many abdominal catastrophes may appear improved for short periods, only to subsequently worsen.

Ⓧ Do not discharge patients with unexplained abdominal pain without explicit discharge instructions, including but not limited to instructions to return for new or worsening symptoms or for persistent pain that does not improve over the next 12 to 24 hours. Explain to your patient that there is a degree of diagnostic uncertainty and that a definitive diagnosis often cannot be reached during the initial visit to the emergency department or urgent care center.

Ⓧ Do not add fiber supplements without an adequate intake of fluids. Otherwise they may exacerbate symptoms.

Ⓧ Do not settle for a specific benign diagnosis in patients for whom you cannot find a clear cause. Do not fail to refer for colonoscopy.

Discussion

The colon performs several complex functions, which include mixing the ileal effluent, fermenting and salvaging the unabsorbed carbohydrate residues, and desiccating the intraluminal contents to form stool. These functions are regulated by neurotransmitters, intrinsic colonic reflexes, and a plethora of learned and reflex mechanisms that govern stool transport and evacuation, most of which are incompletely understood. Constipation may result from structural, mechanical, metabolic, or functional disorders that affect the colon or anorectum, either directly or indirectly. Because there is a significant interaction between the brain and the gut, it is worth emphasizing that neurologic dysfunction may have profound effects on colon function.

Patients who have had two of the following symptoms for at least 12 months fit the criteria for **functional constipation**: straining, lumpy or hard stools, incomplete bowel evacuation or sensation of anorectal blockage at least a quarter of the time, or less than three bowel movements in a week.

For infants to children 16 years of age, the following constitute functional fecal retention: at least 12 weeks of passage of large-diameter stools at intervals of two per week or fewer and/or retentive posturing, avoidance of defecation, and use of both pelvic floor and gluteal muscles. **Functional constipation** is most common in women. Colonic inertia and delayed transit are types of functional constipation caused by decreased muscle activity in the colon. Abnormalities that result in an inability to relax the rectal and anal muscles that allow stool to exit are known as anorectal dysfunction or anismus.

When constipation becomes **chronic** and unresponsive to conventional medical and behavioral treatment, it is necessary to rule out **organic diseases that can present with constipation**. Some of **the more common diseases** include irritable bowel syndrome, diverticulitis, intestinal obstruction, anal fissure, and abdominal tumors. **Metabolic causes** include uremia, hypokalemia, hyponatremia, hypomagnesemia, hypophosphatemia, and hypercalcemia. Endocrine causes include diabetes mellitus and hypothyroidism. **Neuromuscular disorders** that lead to constipation include brain tumors, spinal cord compression, multiple sclerosis, Parkinson disease, cerebral palsy, and stroke or other disorders that cause muscle weakness. **Acute constipation is more often associated with organic disease than is long-standing constipation.** When a particular disorder is suspected, appropriate laboratory studies and colorectal imaging are required.

Flexible sigmoidoscopy and colonoscopy are excellent for identifying lesions that narrow or occlude the bowel. Colonoscopy is the examination of choice in adult patients with constipation who have iron deficiency anemia, a positive guaiac stool test, or a first-degree relative with colon cancer.

In childhood constipation, most difficulties related to defecation are the consequence of painful or psychologically traumatic defecation experiences. **In children younger than 1 year of age**, the possibility of Hirschsprung disease or cystic fibrosis must be considered. However, **in adolescents**, constipation is most commonly a consequence of a learned behavior to suppress the urge to defecate. When specifically asked, adolescents readily admit that they do not use the toilet facilities at school. Repeated suppression of the urge to defecate and stool withholding may be contributing factors to the two colorectal disorders associated with constipation: pelvic floor dysfunction and slow-transit constipation.

A reduction in dietary fiber has been associated with a higher prevalence of constipation in children. Illicit substances, particularly opiates such as heroin and products that contain oxycodone and hydrocodone, are used by approximately 10% of high school seniors nationwide. These substances may cause or exacerbate constipation. Therefore abuse of these substances should be included in the differential diagnosis of the constipated adolescent patient. In addition, constipation is among the most frequently identified concerns in **patients who have anorexia nervosa and bulimia**. Many patients with eating disorders are distressed by and preoccupied with their infrequent bowel movements.

Occult constipation should be considered in **children with recurrent abdominal pain**. Because reporting of stool patterns by children is unreliable, rectal examination should be considered in those with recurrent abdominal pain.

IBS is a common condition in adults and adolescents. There is a significant female predominance in those patients who present to physicians with this condition. Patients with IBS view minor illnesses, such as colds and the flu, more seriously and consult physicians more frequently than do patients who do not have IBS.

Discussion continued

IBS is a heterogeneous disorder with diverse clinical presentations and multiple pathogenic mechanisms. Its exact pathophysiology remains undefined. The three most important contributing factors seem to be hypersensitivity of the gut, altered motility, and psychosocial dysfunction. Changes in intestinal microflora, including small intestinal bacterial overgrowth, carbohydrate malabsorption, and the development of gluten sensitivity or food-specific antibodies are currently being investigated as potential causes. Gastrointestinal infections may act as a triggering factor in a subgroup of patients. Patients with IBS may present with diarrhea, constipation, or a combination of urgency, pain, gas, and bloating. Symptoms are not constant over time. There is temporal fluctuation, with flare-ups alternating with periods of relative well-being in most patients. The type of bowel complaint and predominance of specific symptoms may also vary over time.

Patients who are allergic to gliadin (a constituent of rye, barley, and wheat) may present with symptoms that are indistinguishable from IBS. This condition, known as celiac disease or celiac sprue, can cause a variety of symptoms, including rancid gas, oily or floating stools, bloating, and constipation or diarrhea. Consultation with a gastroenterologist should be obtained prior to starting the patient on a gluten-free diet.

Infant colic can be distressing to parents whose infant is inconsolable during crying episodes. Colic is a diagnosis of exclusion that is made after performing a careful history and physical examination to rule out less common organic causes. Treatment is limited. Feeding changes are sometimes advised. Medications available in the United States have not been proven to be effective in the treatment of colic, and most behavioral interventions have not been proven to be clearly more effective than placebo. The cause of infantile colic remains unclear.

Colic attacks usually start when an infant is 7 to 10 days old and increase in frequency for the next 1 to 2 months. They tend to be worse in the late afternoon and evening and subside by the age of 3 to 4 months. Colicky infants have attacks of screaming in the evening with associated motor behaviors, such as a flushed face, furrowed brow, and clenched fists. The legs are pulled up to the abdomen, and the infants emit a piercing, high-pitched scream. Crying occurs in prolonged bouts and is unpredictable and spontaneous. It appears to be unrelated to environmental events. The child cannot be soothed, even by feeding. These episodes do not just happen suddenly one night when the infant is 6 to 8 weeks old. In that situation, look for some other acute problem, such as intussusception, corneal abrasion, incarcerated hernia, clothing that may be pinching or pricking, or a digital hair tourniquet. A history of apnea, cyanosis, or struggling to breathe may suggest previously undiagnosed pulmonary or cardiac conditions. Lethargy, poor skin perfusion, and tachypnea suggest a serious underlying problem. A rectal temperature greater than 100.4 °F (38 °C) or poor weight gain suggests infection, a gastrointestinal disorder, or nervous system disorder and requires further workup. During the examination, the infant's clothing should be removed to facilitate inspection of the skin, to eliminate any irritation to the skin, and to check for any evidence of trauma or abuse. The examination itself may reassure the parents. Organic causes are found in less than 5% of infants presenting with excessive crying. However, if the child is not "awake and calm" for a reasonable period, consider hospital admission with a complete diagnostic workup.

Laboratory tests and radiographic examinations usually are unnecessary if the child is gaining weight and has a normal physical examination without worrisome symptoms.

At 1-year follow-up, a group of colicky infants compared with noncolicky infants showed no differences in behavior in nine dimensions assessed by means of the Toddler Temperament Scale.

Suggested Readings

Arce, D. A., Ermocilla, C. A., & Costa, H. (2002). Evaluation of constipation. *American Family Physician, 65*, 2283–2290.

Clifford, T. J., Campbell, K., Speechley, K. N., et al. (2002a). Infant colic. *Archives of Pediatrics and Adolescent Medicine, 156*, 1183–1188.

Clifford, T. J., Campbell, K., Speechley, K. N., et al. (2002b). Sequelae of infant colic. *Archives of Pediatrics and Adolescent Medicine, 156*, 1123–1128.

Dalrymple, J., & Bullock, I. (2008). Diagnosis and management of irritable bowel syndrome in adults in primary care: Summary of NICE guidance. *BMJ*, *336*, 556–558.

Drossman, D. A., & Hasler, W. L. (2016). Rome IV—functional GI disorders: Disorders of gut-brain interaction. *Gastroenterology*, *150*(6), 1257–1261.

Eidlitz-Markus, T., Mimouni, M., Zaharia, A., et al. (2004). Occult constipation: A common cause of recurrent abdominal pain in childhood. *The Israel Medical Association Journal*, *6*, 677–680.

Ford, A. C., Moayyedi, P., Chey, W. D., et al. (2018). American college of gastroenterology monograph on management of irritable bowel syndrome. *American Journal of Gastroenterology*, *113*(1), S1–S18.

Ford, A. C., Moayyedi, P., Lacy, B. E., et al. (2014). American college of gastroenterology monograph on the management of irritable bowel syndrome and chronic idiopathic constipation. *American Journal of Gastroenterology*, *109*, S2–S26.

Ford, A. C., Talley, N. J., Schoenfeld, P. S., et al. (2009). Efficacy of antidepressants and psychological therapies in irritable bowel syndrome: Systematic review and meta-analysis. *Gut*, *58*, 367–378.

Keefe, M. R., Lobo, M. L., & Froese-Fretz, A. (2006). Effectiveness of an intervention for colic. *Clinical Pediatrics*, *45*, 123–133.

Kilgour, T., & Wade, S. (2005). Infantile colic. *Clinical Evidence*, *13*, 362–372.

Lehtonen, L., Korhonen, T., & Korvenranta, H. (1994). Temperament and sleeping patterns in colicky infants during the first year of life. *Journal of Developmental and Behavioral Pediatrics*, *15*, 416–420.

Loening-Baucke, V. (2005). Prevalence, symptoms, and outcome of constipation in infants and toddlers. *The Journal of Pediatrics*, *146*, 359–363.

Pimentel, M., Lembo, A., Chey, W. D., et al. (2011). Rifaximin therapy for patients with IBS without constipation. *New England Journal of Medicine*, *364*, 22–32.

Rao, S. (2003). Constipation: Evaluation and treatment. *Gastroenterology Clinics of North America*, *32*, 659–683.

Reijneveld, S. A., van der Wal, M. F., Brugman, E., et al. (2004). Infant crying and abuse. *Lancet*, *364*, 1340–1342.

Roberts, D. M., Ostapchuk, M., & O'Brien, J. G. (2004). Infantile colic. *American Family Physician*, *70*, 735–740.

Savino, F., Cordisco, L., Tarasco, V., et al. (2010). *Lactobacillus reuteri* DSM 17938 in infantile colic: A randomized, double-blind, placebo-controlled trial. *Pediatrics*, *126*, e526–e533.

Tabbers, M. M., Dilorenzo, C., Berger, M. Y., et al. (2014). Evaluation and treatment of functional constipation in infants and children: Evidence-based recommendations from ESPGHAN and NASPGHAN. *Journal of Pediatric Gastroenterology and Nutrition*, *58*(2), 258–274.

Turner, T. L., & Palamountain, S. (n.d.). Infantile colic: Clinical features and diagnosis. UptoDate. http://www.uptodate.com.

Turner, T. L., & Palamountain, S. (n.d.). Infantile colic: Management and outcome. UptoDate. http://www.uptodate.com.

Wald, A. (n.d.a). Pathophysiology of irritable bowel syndrome. UpToDate. http://www.uptodate.com.

Wald, A. (n.d.b). Treatment of irritable bowel syndrome in adults. UpToDate. http://www.uptodate.com.

Youssef, N. N., Sanders, L., & Di Lorenzo, C. (2004). Adolescent constipation: Evaluation and management. *Adolescent Medicine Clinics*, *15*, 37–52.

Diarrhea

(Acute Gastroenteritis)

Presentation

Complaints may range from occasional stool that is not well formed to acute, copious diarrhea that produces profound dehydration and shock. Patients with inflammatory or infectious diarrhea often present with fever, tenesmus (the frequent urge to defecate), abdominal pain, and hemoccult-positive stool. These conditions usually cause a more severe form of diarrhea and require more careful assessment and more aggressive treatment. Noninflammatory diarrhea is usually watery, milder, without significant fever, with only mild abdominal cramping, and without blood or leukocytes in the stool. Nausea and vomiting can occur with both forms of diarrhea (see Chapter 76).

What to Do

✓ **Ask specifically** about the frequency of stools, the volume (much liquid implies a defect in absorption in the small bowel, whereas tenesmus producing little more than mucus implies inflammation of the rectosigmoid wall), the character (color, odor, blood, or mucus), and the consistency (waterlike or just loose stool). Ask about travel, medications (including antibiotics), residence, daycare attendance, pregnancy status, immunosuppression, consumption of unpasteurized dairy products or undercooked meat or fish, similar symptoms previously, and nocturnal symptoms (rare with functional disease).

✓ **Physical examination** should focus on signs of moderate or severe dehydration and signs of systemic toxicity. Excessive volume loss can be detected by abnormal vital signs, including fever, tachycardia, and orthostatic changes. **When dehydration is suspected, obtain a urinalysis and weigh pediatric patients.** Any symptoms or fall in blood pressure or increase in pulse rate of more than 20 beats per minute after standing for a minute suggests hypovolemia. **Urine specific gravity of 1.020 or greater also suggests hypovolemia, and ketones of 2 or greater suggest starvation ketosis.**

✓ Loss of skin turgor and dryness of mucosal membranes are also signs of dehydration. Physical signs in infants and small children may include ill appearance, sunken fontanel, sunken eyes, decreased tears, dry mouth, cool extremities, delayed capillary refill, and a weak cry.

✓ **The presence of peritoneal signs or persistent focal tenderness on abdominal examination** may suggest an infection with an invasive enteric pathogen or a cause requiring urgent surgical evaluation and management.

✓ **Perform a rectal examination and obtain a sample of stool for occult blood testing and for Wright or Gram staining.** If the rectal ampulla is empty, you can still swab the mucosa and may get an even better specimen for stool culture when required. **Stool cultures for enteropathogens need only be obtained when there is a suspected community outbreak, involvement of food handlers, special populations (pregnant women, the immunocompromised, the elderly, or those with significant comorbidities who appear ill), temperature greater than 38.5 °C, severe or prolonged diarrheal illnesses (generally >1–2 weeks in duration), and bloody diarrhea (including Shiga toxin–producing *Escherichia coli*). A spontaneous specimen is also good.**

✅ **If the patient has been on antibiotics within the past 2 months, test the stool for** *Clostridium difficile* **toxin.**

✅ **In pediatric patients with associated vomiting and decreased oral intake, consider checking point-of-care blood glucose.**

✅ **Severe acute diarrhea** warrants immediate medical evaluation and possible hospitalization. The criteria for severe acute diarrhea requiring diagnostic evaluation include volume depletion, fever, six or more stools in 24 hours, an illness lasting longer than 48 hours, significant abdominal pain in individuals older than 50 years of age, and diarrhea in special populations (the elderly, pregnant women, or the immunocompromised). The very young and the very old are at greater risk for developing significant fluid loss, with its attendant complications. In patients with inflammatory bowel disease (IBD), it is important to send stool studies to help rule out an infectious process and differentiate this from an IBD flare.

✅ **If the adult patient is not seriously ill but has a fever higher than 38.5 °C (101.3 °F), the stool is positive for occult blood, or there are any white blood cells (stool leukocytes) in a 400× field, assume the problem is invasive or inflammatory (e.g., *Campylobacter* organisms, *Salmonella*, *Shigella*, enterohemorrhagic and enteroinvasive *E. coli*, *Entamoeba*, ulcerative colitis, and cytotoxic organisms such as *C. difficile* or *Entamoeba histolytica*). If there is no risk for *C. difficile*, and there is no suspicion for enterohemorrhagic *E. coli* or fluoroquinolone-resistant *Campylobacter* infection, prescribe ciprofloxacin (Cipro), 500 mg twice a day for 3 to 5 days, and schedule follow-up.**

✅ Because there are reasonable concerns about a possible association between hemolytic-uremic syndrome and antibiotic administration to children, **many authorities believe that children with infectious diarrhea should not be treated empirically;** rather, treatment should be based on culture results. Ask the patient to bring a fresh stool sample in a specimen cup at follow-up if the diarrhea persists, in case it needs to be sent for culture or examined for ova and parasites.

✅ **If there are no white blood cells on microscopic examination of the stool or the stool is negative for occult blood, assume the diarrhea results from a virus or toxin.**

✅ **Afebrile adult patients with limited diarrhea require no diagnostic studies or treatment other than fluid and electrolyte replacement. These patients will not benefit from antibiotics and require follow-up only if they have continued diarrhea, abdominal pain, or fever.**

✅ **Adult patients who feel sick and appear to be dehydrated will benefit from rapid rehydration with intravenous (IV) 0.9% NaCl or lactated Ringer solution (1–2 L over an hour for an adult with normal cardiovascular and renal function).** Patients who are not vomiting can often be rehydrated by drinking plenty of fluids, such as diluted fruit juices. To replace lost electrolytes, have them eat foods such as saltine crackers, soups, or broth.

✓ **Oral rehydration solutions generally are unnecessary in adults younger than 65 years. When an oral rehydration solution is required, do not use sports drinks** (e.g., Gatorade) because they often contain too much sugar and insufficient salt. If oral rehydration solutions (e.g., Rehydralyte) are unavailable, a less ideal substitute can be prepared by adding 0.5 teaspoon of table salt, 0.5 teaspoon of baking soda, and 4 tablespoons of sugar to 1 L of purified water.

✓ **Both classes of diarrhea (inflammatory and noninflammatory) are best treated with absorbent bulk laxatives such as methylcellulose (Citrucel), using one heaping tablespoon in 8 oz of water three to four times a day.**

✓ **Loperamide (Imodium) often limits symptoms to 1 day. It has antimotility and antisecretory effects and is taken as 4 mg after the first loose stool, followed by 2 mg after each subsequent loose stool to a maximum of 16 mg for 2 days. Do not use antimotility agents if there is a suspicion for *C. difficile* or concern for enterohemorrhagic *E. coli*, because this may facilitate development of hemolytic uremic syndrome. Antimotility agents are suggested for symptomatic patients with absent or low-grade fever and nonbloody stools.**

✓ A chewable loperamide-simethicone combination product has been shown to provide faster and more complete relief of acute, nonspecific diarrhea and associated gas-related abdominal discomfort than either of its components provided alone. Loperamide may be used in pregnant women but should not be used at all in children with inflammatory diarrhea or who are younger than 2 years of age.

✓ **For travelers without signs of invasive or inflammatory diarrhea, give a single dose of ciprofloxacin (Cipro), 500 mg, or norfloxacin (Noroxin), 400 mg orally, to reduce the duration and severity of symptoms.** If symptoms persist or the diarrhea is severe or associated with high fever or bloody stools, prescribe ciprofloxacin, 500 mg twice a day, or norfloxacin, 400 mg three times a day for 3 days. **Azithromycin (Zithromax), 10 mg/kg daily for 3 days, can be used for children, or 500 mg daily for 1 to 3 days can be used in pregnant women and for other adults with quinolone-resistant *Campylobacter*.**

✓ **Probiotics** (*Lactobacillus* preparations [Culturelle Probiotic, Colon Health Probiotic Caps] and yogurt) can also be used; they have efficacy in nonspecific pediatric diarrhea as well as traveler's diarrhea.

✓ **With infants and small children, oral rehydration therapy should be the main treatment. Enteral rehydration by the oral or nasogastric route is as effective as, if not better than, IV rehydration.** Have the parents give an oral rehydration mixture with the goal of replacing the fluid lost. For every one cup of diarrhea lost, give a cup of the following recipe:

○ ½ to 1 cup precooked baby rice cereal

○ 2 cups water

○ ¼ tsp salt

○ Mix the rice cereal, water, and salt together until the mixture thickens but is not too thick to drink. Be sure the ingredients are well mixed. A pinch of the artificial sweetener aspartame (Equal) can be added to make it more palatable. Have the parents give the mixture by spoon often and have them offer these children as much as they will accept (every minute if they will accept it). Instruct the parents that if the child is vomiting, wait 20 minutes and then offer the mixture again in small amounts (½–1 tsp) every few minutes. Ondansetron (Zofran ODT) can be used in this situation as an antiemetic. Bananas or other nonsweetened, mashed fruit can help provide potassium.

✓ **Alternatively, one can give commercial rehydration fluids, such as Rehydralyte, Ricelyte, or Pedialyte, which are sold in drugstores.** When parents are sent home with the child, set a specified amount of time that they should continue to try oral rehydration before coming back to see you. From 4 to 6 hours is a reasonable time period, depending on the age of the child and the degree of dehydration and illness. They should also come back for a recheck if there are more than 10 to 15 stools, minimal urination, or a general worsening of the child's appearance.

✓ **An alternative to voluntary oral rehydration in infants and children who are moderately dehydrated is the use of rapid nasogastric hydration. Patients can be given standard oral rehydration solution down a nasogastric tube of appropriate size administered at a rate of 50 mL/kg of body weight, delivered over 4 hours.**

✓ Infants can become severely dehydrated in short order with viral diarrhea. More severely ill children may benefit from intravenous therapy with normal saline administered at the same rate of 20 to 40 mL/kg over 2 to 4 hours.

✓ **Involve the parents in the decision regarding the method of fluid replacement.**

✓ **During or after diarrhea, children should be given frequent small meals (six or more times a day) and actively encouraged to eat. Nursing infants should continue to breastfeed on demand, and infants and older children should be offered their usual food.** Parents should use well-cooked staple starches that can be easily digested, such as rice, corn, potatoes, or noodles in a soft mashed form. Infants should be given a thick porridge or semiliquid pulp. Milk products and cereals are usually well tolerated.

✓ As soon as an adequate degree of rehydration has been achieved, the diet can be advanced quickly as tolerated, and the usual diet should be started at the earliest opportunity.

✓ All patients with severe dehydration may require large amounts of IV fluids and occasionally must be admitted to the hospital.

What Not to Do

✗ Do not omit the rectal examination, which may disclose a fecal impaction or rectal abscess.

✗ Do not obtain unnecessary stool cultures. It has been estimated that routine stool cultures are positive in only 2% of patients, and most cases of diarrhea in the United States are self-limited and will resolve spontaneously. Follow suggestions for sending stool cultures listed earlier.
Sending stool samples for ova and parasites is usually only recommended for community or daycare outbreaks, patients with ongoing diarrhea (with or without recent travel), patients who are homosexual men, or if there is bloody diarrhea with a paucity of fecal white blood cells.

(X) Do not stop or reduce breastfeeding when a baby has diarrhea. Infants with diarrhea should be breastfed as often and for as long as they want.

(X) Do not restrict children or adults from having milk or milk products. Despite the potential for lactose intolerance, clinical evidence of lactase deficiency is uncommon, and most individuals can tolerate nonhuman milk without difficulty.

(X) Do not give or recommend sugary drinks such as Gatorade, sweetened commercial fruit drinks, cola drinks, or apple juice if there is significant dehydration. These may cause an osmotic diarrhea and a net loss of fluid. Clear liquids are also not recommended as a substitute for oral rehydration solutions.

(X) Do not confuse influenza with stomach flu. Influenza with fever, body aches, cough, and fatigue almost never causes symptoms in the stomach and intestines.

(X) Do not overlook the possibility of acute appendicitis or ischemic bowel disease in those patients with suspicious physical findings or significant risk factors.

(X) Do not have patients use diphenoxylate with atropine (Lomotil). It has central nervous system (CNS) effects that are dangerous if a child accidentally ingests it. It also has unpleasant cholinergic effects.

(X) Do not make the diagnosis of gastroenteritis when the patient is only vomiting. The vomiting may be due to a surgical or nongastrointestinal cause that may possibly be life threatening.

Discussion

Acute infectious gastroenteritis is a common cause of vomiting and diarrhea in the United States. Most patients respond well to symptomatic therapy only. Laboratory testing should be reserved for patients with high fever and bloody or prolonged diarrhea, for the immunocompromised, for suspected cases of antibiotic-associated diarrhea, and for suspected community outbreaks. Empiric antibiotic therapy is generally accepted in adults with fever and hemoccult-positive stool.

Common causes of inflammatory diarrhea include invasive or toxin-producing organisms, such as *Campylobacter jejuni, C. difficile,* enterohemorrhagic and enteroinvasive *E. coli, Shigella* sp., nontyphi *Salmonella* sp., and *E. histolytica.* Consider pet reptiles, rodents, and dogs as a possible source of *Salmonella* and other forms of infectious diarrhea.

Patients with recent antibiotic exposure who present with diarrhea are at risk for antibiotic-associated diarrhea. Most commonly, these patients are afflicted with *C. difficile* infection, and they should be evaluated specifically for

***C. difficile* toxins A and B. Always suspect *C. difficile* as the cause of diarrhea in patients who have been in the hospital for longer than 2 weeks, whatever the reason. Also, inpatients who receive proton-pump inhibitors and the elderly are at increased risk for *C. difficile* diarrhea. First-line therapy consists of vancomycin, 125 mg orally every 6 hours for 10 to 14 days, as well as discontinuation of the precipitating antibiotic (if possible).**

Second-line therapy consists of metronidazole (Flagyl), 500 mg orally three times a day for 10 to 14 days.

Viruses commonly cause diarrhea, but it is rarely severe. Associated symptoms are abrupt onset of nausea and abdominal cramps, followed by vomiting or diarrhea. Fevers occur in approximately 50% of affected individuals. Headache, myalgias, upper respiratory symptoms, and abdominal pain are common. Stool studies are negative for fecal leukocytes and blood. Common causes include norovirus, rotavirus, and enteric adenovirus. Other causes of noninflammatory diarrheas include

Giardia lamblia, Cryptosporidium parvum, Vibrio cholerae, and enterotoxigenic *E. coli.*

Travelers' diarrhea usually begins within the first week of travel and usually resolves without consequence after 3 to 5 days. In most cases, however, symptoms are severe enough to force a change of itinerary or result in confinement to bed. In 1% of cases, hospitalization is necessary.

High-risk regions include the developing countries of Latin America, Africa, Asia, and parts of the Middle East. Areas of intermediate risk include China, southern Europe, Israel, South Africa, Russia, and several Caribbean islands (especially Haiti and the Dominican Republic).

High-risk foods include uncooked vegetables and unpeeled fresh fruit, raw or undercooked meat or seafood (particularly shellfish), and salads. Ice, tap water, and unpasteurized milk carry an increased risk for infection. Safe drinks include bottled carbonated beverages, beer or wine, and boiled or bottled water. Meals eaten in a private home carry reduced risk compared with those eaten in a restaurant. Food from street vendors is particularly risky.

Traveler's diarrhea often cannot be avoided. If these patients are seen by you, they should be treated like any other patient who presents with diarrhea. For patients who are managed in the pretravel period, chemoprophylaxis is generally discouraged. It is most appropriate to prepare the traveler for prompt self-treatment at the first sign of illness using a combination of an antimotility agent (usually loperamide), about eight doses/person, and an antibiotic (usually a fluoroquinolone), six doses/person, both of which can be obtained prior to departure and carried during travel. Consider azithromycin if the patient is traveling with children or a pregnant adult (see regimen earlier in the chapter). If symptoms resolve within 24 hours of initiating therapy, no further treatment is necessary. If diarrhea persists after 1 day, treatment should be continued for 1 or 2 more days.

Rifaximin (Xifaxan), 200 mg orally three times a day for 3 days, is a nonabsorbed oral antibiotic that has been approved for treatment of traveler's diarrhea, but it is not effective against infections associated with fever or blood in the stool or those caused by *Campylobacter.* It has fewer adverse effects and drug interactions than systemic antibiotics, but it cannot be taken during pregnancy. For severe diarrhea, the fluoroquinolones or azithromycin remain the preferred antibiotics.

Acute bloody diarrhea is a frightening symptom that has been associated with *E. coli* 0157:H7 and other Shiga toxin–producing *E. coli* infections, illnesses occasionally complicated by the development of hemolytic-uremic syndrome and death. Suspect this in patients who lack high fever and who have abdominal tenderness and pain with bloody diarrhea. It is recommended that stool samples be cultured for patients with acute bloody diarrhea. Antibiotics and antimotility agents should be avoided in patients with suspected or proven infection with enterohemorrhagic *E. coli.*

It can be useful if acute care practitioners report any suspected infectious outbreaks to public health departments.

Patients with prolonged noninflammatory symptom complexes, especially those who have traveled to endemic areas, may benefit from stool evaluation for parasites. For patients with persistent diarrhea (lasting >1 week), an empirical trial of metronidazole or nitazoxanide for a protozoal infection is sometimes considered.

The treatment of diarrhea in immunocompromised patients is essentially the same as that for normal hosts, but such patients may require prolonged courses of antimicrobial therapy and often require subspecialty consultation.

Noninfectious causes of acute diarrhea include inflammatory bowel disease (most often ulcerative colitis, but diarrhea can also be seen with Crohn disease). Symptoms include diarrhea with mucus, rectal bleeding, and abdominal pain.

Medications are another noninfectious cause. The most common medications responsible for acute diarrhea are laxatives, antacids containing calcium or magnesium, colchicine, antibiotics, sorbitol gums, and enteral tube feedings (especially if hypertonic). Diarrhea usually resolves after cessation of the medication.

Other noninfectious causes of diarrhea that need to be considered are pelvic abscess in the area of the rectosigmoid, intestinal ischemia in the elderly, partial small bowel obstruction, obstipation/fecal impaction, or acute appendicitis.

Gastroenteritis is probably the most common diagnosis in missed appendicitis cases. Children with acute appendicitis present with a much higher incidence of diarrhea than

those in other age groups, but diarrhea can accompany acute appendicitis at any age. Consider using advanced imaging (ultrasonography or, if that fails to be diagnostic, computed tomography [CT] scan) early in equivocal cases.

When inflammatory diarrhea is recurrent, suspect a noninfectious cause such as inflammatory bowel disease.

In the pregnant patient who has diarrhea and systemic illness, consider listeriosis.

Ordinary stool cultures only identify *Campylobacter, Shigella, Salmonella, Aeromonas,* and *Yersinia. Aeromonas* and *Yersinia* may be missed on testing unless specifically sought. Testing for other pathogens, such as *Vibrio* sp., enterohemorrhagic *E. coli* 0157:H7, and other Shiga toxin–producing bacteria, requires special media.

Routine laboratory tests (complete blood count [CBC], electrolytes, renal function) are generally neither helpful nor indicated in making a diagnosis. These tests may be useful as indicators of severity of disease, especially in the elderly or the very young, but your clinical impression is more important.

When methylcellulose (Citrucel) is recommended, patients may remind you that they have diarrhea, not constipation. Because these bulk agents absorb water in the gut lumen, however, they can relieve both problems and obviate the rebound constipation often produced by the narcotic and binding agents also used to treat diarrhea.

Older patients medicated for pain or psychosis can develop a fecal impaction, which can also present as diarrhea. **Irritable bowel syndrome, food allergy, lactose intolerance, and parasite infestation can produce relapsing diarrhea,** but the pattern may only become apparent on follow-up.

Suggested Readings

Atherly-John, Y. C., Cunningham, S. J., Crain, E. F., et al. (2002). A randomized trial of oral vs intravenous rehydration in a pediatric emergency department. *Archives of Pediatric and Adolescent Medicine, 156,* 1240–1243.

Brown, T. (2003). Update on emerging infections: News from the centers for disease control and prevention. norovirus activity—United States, 2002. *Annals of Emergency Medicine, 42,* 417–422.

Chitkara, Y. K. (2005). Limited value of routine stool cultures in patients receiving antibiotic therapy? *American Journal of Clinical Pathology, 123,* 92–95.

Cohen, M. B., Mezoff, A. G., Laney, D. W., et al. (1995). Use of a single solution for oral rehydration and maintenance therapy of infants with diarrhea and mild to moderate dehydration. *Pediatrics, 95,* 639–645.

Dial, S., Alrasadi, K., Manoukian, C., et al. (2004). Risk of *Clostridium difficile* among hospital inpatients prescribed proton pump inhibitors: Cohort and case-control studies. *Canadian Medical Association Journal, 171,* 33–38.

Diemert, D. J. (2002). Prevention and self-treatment of travelers' diarrhea. *Primary Care, 29,* 843–855.

Ericsson, C. D., DuPont, H. L., Mathewson, J. J., et al. (2001). Optimal dosing of ofloxacin with loperamide in the treatment of non-dysenteric travelers' diarrhea. *Journal of Travel Medicine, 8,* 207–209.

Feldman, M., Friedman, L., & Brandt, L. (2010). *Sleisenger and Fordtran's gastrointestinal and liver disease* (9th ed.). St. Louis, MO: Elsevier.

Fonseca, B. K., Holdgate, A., & Craig, J. C. (2004). Enteral vs intravenous rehydration therapy for children with gastroenteritis. *Archives in Pediatric and Adolescent Medicine, 158,* 483–490.

Gore, J. I., & Surawicz, C. (2003). Severe acute diarrhea. *Gastroenterology Clinics of North America, 32,* 1249–1267.

Grunenberg, N. (2003). Is gradual introduction of feeding better than immediate normal feeding in children with gastroenteritis? *Archives of Disease in Childhood, 88,* 455–457.

Kaplan, M. A., Prior, M. J., Ash, R. R., et al. (1999). Loperamide-simethicone vs loperamide alone, simethicone alone, and placebo in the treatment of acute diarrhea with gas-related abdominal discomfort. *Archives of Family Medicine, 8,* 243–248.

Karras, D. J., Ong, S., Moran, G. J., et al. (2003). Antibiotic use for emergency department patients with acute diarrhea: Prescribing practices, patient expectations, and patient satisfaction. *Annals of Emergency Medicine, 42*, 835–842.

LaRocque, R., & Harris, J. B. (n.d.). Approach to the adult with acute diarrhea in resource-rich settings. UptoDate. http://www.uptodate.com.

Leibovitz, E., Janco, J., Piglansky, L., et al. (2000). Oral ciprofloxacin vs intramuscular ceftriaxone as empiric treatment of acute invasive diarrhea in children. *The Pediatric Infectious Disease Journal, 19*, 1060–1067.

Margolis, P. A., Litteer, T., Hare, N., et al. (1990). Effects of unrestricted diet on mild infantile diarrhea. *American Journal of Diseases of Children, 144*, 162–164.

Nager, A. L., & Wang, V. J. (2002). Comparison of nasogastric and intravenous methods of rehydration in pediatric patients with acute dehydration. *Pediatrics, 109*, 566–572.

Phin, S. J., McCaskill, M. E., Browne, G. J., & Lam, L. T. (2003). Clinical pathway using rapid rehydration for children with gastroenteritis. *Journal of Paediatrics and Child Health, 39*, 343–348.

Porter, S. C., Fleisher, G. R., Kohane, I. S., et al. The value of parental report for diagnosis and management of dehydration in the emergency department. *Annals of Emergency Medicine, 41*, 196–205.

Reid, S. R., & Bonadino, W. A. (1996). Outpatient rapid intravenous rehydration to correct dehydration and resolve vomiting in children with acute gastroenteritis. *Annals of Emergency Medicine, 28*, 318–323 (editorial 353–354).

Salam, I., Katelaris, P., Leigh-Smith, S., & Farthing, M. J. (1994). Randomized trial of single-dose ciprofloxacin for traveller's diarrhoea. *Lancet, 344*, 1537–1539.

Sandhu, B. K. (2001). European Society of Paediatric Gastroenterology, Hepatology and Nutrition working group on acute diarrhoea: Rationale for early feeding in childhood gastroenteritis. *Journal of Pediatric Gastroenterology and Nutrition, 33*(2), S13–S16.

Schroeder, M. S. (2005). *Clostridium difficile*–associated diarrhea. *American Family Physician, 71*, 921–928.

Shane, A. L., Mody, R. K., Krump, J. K., et al. (2017). 2017 Infectious Diseases Society of America clinical practice guidelines for the diagnosis and management of infectious diarrhea. *Clinics in Infectious Disease, 65*, e45–e80. https://academic.oup.com/cid/article/65/12/e45/4557073.

Sigel, D., Cohen, P. T., Neighbor, M., et al. (1987). Predictive value of stool examination in acute diarrhea. *Archives of Pathology and Laboratory Medicine, 111*, 715–718.

Spandorfer, P. R., Alessandrini, E. A., Joffe, M. D., et al. (2005). Oral versus intravenous rehydration of moderately dehydrated children. *Pediatrics, 115*, 295–301.

Steffen, R., Collard, F., & Tornieporth, N. (1999). Epidemiology, etiology, and impact of traveler's diarrhea in Jamaica. *Journal of the American Medical Association, 281*, 811–817.

Steiner, M. J., DeWalt, D. A., Byerley, J. S., et al. (2004). Is this child dehydrated? *Journal of the American Medical Association, 291*, 2746–2754.

Enterobiasis

(Pinworm, Seatworm, Threadworm)

Presentation

The patient complains of severe perianal and/or vaginal irritation and itching, which is worse at night and may contribute to insomnia or superinfection of the excoriated perianal skin. Children may exhibit only perianal pruritus and nocturnal restlessness. Rarely, more serious disease can result, including weight loss, urinary tract infection, and appendicitis. Often an entire family is affected.

What to Do

✓ Examine the anus to rule out other causes of itching, such as rectal prolapse, fecal leakage, hemorrhoids, lice (pediculosis), fungal infections (tinea or candidiasis), or bacterial infections (erythrasma) (see pruritus ani in Discussion box, Chapter 66).

✓ **Look for the little white wiggling pinworms directly (especially if the patient comes in at night) and also by pressing the sticky side of cellophane tape wrapped around a tongue blade (sticky side up) to the perianal skin several times. Remove the tape and place it sticky side down on a glass slide. Examine the tape, under the low power of the microscope, for female worms** (only 5% of infected persons have eggs in their stool) approximately 1 cm long, 0.5 mm in diameter, with pointed tails (Fig. 70.1). Adult male pinworms are shorter (2.5 mm in length) and have a blunt tail. (Use shiny rather than "invisible" tape, because the latter's rough surface makes microscopy difficult.) To increase this test's sensitivity to approximately 90%, it should be conducted right after the patient awakens on at least 3 consecutive days.

✓ **If you see pinworms or still suspect them, administer one oral dose of pyrantel pamoate, 11 mg/kg (maximum 1 g), to all family members. This can be obtained over the counter as Pin-X, Pin-Rid, and Reese's Pinworm Medicine (oral suspension 250 mg/5 mL). This should be repeated in 2 weeks. This treatment has lower efficacy and greater side effects (vomiting, diarrhea, anorexia, and nausea) than the medications available by prescription.**

✓ **Two prescription medications are mebendazole (Vermox), 100-mg chewable tablet once orally (not for children <2 years of age), and albendazole (Albenza), 400 mg in adults or 10 mg/kg in children as a single dose. Both of these prescription medications should be repeated after 2 weeks.** All three of these medications are considered unsafe during pregnancy.

✓ Explain to all concerned that this is not a dangerous infection and should be eradicated from the whole family after one or two treatments. Have the family clean all bedrooms and bedding. Explain that thorough hand washing is important because pinworms are transmitted by direct anus-to-mouth spread, by direct contact with dirty linens or clothing, or by dirty hands contaminating food during its preparation or consumption.

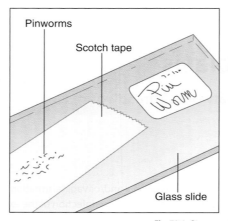

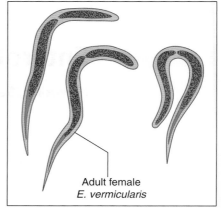

Fig. 70.1 Pinworm examples.

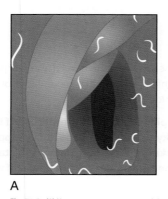

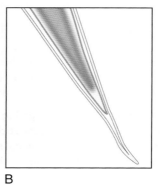

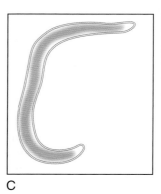

A   B   C

Fig. 70.2 (A) Numerous pinworms scattered throughout the colon as seen with colonoscopy. (B) The adult female worm with a long, pointed tail. (C) The adult male pinworm is short with a blunt tail. (Adapted from Faruqi, S., Ahmed, I., & Membreno, F. [2003]. Pinworms. *Gastrointestinal Endoscopy, 57,* 566.)

Discussion

There is evidence of pinworm infection that dates back to Roman-occupied Egypt (30 BC to AD 395). *Enterobius vermicularis* is also the oldest and most common parasite for which we have direct evidence in the New World, with fecal samples positive for pinworm ova from the American Southwest dating back 10,000 years. The pinworm, threadworm, or seatworm is a nematode, or roundworm, with the largest geographic range of any helminth. It is the most prevalent nematode in the United States. Humans are the only known host, and perhaps 10% of the US population may harbor pinworms, especially children.

Adult worms are quite small: Males range in size from 2 to 5 mm, and females measure 8 to 13 mm (Fig. 70.2). The worms live primarily in the cecum of the large intestine, from which the gravid female migrates at night to lay up to 15,000 eggs on the perineum. The eggs can be spread by the fecal–oral route to the original host and new hosts. In this manner, an entire family can become infected. Ingested eggs hatch in the duodenum, and larvae mature during their migration to the large intestine.

Fortunately, most eggs desiccate and die within 72 hours. In the absence of host autoinfection, infestation usually lasts only 4 to 6 weeks. Egg deposition causes perineal, perianal, and vaginal irritation. The patient's constant itching in an attempt to relieve irritation can lead to potentially debilitating sleep disturbance.

(continued)

Discussion continued

Direct visualization of the white-appearing adult worms or microscopic detection of worms or eggs using the cellophane tape test confirms the diagnosis.

Pruritus ani has many causes, of which pinworm is just one. Consider diet (coffee, tea, chocolate, citrus), malignancy, anal fistulas, other infections (yeast, sexually transmitted diseases [STDs], *Corynebacterium*), psoriasis, Paget disease, or even incomplete cleansing postdefecation as you evaluate the patient with this complaint.

Suggested Readings

Centers for Disease Control and Prevention. (2019). Parasites—enterobiasis (also known as pinworm infection). https://www.cdc.gov/parasites/pinworm/index.html.

Horne, P. D. (2002). First evidence of enterobiasis in ancient Egypt. *The Journal of Parasitology*, *88*, 1019–1021.

Kucik, C. J., Martin, G. L., & Sortor, B. V. (2004). Common intestinal parasites. *American Family Physician*, *69*, 1161–1168.

Esophageal Food Bolus Obstruction

(Steakhouse Syndrome)

Presentation

The patient develops symptoms either immediately after swallowing a large mouthful of food (usually inadequately chewed meat) or as the result of intoxication, wearing dentures, or being too embarrassed to spit out a large piece of gristle. The patient often develops substernal chest pain that may mimic the pain of a myocardial infarction. This discomfort increases with swallowing and is followed by retention of salivary secretions, which, unlike infarction, leads to drooling. The patient usually arrives with a receptacle under the mouth, into which he's been repeatedly spitting. At times these secretions will cause paroxysms of coughing, gagging, or choking. Often the patient can readily tell you where the food has become stuck by pointing to the lower esophagus.

What to Do

✓ **Complete a history and physical examination.** If an esophageal perforation is suspected because of severe pain and diaphoresis after swallowing a sharp object, such as a bone, take posteroanterior and lateral radiographs of the neck and chest, looking for subcutaneous emphysema, pneumomediastinum, pneumothorax, and pleural effusion. If these are negative, but a high level of suspicion remains, a contrast study using a low-osmolality iodinated contrast agent (such as Amipaque, Omnipaque, or Hexabrix) should be performed. These agents are much less likely to cause problems if they contaminate the mediastinum or are accidentally aspirated. If a high suspicion for perforation is still present, despite a negative swallowing study, a computed tomography (CT) scan may be obtained, which may show air around the mediastinum or esophagus or a mediastinal air–fluid level.

✓ **When there is only mild pain or discomfort and the patient is troubled by drooling and the spitting of saliva, offer to insert a small nasogastric tube to the point of obstruction and attach it to low intermittent suction. This insertion will assist the patient in handling excess secretions and reduce the risk for aspiration.** The patient may prefer to keep spitting to avoid the discomfort of nasogastric tube insertion.

✓ **Provide adequate pain relief, when necessary, with a parenteral analgesic such as ketorolac (Toradol) or intravenous (IV) acetaminophen (Ofirmev). Opiate analgesia with morphine or fentanyl may be necessary.**

✓ If the history and physical findings are ambiguous, but there remains a question of esophageal obstruction, give 5 mL of dilute barium PO and obtain radiographs of the chest to locate the foreign body. **When the history and physical findings are classic for a meat**

impaction in the esophagus, there is no need to perform a barium swallow, which may later obscure the view for a consulting endoscopist.

✅ **Give 0.5 to 1 mg of glucagon intravenously to decrease lower esophageal sphincter pressure (infuse slowly to prevent nausea and vomiting). This decrease in pressure will sometimes allow passage of a food bolus.** Even if given slowly, glucagon frequently induces severe nausea. Consider giving a dose of an antiemetic such as ondansetron (Zofran) or metoclopramide (Reglan) prophylactically with the glucagon. If there is no response to glucagon, repeat every 5 to 10 minutes for one to two additional doses. The success rate of this technique is low (only 20–40%) and will be of no value in an impaction of the upper two-thirds of the esophagus. The side effects of this drug include nausea, vomiting, and hyperglycemia. The hyperglycemia is transient and of no clinical significance and does not require monitoring. Adding diazepam (Valium) to this medication does not improve its effectiveness.

✅ **An alternative intravenously drug is metoclopramide (Reglan), 10 mg.** Additional modes of therapy include the use of sublingual nitroglycerin or nifedipine to relax the lower esophageal sphincter, but they are not usually as effective as IV glucagon, which itself is of questionable efficacy.

✅ **Another method of passing a lower esophageal meat impaction (of <6 hours) into the stomach, if glucagon has failed and there are no signs of esophageal perforation, is to have the patient sit up and drink 100 mL of a carbonated beverage or EZ gas (sodium bicarbonate, citric acid, simethicone), followed by 240 mL of water. EZ gas (also known as Carbex) is sometimes found in the radiology department if it is not available in the pharmacy.** Another alternative is to use 15 mL of tartaric acid (18.7 g/100 mL), followed by 15 mL of sodium bicarbonate (10 g/100 mL). When these components are combined in the esophagus, **carbon dioxide is produced, which distends the esophagus and, when successful, propels the impacted meat into the stomach. The patient will be able to report when the impaction has been relieved; he/she will know immediately or the next time he/she attempts to swallow something. (It should be noted that a complication rate of 3% has been reported using this technique. Reported complications include aspiration and vomiting with an esophageal tear.)**

✅ **If the food does not pass spontaneously or with medication, flexible esophagoscopy is the treatment of choice, and a gastroenterologist or surgeon should be consulted**. If the patient is very symptomatic and not handling secretions or is unable to tolerate liquids by mouth, esophagoscopy should happen emergently. If the patient is handling secretions and is not in distress, the procedure may be delayed up to 12 hours; however, the endoscopist should be consulted to determine ideal timing. If a decision is made to delay endoscopy, the patient should remain in the emergency department or be admitted to the hospital until the obstruction is relieved.

✅ **If flexible esophagoscopy is not available, rigid esophagoscopy performed by an ear-nose-throat (ENT) specialist is an alternative option.**

✅ **Be aware that the standard methods for disimpaction outlined earlier may be ineffective or hazardous in the management of food lodged in a metallic esophageal stent.**

✅ When removal of the food bolus has been successful, early medical follow-up should be provided for a comprehensive evaluation of the esophagus as patients often have underlying pathology such as Schatzki rings, esophageal strictures, achalasia, or tumors.

✓ Patients who have experienced a prolonged obstruction or do not have complete resolution of all their symptoms should be admitted to the hospital for further observation and management.

What Not to Do

✗ Do not ignore a patient's claims of a foreign body stuck in the esophagus. The patient is usually right.

✗ Do not obtain plain radiograph films for routine food bolus impactions. They are of very limited value unless a large bone has been ingested.

✗ Do not blindly try to force the food bolus down with the Ewald tube or any other catheter or dilator. This may cause an esophageal tear or perforation. Endoscopists have successfully used an endoscopic push technique, but this has been under direct visualization in a controlled manner.

✗ Do not use meat tenderizers or oral enzymes, such as papain, trypsin, or chymotrypsin. This treatment is slow and ineffective and may possibly carry a risk for enzyme-induced esophageal perforation.

✗ Do not discharge a patient prior to removal of the obstruction. The risks of delayed follow-up are too high.

✗ Do not attempt to remove a hard, sharp esophageal foreign body using any of the abovementioned techniques. These techniques very likely will cause an esophageal injury.

✗ Do not give glucagon to patients with pheochromocytoma or insulinoma. It may cause a pheochromocytoma to release catecholamines, or the secondary hyperglycemia may cause an insulinoma to secrete excess insulin and produce hypoglycemia.

✗ Do not use barium-impregnated cotton balls to detect esophageal foreign bodies. If a foreign body is present, they will obscure the view for the endoscopist.

✗ Do not fail to refer a patient in whom a food bolus has passed to an endoscopist, to rule out malignancy or other underlying pathology and to facilitate dilation of any strictures that may be found.

Discussion

Patients who experience a food bolus obstruction of the esophagus are usually older than 60 years of age and often have an underlying structural lesion. Meat impaction occurs most frequently in the distal esophagus. One of the more common lesions is a benign stricture secondary to reflux esophagitis. Another abnormality, the classic Schatzki ring (distal esophageal mucosal ring), especially above a hiatal hernia, may present with the so-called steakhouse or café coronary syndrome, in which obstruction occurs and is relieved spontaneously.

Other associated problems include postoperative narrowing, neoplasms, and esophageal webs, as well as motility disorders, neurologic disease, and collagen vascular disease. Eosinophilic esophagitis is an increasingly recognized syndrome causing esophageal spasm in response to certain foods (a hypersensitivity reaction) with bolus obstruction. It has been described as "asthma of the esophagus."

Meat impacted in the proximal two thirds of the esophagus is unlikely to pass and

(continued)

Discussion continued

should be removed as soon as possible. Meat impacted in the lower third frequently does pass spontaneously if given enough time, and the patient can safely wait, under medical observation, up to 12 hours before extraction.

Even if a meat bolus does pass spontaneously, endoscopy must still be done later to assess the almost certain (80–90%) chance of an underlying disease. In the great majority of these cases, the underlying disease will be benign.

Flexible endoscopy is the mainstay of esophageal foreign-body removal. Reported success rates are high, with few reported complications. Ideally, food impactions should be removed within about 12 hours of presentation. Early removal is recommended because of local pressure-induced ischemia that may occur secondary to the food bolus.

Chicken bones are the foreign bodies that most often cause esophageal perforation in adults.

Suggested Readings

Blair, S. R., Graeber, G. M., Cruzzavala, J. L., et al. (1993). Current management of esophageal impactions. *Chest*, *104*, 1205–1209.

Chae, H. S., Lee, T. K., Kim, Y. W., et al. (2002). Two cases of steakhouse syndrome associated with nutcracker esophagus. *Diseases of the Esophagus*, *15*, 330–333.

Lacy, P. D., Donnelly, M. J., McGrath, J. P., et al. (1997). Acute food bolus impaction: Aetiology and management. *Laryngology and Otology*, *111*, 1158–1161.

Lao, J., Bostwick, H. E., Berezin, S., et al. (2003). Esophageal food impaction in children. *Pediatric Emergency Care*, *19*, 402–407.

Lee, J., & Anderson, R. (2005). Best evidence topic report. Effervescent agents for oesophageal food bolus impaction. *Emergency Medicine Journal*, *22*, 123–124.

Rice, B. T., Spiegel, P. K., & Dombrowski, P. J. (1983). Acute esophageal food impaction treated by gas-forming agents. *Radiology*, *146*, 299–301.

Singer, A. J., & Konia, N. (1999). Comparison of topical anesthetics and vasoconstrictors vs lubricants prior to nasogastric intubation: A randomized, controlled trial. *Academy of Emergency Medicine*, *6*, 184–190.

Tibbling, L., Bjorkhoel, A., Jansson, E., & Stenkvist, M. (1995). Effect of spasmolytic drugs on esophageal foreign bodies. *Dysphagia*, *10*, 126–127.

Triadafilopoulos, G. (2019). Ingested foreign bodies and food impactions in adults. UptoDate. https://www.uptodate.com/contents/ingested-foreign-bodies-and-food-impactions-in-adults.

Weinstock, L. B., Shatz, B. A., & Thyssen, S. E. (1999). Esophageal food bolus obstruction: Evaluation of extraction and modified push techniques in 75 cases. *Endoscopy*, *31*, 421–425.

Foreign Body, Rectal

Presentation

Rectal foreign bodies may present with abdominal pain, anorectal pain, obstipation, acute urinary retention, or blood or mucous discharge from the rectum. Such foreign bodies are often difficult to diagnose because the history may not be offered by the patient unless directly asked. Sometimes the patient will not volunteer that any object has been inserted or will give outlandish explanations, such as having sat or fallen onto the object. When interviewed privately in a nonjudgmental manner, however, the patient will usually give an accurate account of the foreign body.

Rectal foreign bodies most commonly are found when an object, such as a dildo or vibrator, is inserted into the rectum by the patient or a partner for sexual stimulation; it then causes pain or bleeding or becomes irretrievable. Presentation is frequently delayed by embarrassment, or prior attempts on the part of the patient to remove the object.

Rectal foreign bodies also are found with practices such as "body packing," wherein illicit drugs are packed in latex condoms or plastic bags for illegal transport. Rupture of these packets may lead to profound toxicity and death.

Less often, medical instruments, such as enema tips or thermometers, become lodged in the rectum.

What to Do

✓ Try to determine how long the foreign body has been lodged and if any attempts at removal have been made. Ask specifically about any assault or rape and respond accordingly. Give special consideration to the psychiatric patient.

✓ **The diagnosis of a rectal foreign body can usually be made from the history alone. Perform an abdominal and rectal examination but defer the rectal examination if the foreign body is suspected to be dangerously sharp.**

✓ **If there are signs of peritoneal inflammation** (i.e., rebound tenderness or pain with movement) or blood on rectal examination, suspect a perforation of the bowel, start appropriate intravenous (IV) lines, draw blood for laboratory analysis, obtain flat and upright abdominal radiographs to look for free air, notify surgical consultants, and administer IV antibiotics. Surgical consultation should also be obtained in all cases of nonpalpable rectal foreign bodies.

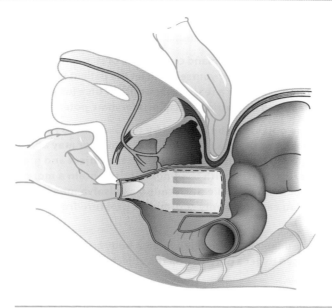

Fig. 72.1 Removal of a foreign body from the rectum. (With permission from Coates, W. C. [2018]. Disorders of the anorectum. In: *Rosen's emergency medicine: Concepts and clinical practice* [9th ed., pp. 1166–1177 (fig. 86.9)]. St. Louis, MO: Elsevier.)

✅ **If there are no signs of perforation, flat and upright abdominal films may still be obtained to help define the location, nature, size, and number of foreign objects (as well as to reveal unsuspected free air).**

✅ Those objects that lie in the low or middle rectum, up to a level of 10 cm, most often can be removed transanally.

✅ **When there is no suspicion of a bowel perforation, provide procedural sedation to help in the removal of the foreign body (see Appendix E).**

✅ **Place the patient on the side in the Sims position or place the patient in the lithotomy position, which will allow for manual suprapubic pressure thereby assisting in the foreign-body removal (Fig. 72.1). If anal discomfort persists, instill lidocaine jelly for mucosal anesthesia or locally infiltrate 1% lidocaine with epinephrine into the anal sphincter. In general, a perianal nerve block similar to that used for anorectal surgery works quite well.** Some authors favor using lidocaine (Xylocaine) 1% with epinephrine and bupivacaine 0.5% with epinephrine in a 50:50 mix. A superficial block and then an intersphincteric block circumferentially around the anal verge can be performed. Finally, to ensure the greatest degree of anesthesia, a pudendal nerve block can be performed. The branches of the pudendal nerve that innervate the anal sphincter complex approach the sphincter complex from a posterolateral location. A pudendal nerve block is done by infiltrating the tissues deeply in a fanlike technique approximately 1 cm medial to the ischial tuberosities in the posterolateral location bilaterally. Approximately 2 to 5 mL of the local anesthetic mix is used on each side. **Always inform the patient that after any local infiltration into the anal sphincter there may be transient fecal incontinence.**

✅ **The method of removal must be individualized, depending on the size, shape, consistency, and fragility of the object.** Objects that are commonly retrieved include fruits and vegetables, household items, especially those whose dimensions resemble the penis, and items purchased specifically with an anal erotic intent.

✅ **Individual situations demand creative use of standard medical instruments and supplies. Set a time limit for yourself, and let the patient know that if the foreign body cannot be removed within a reasonable length of time (usually 10–20 minutes), it will have to be removed in a setting that allows for more potent anesthetics.**

✅ **When the object can be reached by the examining finger and is of a nature that will allow it to be grasped, a lax anal sphincter may allow slow insertion of as much of a gloved hand as possible to grab the object and gradually extricate it. For instance, perforate fruit with the fingertips to obtain a more effective grasp. Having the patient bear down while performing a Valsalva maneuver may help to "deliver" the object. You can also apply suprapubic pressure from above with your free hand** (see Fig. 72.1).

✅ **If you are unable to pull out the foreign body by hand, the following are techniques that can be used to get a purchase on the object and break the vacuum behind it:**

○ **Slide a large Foley catheter with a 30-mL balloon past the object, inflate the balloon, and apply traction to the catheter. (This can be used in conjunction with any of the other techniques.) Two catheters may occasionally be needed, and air should be instilled through the lumen of the catheter to break the vacuum** (Fig. 72.2). **Alternatively, an endotracheal tube can be passed beyond the foreign body, the cuff inflated, and air gently insufflated down the tube.**

○ **Under direct visualization with an anoscope or a vaginal speculum, attempt to grasp the object with a tenaculum, sponge forceps, Kelly clamp, or tonsil snare** (Fig. 72.3). **Brittle objects, especially glass, should be grasped gently, with rubber tubing or gauze covering the metal surfaces of any clamp or forceps.**

○ **An open object, such as a jar or bottle, can be filled with wet plaster, into which a tongue blade can be inserted like a Popsicle stick. When the plaster hardens, traction can be applied to the tongue blade** (Fig. 72.4). **Alternatively, inflation of a Sengstaken-Blakemore tube balloon inside a jar may provide the traction needed to extract the object.**

○ You may be able to place a screw in some objects, which may allow you to grab them and apply traction. Other objects may have to be cut in sections to be removed.

○ **Forceps or soup spoons can be used to deliver a round object** (Fig. 72.5). **When available, an obstetric vacuum extractor may be even more effective for removing round foreign bodies of compatible size and texture** (Fig. 72.6). **Magnets are sometimes useful to help extract metal objects.**

✅ As the object is being removed, the speculum or anoscope should be removed along with it so that the foreign body does not have to fit through these instruments.

✅ With an object that is too high to reach, the patient can be admitted and sedated for removal over the next 6 to 12 hours.

✅ When the object cannot be removed because of patient discomfort or sphincter tightness, removal must be accomplished in the operating room under spinal or general anesthesia.

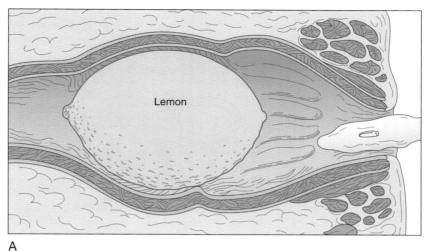

A

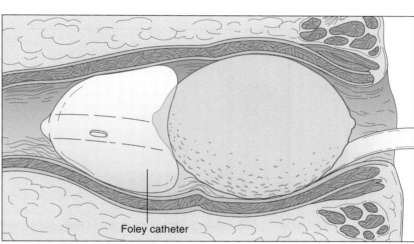

B

Fig. 72.2 The Foley catheter technique is used to break a vacuum behind an object.

⊘ When blood is present in the rectum, when pain is severe or persistent, when there is fever or rectal discharge, or when the object is capable of doing harm to the bowel, proctoscopic evaluation should be performed after removal of the foreign body to rule out rectal injury. Superficial nonbleeding rectal injuries may be left alone. Those that are bleeding or that involve the muscular wall require repair.

⊘ **When pain persists or there is any lingering suspicion of a bowel perforation, keep the patient for 24 hours of observation and consider performing a water-soluble contrast enema study. If there are any postprocedural problems, surgical consultation is recommended.**

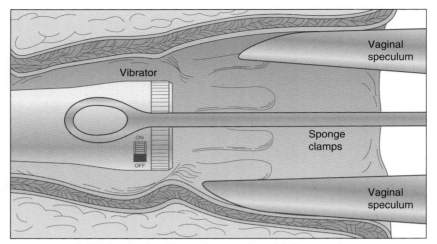

Fig. 72.3 Grasp the object with a tenaculum, sponge forceps, Kelly clamp, or tonsil snare.

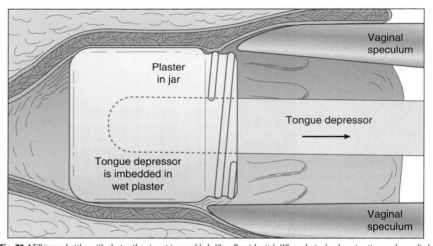

Fig. 72.4 Fill jars or bottles with plaster, then insert tongue blade like a Popsicle stick. When plaster hardens, traction can be applied.

✅ **When the foreign body is extracted without difficulty and the potential for bowel injury is minimal**, proctoscopic evaluation is probably unnecessary, and the patient can be discharged after a reasonable period of observation.

✅ **Consider recommending sexual or psychological counseling.**

What Not to Do

❌ Do not pressure the patient into giving you an accurate story. The patient may be embarrassed, and intimidation will not help.

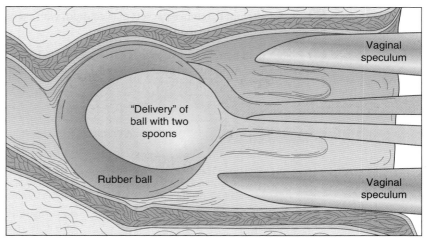

Fig. 72.5 Round objects can be removed with forceps or soup spoons.

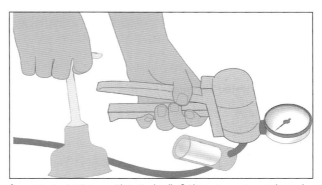

Fig. 72.6 Equipment for soft-cup vacuum extraction: cup with traction handle, fluid trap, vacuum gauge, and manual vacuum pump. (Adapted from Putta, L. V., & Spencer, J. P. [2000]. Assisted vaginal delivery using the vacuum extractor. *American Family Physician, 62*, 1316–1320.)

Ⓧ Do not use enemas or cathartics to help speed the removal of these objects. These treatments are not likely to be effective and may actually cause harm.

Ⓧ Do not attempt to remove a rectal foreign body in a patient who is having severe abdominal pain or who has signs of a bowel perforation.

Ⓧ Do not attempt to remove a rectal foreign body from a patient whose rectal pain and spasm are severe and cannot be overcome with the infiltration of local anesthetic. These patients will require regional or general anesthesia.

Ⓧ Do not push the object higher into the colon while attempting to remove it.

Ⓧ Do not blindly grab for an object with a tenaculum or other such device. This can itself lead to a perforation.

Ⓧ Do not attempt to remove fragile objects that are likely to shatter or sharp, jagged objects, such as broken glass, through the rectum. These should only be removed under anesthesia in surgery.

⊗ Do not attempt to remove packets of illicit drugs with clamps or sharp medical instruments, because spillage can lead to toxicity and death.

⊗ Do not send home a patient who is having continued pain. Admit the patient and observe for peritoneal signs, increased pain, fever, and a rising white blood cell count.

Discussion

Anorectal foreign bodies can be either ingested orally or inserted anally. Although the vast majority are inserted for autoerotic purposes, they may have been placed iatrogenically or as a result of assault or trauma. Ingested objects are rarely a cause of entrapped rectal foreign bodies. Most often these are bones that become impaled in the anal canal. Iatrogenic foreign bodies include thermometers, enema tips, and catheters. Objects placed as a result of assault, trauma, or eroticism represent a diverse collection (e.g., sex toys, tools, wire hangers and instruments, bottles/cans/jars, poles/pipes/tubing, fruits and vegetables, stones, balls, balloons, light bulbs, flashlights).

Most of these rectal foreign bodies can be removed safely in the emergency department or acute care clinic. Relaxation is essential, and sedation is usually necessary if retrieval is to be successful. Some practitioners quite reasonably forgo radiographs before manipulation if the patient is free of pain and fever and if the object is benign.

Suggested Readings

Coates, W. C. (2018). Disorders of the anorectum. In *Rosen's emergency medicine: Concepts and clinical practice* (9th ed.) (pp. 1166–1177). St. Louis, MO: Elsevier. [fig. 86.9].

Couch, C. H., Tan, E. G. C., & Watt, A. G. (1986). Rectal foreign bodies. *Medical Journal of Australia, 144,* 512–515.

Hellinger, M. D. (2002). Anal trauma and foreign bodies. *Surgery Clinics of North America, 82,* 1253–1260.

Putta, L. V., & Spencer, J. P. (2000). Assisted vaginal delivery using the vacuum extractor. *American Family Physician, 62,* 1316–1320.

Rodriguez-Hermosa, J. I., Codina-Cazador, A., Ruiz, B., et al. (2007). Management of foreign bodies in the rectum. *Colorectal Disease, 9,* 543–548.

Steele, S., & Goldberg, J. (n.d.). Rectal foreign bodies. Upto Date. http://www.uptodate.com.

Foreign Body, Swallowed

Presentation

Parents bring in a young child (usually between the ages of 6 months and 6 years) shortly after the child has swallowed a coin, safety pin, or toy. The child may be asymptomatic or have recurrent or transient symptoms of choking, gagging, vomiting, drooling, dysphagia, pain, or a foreign-body (FB) sensation. Stridor or dyspnea resulting from tracheal compression may occur in young children. Disturbed or cognitively impaired adults may be brought from mental health facilities to the hospital on repeated occasions, at times accumulating a sizable load of ingested material. Impacted esophageal foreign bodies are more likely to cause the symptoms described, whereas **gastric foreign bodies are usually asymptomatic**.

What to Do

✅ Many patients are able to give a clear history of FB ingestion; however, young children, psychotic persons, and the cognitively impaired may be unable to give an accurate history.

✅ **Ask capable patients about their symptoms and examine them**, looking for signs of airway obstruction (e.g., coughing, wheezing), bowel obstruction, or perforation (e.g., vomiting, subcutaneous emphysema, chest pain, melena, abdominal pain, abnormal bowel sounds).

✅ **When a FB ingestion is suspected, obtain posteroanterior and lateral radiographic views of the throat and chest to at least the midabdomen to determine if indeed anything was ingested or if the foreign body has become lodged or produced an obstruction. In small children, this should include the area from the nasopharynx to the upper abdomen, which can often be done with a single large radiographic plate. A lateral view will not be necessary if the foreign body is in the stomach.**

✅ **Keep in mind that the patient may have ingested a foreign body that is not radiopaque, therefore negative x-rays do not rule out an ingested foreign body. When dealing with a potentially hazardous radiolucent foreign body, it may be necessary to obtain a computed tomography (CT) scan to visualize the object's location.**

✅ **In an attempt to reduce the patient's exposure to ionizing radiation, it is reasonable to try identifying a radiopaque or radiolucent foreign body using ultrasound. Be aware** that although ultrasonography is useful for identifying retained foreign bodies in soft tissue or in the vagina, this modality is less useful for detecting foreign bodies in the gastrointestinal (GI) tract because the object may be obscured by bowel gas. Gastric foreign bodies may be identified by ultrasonography if anechoic fluid is present in the stomach, which allows an acoustic shadow to be seen. Failure to visualize a foreign body does not rule out the presence of one.

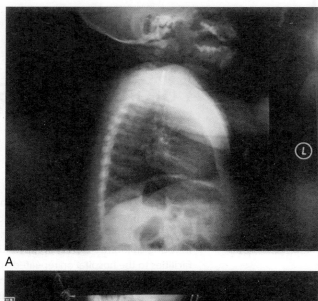

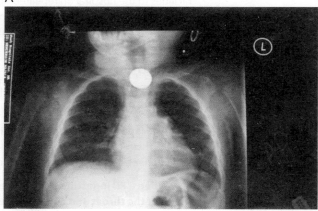

Fig. 73.1 Posteroanterior and lateral combined radiograph views of the chest and neck revealing an upper esophageal coin. (Adapted from Nicholson, J. [2005, April]. Occult ingestion of foreign body. *Emergency Physician Monthly*.)

A coin located in the proximal esophagus will be oriented in the coronal plane on an anteroposterior projection (Fig. 73.1). Tracheal foreign bodies align in the sagittal plane on a lateral projection due to the shape of the tracheal rings. Button batteries, which can be hazardous, can be differentiated from a simple coin by their double-ring appearance on radiographs.

A foreign body with sharp edges or a blunt foreign body lodged in the esophagus for more than 1 day should be removed endoscopically because it is likely to cause a perforation and is still accessible. Button or disk batteries that are impacted in the esophagus can rapidly cause tissue necrosis and perforation and therefore must be removed on an emergent basis. Once a button battery has cleared the esophagus, it will usually traverse the remainder of the GI tract without difficulty and would only need to be removed if there were signs and symptoms of GI injury, if the battery was larger than 20 mm in diameter, or if it failed to pass the pylorus after 48 hours.

✅ **Many sharp, pointed, and elongated foreign bodies should be removed even if they have passed into the stomach.** Examples include toothpicks, medication blister packs, open safety pins, toothbrushes, plastic bag clips, and elongated nails and wires. Foreign bodies longer than 6 cm in children (3 cm in infants) and 10 cm in adults should be removed. **Toothpicks are shorter than this, but they are associated with a high incidence of perforation. Plastic bag clips and sharp plastic holiday confetti** have a propensity to attach to the folds of the small bowel with subsequent small bowel ulceration and the potential for hemorrhage, perforation, and healing with fibrosis and obstruction.

✅ **A single magnetic foreign body will generally pass without incident if it is small. However, if more than one magnetic foreign body were ingested, these generally will require removal.** There is a risk of perforation if two magnets in adjacent bowel loops are attracted to one another, as this will cause pressure in the walls of the loops of bowel in between the two magnets.

✅ **A child who is brought in immediately after ingesting a coin and is asymptomatic but has a coin impacted in the upper or lower esophagus can initially be fed soft bread with clear fluids and observed for several hours to see if the coin will spontaneously pass into the stomach.** If this is unsuccessful, consult with the parents, along with a pediatric endoscopist, regarding further observation for up to 24 hours as an outpatient or inpatient, or possibly performing endoscopic removal as soon as possible.

✅ **When a coin or other smooth object has been lodged in the upper esophagus of a healthy asymptomatic child for less than 24 hours (as seen in Fig. 73.1), and endoscopy is not readily available and the parents are supportive about avoiding general anesthesia, the object can often be removed using a simple Foley catheter technique.** When available, this can be performed under fluoroscopy, although, to avoid this radiation, it can be safely performed as a blind procedure. With the patient mildly sedated (e.g., midazolam [Versed], 0.5 mg/kg per rectum, intranasally or orally, with 30 min allowed for absorption), position the child with the head down (Trendelenburg) and prone to minimize the risk for aspiration. Alternatively, consider ketamine for procedural sedation (see Appendix E). Have a functioning laryngoscope, Magill forceps, and airway equipment at hand. Test the balloon of a Foley catheter (8–12 Fr) to ensure that it inflates symmetrically. Lubricate the catheter with water-soluble jelly and insert it through the nose into the esophagus to a point distal to the foreign body. Inflate the balloon with 5 mL of air and apply gentle traction on the catheter until the foreign body reaches the base of the tongue. Terminate the procedure if you encounter any resistance. The patient will reflexively gag, cough, or spit out the foreign body. Immediately deflate the balloon and remove the catheter (Fig. 73.2). If a first attempt at removal fails, consult an endoscopist. When removal is successful, repeat the radiograph to be sure that there are no additional coins, and discharge the patient after a brief period of observation.

✅ **Also, when there is parental support, esophageal bougienage is a safe, effective, and inexpensive method to advance coins or smooth objects from the distal esophagus into the stomach without sedation.** After topical anesthesia of the throat, wrap the patient in a bed sheet with arms at the side and have an assistant hold the child upright. Advance a well-lubricated, blunt, round-tipped Hurst-type esophageal dilator through the mouth and esophagus into the stomach, then remove it. Obtain a postprocedure radiograph of the chest and upper abdomen to document the location of the foreign body. Esophageal bougienage should be limited to witnessed ingestions of a single coin lodged for less than 24 hours with no

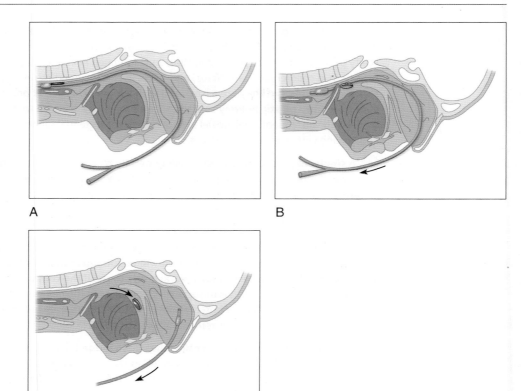

A

B

C

Fig. 73.2 Foley catheter technique.

previous history of esophageal foreign body, disease, or surgery and no respiratory compromise. Dilator size should be 28 Fr for ages 1 to 2, 32 Fr for ages 2 to 3, 36 Fr for ages 3 to 4, 38 Fr for ages 4 to 5, and 40 Fr for those older than 5 years of age. These two rapid, simple, cost-effective techniques have been shown in the past to be safe and effective. Because of the lack of direct visual control and the potential for injury or aspiration, however, many clinicians forgo these procedures and take advantage of the widespread availability of flexible endoscopy when dealing with esophageal foreign bodies.

✓ **Foreign bodies of the esophagus are more difficult to remove when prolonged impaction leads to mucosal edema, swelling, and necrosis.** It is for this reason that Foley catheter manipulation and bougienage are not recommended for coins that have been entrapped for more than 24 hours.

✓ **Children with distal esophageal coins may be safely observed up to 24 hours before an invasive removal procedure, because most will spontaneously pass the coins.**

✓ **When an FB has passed into the stomach and there are no symptoms or hazardous circumstances that demand immediate removal, discharge the patient with instructions to**

return for reevaluation in 3 to 4 days (2 days with button batteries) or sooner if the child develops nausea, vomiting, fever, abdominal pain, rectal pain, or rectal bleeding.

✓ For potentially hazardous radiopaque objects, repeat radiographs every 3 to 4 days to confirm that passage of the object is necessary. This would not be required for small, smooth objects such as coins.

✓ **All subdiaphragmatic coins seem to pass without incident.** Metal detectors can be used to follow the elimination of metallic foreign bodies without further radiation exposure. Having parents sift through stools is often unproductive. (One missed stool negates days of hard work.) It may be helpful to give a bulk laxative to help decrease the intestinal transit time.

What Not to Do

✗ Do not use ipecac for FB ingestions. Emesis is effective for emptying the stomach of liquid but not for removing foreign bodies from the esophagus or stomach. It may even result in regurgitation of a gastric disk battery into the esophagus, where it will be much more hazardous.

✗ Do not forcefully remove an esophageal foreign body, especially if it is causing pain. This removal may lead to injury or perforation.

✗ Do not worry about the corrosive properties of pennies minted in the United States since 1982—that is, with a high (97.5%) zinc content. Although concerns have been raised in the medical and popular press, they are not associated with any more esophageal mucosal injuries than other coins.

✗ Do not automatically assume that an ingested foreign body should be surgically removed. Most potentially injurious foreign bodies pass through the alimentary tract without mishap. Operate only when the patient is actually being harmed by the swallowed foreign body or when there is evidence that it is not moving down the alimentary tract.

✗ Do not miss additional coins after removing one from the proximal esophagus. Take a repeat radiograph after removal of one coin.

✗ Do not routinely refer children with esophageal coins for an additional investigation to look for underlying disease. This is a common occurrence in normal children.

✗ Do not ignore the potential hazards of button battery ingestions (see Discussion box, later). Button batteries in the esophagus demand emergent removal.

✗ In the patient who presents with food (usually meat) bolus impaction, never use meat tenderizer.

Discussion

Older children and fully conscious, communicative adults may be able to identify the material swallowed and point to the location of the discomfort. Localization of the level of impaction, however, is often not reliable. In many instances, the ingestion goes unrecognized or unreported until the onset of symptoms, which may be remote from the time of ingestion. Young children, the cognitively impaired, or psychiatric patients may present with choking, refusal to eat, vomiting, drooling, wheezing, blood-stained saliva, or respiratory distress.

FB ingestion is most common in children 6 months to 6 years of age, who comprise 75% to 80% of all cases. Coins are the most common foreign bodies in children. Others in children include fish bones, marbles, buttons, button batteries, screws, pins, paper clips, crayons, pen and bottle caps, magnets, and small toys. In adults, meat boluses, bones, coins, dentures, fruit pits, and toothpicks are commonly encountered. Ingestion of foreign objects occurs most often in edentulous adults and in individuals with psychiatric conditions, cognitive impairment, or chemical dependency. Intentional ingestion of various foreign bodies is encountered commonly in prisoners and patients with psychiatric disorders.

Although most coins swallowed by healthy children pass through the GI tract without difficulty, patients with previous GI tract surgery or congenital gut malformations are at increased risk for obstruction or perforation. As with coins, most other swallowed foreign bodies in children and adults will traverse the GI tract without difficulty and require no intervention.

The narrowest and least distensible strait in the GI tract is usually the cricopharyngeus muscle at the level of the thyroid cartilage. Next narrowest is usually the pylorus, followed by the lower esophageal sphincter and the ileocecal valve. Thus anything that passes the throat will probably pass through the anus as well (although all of these sites are potential locations for FB impaction). In general, foreign bodies below the diaphragm should be left alone. Exceptions to this include foreign bodies that are sharp or shaped in such a way that they are not likely to pass, as well as multiple magnets.

High-powered magnets are becoming increasingly common in toys and other household objects. When two or more magnets are ingested, especially at different times, there is a risk of perforation, obstruction, pressure necrosis, and fistulas as pressure can build on the walls of adjacent bowel loops in between two magnets attracted to one another.

Complications are related to the type of foreign body and are more common if it remains entrapped more than 24 hours. These include inconsequential mucosal scratches or abrasions, lacerations, esophageal stricture, esophageal necrosis, retropharyngeal abscess formation, hemorrhage, obstruction, and perforation.

A significant portion of children with esophageal foreign bodies are asymptomatic; therefore any child suspected of ingesting a foreign body requires radiography to document whether it is present and, if so, where it is located. However, radiolucent objects will not appear on x-rays.

Large button batteries (the size of quarters) have become stuck in the esophagus, eroded through the esophageal wall, and produced fatal exsanguination. Severe esophageal damage and perforation can occur within a few hours. Some serious complications can occur days or weeks after the initial ingestion.

The smaller variety and batteries that have passed into the gut have not posed such a danger. A button battery lodged in the esophagus should be considered a true emergency and removed immediately by an endoscopist. A button battery found in the stomach should be allowed to pass spontaneously. **Smaller batteries** need only weekly radiographic follow-up; the larger ones should be checked every 48 hours. Failure to pass the pylorus within 2 days is an indication for endoscopic removal. The maximum GI transit time for such foreign bodies in children is 5 days.

Any child with respiratory distress should have the coin removed promptly. Time will probably not allow this to be done under ideal conditions in the operating room. Rapid removal using a McIntosh laryngoscope blade to expose the esophageal entrance and then extracting the coin from the esophagus has been described. Ketamine has been shown to be effective without significant complications in one study that demonstrated its use in the removal of esophageal foreign bodies in pediatric patients. Under critical conditions, combining these two modalities may be quite helpful.

In adults, esophageal foreign body obstruction is most typically caused by a meat bolus impaction. The upper esophageal sphincter, level of the

Discussion continued

aortic arch, or the diaphragmatic hiatus are all anatomically narrow, and a food bolus may therefore become impacted at any of these sites. Patients with total obstruction, who have inability to pass their secretions, should be treated within 12 hours because of the risk of pulmonary aspiration. A trial of glucagon 1.0 mg intravenously, administered slowly to avoid nausea and vomiting, may be used in attempt to relax the esophagus. If this is ineffectual, endoscopy allows removal of the impacted food bolus, as well as evaluation of concomitant causative conditions such as esophageal carcinoma, stricture, achalasia, or eosinophilic esophagitis. Patients who pass a food bolus without endoscopy should be referred for later endoscopy to evaluate for causative conditions. See Chapter 71 for additional information on esophageal food impaction.

Suggested Readings

Binder, L., & Anderson, W. A. (1984). Pediatric gastrointestinal foreign body ingestions. *Annals of Emergency Medicine, 13*, 112–117.

Cantu, S., & Conners, G. P. (2001). Esophageal coins: Are pennies different? *Clinics in Pediatrics, 40*, 677–680.

Connors, G. P. (1997). A literature-based comparison of three methods of pediatric esophageal coin removal. *Pediatric Emergency Care, 13*, 154–157.

Connors, G. P., Chamberlain, J. M., & Ochsenschlager, D. W. (1995). Symptoms and spontaneous passage of esophageal coins. *Archives of Pediatric and Adolescent Medicine, 149*, 36–39.

Dokler, M. L., Bradshaw, J., Mollitt, D. L., et al. (1995). Selective management of pediatric esophageal foreign bodies. *The American Journal of Surgery, 61*, 132–134.

Duncan, M., & Wong, R. K. H. (2003). Esophageal emergencies: Things that will wake you from a sound sleep. *Gastroenterology Clinics of North America, 32*, 1035–1052.

Eisen, G. M., Baron, T. H., Dominitz, J. A., et al. (2002). Guideline for the management of ingested foreign bodies. *Gastrointestinal Endoscopy, 55*, 802–806.

Emslander, H. C., Bonadio, W., & Klatzo, M. (1996). Efficacy of esophageal bougienage by emergency physicians in pediatric coin ingestion. *Annals of Emergency Medicine, 27*, 726–729.

Gilger, M., & Jain, A. (2019). Foreign bodies of the esophagus and gastrointestinal tract in children. UptoDate. https://www.uptodate.com/contents/foreign-bodies-of-the-esophagus-and-gastrointestinal-tract-in-children.

Ginaldi, S. (1985). Removal of esophageal foreign bodies using a Foley catheter in adults. *American Journal of Emergency Medicine, 3*, 64–66.

Gracia, C., Frey, C. F., & Bodai, B. I. (1984). Diagnosis and management of ingested foreign bodies: A ten-year experience. *Annals of Emergency Medicine, 13*, 30–34.

Hodge, D., Tecklinburg, F., & Fleisher, G. (1985). Coin ingestion: Does every child need a radiograph? *Annals of Emergency Medicine, 14*, 443–446.

Hostetler, M. A., & Barnard, J. A. (2002). Removal of esophageal foreign bodies in the pediatric ED: Is ketamine an option? *American Journal of Emergency Medicine, 20*, 96–98.

Mahafza, T. M. (2002). Extracting coins from the upper end of the esophagus using a Magill forceps technique. *international Journal of Pediatric Otorhinolaryngology, 62*, 37–39.

Schunk, J. E., Harrison, M., Corneli, H. M., et al. (1994). Fluoroscopic Foley catheter removal of esophageal foreign bodies in children: Experience with 415 episodes. *Pediatrics, 94*, 709–714.

Silva, R. G., & Ahluwalia, J. P. (2005). Asymptomatic esophageal perforation after foreign body ingestion. *Gastrointestinal Endoscopy, 61*, 615–619.

Soprano, J. V., Fleisher, G. R., & Mandl, K. D. (1999). The spontaneous passage of esophageal coins in children. *Archives of Pediatric and Adolescent Medicine, 153*, 1073–1076.

Triadafilopoulos, G. (2019). Ingested foreign bodies and food impactions in adults. UptoDate. https://www.uptodate.com/contents/ingested-foreign-bodies-and-food-impactions-in-adults.

Uyemura, M. C. (2005). Foreign body ingestion in children. *American Family Physician*, *72*, 287–291.

Wright, C. C., & Closson, F. T. (2013). Updates in pediatric gastrointestinal foreign bodies. *Pediatric Clinics of North America*, *60*(5), 1221–1239.

Hemorrhoids

(Piles)

Presentation

Patients with external hemorrhoids (Fig. 74.1) generally complain of a painful anal lump of sudden onset, which may become intense in severity. This type of pain, in most instances, represents a thrombosed hemorrhoid, which will appear to be purple and is located within the anal canal. It may have been precipitated by straining during defecation, heavy lifting, or pregnancy, but in most cases, there will be no definite preceding event. The external hemorrhoidal swelling is caused by thrombosis of the venous complex. It is very tender to palpation and usually does not bleed unless there is erosion of the overlying skin.

More commonly, patients with internal hemorrhoids (Fig. 74.2) usually seek help because of painless (or nearly painless) bright red bleeding during or after defecation. Patients usually notice intermittent spotting on toilet tissue or blood dripping into the toilet bowl, or both. Blood may be admixed with stool, or blood may appear as streaks on the stool. A prolapsed internal hemorrhoid appears as a protrusion of painless, moist red tissue covered with rectal mucosa at the anal verge. Prolapsed internal hemorrhoids may become strangulated and thrombosed, and thus painful.

Fecal seepage or soiling and a mucoid discharge are most often associated with internal hemorrhoids but may also occur with external lesions. This can cause pruritus, which may be another reason for patients to seek medical care.

What to Do

✅ **If the problem is rectal bleeding** (which in most cases is minimal), it should be approached as with any other gastrointestinal (GI) bleeding. The amount of bleeding should be quantified with orthostatic vital signs and a hemoglobin and hematocrit. It should be noted that both hemoglobin and hematocrit may lag behind blood loss and be falsely reassuring in heavy bleeding. When there is evidence of severe hemorrhage, rapid volume replacement and early surgical consultation should be initiated.

✅ **A detailed history** will help establish the diagnosis of hemorrhoids. The color and character of anorectal bleeding and any relief the patient may have obtained from reducing a prolapsed hemorrhoid back into the anal canal may lead to the diagnosis.

✅ **An adequate physical examination** should include careful inspection, palpation, and digital examination. Anoscopy and proctosigmoidoscopy should be performed as soon as possible when there is rectal bleeding. However, evidence of hemorrhoidal bleeding does not exclude other causes of rectal bleeding such as colorectal cancer; therefore a complete colonic

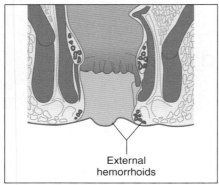

Fig. 74.1 External hemorrhoid.

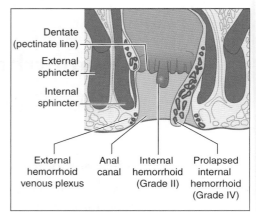

Fig. 74.2 Internal hemorrhoid.

evaluation should be done at some point in those who are at risk, based on family history, or who are at an age for colonic screening evaluation. Young patients in whom hemorrhoids are the obvious source of bleeding may not require more than a digital rectal examination and anoscopy.

✅ **For nonthreatening rectal bleeding from hemorrhoids, the initial management should include a high-fiber diet, stool softeners, and bulk laxatives, and the patient should be instructed to spend less time sitting and straining during bowel movements.** Patients also should be taught not to neglect their first urge to defecate; those who are troubled with constipation should be given an osmotic laxative (see Chapter 68).

✅ Prolapsed or strangulated internal hemorrhoids warrant surgical consultation and possible hospital admission.

✅ **If the problem is mild pain**, the rectum should be examined using a topical anesthetic (lidocaine jelly) as a lubricant. First, look for thrombosed external hemorrhoids and prolapsed internal hemorrhoids, which may become thrombosed, edematous, or strangulated. Have the patient perform a Valsalva maneuver as you provide traction on the skin of the buttocks to evert the anus. Examine the posterior mucosa for anal fissures. After the topical anesthesia has taken effect, complete the digital rectal examination, looking for evidence of rectal abscesses or other masses. Internal hemorrhoids are usually not palpable unless they have prolapsed.

✅ If topical mucosal anesthetic does not give enough relief to permit examination, follow with subcutaneous injection of 5 to 10 mL of 1% lidocaine with epinephrine or ropivacaine 0.5% with epinephrine for extended pain relief.

✅ **If topical anesthetics on the rectal mucosa help control the pain, provide more of the same, perhaps also with some added corticosteroid for anti-inflammatory effect such as hydrocortisone (Anusol-HC cream). Suppositories are convenient but may not deliver the medication where it is needed; so, prescribe hydrocortisone cream or hydrocortisone/ pramoxine foam (Proctofoam-HC) applied externally rather than internally. Corticosteroid preparations are particularly helpful with anal pruritus.**

✅ **Pain may also be relieved by reducing sphincter spasm. Prescribe topical nifedipine 0.2% or diltiazem gel 2% with lidocaine gel 1.5% to be applied every 12 hours.** Topical glyceryl trinitrate 0.2% or nitroglycerin ointment can be substituted for the diltiazem and nifedipine, but many patients are unable to tolerate the headaches that frequently occur. (These prescriptions often need to be filled at a compounding pharmacy.)

✓ **Instruct the patient to treat lesser pain and itching with witch hazel compresses, a low-potency steroid cream, good anal hygiene, and ice packs followed by warm sitz baths or hot compresses. A sitz bath may be the most effective of these therapies;** it consists of a warm-water (40° C) bath that relieves tissue edema and sphincter spasm. **Zinc oxide paste or petroleum jelly may ease defecation and soothe itching. Prevent constipation by using bulk laxatives (i.e., bran, methylcellulose, polycarbophil)** (see Chapter 68) **and stool softeners (docusate [Colace], 50–100 mg four times a day), and arrange follow-up.** Inform the patient that some hemorrhoids may recur and require surgical removal.

✓ **Small, ulcerated, external hemorrhoids** usually do not require any treatment for hemostasis. Bulk laxatives and gentle cleansing are generally all that is required. Occasionally, patients present several days after an external hemorrhoid has thrombosed with a small gush of dark blood because of a ruptured pile. This may continue to ooze for 1 to 2 days. With or without rupture, if the pain has subsided, all that is required is reassurance and the general measures described previously. Inform the patient that symptoms should resolve in approximately 2 weeks.

✓ **When an acutely thrombosed external hemorrhoid is engorged and causing severe pain, and there are no anticipated bleeding problems, the hemorrhoid should be incised to provide pain relief. Consider using procedural sedation** (see Appendix E). Apply an ice pack for 15 minutes; then, using the smallest needle available, inject around it and infiltrate the dome of the mass with a local anesthetic to allow for examination and excision. **As described previously, use lidocaine or ropivacaine with epinephrine. Have an assistant spread the buttocks. The thrombus may be enucleated through an elliptic incision over the anal mucosa. Make the elliptic incision around the clot but not past the cutaneous layer or past the anal verge. Dark locular clots can be broken up by inserting a straight hemostat into the wound and spreading the tips, thereby allowing the clots to be expressed. Pain relief from this simple surgical technique can be dramatic, but excision is not effective unless the entire thrombosed clot is completely removed** (Figs. 74.3 and 74.4). Apply a compression dressing and tape the buttocks together for 12 hours to minimize bleeding. Occasionally, a topical hemostatic such as Surgifoam or Gelfoam may be needed to help control oozing. The patient can then begin the nonsurgical treatment described previously. Schedule a follow-up examination in 2 days. Nonsteroidal anti-inflammatory drugs (NSAIDs) and acetaminophen (Tylenol) are the postprocedure analgesics of choice. If possible, avoid narcotic analgesia, as this will worsen constipation.

What Not to Do

✗ Do not labor to reduce prolapsed internal hemorrhoids unless they are part of a large rectal prolapse with some strangulation. Everything may prolapse again when the patient stands or strains. Bulky but asymptomatic hemorrhoids should be left alone. Treatment is directed toward symptom control, not appearance, until definitive care is received.

✗ Do not traumatize the patient when doing an examination. Be cautious, as the pain may be intense.

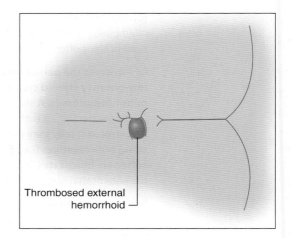

Thrombosed external
hemorrhoid —

Fig. 74.3 Thrombosed external hemorrhoid.

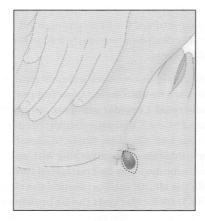

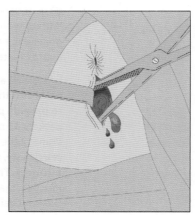

Fig. 74.4 Thrombosed
hemorrhoid excision.

(X) Do not miss infectious, neoplastic, and other anorectal pathologic conditions that can resemble or coexist with hemorrhoids. Consider rectal prolapse, polyps, carcinoma, hypertrophied anal papilla, skin tags, fissure, fistula, and perianal abscess in the differential diagnosis.

(X) Do not excise a thrombosed hemorrhoid when the patient has a bleeding abnormality, is taking an anticoagulant or daily aspirin, or has increased portal venous pressure.

(X) Do not allow patients to use hydrocortisone topical therapy for longer than 7 to 10 days. Prolonged use can lead to mucosal atrophy.

(X) Do not have the patient sit on a doughnut-shaped cushion. This may increase venous congestion.

Discussion

The word *hemorrhoid* comes from the Greek *hemo* ("blood") plus *rrhoos* ("flowing"). The word *piles* comes from the Latin *pila* ("ball"). As a disease entity, hemorrhoids have been reported to plague the human race since the earliest history.

Three-quarters of Americans have hemorrhoids at some point in their lifetime. Predisposing factors include heredity, age, portal hypertension, anal sphincter tone, occupation, low-fiber diet, obesity, diarrhea, straining to defecate, and pregnancy.

The submucosal tissue within the anal canal is made up of a discontinuous series of vascular cushions that contribute to continence by partially occluding the anus. The three main cushions are found in the left lateral, right anterior, and right posterior positions. These vascular cushions may also protect the anal canal from injury by filling with blood during defecation. The deterioration of supporting tissue to the vascular cushions in the anal canal produces venous distention, erosion, bleeding, and thrombosis. Several theories have been postulated regarding the etiology of hemorrhoids; however, the precise cause is still unknown.

Hemorrhoids are classified according to location and degree of prolapse. The dentate line separates internal from external hemorrhoids. Internal hemorrhoids arise proximal to the dentate line and are covered by mucosa. External hemorrhoids are located distal to the dentate line and are covered by squamous epithelia that contain numerous somatic pain receptors. External skin tags, which represent residual excess skin associated with previous thrombosis of external hemorrhoids, or which can be associated with anal fissures or Crohn disease, are often confused with external hemorrhoids, but they are not hemorrhoids.

There is no widely used classification system for grading external hemorrhoids, but **internal hemorrhoids are graded from I to IV**. First-degree internal hemorrhoids do not protrude, cannot be palpated by digital examination, and require anoscopy for diagnosis. Second-degree hemorrhoids protrude with straining or defecation but reduce spontaneously. Third-degree hemorrhoids prolapse with straining or defecation and require manual reduction. Fourth-degree hemorrhoids are irreducibly prolapsed and may strangulate.

External hemorrhoids are usually small and cause pain only when they are acutely thrombosed. Internal hemorrhoids are usually painless, and patients generally present with painless bleeding or a bloody mucoid discharge, often associated with their prolapse, anal soiling, and (occasionally) pruritus.

Elastic banding techniques, which have become one of the most frequently applied methods of treatment of internal hemorrhoids, can be 80% to 90% curative for lesions of second, third, and fourth degrees. This technique is associated with a low complication rate (<2%). When treating patients with bleeding diatheses, both internal and external hemorrhoids are best treated by means of surgical resection.

The diagnosis of hemorrhoids may cover a variety of minor ailments of the anus that may or may not be related to the hemorrhoidal veins (vascular cushions). **Anal and perianal itching** can be caused by dermatologic conditions, such as psoriasis, eczema, lichen planus, and allergic dermatitis (see pruritus ani in Discussion box, Chapter 66). Infections of the anal and perianal area include abscess, herpes simplex, scabies, candidiasis, erythrasma, and pinworms (see Chapter 70). Perianal itching can also be the result of diabetes, leukemia, aplastic anemia, thyroid disease, hyperbilirubinemia, and precancerous and cancerous lesions. Punch biopsy may be indicated when pruritus ani is chronic.

Suggested Readings

Bleday, R., & Breen, E. (2019a). Hemorrhoids: Clinical manifestations and diagnosis. UptoDate. https://www.uptodate.com/contents/hemorrhoids-clinical-manifestations-and-diagnosis.

Bleday, R., & Breen, E. (2019b). *Home and office treatment of symptomatic hemorrhoids*. UptoDate. https://www.uptodate.com/contents/home-and-office-treatment-of-symptomatic-hemorrhoids.

Gopal, D. V. (2002). Diseases of the rectum and anus: A clinical approach to common disorders. *Clinical Cornerstone, 4*, 34–48.

Sardinha, T. C., & Corman, M. L. (2002). Hemorrhoids. *Surgical Clinics of North America, 82*, 1153–1167.

Singultus

(Hiccups)

Presentation

Recurring, unpredictable, clonic contractions of the diaphragm that produce sharp inhalations are known as singultus or more commonly as hiccups. Hiccups are usually precipitated by some combination of laughing, talking, eating, and drinking but may also occur spontaneously. Most cases resolve spontaneously, and patients do not come to a physician's office unless hiccups are prolonged or severe. A bout of hiccups is any episode lasting more than a few minutes. If hiccups last longer than 48 hours, they are considered persistent or protracted. Hiccups lasting longer than 1 month are called intractable.

What to Do

✓ **For a bout of hiccups, stimulate the patient's soft palate by rubbing it with a swab, spoon, catheter tip, or gloved finger, just short of stimulating a gag reflex, and, if necessary, repeat this several times. Alternatively, stimulate the same general area by depositing a tablespoon of granulated sugar at the base of the tongue, in the area of the lingual tonsils, and have the patient let it dissolve (See Video 75.1).** Such maneuvers (or their placebo effect) may abolish simple cases of hiccups. Other simple measures include having the individual bite on a lemon or inhale a noxious agent (e.g., ammonia). You can also have the patient perform a Valsalva maneuver, breath hold, or pull the knees up to the chest and lean forward.

✓ **With persistent and protracted hiccups, look for an underlying cause and ask about precipitating factors or previous episodes.** Drugs that are known to cause hiccups include benzodiazepines, short-acting barbiturates, and dexamethasone. Persistence of hiccups during sleep suggests an organic cause; conversely, if a patient is unable to sleep or if the hiccups stop during sleep and recur promptly on awakening, a psychogenic or idiopathic cause is indicated.

✓ **Obtain a complete history and perform a complete physical examination.** Serious, potentially life-threatening conditions such as myocardial infarction, pericarditis, and aberrant cardiac pacemaker electrode placement are potential sources of persistent hiccups. Look in the ears. (Foreign bodies, such as a hair against the tympanic membrane, can cause hiccups.) Examine the neck (look for thyromegaly and lymphadenopathy), chest, and abdomen, perhaps including an upright chest radiograph, to look for neoplastic, inflammatory, or infectious processes irritating the phrenic nerve or diaphragm. Acute and chronic alcohol intoxication and gastroesophageal reflux or other gastrointestinal disorders should also be considered as potential causes of hiccups.

✓ Perform a neurologic examination, looking for evidence of partial continuous seizures or brain stem lesions. Early multiple sclerosis is thought to be one of the most frequent neurologic causes of intractable hiccups in young adults.

✅ **Routine laboratory evaluation** is not always needed in a simple bout of hiccups but may include a complete blood count (CBC) with differential (looking for infection or neoplasm) and a basic metabolic panel. (Hyponatremia, hypokalemia, hypocalcemia, and uremia can cause persistent hiccups.)

✅ **Additional testing** is not limited to, but may include, an electrocardiogram (ECG), chest computed tomography (CT), and upper endoscopy.

✅ Direct treatment toward the specific illness causing the hiccups, if this is identified.

✅ **If hiccups persist after using simple measures, try chlorpromazine (Thorazine), the only US Food and Drug Administration (FDA)–approved medication for hiccups, 25 to 50 mg orally three or four times a day.** (The same dose may be given intravenously [IV] or intramuscularly [IM].) To avoid or minimize hypotension, consider giving a bolus, 500 to 1000 mL, of IV normal saline. Chlorpromazine is contraindicated in elderly patients with dementia. Side effects include dystonic reaction, drowsiness, and the risk of tardive dyskinesia. **Alternatively, haloperidol (Haldol), 2 to 5 mg IM, followed by 1 to 4 mg orally three times a day for 2 days may be equally effective, with less potential for hypotension. Another approach is to use metoclopramide (Reglan), 10 mg orally three or four times a day, followed by a maintenance regimen of 10 to 20 mg orally three to four times a day for 10 days. Reglan and Haldol are also associated with tardive dyskinesia but may be less expensive than Thorazine with less frequent side effects.**

✅ **For intractable hiccups**, phenytoin (Dilantin), valproic acid (Depakote), or carbamazepine (Tegretol) can be given in typical anticonvulsant doses. Alternatively, baclofen (a centrally acting muscle relaxant) can be prescribed at 10 to 20 mg two or three times a day with gabapentin (Neurontin) as an add-on, if necessary, especially in patients with solid malignancies.

✅ There are some reports of acupuncture or hypnosis being efficacious; these can be tried if the aforementioned are unsuccessful.

✅ **Arrange for follow-up and additional evaluation if the hiccups recur or persist.**

What Not to Do

❌ Do not assume hiccups are a benign condition, especially in those patients with a history of coronary artery disease (CAD), prior pacemake placement, or other risk factors for CAD such as diabetes, hypertension, hyperlipidemia, smoking, obesity. Consider at least a screening EKG in these higher-risk patients.

Discussion

The medical term *singultus* apparently originates from the Latin *singult*, which is very descriptive and roughly translates as "the act of catching one's breath while sobbing."

Hiccups result from an involuntary spasmodic contraction of the diaphragm and external intercostal muscles with ensuing quick inspiration.

This is followed by a rapid closure of the glottis, which prevents overinflation of the lungs.

Hiccups are mediated by a reflex arch consisting of the afferent and efferent limbs and supraspinal central connection, which are thought to be independent of the respiratory center in the brainstem. The exact cause remains unclear.

Discussion continued

When there is an organic cause, irritation of the various branches of the vagus nerve are often involved. **Despite a long list of possible causes, in most cases no organic cause can be identified, and a diagnosis of idiopathic chronic hiccups is made.**

Although unlikely, there are potentially serious complications, such as dehydration and weight loss, resulting from the inability to tolerate fluids and food.

Patients who experience syncope with the hiccups should be hospitalized and evaluated for possible life-threatening arrhythmias, which have been reported as both the cause and the effect of hiccups.

Hiccups, in general, are a common malady, and fortunately most bouts are usually transient and benign. Persistent or intractable episodes are more likely to result from serious pathophysiologic processes that affect a component of the hiccup reflex mechanism.

The common denominator among various hiccup cures for brief episodes seems to be stimulation of the glossopharyngeal nerve, but as for every self-limiting disease, there are always many effective cures.

... hold your breath, and if after you have done so for some time the hiccup is no better, then gargle with a little water, and if it still continues, tickle your nose with something and sneeze, and if you sneeze once or twice, even the most violent hiccup is sure to go.

—Eryximachus, the physician to Aristophanes, in Plato's Symposium.

Suggested Readings

Berlin, A. L., Muhn, C. Y., & Billick, R. C. (2003). Hiccups, eructation, and other uncommon prodromal manifestations of herpes zoster. *Journal of the American Academy of Dermatology, 49*, 1121–1124.

Friedman, N. L. (1996). Hiccups: A treatment review. *Pharmacotherapy, 16*, 986–995.

Ge, A. X., Ryan, M. E., Giaccone, G., et al. (2010). Acupuncture treatment for persistent hiccups in patients with cancer. *Journal of Alternative and Complementary Medicine, 16*, 811–816.

Kolodzik, P. W., & Eilers, M. A. (1991). Hiccups (singultus): Review and approach to management. *Annals of Emergency Medicine, 20*, 565–573.

Launois, S., Bizec, J. L., Whitelaw, W. A., et al. (1993). Hiccup in adults: An overview. *European Respiratory Journal, 6*, 563–575.

Lembo, A. (2012). *Overview of hiccups.* UptoDate. http://www.uptodate.com.

Marinella, M. A. (2009). Diagnosis and management of hiccups in the patient with advanced cancer. *Journal of Community and Supportive Oncology, 7*, 122–127.

Nathan, M. D., Leshner, R. T., & Keller, A. P. (1980). Intractable hiccups (singultus). *Laryngoscope, 90*, 1612–1618.

Viera, A. J., & Sullivan, S. A. (2001). Remedies for prolonged hiccups. *American Family Physician, 63*, 1684–1686.

Wagner, M. S., & Stapczynski, J. S. (1982). Persistent hiccups. *Annals of Emergency Medicine, 11*, 24–26.

Vomiting

(Food Poisoning, Gastroenteritis)

Presentation

The patient typically seeks medical care 1 to 6 hours after eating because of severe nausea, vomiting, retching, and abdominal cramps that may progress later into diarrhea. Patients may present with a wide range of findings. Signs and symptoms can range from mild to severe illness. It begins with minor nausea, vomiting, malaise, and diarrhea, progressing to conditions where patients may appear very ill: pale, diaphoretic, tachycardic, orthostatic, and perhaps complaining of paresthesias.

Others may have similar symptoms from eating the same food. The physical examination, however, is often reassuring. There is minimal abdominal tenderness, localized, if at all, to the epigastrium or to the rectus abdominis muscle (which is strained by the vomiting).

What to Do

✅ **Obtain as much historical information as possible and completely examine the patient.** Always consider pregnancy in women of childbearing age who present with vomiting. If there is any suspicion of a more serious underlying disorder (especially in the older patient), perform those tests needed to rule out myocardial infarction, perforated ulcer, aortic aneurysm, bowel obstruction, or any of the catastrophes that can present in a similar fashion. **Always maintain a high index of suspicion for acute appendicitis or other surgical conditions in the patient who presents with abdominal pain and vomiting.**

✅ **In the meantime, rapidly infuse 0.9% NaCl or Ringer lactate solution intravenously (IV) and observe the patient, doing repeated vital sign checks and physical examinations. Fluid and electrolyte replenishment is the mainstay of medical treatment.** In adults who have adequate renal and cardiovascular reserve to handle rapid hydration, 1 to 2 L infused over 60 minutes often provides dramatic improvement of all symptoms.

✅ Patients with risk of acute congestive heart failure require more cautious rehydration. Elderly patients complaining of abdominal pain should be taken very seriously and are more likely to require a comprehensive diagnostic workup.

✅ **The use of antiemetics for acute gastritis or gastroenteritis is somewhat controversial.** With mild symptoms, there is probably no need to add this treatment and incur additional expense as well as risk the potential side effects of some of these drugs. For someone who is actively vomiting, however, these drugs can provide comfort and improve the process of rehydration.

✓ **In adults, ondansetron (Zofran), 4 mg intravenously (IV), is particularly advantageous because it has minimal side effects. Alternatives include prochlorperazine (Compazine), 10 mg, which can also be given IV, along with diphenhydramine (Benadryl), 12.5 to 25 mg,** to help reduce the incidence of extrapyramidal symptoms (such as dystonic reactions and akathisia). Metoclopramide (Reglan) can also be given (slowly to reduce risk of akathisia) in a dose of 10 mg IV. A patient's home medications and risk of QTc prolongation should be considered prior to giving antiemetics if there is concern of causing QTc prolongation and Torsades de pointes. Medications often used for nausea and vomiting that do not prolong the QTc include diphenhydramine (Benadryl) and benzodiazepines.

✓ **Administration of ondansetron in early pregnancy is somewhat controversial, as there is mixed evidence tied to cardiac defects and cleft palate in the fetus. Generally, in pregnant patients in the first trimester, we recommend doxylamine (Unisom), 12.5 to 25 g orally every 6–8 hours, and pyridoxine (vitamin B$_6$), 10 to 25 mg orally every 6–8 hours.**

✓ **For children who are older than 6 months of age, ondansetron (Zofran), 0.15 mg/kg IV, can be given. Ondansetron (although very expensive under the brand name) can also be given as an oral disintegrating tablet (ODT), which is reasonably priced as a generic.** Half of a 4-mg tablet (2 mg) is an appropriate dose for an average 2-year-old (weighing 8–15 kg). The 4-mg tablet can be given to children weighing 16 to 30 kg, and 8 mg can be given to heavier children. **Alternatively, metoclopramide (Reglan), 0.1 to 0.2 mg/kg IV, can be given.**

✓ **If after 1 to 2 hours the pediatric patient is improving and beginning to tolerate oral fluids and has a benign repeat abdominal examination, discharge with instructions to advance the diet over the next 24 hours, starting with an oral rehydration solution,** such as the following recipe from the World Health Organization:

1 cup orange juice

3⁄4 tsp table salt

1 tsp baking soda

4 Tbsp sugar

4 cups water

✓ The child should expect to be eating and feeling well in another 1 or 2 days.

✓ **Children can be rehydrated using the techniques described in Chapter 69.**

✓ If symptoms resolve more slowly, discharge the patient with a single dose of an antiemetic as described earlier.

✓ **Adults with abdominal cramping may be helped with a dose of the antispasmodic dicyclomine (Bentyl), 20 mg intramuscularly or orally (up to four times a day).**

✓ **If cannabinoid-induced hyperemesis syndrome (CHS) is suspected**, capsaicin is recommended as a reasonable first-line treatment approach despite limited clinical evidence regarding its use. Apply capsaicin cream (0.075%) to a 15 × 25-cm area in the periumbilic region of the patient's abdomen, with reapplications every 4 hours. Within a few hours the patient's symptoms of abdominal pain and vomiting should be expected to completely resolve. The patient can be discharged with the tube of capsaicin cream in the event that the symptoms return. You must emphasize to the patient the necessity to stop using marijuana, since it is the only proven cure for CHS.

⊘ **Patients should always be encouraged to return** for further evaluation and treatment if their symptoms return or if pain continues or worsens.

⊘ **If hypotension or other significant signs or symptoms persist**, if the patient cannot tolerate parenteral rehydration, or cannot resume oral intake, the patient may have to be admitted to the hospital for further evaluation and treatment.

What Not to Do

✗ Do not take abdominal pain and vomiting lightly in an elderly patient.

✗ Do not presume food poisoning without a good history for it (i.e., multiple individuals being sickened after eating the same food).

✗ Do not overlook pregnancy as a possible cause of vomiting.

✗ Do not assign blame for the cause of any suspected food poisoning. The information available is almost always circumstantial until public health authorities complete their investigation.

✗ Do not skimp on IV fluids. Monitor vital signs and urinary output and generously replace fluid losses.

✗ Do not pursue expensive laboratory investigations for straightforward cases. Diagnostic tests usually are unnecessary in an otherwise healthy patient who is stable and whose history and physical examination are consistent with acute gastroenteritis.

Discussion

Whenever possible, the cause of vomiting should be ascertained and specific treatment for an underlying cause initiated—particularly when emergent conditions such as central nervous system (CNS) lesions, myocardial infarction, acute abdomen, bowel obstruction, bowel ischemia, and endocrine/metabolic disorders are suspected. As mentioned, **always consider pregnancy in women of childbearing age who present with vomiting.** Consider bowel obstruction if there is distention and pain on abdominal palpation. Feculent vomiting is concerning for large bowel obstruction. Patients may present with a chief complaint of vomiting and, on exam, have nystagmus; these patients should be evaluated and treated for vertigo. Eating disorders must also be considered. In the diabetic, gastroparesis may be the cause.

Patients with CHS and cyclic vomiting syndrome are being seen more frequently in emergency departments (EDs). CHS patients may require treatment for intractable emesis, dehydration, and electrolyte abnormalities. Thought to be a variant of cyclic vomiting syndrome, CHS has become more prevalent with increasing cannabis potency and use,

as enabled by various states having legalized the recreational use of cannabis.

The phases of CHS involve a prodrome, hyperemesis, and recovery. The prodromal phase is notable for early morning nausea, anorexia, fear of vomiting, and abdominal discomfort that can last for days. The hyperemetic phase is characterized by nausea, frequent emesis, and diffuse abdominal pain lasting 24 hours or longer. The recovery phase involves resolution of nausea, emesis, and anorexia. CHS represents a paradox, because the major psychoactive component of marijuana, Δ9-tetrahydrocannabinol, is an effective and widely used antiemetic. Standard antiemetics such as ondansetron and prochlorperazine are some of the most commonly used medications in acute care settings. A recent systematic review of pharmacologic treatment of CHS concluded that these drugs alone are frequently ineffective, and alternative agents used off-label, such as benzodiazepines, haloperidol, and topical capsaicin cream, have the greatest efficacy based mainly on case series and reports. Another important consideration in the ED is that the selected

Discussion continued

agents may be administered parenterally, rectally, sublingually, or topically, because CHS patients may be unable to tolerate oral medication and will often require IV crystalloid hydration and electrolyte correction.

Capsaicin, or 8-methyl-*N*-vanillyl-6-nonenamide, is a chemical found in several species of chili pepper and may be the most effective treatment. Capsaicin is available as a topical cream that produces a sensation of heat on contact with skin. This may help to explain why some of these patients report that hot showers relieve their symptoms. Cessation of cannabis should be emphasized by the treating clinician as the only proven cure for CHS. Patients may be surprised to learn that the root cause for their episodic hyperemesis is long-term cannabis use, which may prevent future attempts at self-treatment with more cannabis.

Many prescription drugs may cause nausea and vomiting, and these will be cured with cessation of the drug; so, take a good medication history, asking about both prescribed and nonprescribed drugs.

In most cases of simple, uncomplicated vomiting with gastroenteritis or foodborne illness, the precise cause need not be determined, and therefore symptomatic treatment is all that is required.

Many of the symptoms accompanying any gastroenteritis seem to be related to electrolyte disturbances and dehydration, which can be substantial even in the absence of copious vomiting and diarrhea. Lactated Ringer solution is considered the choice for IV rehydration by many clinicians because it approximates normal serum electrolytes and can be infused rapidly. Lactated Ringer approximately replaces the electrolytes lost in diarrhea, although normal saline has more of the chloride lost by vomiting. Both work quite well in the acute setting for either diarrhea or vomiting or a combination of the two.

Most food items that cause foodborne illness are raw or undercooked foods of animal origin, such as meat, milk, eggs, cheese, fish, or shellfish. A clearly implicated food source may give a clue to the cause: shellfish suggesting *Vibrio parahaemolyticus;* rice suggesting *Bacillus cereus;* meat or eggs suggesting staphylococci, *Campylobacter* organisms, clostridia, salmonellae, shigellae, enteropathic *Escherichia coli,* or *Yersinia* sp.

Vibrio **bacteria**, so named because they are so motile that they appear to vibrate, are most common in states bordering the Gulf of Mexico. These flagellated bacteria inhabit marine environments and can cause gastroenteritis, wound infections, and septicemia. *V. vulnificus* infection more often follows ingestion of raw or undercooked oysters, and *V. parahaemolyticus* infection is more likely to be associated with eating shrimp or crabs. Fever, chills, and headache, in addition to the gastrointestinal symptoms, are common manifestations of this infection. Patients with liver disease, impaired immune systems, and diabetes are at increased risk for fulminant infections.

B. cereus causes an acute emetic syndrome, most commonly within 1 to 6 hours of ingesting fried rice obtained from a Chinese restaurant. *B. cereus* also causes a less common diarrheal syndrome with an onset of 8 to 16 hours after ingestion. There is no role for antimicrobial therapy in the treatment of these syndromes.

The most common food poisoning seen in most EDs is caused by the heat-stable toxin of staphylococci, which is introduced into food from infections in handlers and grows when the food sits warm. Foods that are frequently incriminated in staphylococcal food poisoning include meat and meat products; poultry and egg products; mayonnaise-containing salads, such as egg, tuna, chicken, potato, and macaroni; bakery products, such as cream-filled pastries and cream pies; and milk and dairy products. Foods containing the toxins usually look and taste normal. Sudden onset of nausea, vomiting, abdominal pain, and watery diarrhea usually occurs 30 minutes to 8 hours after eating contaminated food. Because these symptoms are toxin mediated, antibiotics are not indicated.

Chemical toxins have a similar presentation, but the onset of symptoms may be more immediate. Heavy metal poisoning is a rare cause of gastroenteritis and results from gastric irritation caused by copper, zinc, iron, tin, or cadmium. Accidental ingestion of these substances can occur if a person drinks an acidic or carbonated beverage that came into contact with a metal container or metal tubing. Common symptoms include nausea, vomiting, diarrhea, cramps, and, with copper and tin, a metallic taste that usually occurs 5 to 60 minutes after ingestion. For chemical or heavy metal poisoning, consult with a poison control center for advice on appropriate treatment.

Discussion continued

Other bacterial food poisonings usually present with onset of symptoms later than 1 to 6 hours after eating, less nausea and vomiting, more cramping and diarrhea, and longer courses. See Chapter 69 for management of these predominantly diarrheal illnesses.

Seafood ingestion syndromes, such as ciguatera poisoning and scombroid poisoning, can be distinguished from other forms of foodborne illnesses by symptoms such as perioral numbness and reversal of temperature sensation (ciguatera poisoning) or flushing and warmth (scombroid poisoning). Grouper, red snapper, amberjack, sea bass, and barracuda are the most common species of fish implicated in ciguatera poisoning.

Ciguatoxin is a naturally occurring toxin found in a dinoflagellate *(Gambierdiscus toxicus)* that is consumed by fish. The ciguatoxins become concentrated in these larger fish and are unaffected by normal cooking. Symptoms appear about 5 hours (2–30 hours) after eating toxic fish. The first manifestations of poisoning include abdominal pain, nausea, vomiting, painful defecation, and diarrhea. Pruritus and paresthesias, described as uncomfortable tingling sensations, most often develop in the extremities and mouth and, along with a peculiar sensory reversal of hot and cold, are the symptomatic hallmarks of ciguatera poisoning. Pain, paresthesias, pruritus, and weakness may persist for several weeks, and chronic symptoms have been reported. Successful management of these neurologic symptoms with IV mannitol has been described in the past, but a double-blind randomized trial of mannitol therapy in ciguatera fish poisoning did not support single-dose mannitol as standard treatment. Pruritus can be treated with antihistamines, such as hydroxyzine (Atarax, Vistaril), 25 mg three or four times a day. Treat neuropathic symptoms with gabapentin (Neurontin), 100 mg three to four times a day, titrating up to 800 to 1200 mg three times a day

as needed. Musculoskeletal pain should be treated with an appropriate analgesic. The patient should be instructed to avoid all fish, alcohol, caffeine, and nuts for 6 months because these items may precipitate a recurrence of symptoms.

Scombroid poisoning is caused by improper refrigeration of Scombroidea (bluefin and yellowfin tuna, skipjack, albacore, marlin, and mackerel). Nonscombroid fish, such as mahi-mahi, amberjack, and herring, may also produce this syndrome. Bacterial growth and breakdown of the fish flesh result in the production of histamine and a histamine-like toxin, saurine, neither of which are affected by normal cooking temperatures. These fish either may have a bitter, peppery, or metallic taste or may taste perfectly normal. Symptoms consist of a histamine-like reaction that includes flushing, rash, and hot sensations of the skin and mouth, along with headache, anxiety, dizziness, nausea, vomiting, and diarrhea occurring approximately 10 to 30 minutes after ingestion. Antihistamines, such as hydroxyzine (Atarax, Vistaril), 25 mg one to four times a day, are effective, along with H_2 blockers, such as ranitidine (Zantac), 150 mg twice a day, and, in more severe cases, methylprednisolone (Solu-Medrol), 125 mg IV. Symptoms are self-limited, but medications may be required for several days.

When symptoms are severe with large ingestions of either form of fish poisoning, patients should also be given activated charcoal AD (Superchar), 1 g/kg orally.

Whenever someone suffers any gastrointestinal upset, it is essential to obtain a thorough history pertaining to last food eaten, travel, and potential sick contacts. When the index of suspicion for a foodborne illness is high, this information should be reported to the local health department for definitive diagnosis and epidemiologic management.

Suggested Readings

American College of Obstetricians and Gynecologists. (2018). Practice bulletin—nausea and vomiting of pregnancy. *Obstetrics & Gynecology*, *131*(1), e15–e30.

American Gastroenterological Association. (2001). American Gastroenterological Association medical position statement: Nausea and vomiting. *Gastroenterology*, *120*, 261–263.

Apfel, C. C., Korttila, K., Abdalla, M., et al. (2004). A factorial trial of six interventions for the prevention of postoperative nausea and vomiting. *New England Journal of Medicine*, *350*, 2441–2451.

Berkovitch, M., Mazzota, P., Greenberg, R., et al. (2002). Metoclopramide for nausea and vomiting of pregnancy: A prospective multicenter international study. *American Journal of Perinatology*, *19*, 311–316.

Borowitz, S. M. (2005). Are antiemetics helpful in young children suffering from acute viral gastroenteritis? *Archives of Disease in Childhood*, *90*, 646–648.

Büttner, M., Walder, B., von Elm, E., et al. (2004). Is low-dose haloperidol a useful antiemetic? *Anesthesiology*, *101*, 1454–1463.

Farthing, M., Salam, M. A., Lindberg, G., et al. (2013). Acute diarrhea in adults and children: a global perspective. *Journal of Clinical Gastroenterology*, *47*(1), 12–20.

Moon, A. M., Buckley, S. A., & Mark, N. M. (2018). Successful treatment of cannabinoid hyperemesis syndrome with topical capsaicin. *Society guideline*. *ACG Case Report Journal*, *5*, e3.

Parlak, I., Atilla, R., Cicek, M., et al. (2005). Rate of metoclopramide infusion affects the severity and incidence of akathisia. *Emergency Medicine Journal*, *22*, 621–624.

Reeves, J. J., Shannon, M. W., & Fleisher, G. R. (2002). Ondansetron decreases vomiting associated with acute gastroenteritis: A randomized, controlled trial. *Pediatrics*, *109*, e62.

Richards, J. R. (2018). Cannabinoid hyperemesis syndrome: Pathophysiology and treatment in the emergency department. *Journal of Emergency Medicine*, *54*(3), 354–363.

Scorza, K., Williams, A., Phillips, J. D., & Shaw, J. Evaluation of nausea and vomiting. *American Family Physician*, 76, 76–84.

Schnorf, H., Taurarii, M., & Cundy, T. (2002). Ciguatera fish poisoning: A double-blind randomized trial of mannitol therapy. *Neurology*, *58*, 873–888.

Taylor, L. G., et al. (2017). Antiemetic use among pregnant women in the United States: The escalating use of ondansetron. *Pharmacoepidemiology and Drug Safety*, *26*(5), 592–596.

Vinson, D. R. (2004). Diphenhydramine in the treatment of akathisia induced by prochlorperazine. *Journal of Emergency Medicine*, *26*, 265–270.

World Global Organization (WGO). (2013). *Guideline for acute diarrhea in adults and children—a global perspective*.

PART 7

Urologic Emergencies

■ Laurel B. Plante   ■ Stephen J. Skinner

Blunt Scrotal Trauma

Presentation

Blunt injuries to the scrotum usually occur in patients who are younger than 50 years of age as a result of an athletic injury; a straddle injury; an automobile, motorcycle, or industrial accident; or an assault. Patients present with various degrees of pain, ecchymoses, and swelling as well as faintness, nausea, or vomiting (Fig. 77.1). The symptoms from minor injuries will gradually resolve on their own after 1 to 2 hours. In the more severe injury of testicular rupture, pain is usually severe, and the scrotal sac may appear full, ecchymotic, and very tender.

The presence of both testicular swelling and tenderness suggests more significant testicular injury; however, testicular rupture can be present in the absence of tenderness.

What to Do

✓ Get a clear history of the exact mechanism, the force of the trauma, and the point of maximum impact. Determine if there was any bloody penile discharge or hematuria and whether the patient has any preexisting genital disease, such as previous genitourinary surgery, infection, or mass.

✓ Gently examine the external genitalia with the understanding that intense pain may result in a suboptimal examination. If scrotal swelling is not too severe, try to palpate and assess the intrascrotal anatomy.

✓ **When there is minimal pain and tenderness, with normal anatomy, no further evaluation is necessary.**

✓ **There is a high risk for urethral injury in straddle injuries.** Obtain a urinalysis. If blood is present in the urine (or at the urethral meatus), perform a retrograde urethrogram and obtain urologic consultation.

✓ **After any significant blunt trauma,** when pain or swelling prevents demonstration of normal intrascrotal anatomy, obtain a testicular color Doppler ultrasonograph to help determine the

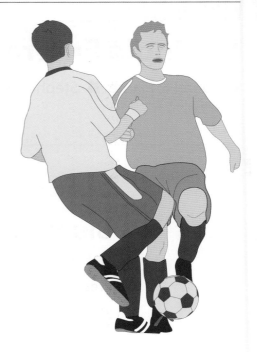

Fig. 77.1 Blunt injury to the scrotum.

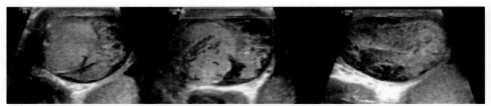

Fig. 77.2 Ultrasound images of right testis showing *(from left to right):* injured testis, Doppler view of injured testis, and right extratesticular hematoma. (With permission from Moynihan, M. J., Manganiello, M. [2020]. Bilateral testes fractures from blunt scrotal trauma. *Urology Case Reports, 28,* 101026.)

need for urologic consultation and operative intervention. Ultrasonography is the gold standard diagnostic tool with excellent sensitivity and specificity (Fig. 77.2).

⊘ **Scrotal hematomas** can involve the testis, epididymis, or scrotal wall. Patients with intratesticular hematomas fare poorly without exploration; 40% of these hematomas result in testicular infection or necrosis, which often requires orchiectomy. **Scrotal exploration is warranted if there is compelling evidence of testicular fracture or rupture on scrotal sonography or physical examination.** It is most appropriate to explore a grossly abnormal scrotum without ultrasonography when the index of suspicion is high. This should occur when there is a clinical hematocele. This may be evidenced by persistent moderate to severe pain, tender ecchymotic fullness of the scrotal sac, and a testicle that feels enlarged and/or irregular or is difficult to palpate. The presence of a large hematocele on ultrasonography is another

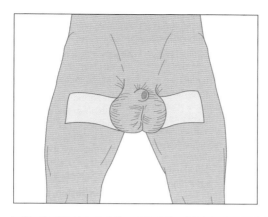

Fig. 77.3 Scrotal support.

indication for exploration. In one study, all patients with operatively confirmed testicular rupture had a combination of the following ultrasound features: the presence of hematocele, disruption of the tunica albuginea, and/or extrusion of the seminiferous tubules.

✅ Small hematoceles, epididymal hematomas, or contusions of the testis generally pose little risk to the patient and do not require surgical exploration.

✅ **All posttraumatic lesions should be followed to demonstrate sonographic resolution, because 10% to 15% of testicular tumors first present after an episode of scrotal trauma.**

✅ **Simple superficial scrotal lacerations** can be closed using Vicryl absorbable suture or tissue adhesive (Dermabond).

✅ **When emergent urologic intervention is not required,** provide analgesia (consider nonsteroidal anti-inflammatory drugs [NSAIDs], bed rest, scrotal support, a cold pack, and urologic follow-up) (Fig. 77.3).

✅ Patients should always be instructed to return immediately if pain increases, becomes severe, or is accompanied by vomiting or lightheadedness.

What Not to Do

❌ Do not miss testicular torsion, which is associated with minor to moderate blunt trauma approximately 20% of the time. (See symptoms and signs of testicular torsion in Chapter 79.)

❌ Do not miss the rare traumatic testicular dislocation that results in an "empty scrotum." In most cases (80.2%), a traumatic dislocation of the testis (TDT) occurred after a motorcycle accident. The main mechanism of TDT is a direct force propelling the testis out of the scrotum, after rupture of the fasciae of the spermatic cord.

   The most common site of dislocation is the superficial inguinal pouch (almost 50% of all cases). Other less common sites of TDT are as follows: pubic (18%), penile (8%), canalicular (8%), truly abdominal (6%), perineal (4%), acetabular (4%), and crural (2%).
   Immediate urology consultation is required.

❌ Do not discharge a patient until he can demonstrate the ability to urinate.

Discussion

Blunt testicular trauma occurs from a direct blow to the testes with impingement against the symphysis pubis or ischial ramus. Trauma can result in contusion, hematoma, fracture, rupture, or (rarely) dislocation of the testis. Testicular rupture is a surgical emergency. More than 80% of ruptured testes can be saved if surgery is performed within 72 hours of injury. Complications of testicular trauma include testicular atrophy, infection, infarction, and infertility, which are much more likely with nonoperative management of serious injuries.

If Doppler studies demonstrate a serious injury, early exploration, evacuation of hematoma, and repair of testicular rupture tend to result in an earlier return to normal activity, with less risk for testicular atrophy, infection, infarction, and infertility.

Sonographic findings in testicular rupture include interruption of the tunica albuginea; contour abnormality; a heterogeneous testis with irregular, poorly defined borders; scrotal wall thickening; and a large hematocele. A heterogeneous parenchymal echo pattern with loss of testicular contour is highly sensitive (100%) and specific (93.5%) for testicular rupture or testicular torsion.

The sonographic appearance of hematomas varies with time. Acute hematomas appear hyperechoic and subsequently become complex, with cystic components. Color Doppler sonography in posttraumatic patients may reveal focal or diffuse hyperemia of the epididymis, which represents traumatic epididymitis.

In conclusion, patients presenting after blunt scrotal trauma with clinical hematocele should progress directly to exploration. The remainder should undergo scrotal ultrasonography. Those with large hematoceles or suspected rupture on ultrasonography should also proceed to exploration. Those without hematocele, a clearly distinct tunica albuginea, and a lack of fracture planes within the testes are a subgroup that can be successfully treated conservatively.

Suggested Readings

Bhatt, S., & Dogra, V. S. (2008). Role of US in testicular and scrotal trauma (review). *Radio Graphics, 28*, 1617–1629.

Chandra, R. V., Dowling, R. J., Ulubasoglub, M., et al. (2007). Rational approach to diagnosis and management of blunt scrotal trauma. *Urology, 70*, 230–234.

Dogra, V., & Bhatt, S. (2004). Acute painful scrotum. *Radiology Clinics of North America, 42*, 349–363.

Ko, S., Ng, S., Wan, Y., et al. (2004). Testicular dislocation: An uncommon and easily overlooked complication of blunt abdominal trauma. *Annals of Emergency Medicine, 43*, 371–375.

Moynihan, M. J., & Manganiello, M. (2020). Bilateral testes fractures from blunt scrotal trauma. *Urology Case Reports, 28*, 101026.

Rosenstein, D., & McAninch, J. W. (2004). Urologic emergencies. *Medicine Clinics of North America, 88*, 495–518.

Zavras, N., Siatelis, A., Misiakos, E., et al. (2014). Testicular dislocation after scrotal trauma: A case report and brief literature review. *Urology Case Reports, 2*(3), 101–104.

Colorful Urine

Presentation

Patients may complain of or be frightened about the color of their urine. Color may be one component of some urinary complaint, or the color may be noted incidentally on urinalysis.

What to Do

✅ Ask about symptoms of urinary urgency, frequency, and painful urination. Include questions about flank or abdominal pain as well as recent ingestion of any food colorings, over-the-counter (OTC) or prescription medications, or diagnostic dyes. Ascertain the circumstances surrounding the change of urine color: Did the color appear only after the urine contacted the container or the water in the toilet bowl? Did the urine have to sit in the sun for hours before the color appeared?

✅ **Obtain a fresh urine sample for analysis.**

✅ **Persistent foam suggests protein (yellow foam, bilirubin),** which should also show up on a dipstick test.

✅ **With red or tea-colored urine, a positive dipstick for blood implies the presence of red cells, free hemoglobin, or myoglobin,** which can be double-checked by examining the urinary sediment for red cells and the serum for hemoglobinemia. In patients with normal renal function, hemoglobinuria can be distinguished from myoglobinuria by drawing a blood sample, spinning it down, and looking at the serum. **Free hemoglobin produces a pink serum that will test positive with the dipstick. Myoglobin is cleared more efficiently by the kidneys, usually leaving clear serum that tests negative with the dipstick.** Consider sending the urine for microscopic urinalysis to determine the presence of red blood cells.

✅ **If the urine is red and acidic but does not contain hemoglobin, myoglobin, or red blood cells, suspect an indicator dye, such as phenolphthalein (the former laxative in Ex-Lax),** in which case the red should disappear when the urine is alkalinized with a few drops of potassium hydroxide (KOH).

✅ **Fourteen percent of individuals who eat beets produce reddish urine** because of the excretion of the pigment betalain. **Blackberries can turn acidic urine red, whereas rhubarb, anthraquinone laxatives, and some diagnostic dyes will redden urine only when it is alkaline.**

✅ **Orange urine may be produced by phenazopyridine (Pyridium) or ethoxazene (Serenium),** both of which are used as urinary tract anesthetics to diminish dysuria. **Rifampin will also turn urine orange, as will carrots, rhubarb, beets, aloe, riboflavin, vitamin A, and vitamin B_{12}.**

✅ **Blue or green urine may be caused by a blue dye, such as methylene blue, a component in several medications (Trac Tabs, Urised, Uroblue)** used to reduce symptoms of cystitis. **A blue pigment may also be produced by *Pseudomonas* infection. Food Dye and Color Blue Number 1 (FD & C Blue No. 1) has been reported to be absorbed from the gastrointestinal (GI) tract in some patients sufficiently to cause the urine to be dark green.**

✅ **Intermittent passage of milky white urine possibly associated with dysuria, urinary frequency, urgency, or retention may be due to the rare condition of chyluria, where chyle is excreted into the urine, often turning it milky white.** Chyle is the lymphatic fluid composed of chylomicrons that predominantly contains albumin, fibrin, emulsified lipids, cholesterol, and triglycerides absorbed from the intestinal lacteals and that normally drains into the thoracic duct. Pathologic obstructions, valvular insufficiency, or abnormal communications can result in retrograde flow of this lymphatic fluid into the renal lymphatics and then into the urinary tract.

Examination of urine in standing test tubes shows layering with fat on top, a middle layer of fibrin clots, and cells with debris on the bottom. Urinalysis will often show varying degrees of proteinuria and hematuria, and additional testing for urinary chylomicrons will be positive. Initial imaging may include ultrasonography or computed tomography to assess for obstruction.

Patients who present to the emergency department (ED) or clinic with this condition often present with urinary retention, and the initial management should include relief of the obstruction, basic laboratory evaluations for common causes of chyluria, and consultation with urology to determine the likelihood of recurrence and the potential need for inpatient evaluation versus close outpatient follow-up.

✅ **In the critically ill patient requiring enteral feeding,** the practice of adding colored dye (including FD & C Blue No. 1) to the tube feeding to quickly detect occult aspiration can also cause urine discoloration.

✅ **Purple urine bag syndrome (PUBS)** is a term that has been used to describe the purple discoloration of the collecting bag and tubing that occurs rarely and is predominantly found in elderly bedridden women with chronic urinary catheterization, alkaline urine, and constipation. No specific cause has been found, and it appears to be a benign condition. PUBS has not been demonstrated to have any implication other than the possibility of a urinary tract infection and has not been proven to change the prognosis of patients.

✅ **Brown or black urine (not resulting from myoglobin or bilirubin) may be caused by l-dopa, melanin, phenacetin, or phenol poisoning as well as anthraquinones mentioned previously.** Metabolites of the antihypertensive methyldopa (Aldomet) may turn black on contact with bleach (which is often present in toilet bowls). **Phenytoin (Dilantin) and the statins (Lipitor, Lescol, Mevacor, Pravachol, and Zocor) are also potential causative agents.**

✅ **Contamination with povidone-iodine (Betadine)** solution or douche can turn urine brown.

✅ **Melanin and melanogen, found in the urine of patients with melanoma**, will darken standing urine from the air-exposed surface downward.

What Not to Do

ⓧ Do not allow the patient to alter the urine factitiously. Have someone observe urine collection and inspect the specimen at once.

ⓧ Do not let a urine dipstick sit too long in the sample (allowing chemical indicators to diffuse out) or hold the dipstick vertically (allowing chemicals to drip from one pad to another and interfere with reagents).

ⓧ Do not be misled by dye in urine interfering with dipstick indicators. Pyridium can make a dipstick appear falsely positive for bilirubin, while contamination with hypochlorite bleach can cause a false-positive test for hemoglobin. In addition, the urobilinogen dipstick test is not adequate for diagnosing porphyria.

Discussion

Porphyrins or eosin dyes fluoresce under ultraviolet light. Eosin turns urine pink or red but fluoresces green.

Automobile radiator antifreeze contains fluorescein, to help locate leaks with ultraviolet light. Because this dye is excreted in the urine, green fluorescence can be a clue to ethylene glycol poisoning.

Suggested Readings

Baran, R. B., & Rowles, B. (1973). Factors affecting coloration of urine and feces. *Journal of the American Pharmacy Association, 13*, 139–142.

Carpenito, G., & Kurtz, I. (2002). Green urine in a critically ill patient. *American Journal of Kidney Disease, 39*, e20.

Seak, C. K., Lin, C. C., Seak, C. J., et al. (2010). A case of black urine and dark skin—cresol poisoning. *Clinical Toxicology (Philadelphia), 48*, 959–960.

Shah, U. H., Ngoc, H., & Gupta, S. (2020). Milky white urine after relief of urinary retention. *Journal of Emergency Medicine, 58*(3), e149–e152.

Su, H. K., Lee, F. N., Chen, B. A., et al. (2010). Purple urine bag syndrome. *Emergency Medicine Journal, 27*, 714.

Vallejo-Manzur, F., Mireles-Cabodevila, E., & Varon, J. (2005). Purple urine bag syndrome. *American Journal of Emergency Medicine, 23*, 521–524.

Epididymitis

Presentation

A male child, adolescent, or adult complains of dull to moderately severe unilateral scrotal pain developing gradually over a period of hours to days and possibly radiating to the ipsilateral lower abdomen or flank. In adult or adolescent males, there may be a history of recent urinary tract infection, urethritis, prostatitis, or prostatectomy (allowing ingress of bacteria), strain from lifting a heavy object, or sexual activity with a full bladder (allowing reflux of urine). Foley catheter drainage, intermittent catheterization, and other forms of urinary tract instrumentation predispose to infection and epididymitis. Drugs, such as amiodarone, also may cause epididymitis (chemical epididymitis), which affects the head of the epididymis only. There may be fever or urinary urgency or frequency. Nausea is unusual.

The epididymis (located posterolateral to the testis) is tender, swollen, warm, and difficult to separate from the firm, nontender testicle. Over time, increasing inflammation can extend up the spermatic cord and fill the entire scrotum, making examinations more difficult, with testicular tenderness, as well as producing frank prostatitis or cystitis. The rectal examination therefore may reveal a very tender, boggy prostate.

What to Do:

✓ **The first priority is to rule out the possibility of testicular torsion.** Key details to elicit on initial history include the onset and duration of the symptoms, including any previous such episodes. Testis torsion typically begins suddenly over a matter of minutes with intense pain, whereas epididymitis typically has a more gradual onset over a period of hours to days with more moderate pain. Associated symptoms, such as nausea and vomiting, seem to be more specific for torsion, whereas dysuria, urgency, and frequency point to an infectious or inflammatory cause, such as epididymitis.

✓ **The age of the patient may also be helpful in the diagnosis** because testis torsion has a bimodal distribution, with peak incidence in early childhood and preadolescence. The incidence of acute epididymitis increases sharply during adolescence, correlating with increased sexual activity.

✓ **The scrotum and its contents should be inspected and palpated.** Patients with epididymitis typically appear more comfortable than those with torsion. The position, axis, and lie of the testis should all be documented. A torsed testis is typically enlarged (because of venous congestion) and lies high within the scrotum and may have rotated transversely, giving its axis a more horizontal appearance (Fig. 79.1). Conversely, the testis has a normal lie and axis in acute epididymitis. **After 24 hours, the scrotal appearance of testicular torsion may be identical to that of epididymitis.**

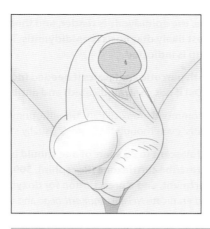

Fig. 79.1. The acute scrotum with testicular torsion. Note the horizontal lie and elevated position of the right testis. (Adapted from Rosenstein, D., & McAninch, J. W. [2004]. Urologic emergencies. *Medical Clinics of North America, 88,* 495–518.)

✓ **Before palpation of the testicles, the cremasteric reflex should be assessed,** beginning with the unaffected side. This reflex is elicited by lightly stroking the superomedial aspect of the thigh, causing brisk testicular retraction. **Absence of the cremasteric reflex is highly sensitive for testis torsion.**

✓ The testis and spermatic cord should next be gently palpated. A torsed testis is diffusely tender, whereas in acute epididymitis, the pain may be localized to the head of the epididymis and the superior pole of the testis.

✓ **Laboratory evaluation in acute scrotal pain should include obtaining a midstream urinalysis, Gram stain, and urine culture.** Presence of pyuria or bacteriuria suggests epididymitis but does not confirm the diagnosis or rule out testicular torsion.

✓ **All patients suspected of epididymitis** should have an appropriate specimen analyzed **for gonococcal and chlamydial urethritis.** Culture, nucleic acid hybridization tests, and nucleic acid amplification tests (NAATs) are available. Culture and nucleic acid hybridization tests require a urethral swab, whereas NAATs can be performed on a urine sample (which is the preferred modality).

✓ **If the clinical diagnosis strongly suggests testis torsion, there should be no delay in obtaining further testing. Urologic consultation should be obtained immediately to provide expeditious surgical exploration.** Cooling of the affected testicle with an ice pack while awaiting surgery may decrease the ischemic insult. **Manual reduction of a torsed testis can be attempted with or without narcotic analgesia.** Successful detorsion alleviates acute symptoms and may obviate emergent exploration; however, it is not a definitive treatment. Testes usually, but not always, torse in an inward direction. Manual detorsion should proceed with turning the testicle in an outward direction (as in "opening a book") or in the direction that the clinician would supinate the hands when approaching the patient from the feet. With successful detorsion, there will be release and elongation of the cord, followed by a marked diminution in symptoms. If pain increases or the spermatic cord shortens, stop and attempt the maneuver in the reverse direction. **As mentioned, successful manual reduction is not a definitive treatment and should soon be followed by elective orchidopexy.**

✅ **If the testis has a normal lie, the epididymis is tender, and there is a positive cremasteric reflex, then the most likely diagnosis is epididymitis. Testicular torsion is doubtful, and no further workup is indicated.**

✅ **Patients may be treated with narcotic analgesics if needed (nonsteroidal antiinflammatory drugs [NSAIDs] if not contraindicated) and antibiotics.**

✅ Most pediatric urologists recommend amoxicillin or trimethoprim–sulfamethoxazole for the prepubertal male with epididymitis, even though the urine is usually sterile.

✅ **The sexually active male adolescent to 35 years of age should be treated for a presumed sexually transmitted disease. Prescribe ceftriaxone (Rocephin), 500 mg intramuscularly (IM), in the clinic or emergency department, and a prescription for doxycycline (Vibramycin), 100 mg twice daily for 7 days,** should eradicate *Neisseria gonorrhoeae* and *Chlamydia trachomatis*. An alternative treatment is a single 240mg IM dose of gentamicin with a single 2g oral dose of azithromycin. (Counsel the patient that they may experience nausea, vomiting, or diarrhea with this dose of azithromycin.)

✅ **Sexually active males who perform insertive anal intercourse should be treated for chlamydia, gonorrhea, and enteric organisms with ceftriaxone, 500 mg IM for one dose, followed by levofloxacin (Levaquin), 500 mg once daily for 10 days, or ofloxacin, 300 mg twice daily for 10 days.**

✅ **In men older than 35 years of age who have suspected epididymitis from enteric organisms, use levofloxacin (Levaquin), 500 mg once daily for 10 days, or ofloxacin, 300 mg twice daily for 10 days.**

✅ Epididymitis secondary to chronic use of amiodarone responds only to discontinuation or reduction of dosage.

✅ **Arrange for 2 to 3 days of strict bed rest with the scrotum elevated.** The patient should use an athletic supporter when up, soak in warm tub baths, and obtain urologic follow-up within several days. For the first 72 hours, cool packs may be helpful.

✅ **Always warn patients or parents of the possibility of intermittent torsion and the need to return immediately if severe or worsening pain develops.**

✅ All prepubertal males with confirmed epididymitis should have close follow-up and consideration for referral to a pediatric urologist because of the high incidence of an underlying anatomic abnormality.

✅ **If there is any doubt about the diagnosis because of an atypical history and/or indistinct physical findings, perform an emergent testicular color Doppler ultrasound study. Epididymitis will show a normal or increased blood flow to the testis and epididymis, whereas torsion will show low or no flow.**

✅ **One needs to keep in mind that the testicle may spontaneously detorse before ultrasonography is performed, yielding a normal study or one with postischemic increased flow in a patient still at risk for further episodes of torsion. When the study is nondiagnostic, urologic consultation is required.** Unless you are absolutely certain that your patient does not have testicular torsion, you must insist that the urologist see him as soon as possible.

✓ If the patient is toxic and febrile, have the patient admitted, give antibiotics intravenously, and suspect testicular and/or epididymal abscess.

What Not to Do:

✗ Do not miss testicular torsion. It is far better to have the urologist explore the scrotum and find epididymitis than to delay and lose a testicle to ischemia (which can happen in only 4–6 hours). Half of symptomatic males describe previous similar transient episodes of scrotal pain, consistent with intermittent torsion/detorsion. When torsion is strongly suspected, do not delay the management of the case by waiting for the results of ancillary tests.

✗ Do not perform an incomplete manual detorsion of a testicle with a twist greater than or equal to 720 degrees. Partial detorsion may relieve symptoms and improve the examination but not relieve the ischemia. Continue to rotate the testicle one to three turns until the patient is pain free with a normal testicular lie.

✗ Do not overlook the testicular examination in any male with abdominal pain. In some instances of testicular torsion, a gradual onset of testicular and abdominal pain is the primary complaint.

✗ Do not rely on white blood cell counts and urinalysis to help make the diagnosis of acute epididymitis. Although a urinalysis should be performed in all patients with suspected epididymitis, most patients with epididymitis have normal urinalysis.

Discussion

Epididymitis is the most common cause of acute scrotum in adolescent boys and adults. Sexually transmitted *C. trachomatis* and *N. gonorrhoeae* are common pathogens in men younger than 35 years. In prepubertal boys and men older than 35 years of age, the disease is most frequently caused by *Escherichia coli* and *Proteus mirabilis*.

Prehn described the clinical differentiation of scrotal pain associated with epididymitis and acute torsion. Pain is relieved when the affected hemiscrotum is elevated in epididymitis. The elevation takes the weight of the testis off the epididymal suspension **(a positive Prehn sign). A positive Prehn's sign supports the diagnosis of epididymitis, but it is unreliable in differentiaitng between torsion and epididymitis.**

Epididymitis first affects the tail of the epididymis and then spreads to involve its body and head. Orchitis develops in 20% to 40% of cases by direct spread of infection, thereby leading to testicular swelling and tenderness (epididymo-orchitis) similar to that seen with testicular torsion.

Unlike testicular torsion, torsion of an appendage testis is a self-resolving, benign process and is usually much less painful than epididymitis or testicular torsion, but it is often confused with these two entities. Although appendices can be found on the testicle, epididymis, or spermatic cord, it is usually the appendix found on the testicle (appendix testis) that is prone to torsion.

The most important aspect of the physical examination is pain and tenderness localized to the region of the appendix testis (usually superior lateral testis). Every attempt should be made to have the patient localize the pain. If only a part of the testis is tender, testicular torsion is doubtful. If the epididymis is not tender, epididymitis is also doubtful. The classic "blue dot sign" of an infarcted appendage may be seen through thin scrotal skin if there is a minimal amount of edema and erythema. These cases are managed conservatively, with attention given to pain management. The pain usually resolves in 2 to 3 days with atrophy of the appendix that may eventually calcify. **The role of sonographic examination in torsion of the testicular appendages is to exclude torsion of the entire testicle.**

Testicular torsion causes venous engorgement that results in edema, hemorrhage, and subsequent arterial compromise, which results in testicular

Discussion continued

ischemia. The extent of testicular ischemia depends on the degree of torsion, which ranges from 180 degrees to 720 degrees or more. **Experimental studies indicate that 720-degree torsion is required to occlude the testicular artery. When torsion is 180 degrees or less, diminished flow is seen.** The testicular salvage rate depends on the degree of torsion and the duration of ischemia. A nearly 100% salvage rate exists within the first 6 hours after onset of symptoms, a 70% rate within 6 to 12 hours, and a 20% rate within 12 to 24 hours.

The role of color Doppler and power Doppler sonography in the diagnosis of acute testicular torsion is well established. Torsion may be complete, incomplete, or transient. Cases that show partial or transient torsion present a diagnostic challenge. The ability of color Doppler imaging to diagnose incomplete torsion accurately remains undetermined. The presence of a color or power Doppler signal in a patient with the clinical presentation of torsion does not exclude torsion. **Testicular imaging studies have a 10% to 15% false-negative rate.**

Because of overlapping symptoms, historical findings may be of little use in differentiating epididymitis, testicular torsion, and torsion appendix testis. Physical examination findings are helpful. Patients with testicular torsion are much more likely to have a tender testicle, an abnormal testicular lie, and/or an absent cremasteric reflex when compared with patients with epididymitis. **The presence of the cremasteric reflex is the most valuable clinical finding in ruling out testicular torsion. Color Doppler ultrasonography is extremely helpful in diagnosing the etiology of an acute scrotum, although, at times, diagnostic surgical exploration will be required for making a definitive diagnosis.**

Chronic epididymitis (symptoms >6 weeks) may be associated with granulomatous disease such as tuberculosis and a broad range of noninfectious conditions such as cancer and autoimmune diseases. This requires referral to a urologist for evaluation and management.

Suggested Readings

Beni-Israel, T., Goldman, M., Bar Chaim, S., & Kozer, E. (2010). Clinical predictors for testicular torsion as seen in the pediatric. *American Journal of Emergency Medicine, 28,* 786–789.

Caldamone, A. A., Valvo, J. R., Altebarmakian, V. K., et al. (1984). Acute scrotal swelling in children. *Journal of Pediatric Surgery, 19,* 581–584.

Centers for Disease Control and Prevention. (2010). Sexually transmitted diseases treatment guidelines 2010 *Morbidity and Mortality Weekly Report* (Vol. 59. , 1–110. http://www.cdc.gov/std/treatment/2010/STD-Treatment-2010-RR5912.pdf. RR–12.

Elsevier Point of Care. (2020). *Epididymitis.* Amsterdam, Netherlands: Elsevier BV.

Kadish, H. (2002). The tender scrotum. *Clinics in Pediatric Emergency Medicine, 3,* 55–61.

Kadish, H. A., & Bolte, R. G. (1998). A retrospective review of pediatric patients with epididymitis, testicular torsion, and torsion of testicular appendages. *Pediatrics, 102,* 73–76.

Knight, P. J., & Vassy, L. E. (1984). The diagnosis and treatment of the acute scrotum in children and adolescents. *Annals of Surgery, 200,* 664–673.

Liguori, G., Bucci, S., Zordani, A., et al. (2011). Role of US in acute scrotal pain. *World Journal of Urology, 29,* 639–643.

Rosenstein, D., & McAninch, J. W. (2004). Urologic emergencies. *Medical Clinics of North America, 88,* 495–518.

Wan, J., & Bloom, D. A. (2003). Genitourinary problems in adolescent males. *Adolescent Medicine, 14,* 717–731.

Yang, C., Jr., Song, B., Liu, X., et al. (2011). Acute scrotum in children: An 18-year retrospective study. *Pediatric Emergency Care, 27,* 270–274.

Genital Herpes Simplex

Presentation

The patient may be distraught with severe genital pain, with subsequent outbreak of painful vesicles on the external genitalia that may ulcerate or erode. Alternatively, the patient may just be concerned about paresthesias and subtle genital lesions, may want pain relief during a recurrence, or may be suffering complications such as superinfection or urinary retention. Often, with primary infection, there are associated systemic symptoms such as fever, malaise, myalgias, and headache.

Instead of the classic grouped vesicles on an erythematous base, herpes in the genitals usually appears as groupings of ulcers (2–3 mm in size), representing the bases of abraded vesicles (Figs. 80.1, 80.2, and 80.3). Resolving lesions are also less likely to crust on the genitals. Lesions can be tender and should be examined with gloves on because they shed infectious viral particles. Inguinal lymph nodes may be painful, are usually involved bilaterally, and are not confluent.

What to Do

⊘ Attempt to make a more definitive diagnosis by collecting a specimen from an active lesion.

⊘ **Cell culture and polymerase chain reaction (PCR) are the preferred herpes simplex virus (HSV) tests.** The sensitivity of viral culture is low, especially for recurrent lesions, and declines rapidly as lesions begin to heal. Nucleic acid amplification methods, including PCR assays for HSV deoxyribonucleic acid (DNA), are more sensitive and are increasingly available. Viral culture isolates and PCR amplicons should be typed to determine which type of HSV is causing the infection. Failure to detect HSV by culture or PCR, especially in the absence of active lesions, does not indicate an absence of HSV infection because viral shedding is intermittent. Cytologic detection of cellular changes associated with HSV infection is an insensitive and nonspecific method of diagnosing genital lesions (i.e., Tzanck preparation) and therefore is not reliable. Although a direct immunofluorescence (IF) assay using fluorescein-labeled monoclonal antibodies is also available to detect HSV antigen from genital specimens, this assay lacks sensitivity.

⊘ Strongly consider testing for coinfections such as chlamydia, gonorrhea, syphilis, and human immunodeficiency virus (HIV).

⊘ **For the immunocompetent patient, prescribe acyclovir (Zovirax), 400 mg three times a day for 7 to 10 days. Alternative treatment regimens include famciclovir (Famvir), 250 mg three times a day for 7 to 10 days, and valacyclovir (Valtrex), 1000 mg twice daily for 7 to 10 days.**

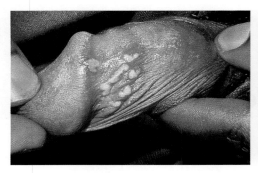

Fig. 80.1 Herpes genitalis in a male patient. (Adapted from White, G. M., & Cox, N. H. [2006]. *Diseases of the skin* [2nd ed.]. St. Louis, MO: Mosby.)

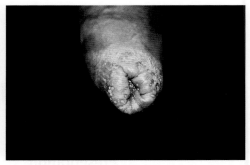

Fig. 80.2 Primary genital herpes in a male patient. (Adapted from Bolognia, J., Jorizzo, J., & Rapini, R. [2003]. *Dermatology.* St. Louis, MO: Mosby.)

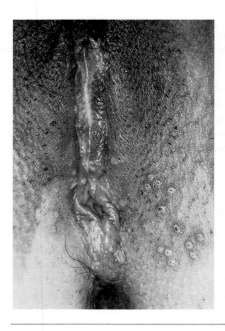

Fig. 80.3 Primary genital herpes in a female patient. (Adapted from Bolognia, J., Jorizzo, J., & Rapini, R. [2003]. *Dermatology.* St. Louis, MO: Mosby.)

◯ **For recurrent infections, prescribe any of the following choices: acyclovir, 400 mg three times a day for 5 days, or 800 mg twice daily for 5 days, or 800 mg three times a day for 2 days; famciclovir, 1000 mg twice daily for 1 day; or valacyclovir, 1000 mg daily for 5 days.**

◯ **With pain**, if there are no contraindications, prescribe adequate antiinflammatory or narcotic analgesics for pain. Try cool compresses and sitz baths for additional comfort.

◯ **Warn the patient of the following:**

　　◯ Lesions and pain can be expected to last 2 to 3 weeks during the initial attack (usually less in recurrences).

○ Although acyclovir reduces viral shedding, patients should assume they are contagious whenever there are open lesions (and can potentially transmit the virus at other times as well). Men with HSV infection should be counseled and advised to use barrier contraceptive methods during intercourse.

○ The patient should be careful about touching lesions and washing hands, because other skin can be inoculated.

○ Recurrences can be triggered by any sort of local or systemic stress and will not be helped by topical acyclovir.

○ **Suppressive therapy should be considered for patients who have more than four to six episodes per year or to reduce transmission in couples where one partner is HSV-2 positive.** This therapy can reduce the frequency of recurrences by 70% to 80%. Prescribe acyclovir, 400 mg twice daily; famciclovir, 250 mg twice daily; or valacyclovir, 500 mg to 1 g once. Because the number of recurrences decreases over time, it is wise to discuss discontinuation of suppressive therapy annually with patients.

What Not to Do

🚫 Do not confuse these lesions with the painless, raised genital ulcer of syphilis or the erosive lesions of Stevens-Johnson syndrome, which will also involve at least one other mucous membrane, such as oral mucosa, pharynx, larynx, lips, or conjunctiva.

🚫 Do not delay starting treatment pending culture results. Treatment is more effective if started earlier in the course of the infection.

Discussion

Genital herpes is a sexually transmitted disease caused by the human herpesviruses HSV-1 and HSV-2. Infection is transmitted by direct contact with infected mucosa or secretions, and the incubation period averages 4 days (range, 2–12 days). Infection is spread by vaginal, anal, or oral sex with someone who has the disease. Most people with the infection have no or mild symptoms. The peak incidence of primary infection occurs in young sexually active adults. Antiviral treatment should be offered for primary or recurrent infections to reduce the active period of viral shedding and symptoms.

In men, painful vesicular lesions occur on the penile shaft, glans, and prepuce. Men who practice receptive anal intercourse can develop HSV proctitis with pain, tenesmus, and rectal discharge. In women, painful vesicular lesions on an erythematous base, often bilateral, may be seen on labia, vulva, perineum, perianal areas, or internal genitalia. Bilateral, tender, inguinal adenopathy is more common with primary HSV episodes than with recurrences.

The natural history of herpetic vesicles involves stages of ulceration, crust formation, and resolution over a period of 1 to 2 weeks (sometimes longer in primary infection). Latent infection is established in dorsal root ganglia indefinitely, and recurrent infection is common. Within 12 months of the initial HSV-2 episode, 90% of patients have had at least one recurrence, and approximately 40% have had six or more recurrences. Fortunately, recurrences tend to decrease over time. These infections are generally milder in terms of duration, extent of lesions, and pain and may be associated with a prodrome of itching or burning pain. There is no cure for genital herpes.

HSV-1 commonly affects mouth, gums, and lips but can also cause anogenital infection. HSV-2 commonly affects the anogenital region but can also cause oral infection. HSV-2 is the cause of approximately 80% of genital ulcer disease in the United States. Diagnosis of herpes infection can be made largely on clinical grounds with a typical history and physical

(continued)

Discussion continued

examination, although typical symptoms and signs are absent in many infected patients.

Serologic testing is generally not recommended for primary diagnosis, but type-specific serologic testing for HSV may be useful for a definitive diagnosis in patients who have symptomatic disease in the healing stages or in recurrent infections when cultures of lesions are less likely to yield the virus. Also, in some cases, HSV serotyping may influence prognosis, treatment, and counseling. The Centers for Disease Control and Prevention (CDC) recommends glycoprotein G tests, which have a high sensitivity (80–98%) and specificity (>96%). Those tests include POCkit HSV-2 (Diagnology, Research Triangle Park, Durham, NC) and HerpeSelect-1 and 2 ELISA and HerpeSelect 1 and 2 Immunoblot (Focus Technologies, Cypress, CA).

All the acyclic nucleoside analogue antiviral agents (acyclovir, valacyclovir, famciclovir) are equally effective in the treatment of an acute first episode of genital herpes infection and in the episodic treatment of recurrent herpes. Acyclovir is the least expensive regimen but is less convenient and must be taken more often than valacyclovir and famciclovir.

Counseling is an important part of the management of genital herpes infection. Key points to make when counseling patients should include the potential for recurrences and the effectiveness of antiviral medication for the treatment of recurrences. Because HSV infection may initially be asymptomatic, a symptomatic episode does not necessarily mean that the patient's current partner is not monogamous. Patients should be counseled regarding the possibility of transmission during periods of asymptomatic viral shedding and the need to abstain from sexual activity with uninfected partners when lesions or prodromal symptoms are present. They should also be encouraged to use condoms. They should be advised that the risk for HSV transmission to an uninfected partner is not completely eliminated by taking these precautions and that genital ulcer disease increases the risk for transmission of HIV.

The diagnosis of genital herpes can be emotionally devastating to a young man or woman who is infected. Although it is advisable for patients to inform future sexual partners about their infection, it is also understandable that discussing this with a future partner can be difficult. It is very important for the physician caring for these patients to provide appropriate nonjudgmental psychological as well as medical support.

Currently, there is no role for topical acyclovir in the treatment of genital herpes.

Suggested Readings

Benedetti, J., Corel, L., & Ashley, R. (1994). Recurrence rates in genital herpes after symptomatic first-episode infection. *Annals of Internal Medicine, 121,* 847–854.

Centers for Disease Control and Prevention. (n.d.). Genital herpes—STD information from CDC. https://www.cdc.gov/std/Herpes/

Centers for Disease Control and Prevention. (2010). Sexually transmitted diseases treatment guidelines, 2010. *Morbidity and Mortality Weekly Report, 59*(RR-12), 1–110. http://www.cdc.gov/std/treatment/2010/STD-Treatment-2010-RR5912.pdf

Diaz-Mitoma, F., Sibbald, G., Shafran, S. D., et al. (1998). Oral famciclovir for the recurrent suppression of recurrent genital herpes. *Journal of the American Medical Association, 280,* 887–892.

Elsevier Point of Care. (2020). *Genital herpes infection.* Amsterdam, Netherlands: Elsevier BV.

Kodner, C. (2003). Sexually transmitted infections in men. *Primary Care, 30,* 173–191.

Merin, A., & Pachankis, J. E. (2011). The psychological impact of genital herpes stigma (review). *Journal of Health Psychology, 16,* 80–90. Epub.

Rimsza, M. E. (2005). Sexually transmitted infections: New guidelines for an old problem on the college campus. *Pediatric Clinics of North America, 52,* 217–228.

Warren, T., & Ebel, C. (2005). Counseling the patient who has genital herpes or genital human papillomavirus infection. *Infectious Disease Clinics of North America, 19,* 459–476.

Phimosis and Paraphimosis

Presentation

Phimosis is the inability to retract the foreskin over the glans and is usually the result of a contracted preputial opening (Fig. 81.1). Patients with phimosis may seek acute medical care when they develop signs and symptoms of infection, such as pain and swelling of the foreskin and a purulent discharge. Pediatric patients with acute phimosis are either fussy or complain of penile pain over hours to days. Children also may develop hematuria or urinary retention because of obstruction or dysuria. On physical examination, the physician discovers a tender foreskin that is not easily retracted.

Paraphimosis occurs when a tight foreskin cannot be replaced into its normal position after it is retracted behind the glans. The tight ring of preputial skin (phimotic ring), which is caught behind the glans, creates a venous and lymphatic tourniquet that leads to edematous swelling of the foreskin and glans. It usually presents as a swollen tender penis with a large ventral penile-skin bulge and multiple folds just under the glans (Figs. 81.2 and 81.3).

What to Do

✅ **When either of these conditions becomes painful,** provide adequate analgesia with oral or parenteral medication. **A penile nerve block may be required.** Using a 30-gauge needle, inject 1% lidocaine (Xylocaine) approximately 1 cm distal to the base of the penis, where it exits beneath the pubic arch at the 10-o'clock and 2-o'clock positions of the dorsum of the penis. Use caution not to inject intravascularly. If this does not provide adequate anesthesia, a ring block can be performed around the entire circumference of the base of the penis.

✅ **For paraphimosis, squeeze the glans firmly for at least 10 minutes to reduce the edematous swelling.** Wrap the shaft and swollen glans with a gauze pad followed by a 2-inch elastic bandage to produce constant, gentle compression. **After 10 to 15 minutes, remove the bandage, push the glans proximally, and slide the prepuce back over the glans** (Fig. 81.4). An alternative approach for reducing the swelling is to apply an ice-filled surgical glove for 5 minutes.

✅ **If manual reduction fails and the penis does not regain its normal uncircumcised appearance, anesthetize the dorsal foreskin and carefully grasp the foreskin with nonserrated clamps and pull it over the glans penis. If this is unsuccessful, crush the dorsal foreskin with a straight hemostat along the midline and then make a linear incision through this crushed skin track. This incision will relieve the constricting band.** The foreskin is then repositioned over the glans and, when possible, sutured in place. **Paraphimosis is a medical emergency;** failure to reduce the foreskin can lead to preputial necrosis and gangrene.

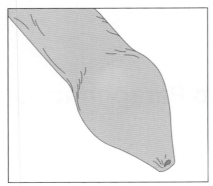

Fig. 81.1 Phimosis.

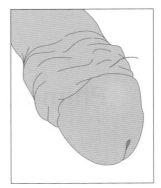

Fig. 81.2 Paraphimosis.

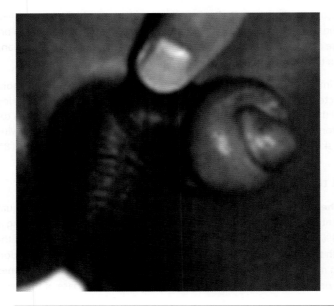

Fig. 81.3 Paraphimosis. (Adapted from McGrath, N., Howell, J. M., & Davis, J. E. [2011]. Pediatric genitourinary emergencies. *Emergency Medicine Clinics of North America, 29*, 655–666.)

✅ **If the phimosis patient has secondary urinary obstruction, catheterize the urethra with a small-gauge catheter. If you cannot find the urethral meatus, try using a small nasal speculum or hemostat to widen the opening or anesthetize the dorsal foreskin, and carefully incise the constricting tissue with a vertical incision (dorsal slit) to allow retraction.**

✅ **Treating phimosis usually involves the management of acute infection.** Frequent hot compresses or soaks are needed, along with antibiotics. Topical antibiotics, such as mupirocin (Bactroban), may be adequate when poor hygiene leads to infection in the pediatric patient. Sexually transmitted diseases should be suspected and treated appropriately in adolescents and

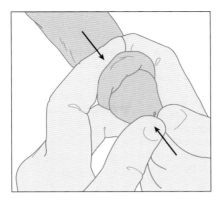

Fig. 81.4 Manual reduction of paraphimosis by counterpressure between thumbs and fingers.

adults (see Chapter 83). Candidal infections, with their typical white cheesy exudate, are often associated with diabetes mellitus and can be treated with a single dose of fluconazole (Diflucan), 200 mg by mouth.

✓ **When infection is not a problem, phimosis can be successfully treated with a steroid cream** (1% hydrocortisone, 0.1% triamcinolone, or 0.05% betamethasone), **four times daily, with a gentle stretch on the foreskin for 2 to 6 weeks.** Successful treatment response may be seen up to 12 weeks. After the phimosis resolves, the foreskin should be retracted daily to prevent recurrence.

✓ **Be aware that it is common for young children to have a physiologic phimosis that usually resolves by the age of 5 years. It is important to distinguish between a physiologic and a pathologic phimosis when evaluating the pediatric patient.** Physiologic phimosis can be distinguished by the absence of meatal scarring, infection, and pouting or flowering of the distal foreskin with retraction.

✓ Instruct parents in the technique and importance of proper cleaning of their son's prepuce. Always thoroughly clean the area but do not forcibly retract the foreskin for cleaning, which can lead to tears and scarring. Only clean under the foreskin when it has demonstrated the ability to retract. Have parents place the child in a tub of warm water to alleviate dysuria.

✓ **In both paraphimosis and phimosis, follow-up care should be provided. When swelling and inflammation subside, circumcision should be considered.**

What Not to Do

✗ Do not confuse paraphimosis with, or overlook, a circumferential foreign body (such as a hair tourniquet or rubber band).

✗ Do not attempt forced retraction when treating phimosis. Forceful retraction causes future adhesions and strictures.

✗ Do not obtain unnecessary studies. Diagnosis is made by history and physical examination, although a radiograph or ultrasound may be useful if a constricting foreign body is suspected.

Discussion

Poor hygiene and chronic inflammation are the usual causes of stenosing fibrosis of the preputial opening. It can be normal for boys up to 5 years of age not to be able to retract the foreskin completely. Repeated inflammation, even through tension on a minimally restrictive aperture from normal erections, may exacerbate the fibrosis and lead to phimosis. Vitamin E cream and topical steroid ointments may help soften a phimotic ring. When phimosis results in acute urinary retention, the tip of a hemostat can be inserted into the scarred end of the foreskin and gently opened, allowing the patient to void satisfactorily until urologic consultation can be obtained.

In the case of neglected paraphimosis, arterial occlusion may supervene, and ischemia, skin necrosis, and, eventually, gangrene of the glans develop. One common iatrogenic cause of paraphimosis is negligence in reducing the foreskin after retracting it to clean the glans and insert a Foley catheter.

Suggested Readings

Chamberlin, J. D., Dorgalli, A., Abdelhalim, C. A., Davis-Doa, C. L., Chalmers, M. S., Kelly, Z. T., ... Khoury, A. E. (2019). Randomized open-label trial comparing topical prescription triamcinolone to over-the-counter hydrocortisone for the treatment of phimosis. *Journal of Pediatric Urology, 15*(4), 388 e1–e5.

Elsevier Point of Care. (2018). *Phimosis.* Amsterdam, Netherlands: Elsevier BV.

Mackway-Jones, K., & Teece, S. (2004). Best evidence topic reports: Ice, pins, or sugar to reduce paraphimosis. *Emergency Medicine Journal, 21,* 77–78.

McGrath, N., Howell, J. M., & Davis, J. E. (2011). Pediatric genitourinary emergencies. *Emergency Medicine Clinics of North America, 29,* 655–666.

Tanaka, S., & Brock, J. W., III. (2011). Pediatric urologic conditions, including urinary infections. *Medical Clinics of North America, 95,* 1–13.

Wan, J., & Bloom, D. A. (2003). Genitourinary problems in adolescent males. *Adolescent Medicine, 14,* 717–731, viii.

Prostatitis, Acute Bacterial

Presentation

A man complains of acute onset of malaise, fever, chills, and perineal, rectal, or low back pain. He also may have dysuria, urinary urgency and frequency, and signs of obstruction to urinary flow, ranging from a weak stream to urinary retention. There may be painful ejaculation and hematospermia. On gentle examination, the prostate is swollen, hot, and exquisitely tender. The infection may spread from or into the contiguous urogenital tract (epididymis, bladder, urethra) or the bloodstream.

Patients with chronic bacterial prostatitis will have similar recurrent symptoms without fever and with a more normal but possibly tender prostate.

What to Do

✅ **Perform a rectal examination and, only once, gently palpate the prostate to see if it is tender, swollen, edematous, warm, fluctuant, or boggy.**

✅ For patients who appear to be toxic with systemic symptoms, consider hospital admission for intravenous (IV) antimicrobials. An aminoglycoside and β-lactam combination or a fluoroquinolone may be administered, along with IV hydration. Gentamicin (Garamycin), 1 to 1.5 mg/kg IV three times a day can be added. Alternatively, give levofloxacin (Levaquin), 750 mg IV once daily, or ciprofloxacin, 400 mg IV twice daily.

✅ Men younger than 35 years of age, men who have sex with men, and men who engage in high-risk sexual behaviors should be presumptively treated for sexually transmitted infections (STIs) to cover both *Neisseria gonorrhoeae and Chlamydia trachomatis* (see Chapter 83).

✅ **Evaluate and treat for possible associated urinary retention** (see Chapter 84). In severe cases, a suprapubic catheter may be preferable to a Foley catheter for bladder decompression and urinary drainage because it avoids trauma to the prostate with resulting pain and hematogenous spread of infection.

✅ **Culture the urine** to help identify the organism responsible. (This will usually identify the organism involved in acute bacterial prostatitis.) **Test for STIs,** such as gonorrhea or chlamydia, with a nucleic acid amplification test.

✅ **For the nontoxic patient, empiric therapy should be started. Typical regimens include ciprofloxacin (500 mg by mouth twice a day) or levofloxacin (500 mg by mouth once a day) for 4 to 6 weeks. Alternatively, a less expensive regimen is trimethoprim-sulfamethoxazole (Bactrim DS) by mouth twice daily for 4 to 6 weeks. The long duration of treatment is necessary to penetrate deep prostatic tissues.**

For pain and fever, prescribe nonsteroidal antiinflammatory drugs (NSAIDs) if there are no contraindications. If the patient needs narcotics, add stool softeners to prevent constipation.

Arrange for urologic follow-up.

What Not to Do

Do not massage or repeatedly palpate the prostate. Rough treatment is unlikely to help drain the infection or produce the responsible organism in the urine but is likely to extend or worsen a bacterial prostatitis or to precipitate bacteremia, urosepsis, or septic shock.

Discussion

Prostatitis is a common condition in men that encompasses a spectrum of disease ranging from acute infection of the prostate requiring immediate antibiotic therapy (acute bacterial prostatitis) to subacute recurrent infection of the prostate (chronic bacterial prostatitis) to nonbacterial chronic prostatic inflammation and pelvic pain syndromes. Immediate treatment is required for acute bacterial prostatitis associated with signs of sepsis, prostatic abscess, or acute urinary retention.

Risk factors for acute bacterial prostatitis include chronic indwelling urinary catheters, diabetes, cirrhosis, immunosuppression, and intermittent urinary self-catheterization.

Acute and chronic bacterial prostatitis is treated with empiric antibiotic therapy (e.g., oral fluoroquinolone or sulfamethoxazole-trimethoprim, IV ampicillin plus gentamicin), which is tailored to culture and sensitivity results once available.

For the treatment of bacterial prostatitis, only trimethoprim and the fluoroquinolones possess both the appropriate bactericidal activity and the ability to diffuse into the prostate. Levofloxacin shows particularly good penetration into prostatic tissue.

Blood in the ejaculate or painful ejaculation may cause a patient to come to an acute care facility. These symptoms may be a sign of inflammation in the prostate and epididymis or, especially in younger males, may simply be a self-limiting sequela of vigorous sexual activity.

The diagnosis of acute prostatitis largely relies on clinical signs and symptoms and a limited number of laboratory findings. Prostate-specific antigen (PSA) levels may be elevated in both acute and chronic bacterial prostatitis but need not be obtained on initial evaluation. Men who present with an elevated PSA level and findings of prostatitis should be given a course of antibiotics followed by a repeat PSA measurement before any biopsy is performed.

Suggested Readings

David, R. D., DeBlieux, P. M. C., & Press, R. (2005). Rational antibiotic treatment of outpatient genitourinary infections in a changing environment. *The American Journal of Medicine, 118*(Suppl. 7A), 7S–13S.

Elsevier Point of Care. (2019). *Prostatitis*. Amsterdam, Netherlands: Elsevier BV.

Hua, V. N., & Schaeffer, A. J. (2004). Acute and chronic prostatitis. *Medical Clinics of North America, 88*, 483–494.

Krieger, J. N. (2003). Prostatitis revisited: New definitions, new approaches. *Infectious Disease Clinics of North America, 17*, 395–409.

Ramakrishnan, K., & Salinas, R. C. (2010). Prostatitis: Acute and chronic (review). *Primary Care, 37*, 547–563, viii–ix.

Sharp, V. J., Takacs, E. B., & Powell, C. R. (2010). Prostatitis: Diagnosis and treatment (review). *American Family Physician, 82*, 397–406.

Urethritis

(Drip, Clap)

Presentation

A man complains of dysuria, a burning discomfort along the urethra, pruritus of the urethral meatus, and/or a urethral discharge. A copious, thick yellow-green discharge that stains underwear is characteristic of gonorrhea, whereas a thinner mucopurulent or white scant discharge with milder symptoms is characteristic of *Chlamydia*. These symptoms may be transient.

Urethritis in a woman may be asymptomatic or indistinguishable from cystitis or vaginitis. It may manifest as urinary tract infection (UTI) symptoms with a low concentration of bacteria on urine culture or tenderness localized to the distal periurethral area of the anterior vaginal wall. Female patients may not be able to distinguish urethral discharge from vaginal discharge. In addition to increased vaginal discharge, women who develop cervicitis may have intermenstrual bleeding, especially postcoital spotting or dyspareunia and cervical friability.

What to Do

✓ **Obtain a sexual history** that includes number of contacts, gender of contacts, anal/ oral practices, and symptoms or illnesses in partners. Determine the color, consistency, and quantity of any discharge as well as any accompanying symptoms, such as genital or abdominal discomfort, dyspareunia, and dysuria.

✓ Examine the entire genital area for lesions, and check undergarments for discharge staining. Palpate testes and epididymides for any mass or tenderness, or, in the case of a female patient, perform a complete pelvic examination, looking for discharge and cervical motion tenderness. **Keep in mind the female patient can often be asymptomatic, and the absence of discharge does not rule out infection.**

✓ Have the male patient milk the ventral surface of his penis to produce any discharge at the urethral meatus. (If discharge is scant, this should be attempted 1 to 2 hours after last voiding.)

✓ **In men**, **nucleic acid amplification tests (NAATs)** are preferred for the detection of *C. trachomatis* and *Neisseria gonorrhoeae,* and urine is the preferred specimen.

✓ In addition to these tests or when NAATs are not available, obtain a Gram stain of any urethral discharge, looking for Gram-negative diplococci inside white cells, which indicate gonococcal infection. (Their absence does not rule out the possibility.) Urethritis in men is confirmed by any of the following:

- ○ The presence of mucopurulent or purulent discharge
- ○ Two or more white blood cells (WBCs) per oil-immersion field on a Gram stain of urethral secretions
- ○ Ten or more WBCs per high-power field on microscopic examination of first-void urine

○ Positive leukocyte esterase test on first-void urine

○ If point-of-care diagnostic tools (e.g., Gram, methylene blue [MB] or gentian violet [GV] stain microscopy, first-void urine with microscopy, and leukocyte esterase) are not available, drug regimens effective against both gonorrhea and chlamydia should be administered empirically.

✓ **In female patients, order a urine or blood test to rule out pregnancy.**

✓ **Examine the urine sediment for swimming protozoa, implying infection with *Trichomonas vaginalis* (Chapter 94), best treated with metronidazole (Flagyl), 2 g by mouth once or 500 mg twice daily for 7 days. Always warn the patient of the interaction between Flagyl and alcohol.**

✓ **Endocervical swabs from women and urethral swabs or urine specimens from men can be used to detect *C. trachomatis* and *N. gonorrhoeae* by using NAATs.** NAATs do not require viable organisms, they are substantially more sensitive than previous tests, and the same specimen can be used to test for both organisms. When obtaining a urine sample from men, it is important to obtain either a first-void urine (first in the morning) or, more realistically, a first-catch urine. This is the initial portion of the urinary stream (generally up to the first 20 mL), and it must be collected without precleaning the urethral meatus. For better sensitivity, there should be at least 1 hour after the previous micturition that day. **When a NAAT is not available or not economical, nucleic acid hybridization assays can be used to detect *C. trachomatis* or *N. gonorrhoeae*.** The Gen-Probe PACE 2 (Gen-Probe, San Diego, CA) and the Digene Hybrid Capture II (Gen-Probe) assays can detect both organisms in a single specimen. These tests are less sensitive than NAATs.

✓ **Cultures can be performed when transport and storage conditions are conducive to maintaining the viability of *N. gonorrhoeae* and *C. trachomatis*, especially when an isolate is needed (e.g., sexual abuse or treatment failure) and for monitoring of antimicrobial resistance.** Cultures for *N. gonorrhoeae* have a high sensitivity and specificity and low cost, whereas *C. trachomatis* cell cultures have a relatively low sensitivity at a relatively high cost.

✓ **Order a serologic test for established syphilis.** Further antibiotic treatment is required if the rapid plasma reagin (RPR) or Venereal Disease Research Laboratory (VDRL) test is positive.

✓ **Empirical treatment must be considered in ALL symptomatic patients whose behavior puts them at risk for sexually transmitted infections (STIs), those who may be lost to follow-up, and those who have a history of recent exposure to an infected partner, regardless of their symptoms.** Dual treatment of *C. trachomatis* and *N. gonorrhoeae* should be provided when an empirical treatment is instituted.

✓ **Dual treatment is indicated** for the initial management of urethritis or cervicitis unless a sensitive laboratory technology is used to rule out *C. trachomatis* and/or *N. gonorrhoeae*.

✓ **To treat *N. gonorrhoeae*, give ceftriaxone (Rocephin), 500 mg once intramuscularly (preferred treatment).**

✓ **To treat *C. trachomatis*, give doxycycline (Doryx), 100 mg by mouth twice daily for 7 days (preferred treatment), or consider giving azithromycin (Zithromax), 2 g once by mouth. (Azithromycin provides prophylaxis for syphilis.)**

✓ When ceftriaxone cannot be used for treating urogenital or rectal gonorrhea because of cephalosporin allergy, a single 240 mg IM dose of gentamicin plus a single 2 g oral dose of azithromycin is an option. Gastrointestinal symptoms, primarily vomiting within 1 hour of dosing, have been reported among 3%–4% of treated persons (26). If administration of IM ceftriaxone is not available, a single 800 mg oral dose of cefixime is an alternative regimen.

However, cefixime does not provide as high, or as sustained, bactericidal blood levels as does ceftriaxone and demonstrates limited treatment efficacy for pharyngeal gonorrhea.

✓ **Because of the changing patterns of antibiotic resistance, always check for the latest CDC antimicrobial guidelines for the treatment of all STIs.**

✓ Diagnosis and treatment of cervicitis in pregnant women does not differ from that in women who are not pregnant.

✓ To treat recurrent and persistent urethritis, give metronidazole (Flagyl), 2 g once by mouth, or tinidazole 2 g once orally, plus azithromycin, 2 g once orally. **Patients should be instructed to refrain from sexual intercourse until 7 days after therapy is completed.**

✓ **Treat sexual partners** of patients known or suspected to have a STI with the same antibiotic regimen. (Cultures may be omitted.) These patients should refer all sexual partners within the preceding 60 days for evaluation and treatment; a specific diagnosis may facilitate partner referral. In cases where gonococcal expedited partner therapy (provision of prescriptions or medications for the patient to take to a sex partner without the health care provider first examining the partner) is permissible by state law and the partner is unable or unlikely to seek timely treatment, the partner may be treated with a single 800 mg oral dose of cefixime, provided that concurrent chlamydial infection in the patient has been excluded. Otherwise, the partner may be treated with a single oral 800 mg cefixime dose plus oral doxycycline 100 mg twice daily for 7 days.

✓ Federal and state reporting regulations should be followed, with subsequent tracking of sexual contacts by state infection control boards.

✓ **Patients should be instructed to return if symptoms persist or recur.**

✓ **Test-of-cure is not recommended as a routine procedure** after therapy for *C. trachomatis* or *N. gonorrhoeae* infection with first-line Centers for Disease Control and Prevention (CDC)–recommended treatment regimens, however, for persons with pharyngeal gonorrhea, a test-of-cure is recommended, using culture or nucleic acid amplification tests 7–14 days after initial treatment, regardless of the treatment regimen.

✓ **Instruct the patient on the correct use of the condom to help prevent reinfection.**

What Not to Do

✗ Do not assume the dysuria is due to a simple UTI and treat inappropriately. When there are risk factors, be liberal with testing for STIs.

✗ Do not perform Gram-stain testing for *N. gonorrhoeae* infection among women. The sensitivity of endocervical specimens is lower than that of urethral specimens from men with symptomatic gonorrhea, and adequate specificity requires a skilled microscopist.

✗ Do not send off a serologic test for syphilis without following up on the results.

Discussion

Common causative organisms for urethritis and cervicitis are *N. gonorrhoeae* and *C. trachomatis*. *Ureaplasma urealyticum, Mycoplasma hominis, M. genitalium*, and *T. vaginalis* also are implicated in these clinical conditions. Although they are easily eradicated if treated early, some of these infections have been linked to serious reproductive health consequences, more systemic effects

(continued)

Discussion continued

such as disseminated gonococcal infections and Reiter syndrome, and facilitation of human immunodeficiency virus (HIV) transmission. *M. genitalium* accounts for 15% to 25% of nongonococcal urethritis (NGU) cases in the United States. However, US Food and Drug Administration (FDA)–cleared diagnostic tests for *M. genitalium* are not available.

N. gonorrhoeae, a gram-negative diplococcus, is a major cause of pelvic inflammatory disease (PID), ectopic pregnancy, and infertility. *C. trachomatis*, an obligate intracellular bacterium, is the most common sexually transmitted bacterial pathogen in the United States and worldwide and is a leading cause of PID. The prevalence of both infections is higher among ethnic minorities and the poor. Age-specific rates are highest among girls and women 15 to 24 years of age and men 20 to 24 years of age. Both *ureaplasma* and *mycoplasma* have been isolated in cases of PID and NGU. Recent studies have reported serious consequences of **trichomoniasis**, including increased perinatal mortality and increased HIV transmission. **There is increasing evidence that *T. vaginalis* is a common cause of NGU in men.** Diagnostic and treatment procedures for these organisms are reserved for situations in which these infections are suspected (e.g., contact with trichomoniasis, urethral lesions, or severe dysuria and meatitis, which might suggest genital herpes) or when NGU is not responsive to recommended therapy.

Infections at any one site of the genitourinary tract produce poorly localizing symptoms, particularly in women, which may result in delayed diagnosis or misdiagnosis. Failure to recognize the causal relationship between symptoms of dysuria and STIs by patients and clinicians often results in failure to seek timely diagnosis and treatment. Longer duration and more gradual onset of dysuria may suggest *C. trachomatis* infection, whereas sudden onset of symptoms and hematuria suggest bacterial infection.

Disseminated gonorrhea with arthritis and dermatitis presents with fever, chills, and migratory polyarticular arthritis; a characteristic petechial necrotic pustular or tender papular rash of the distal extremities; and tenosynovitis of extensor tendons of the hands, wrists, or ankle tendons. This represents a more serious infection requiring a more comprehensive evaluation, extended parenteral antibiotic therapy, and hospitalization for all but the mildest cases.

Reiter syndrome is a triad of arthritis, urethritis, and conjunctivitis with associated skin lesions. The pathogenesis is unclear, but *C. trachomatis* has been implicated strongly along with other bacterial organisms. Treatment of Reiter syndrome consists of antimicrobial therapy against *Chlamydia*, nonsteroidal antiinflammatory drugs (NSAIDs), steroid injections of the affected joints, and topical steroids for uveitis.

The CDC updates treatment recommendations every few years, incorporating changes in antibiotics and sensitivity.

Suggested Readings

Augenbraun, M., Bachmann, L., Wallace, T., et al. (1998). Compliance with doxycycline therapy in sexually transmitted disease clinics. *Sexually Transmitted Diseases*, *25*, 1–4.

Bremnor, J. D., & Sadovsky, R. (2002). Evaluation of dysuria in adults. *American Family Physician*, *65*, 1589–1596.

Brill, J. R. (2010). Diagnosis and treatment of urethritis in men. *American Family Physician*, *81*, 873–878.

Centers for Disease Control and Prevention. (2015). *Sexually transmitted diseases (STDs): 2015 STD treatment guidelines*. http://www.cdc.gov/std/treatment/2015/.

Chen, J. C. (2004). Update on emerging infections: News from the Centers for Disease Control and Prevention. *Morbidity and Mortality Weekly*, *53*, 197–198.

Kodner, C. (2003). Sexually transmitted infections in men. *Primary Care*, *30*, 173–191.

Sancta St. Cyr, MD1; Lindley Barbee, MD1,2; Kimberly A. Workowski, MD1,3; Laura H. Bachmann, MD1; Cau Pham, PhD1; Karen Schlanger, PhD1; Elizabeth Torrone, PhD1; Hillard Weinstock, MD1; Ellen N. Kersh, PhD1; Phoebe Thorpe, MD1; Update to CDC's Treatment Guidelines for Gonococcal Infection, 2020 Weekly / December 18, 2020 / 69(50);1911–1916.

Simpson, T., & Oh, M. K. (2004). Urethritis and cervicitis in adolescents. *Adolescent Medicine Clinics*, *15*, 253–271.

Stamm, W. E., Hicks, C. B., Martin, D. H., et al. (1995). Azithromycin for empirical treatment of the nongonococcal urethritis syndrome in men. *Journal of the American Medical Association*, *274*, 545–549.

Taylor, B. D., & Haggerty, C. L. (2011). Management of *Chlamydia trachomatis* genital tract infection: Screening and treatment challenges. *Infection and Drug Resistance*, *4*, 19–29.

Urinary Retention, Acute

Presentation

Urinary retention is a common problem encountered in the emergency department. Acute urinary retention (AUR) presents as a sudden inability to voluntarily void.

The patient, usually male, may complain of increasing dull, low abdominal discomfort or pain and the urge to urinate, without having been able to urinate for many hours. Lower abdominal pain may become severe. Urinary hesitancy, sensation of incomplete voiding, an interrupted or decreased urinary stream, and straining to void are other typical symptoms of obstruction. Flank pain may accompany obstruction that leads to hydroureter and hydronephrosis.

Elderly and debilitated patients may be asymptomatic or have vague discomfort with urinary frequency but small volumes, overflow, or stress incontinence.

A firm, distended bladder can often be palpated between the symphysis pubis and umbilicus, although this can sometimes be masked by body habitus. Rectal examination may reveal an enlarged or tender prostate or suspected tumor, although a prostate that is of normal size and consistency by palpation can still be the cause of urethral obstruction.

What to Do

✅ When there is reasonable confidence that the patient is suffering from urinary retention based on the history and physical examination, prepare the patient for the insertion of a urethral urinary catheter.

✅ **Ultrasonography is useful** in confirming suspected bladder distention and can also determine whether proximal distention is present in the urinary tract. **Automated bladder volume devices** quickly estimate bladder volume and can be useful both on presentation and after attempted decompression. Neither of these modalities should be allowed to substantially delay catheter insertion.

✅ Assist the patient in lying flat on the back. Lying in a supine position will relax the bladder and urethra, therefore making the catheter easier to pass.

✅ **In a male patient, distend the urethra with lidocaine jelly 2% in a catheter-tipped syringe (Uroject, Uro-Jet) and try a Foley catheter (16, 18, or 20 Fr). When there is minimal distress from bladder distension, leave the lidocaine jelly in place 15 to 20 minutes to obtain good mucosal anesthesia before inserting the catheter** (Fig. 84.1). Have the patient or an assistant squeeze the distal penis closed to keep the lidocaine jelly from flowing out.

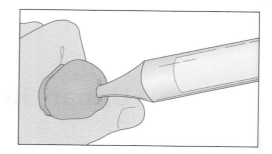

Fig. 84.1 Lidocaine jelly administrator.

✓ **When the patient is very uncomfortable** and after inserting the lidocaine jelly, delay only long enough to provide good aseptic technique, **pass a Foley catheter into the bladder, and collect the urine in a closed collecting system bag.** Reassuring the patient and having him breathe through his mouth may help relax the external sphincter of the bladder and facilitate the passage of the catheter. Hold the penis perpendicular to the body and gently pull it upright to help the catheter pass through the prostate using slow, steady pressure.

✓ **If the problem is negotiating the curve around a large prostate, use a Coudé catheter** because it is designed to match the curvature of the bulbar urethra.

✓ If the bladder still cannot drain, obtain urologic consultation for instrumentation with stylets, sounds, filiforms, and followers, or under emergent conditions consider a percutaneous suprapubic catheterization (but, whenever possible, only in conjunction with a consulting urologist). Suprapubic catheterization can be performed by adequately trained emergency physicians. The bladder must be identified through palpation, and ideally visualized in real time with ultrasound. This catheterization is then accomplished either by using a percutaneous Seldinger technique with passage of a guidewire into the bladder, dilation of the tract, and overwire catheter insertion or by insertion of a trocar, through which a catheter is subsequently placed. A risk unique to the suprapubic approach is bowel injury, occurring with a reported incidence of 2.4% to 2.7%.

✓ **Check renal and urinary function with urinalysis, a urine culture, and serum blood urea nitrogen (BUN) and creatinine determinations along with electrolytes.**

✓ Examine the patient to ascertain the cause of the obstruction. Urinalysis may show hematuria, crystalluria, and/or an elevated pH (>7.5), suggesting the presence of renal calculi. The presence of pyuria, bacteriuria, elevated pH, and/or nitrites suggests infection. Consider obstruction from an internal cause, such as constipation or a mass pressing on the urethra and bladder.

✓ If there is an infection of the bladder, give antibiotics (see Chapter 85).

✓ **If the volume drained is modest (0.5–1.5 L) and the patient is hemodynamically stable, capable of maintaining the catheter, and ambulatory, attach the Foley catheter to a leg bag and discharge the patient for urologic follow-up (and probably catheter removal) the next day or within 3 days.** Microscopic and gross hematuria following decompression are typically benign and self-limited.

✓ If the volume drained is small (100–200 mL), remove the catheter and search for alternate causes of the abdominal mass and urinary urgency.

✓ **When prostatic enlargement (which is a common cause of bladder outlet obstruction in older men) is suspected, α-blocker agents may be helpful, especially in those patients who want to be sent home with a trial without an indwelling urinary catheter. Prescribe alfuzosin (Uroxatral), 10 mg once daily taken with food; doxazosin (Cardura XL), 4 mg once daily at breakfast; or tamsulosin (Flomax), 0.4 mg once daily 30 minutes after eating. These drugs can cause symptomatic hypotension, particularly in patients with ventricular hypertrophy. Giving the first dose at bedtime may help avoid syncope.**

✓ Warn the patient to return if obstructive symptoms recur, and provide early urologic follow-up, ideally within the next 24 to 72 hours.

✓ Those patients with serious infections, ongoing postobstructive diuresis, hemodynamic instability, significant electrolyte abnormalities, or where prolonged obstructive hydroureteronephrosis caused postrenal kidney injury should be hospitalized for fluid and electrolyte replacement and specialist evaluation.

What Not to Do

✗ Do not delay bladder decompression waiting for laboratory results or imaging studies unless there is a special need to know.

✗ Do not attempt blind urethral catheterization in patients with recent urologic surgery or confirmed or suspected urethral trauma.

✗ Do not use stylets or sounds unless you have experience instrumenting the urethra; these devices can cause considerable trauma.

✗ Do not remove the catheter right away if the bladder was significantly distended. Bladder tone will take several hours to return, and the bladder may become distended again.

✗ Do not clamp the catheter to slow decompression of the bladder, even if the volume drained is more than 2 L. This only delays the patient's visit and is of no value.

✗ Do not use bethanechol (Urecholine) unless there is clearly no obstruction or that inadequate (parasympathetic) bladder tone is the only cause of the distention and there is no possibility of gastrointestinal disease.

✗ Do not perform an intravenous pyelogram in patients with compromised renal function. This can cause further renal compromise because of nephrotoxicity.

✗ Do not routinely prescribe prophylactic antibiotics. They lower the incidence of bacteriuria at the expense of selecting out more virulent organisms. Unless the patient is at high risk for the complications of catheter-associated bacteriuria (i.e., renal transplant and granulopenic patients), antibiotic prophylaxis for short-term catheterization is not warranted. A small percentage of low-risk patients with bacteriuria will progress to symptomatic urinary tract infection. However, most will clear spontaneously.

Discussion

Prompt bladder decompression is the mainstay of treatment for nearly all etiologies of AUR. This can be accomplished by urethral or suprapubic catheterization. Both routes have advantages, disadvantages, and contraindications. If imaging studies are unavailable or inconclusive regarding the degree of retention, catheterization can be diagnostic and therapeutic.

Urinary retention is characterized by a urine residual greater than 200 mL after attempted voiding.

Urinary retention may be caused by stones lodged in the urethra or urethral strictures (often from gonorrhea); foreign bodies, including blocked urinary catheters; prostatitis, prostatic carcinoma, or benign prostatic hypertrophy; blood clot, following urologic procedures; and tumor in the bladder.

Any drug with anticholinergic effects or α-adrenergic effects, such as antihistamines, ephedrine sulfate, and phenylpropanolamine, can precipitate urinary retention. Morphine and other narcotics inhibit the voiding reflex and increase the muscle tone of the external sphincter, both of which can contribute to urinary retention. Other drugs that can cause urinary retention are tricyclic antidepressants, detrusor relaxants (e.g., oxybutynin [Ditropan]), and calcium channel blockers.

Neurologic causes include cord lesions, diabetic neuropathy, Parkinson disease, stroke, malignancy that compresses the spinal cord, and multiple sclerosis. Patients with genital herpes or herpes zoster may develop urinary retention from nerve involvement.

Urinary retention has also been reported following vigorous anal intercourse. In addition, anything that causes compression from outside the urinary tract can cause obstruction. Abdominal aneurysms, tumors (primary or metastatic, benign or malignant), pregnancy, ovarian abscess, intraabdominal abscess (e.g., ruptured appendiceal abscess), and large fecal impactions are some examples of extrinsic lesions that can cause obstruction. The urethral catheterization outlined is the appropriate initial treatment for all these conditions.

Sometimes hematuria develops midway through bladder decompression, probably representing loss of tamponade of vessels that were injured as the bladder distended. This should be watched until the bleeding stops (usually spontaneously) to be sure that there is no great blood loss, no other urologic disease responsible, and no clot obstruction.

Postobstructive diuresis is a condition in which elevated renal tract pressure impairs the kidneys' ability to concentrate urine, leading to diuresis when pressure is normalized. It is defined as a urinary output greater than 200 mL for at least 2 hours after decompression, or greater than 3 L in 24 hours. Hemodynamic instability has been reported secondary to volume losses, particularly in patients with decreased intravascular reserve. Patients should be rehydrated orally or intravenously, with some sources advocating replacement of 75% of urinary losses, although high-quality evidence on this topic is lacking. Despite advocacy by some practitioners, there is no evidence that gradual or intermittent decompression decreases the risk of hematuria, hemodynamic instability, hydronephrosis, or postobstructive diuresis compared with immediate decompression.

Suggested Readings

Billet, M., & Windsor, T. A. (2019). Urinary retention. *Emergency Medicine Clinics of North America, 37*(4), 649–660.

Harmanli, O. H., Okafor, O., Ayaz, R., & Knee, A. (2009). Lidocaine jelly and plain aqueous gel for urethral straight catheterization and the Q-tip test: A randomized controlled trial. *Obstetrics & Gynecology, 114*, 547–550.

Lucas, M. G., Stephenson, T. P., & Nargund, V. (2005). Tamsulosin in the management of patients in acute urinary retention from benign prostatic hyperplasia. *British Journal of Urology, 95*, 354–357.

McNeill, S. A., & Hargreave, T. B. (2004). Members of the Alfaur Study Group: Alfuzosin once daily facilitates return to voiding in patients with acute urinary retention. *Journal of Urology, 171*, 2316–2320.

Siderias, J., Guadio, F., Singer, A. J., et al. (2004). Comparison of topical anesthetics and lubricants prior to urethral catheterization in males. *Academic Emergency Medicine, 11*, 703–706.

Urinary Tract Infection, Lower (Cystitis), Uncomplicated

Presentation

The patient (usually female) complains of urinary frequency and urgency, internal dysuria, and suprapubic pain or discomfort. The onset of symptoms is generally abrupt, often causing her to seek care within 24 hours. There may have been some antecedent trauma (sexual intercourse) to inoculate the bladder, and there may be blood in the urine (hemorrhagic cystitis). Usually, there is no labial irritation, external dysuria, or vaginal discharge (which would suggest vaginitis or cervicitis), and no fever, chills, nausea, flank pain, or costovertebral angle tenderness (which would suggest an upper urinary tract infection [UTI] or pyelonephritis).

What to Do

⊘ **Examine a clean-catch urine specimen.** Instruct the patient to wipe the introitus from front to back three times, using three separate wipes, and begin urinating into the toilet before filling the sample cup. In women of childbearing age, send a urine pregnancy test—this will influence the choice of antibiotic and follow-up. Use a dipstick test for leukocyte esterase, send for a urinalysis, or Gram stain a sample of urine. Epithelial (also known as squamous) cells on the microscopic examination are evidence of contamination from the vagina. **The presence of any white blood cells (WBCs) or bacteria in a clean sample confirms the infection.** A positive nitrite on dipstick is helpful, but a negative test does not rule out infection because many bacteria do not produce nitrites. Menses or vaginal discharge makes a clean catch difficult. One technique is to insert a tampon before giving the sample. A better technique is urinary catheterization.

⊘ **If the clinical picture is clearly of an uncomplicated lower UTI in a nonpregnant patient, prescribe nitrofurantoin extended-release capsule (Macrobid), 100 mg orally twice a day for 5 days. Nitrofurantoin is an appropriate choice for first-line therapy because of minimal resistance, and its efficacy is comparable with that of 3 days of trimethoprim/sulfamethoxazole (TMP-SMX).**

⊘ **Alternatively, when local *Escherichia coli* resistance to TMP/SMX is less than 20%, give trimethoprim, 160 mg, plus sulfamethoxazole, 800 mg (Bactrim DS or Septra DS), one tablet orally twice a day for 3 days. It should be noted that when used alone, TMP is as efficacious as TMP-SMX and is associated with fewer side effects.**

⊘ Otherwise, give a 3-day regimen of a quinolone, such as ciprofloxacin (Cipro), 500 mg by mouth twice daily, or Cipro XR, 500 mg once daily; or levofloxacin (Levaquin), 250 mg orally once daily. **The fluoroquinolones should be reserved as antimicrobials of last resort** for acute cystitis due to a US Food and Drug Administration (FDA) warning issued in 2018 regarding the development of mental health side effects, specifically agitation, disorientation, delirium, memory impairment, nervousness, and problems with attention. In addition, the FDA expressed concerns about blood sugar disturbances associated with fluoroquinolone use; later in 2018, the FDA issued a warning about an increased risk of aortic dissection.

✅ **It is important to know local resistance patterns and adjust your antibiotic prescribing accordingly.** Single-dose treatment with two TMP/SMX DS tablets is also effective in the young healthy female but is associated with a higher early recurrence rate.

✅ **In pregnancy, give a 7-day course of nitrofurantoin (Macrodantin), 100 mg orally four times a day, or nitrofurantoin extended release (Macrobid), 100 mg orally twice a day.** Cephalosporins (i.e., cephalexin [Keflex], 250–500 four times a day for 7 days) are alternatives in pregnancy, but not quinolones (or sulfas 2 weeks before delivery because of the potential increased risk for kernicterus). Trimethoprim is contraindicated during the first trimester because of its antifolate properties.

✅ Instruct the patient to drink plenty of liquids (such as cranberry juice) and remain hydrated, but there is no need to drink excessively.

✅ **If the dysuria is severe, also prescribe phenazopyridine (Pyridium), 200 mg three times a day for 2 days only, to act as a surface anesthetic in the bladder.** Warn the patient that it will stain her urine (and possibly clothes) orange.

✅ **Extend antimicrobial therapy to 7 days and obtain cultures when treating a patient who is unreliable, diabetic, symptomatic more than 5 days, older than 50 years of age, or younger than 16 years of age. Also, extend treatment and obtain cultures** for all male patients and for those with an indwelling urinary catheter, renal disease, obstructive urinary tract lesions, recurrent infection, or other significant medical problems. **For male patients and complicated UTIs, cefpodoxime 100 mg twice daily 7 days** provides good coverage.

✅ **If there are no bacteria or few WBCs, no hematuria or suprapubic pain, gradual onset over 7 to 10 days, and a new sexual partner, with a history of vaginal discharge and/or vaginal irritation, the dysuria may be caused by a chlamydial or ureaplasmal urethritis** (see Chapters 83 and 94). Perform a pelvic examination and obtain samples for nucleic acid amplification testing and possible culture. Ask the patient about the use of spermicides or douches, which may irritate the periurethral tissue and cause dysuria. Adolescent females who are screened for both *Chlamydia trachomatis* and UTI have high rates of concurrent disease. Urinary or vaginal symptoms do not differentiate well between these infections. **Clinical diagnosis is imprecise, suggesting that sexually active adolescent females with vaginal or urinary symptoms should be tested for both *C. trachomatis* and UTI.**

✅ **When there is a history of lower UTI symptoms with negative urinalysis, cultures, and workups for sexually transmitted diseases, consider a paraurethral gland infection (sometimes referred to as female prostatitis)** as the cause of this female urethral syndrome. This is usually associated with tenderness at either side of the distal two-thirds of the urethra, adjacent to the urethral meatus (Skene paraurethral glands). During the pelvic examination, press firmly against the posterior and the lateral vaginal walls as a control maneuver to demonstrate the lack of pain with firm palpation. Then, bend the examining index finger forward to compress the paraurethral tissue firmly against the flat backside of the pubic bone. An affected patient will have an abrupt pain response, whereas an unaffected patient may only respond with the sensation of having to void. Treat presumed *Chlamydia* with doxycycline, 100 mg twice a day for 2 to 4 weeks. After an initial treatment failure, older and younger women should be given a quinolone (under the guidance of a urologist or gynecologist) for at least 1 month. Hot sitz baths may provide comfort. It is always wise to presumptively treat for gonorrhea as well with ceftriaxone, 500 mg intramuscularly.

✅ **If there is external dysuria, vaginal discharge, odor, itching, and no frequency or urgency, evaluate for vaginitis** (see Chapters 83 and 94) **with a pelvic examination.**

✅ **With adult UTIs, arrange for follow-up in 2 days if the symptoms have not completely resolved.** If necessary, urine culture and a longer course of antibiotics can be undertaken. Approximately 90% of women are asymptomatic within 72 hours after initiating antimicrobial therapy. A follow-up visit or culture is not required in women who are asymptomatic after therapy. However, UTIs in most men should be considered complicated until proven otherwise.

✅ **Pediatric UTIs** differ from adult UTIs. Pediatric UTIs may indicate a significant genitourinary anomaly, their accurate diagnosis requires invasive collection methods such as suprapubic aspiration or transurethral catheterization in infants and young children, and accurate diagnosis requires a urine culture rather than relying solely on a simple urinalysis. UTIs in children, especially young children, can manifest as nonspecific symptoms (therefore the clinician must maintain a high index of suspicion). Children, especially those younger than 5 years of age, have increased risk for renal scarring after a single UTI. (Therefore it is important to diagnose quickly and to initiate appropriate broad-spectrum antibiotic therapy.)

✅ Although a midstream, clean-catch void can be a reliable method of urine collection in adults and older children, it is usually impossible for preschool children. For older children, patients and parents should be instructed to cleanse the periurethral area well, spread labia or partially retract the foreskin, and allow the initial urine to be wasted before beginning collection in a sterile container. Having girls sit backward on the toilet may facilitate this.

✅ **In small children, transurethral bladder catheterization is the preferred method for obtaining urine by many practitioners and parents.**

✅ **The clues to the diagnosis of UTI in children before culture results include urine nitrite, leukocyte esterase, bacteria, or WBCs. Bacteria on Gram stain are another specific indicator of UTI. The combination of leukocyte esterase, nitrite, and bacteria on microscopy is a sensitive test (sensitivity 99.8%, specificity 70%). The absence of any of these findings on urinalysis and microscopic examination nearly (but not completely) eliminates the diagnosis of UTI.** More than 5 to 10 WBCs per high-powered field on catheter specimen in the presence of a suggestive clinical picture should be presumed to represent a true UTI until proven otherwise by a negative culture.

✅ **For uncomplicated infections in the nontoxic child, prescribe 8 mg/kg/day of TMP/SMX orally divided every 12 hours for 10 days (where local resistance of uropathogens to TMP/SMX is <20%); or cefixime (Suprax), 8 mg/kg/day divided every 12 hours, up to a maximum of 400 mg, for 7 days; or cephalexin (generic), 50 to 100 mg/kg/day divided every 6 hours by mouth for 7 days; or, if the patient is vomiting, ceftriaxone (Rocephin), 50 to 75 mg/kg once daily intravenously or intramuscularly.** Because it is difficult to rule out pyelonephritis in febrile infants with UTI, a full 14-day course of antibiotics is indicated.

✓ Arrange follow-up for all children because a UTI may be the first evidence of underlying urinary tract disease.

What Not to Do

✗ Do not forget to check for pregnancy.

✗ Do not undertake expensive urine cultures for every lower UTI of recent onset in nonpregnant, normal, healthy women with no history of recent UTI or antibiotic use.

✗ Do not use the single-dose or 3-day regimens for a possible upper UTI or pyelonephritis.

✗ Do not rely on gross inspection of the urine sample. Cloudiness is usually caused by crystals, and odors can result from diet or medication.

✗ Do not request a follow-up visit or culture after therapy for a woman's uncomplicated UTI unless her symptoms persist or recur.

Discussion

Lower UTI or cystitis is a superficial bacterial infection of the bladder or urethra. Most of these infections involve *E. coli, Staphylococcus saprophyticus,* or enterococci.

The urine dipstick is a reasonable screening measure that can direct therapy if results are positive. Under the microscope in a clean sediment (free of epithelial cells), 1 WBC per 400 field suggests significant pyuria, although clinicians accustomed to imperfect samples usually set a threshold of 3 to 5 WBCs per field. In addition, *Trichomonas* organisms may be appreciated swimming in the urinary sediment, indicating a different cause for urinary symptoms or associated vaginitis.

In a straightforward lower UTI, urine culture may be reserved for cases that fail to resolve with single-dose or 3-day therapy. In complicated or doubtful cases or with recurrences, a urine culture before initial treatment may be helpful.

Risk factors for UTI in women include pregnancy, sexual activity, use of diaphragms or spermicides, failure to void postcoitally, and history of previous UTI. Healthy women may be expected to suffer

a few episodes of lower UTI in a lifetime without indicating any major structural problem or incurring any long-term medical sequelae, but recurrences at short intervals suggest inadequate treatment or underlying abnormalities.

Young men, however, have longer urethras and far fewer lower UTIs. They probably should be evaluated urologically after just one episode unless they have a risk factor such as an uncircumcised foreskin, human immunodeficiency virus (HIV) infection, or homosexual activity, and they respond successfully to initial treatment. In sexually active men, consider urethritis or prostatitis as the cause. In men who are older than 50 years of age, there is a rapid increase in UTI resulting from prostate hypertrophy, obstruction, and instrumentation.

UTIs among pediatric patients are associated with significantly greater morbidity and long-term sequelae than UTIs among adults, including impaired renal function and end-stage renal disease.

TMP-SMX has been the standard therapy for UTI; however, *E. coli* is becoming increasingly resistant to this medication.

Suggested Readings

Bent, S., Nallamothu, B. K., Simel, D. L., et al. (2002). Does this woman have an acute uncomplicated urinary tract infection? *JAMA*, *287*, 2701–2710.

Chung, A., Arianayagam, M., & Rashid, P. (2010). Bacterial cystitis in women (review). *Australian Family Physician*, *39*, 295–298.

Cooper, K. L., Badalato, G. M., & Rutman, M. P. (2020). Infections of the urinary tract. In: *Campbell-Walsh urology* (12th ed., pp. 1129–1201). Philadelphia, PA: Elsevier.

Gittes, R. F. (2002). Female prostatitis. *Urology Clinics of North America*, *29*, 613–616.

Hoberman, A., Wald, E. R., Hickey, R. W., et al. (1999). Oral versus initial intravenous therapy for urinary tract infections in young febrile children. *Pediatrics*, *104*, 79–86.

Hooten, G. K., & Stamm, W. E. (2001). Increasing antimicrobial resistance and the management of uncomplicated community-acquired urinary tract infections. *Annals of Internal Medicine*, *135*, 41–50.

Huppert, J. S., Biro, F. M., Mehrabi, J., & Slap, G. B. (2003). Urinary tract infection and *Chlamydia* infection in adolescent females. *Journal of Pediatric and Adolescent Gynecology*, *16*, 133–137.

Jou, W. W., & Powers, R. D. (1998). Utility of dipstick urinalysis as a guide to management of adults with suspected infection of hematuria. *Southern Medical Journal*, *91*, 266–269.

Layton, K. L. (2003). Diagnosis and management of pediatric urinary tract infection. *Clinics in Family Practice*, *5*, 367–383.

McKinnell, J. A., Stollenwerk, N. S., Jung, C. W., & Miller, L. G. (2011). Nitrofurantoin compares favorably to recommended agents as empirical treatment of uncomplicated urinary tract infections in a decision and cost analysis. *Mayo Clinic Proceedings*, *86*, 480–488.

Mehnert-Kay, S. A. (2005). Diagnosis and management of uncomplicated urinary tract infections. *American Family Physician*, *72*, 451–456.

Michael, M., Hodson, E. M., Craig, J. C., et al. (2002). Short compared with standard duration of antibiotic treatment for urinary tract infection: A systematic review of randomised controlled trials. *Archives of Disease in Childhood*, *87*, 118–123.

Raz, R., Chazen, B., Kennes, Y., et al. (2002). Empiric use of trimethoprim-sulfamethoxazole (TMP-SMX) in the treatment of women with uncomplicated urinary tract infections, in a geographical area with a high prevalence of TMP-SMX–resistant uropathogens. *Clinics in Infectious Diseases*, *34*, 1165–1169.

Shapiro, T., Dalton, M., Hammock, J., et al. (2005). The prevalence of urinary tract infections and sexually transmitted disease in women with symptoms of a simple urinary tract infection stratified by low colony count criteria. *Academic Emergency Medicine*, *12*, 38–44.

Stamm, W. E., & Hooton, T. M. (1993). Management of urinary tract infections in adults. *New England Journal of Medicine*, *329*, 1328–1334.

Valenstein, P. N., & Koepke, J. A. (1984). Unnecessary microscopy in routine urinalysis. *American Journal of Clinical Pathology*, *82*, 444–448.

Vogel, T., Verreault, R., Gourdeau, M., et al. (2004). Optimal duration of antibiotic therapy for uncomplicated urinary tract infection in older women: A double-blind randomized controlled trial. *Canadian Medical Association Journal*, *170*, 469–473.

PART 8

Gynecologic Emergencies

■ Mariah McNamara ■ Jessica Russell

CHAPTER

Bartholin Abscess

86

Presentation

A female of reproductive age presents for evaluation of vulvar pain and swelling that has developed over the past 2 to 3 days. Pain is increased when walking and sitting. On physical examination in the lithotomy position, there is a unilateral (occasionally bilateral), tender, fluctuant, mildly erythematous swelling at the 4-o'clock or 8-o'clock position within the posterior labium minora (Fig. 86.1).

What to Do

✓ **If the swelling and pain are mild without fluctuance (bartholinitis) or if the abscess is small, the patient can be placed on antibiotics, such as Bactrim or Augmentin PLUS clindamycin (see later), and instructed to take warm sitz baths. Early follow-up should be provided.** Unilateral or bilateral Bartholin gland infection in most cases is not caused by a sexually transmitted infection (STI). In sexually active women with multiple partners, however, consider testing for STI, and treat presumptively if high risk. (One emergency department [ED] study revealed that 10% of ED patients with a Bartholin abscess were infected with *Neisseria gonorrhoeae*.) Treatment for STI should include oral doxycycline, 100 mg twice a day for 7 days, PLUS ceftriaxone 500 mg intramuscularly (IM) once (see Chapter 91).

✓ **When the abscess is painful or is enlarged and fluctuant, a puncture/incision of 0.5 to 1 cm should be made over the medial bulging mucosal surface of the labia minora and the pus evacuated.** First prepare the mucosal surface with povidone-iodine (Betadine) solution. Anesthetize the overlying tissue with lidocaine (Xylocaine) without epinephrine. A No. 11 scalpel blade can be used to make the 0.5-cm stab incision, about 1.5 cm deep, at the area of maximal fluctuance.

✓ **After drainage, loose packing or a Word catheter should be inserted through the incision. For Word catheter insertion, test the catheter to ensure the balloon is intact. Insert it into the cavity and inflate the tip of the catheter with sufficient sterile water or saline to hold it in place (approximately 1.5–3 mL)** (Fig. 86.2). If balloon inflation is not tolerated, deflate

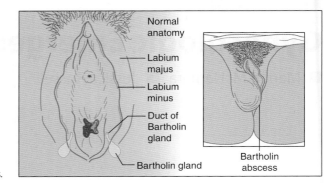

Fig. 86.1 Bartholin abscess.

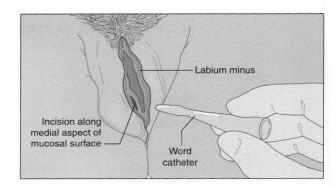

Fig. 86.2 Insertion of Word catheter after catheter incision and drainage.

and reposition the Word catheter before reinflation. The free end of the catheter may then be tucked up into the vagina for comfort. If the initial incision is too large, the Word catheter may fall out.

✅ **Complications are rare and include bleeding, hematoma, scarring, dyspareunia, and persistent or recurrent infection.**

✅ **After drainage**, use of prophylactic antibiotics is not always necessary unless there is significant surrounding cellulitis, signs of systemic illness, multiple comorbidities, concern for methicillin-resistant *Staphylococcus aureus* (MRSA), pregnancy, or immune compromise. The goal of antibiotics is to cover for MRSA, *Streptococcus*, and gram-negative aerobes. **Options include amoxicillin/clavulanate (Augmentin) 875 mg/125 mg twice daily × 7 days, or sulfamethoxazole/trimethoprim (Bactrim) 1 DS tablet twice daily × 7 days PLUS clindamycin 300 mg four times a day × 7 days.** The patient should be instructed to take sitz baths and be provided with mild analgesics for the first 1 to 2 days. **If STI is suspected, treatment, as noted previously, should be administered.**

✅ **Inform the patient that the catheter should stay in place for up to 4 to 6 weeks to allow a permanent tract to form and thereby help prevent recurrent abscess formation.**

✅ Arrange for a follow-up examination within 3 days. Patients should be offered a peripad and be instructed to continue sitz baths and pelvic rest.

✅ If recurrent, repeat incision and drainage (I&D) should be performed, with gynecologic referral and consideration of marsupialization.

What Not to Do

(X) Do not make a drainage incision on the external labium, as this can lead to scarring.

(X) Do not mistake a nontender Bartholin duct cyst, which does not require immediate treatment, for an inflamed abscess.

(X) Do not mistake a more posterior perirectal abscess for a Bartholin abscess. The perirectal abscess requires a different treatment approach.

(X) Do not miss an underlying malignancy; consider biopsy if there is a solid component, if the abscess is unresponsive to treatment, or in postmenopausal patients.

(X) Do not use a Word catheter in latex-allergic patients, as these are often made of latex.

Discussion

Bartholin glands are epithelial secretory glands commonly paired within the labia minora at approximately the 4-o'clock and 8-o'clock positions on the posterolateral aspect of the vestibule. Normally pea sized and draining through a 2.5-cm duct into a fold between the hymenal ring and the labium, obstruction of the gland at the ostium can cause the glands to become cystic due to an accumulation of mucus and subsequently form abscesses when this cyst becomes infected with bacteria and the gland distends with pus. Previous abscesses or cysts are a risk factor for recurrence.

Simple incision and drainage without Word catheter placement may be inadequate and lead to a considerable number of recurrences of abscesses. The Word catheter is an inflatable latex balloon on the tip of a 10-Fr, 5-cm, single-barreled catheter designed to retain itself in the abscess cavity for 4 to 6 weeks to help ensure the development of a tract for continued drainage. It seldom stays in place that long. The size of the incision should be kept less than 1 cm. If the incision is too large when using a Word catheter, the balloon may fall out prematurely.

Iodoform or plain ribbon gauze can be inserted into the incised abscess as a substitute. If a wide opening persists, recurrent infections are not likely to occur, but they are common if the stoma closes.

The most common organisms involved in the development of a Bartholin abscess include *Escherichia coli*, polymicrobial, *Streptococcus* species and *Enterococcus faecalis*. Anaerobic infections are most commonly *Bacteroides fragilis*. Consider a culture if there is a concern for MRSA.

Suggested Readings

Elkins, J. M., Hamid, O. S., Simon, L. V., & Sheele, J. M. (2020). Association of Bartholin cysts and abscesses and sexually transmitted infections. *American Journal of Emergency Medicine*. https://doi.org/10.1016/j.ajem.2020.04.027

Elsevier Point of Care. (2019). *Bartholin cyst and abscess*. Amsterdam, Netherlands: Elsevier BV.

Krissi, H., Shmuely, A., Aviram, A., et al. (2016). Acute bartholin's abscess: Microbial spectrum, patient characteristics, clinical manifestation, and surgical outcomes. *European Journal of Clinical Microbiology & Infectious Diseases*, 35, 443. https://doi.org/10.1007/s10096-015-2557-9.

Mattila, A., Miettinen, A., and Heinonen, P. K. Microbiology of Bartholin's Duct Abscess. *Infectious Diseases in Obstetrics and Gynecology* 1.6 (1994): 265–268. Web.

Owen, J. W., Koza, J., Shiblee, T., et al. (2005). Placement of a word catheter: A resident training model. *American Journal of Obstetrics and Gynecology*, 192, 1385–13872005.

Zeger, W., & Holt, K. (2003). Gynecologic infections. *Emergency Medicine Clinics of North America*, 21, 631–648.

Condylomata Acuminata

(Genital Warts)

Presentation

Patients may complain of perineal itching, burning, pain, and tenderness, although they are commonly asymptomatic, especially with cervical and vaginal involvement. Distinctive fleshy warts can be found on the external genitalia or anus (Figs. 87.1 and 87.2). Lesions are pedunculated or broad-based with pink to gray soft excrescences, with multiple papillae arising from a single base. They occur in clusters or individually and can become friable. In addition to the external genitalia (i.e., the penis, vulva, scrotum, perineum, and perianal skin), genital warts can occur on the uterine cervix as well as in and around the vagina, urethra, anus, and mouth.

What to Do

⊘ External warts seldom require biopsy for diagnosis. Biopsy is needed only when the diagnosis is uncertain, the lesions do not respond to standard therapy, the disease worsens during therapy, the patient is immunocompromised, or warts are pigmented, indurated, fixed, and ulcerated. The differential diagnosis of anogenital warts includes molluscum contagiosum (Figs. 87.3 and 87.4), verruca vulgaris (common nongenital wart), secondary syphilis *(Condyloma lata)* (Fig. 87.5), hypertrophic vulvar dystrophies, and vulvar intraepithelial and invasive neoplasias. Consider atypical, pigmented, intravaginal, cervical, and persistent warts for referral for gynecologic evaluation. Recognition of cervical lesions may require colposcopy.

⊘ **The primary goal of treating visible genital warts is the removal of symptomatic warts. In most patients, treatment can induce wart-free periods.** Treatment of genital warts should be guided by the number, size, site, and morphology of lesions, as well as the preference of the patient, cost, convenience, available resources, and experience of the health care provider. **No definitive evidence suggests that any of the available treatments are superior to the others. Modalities of therapy include physical or chemical destruction, immunologic therapy, or surgical excision.**

⊘ **Because of uncertainty regarding the effect of treatment on future transmission and the possibility for spontaneous resolution, an acceptable alternative for some patients is to forgo treatment and await spontaneous resolution.**

⊘ Most patients have 10 or less genital warts, with a total wart area of 0.5 to 1 cm^2. These warts respond to most treatment modalities. **Many patients require a course of therapy rather than a single treatment. In general, warts located on moist surfaces and/or in intertriginous areas respond better to topical treatment than do warts on drier surfaces.**

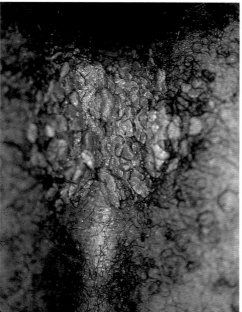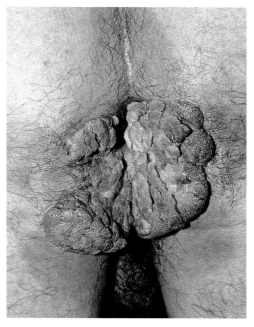

Fig. 87.1 Condylomata acuminata on the perineum. (Adapted from Black, M., McKay, M., Braude, P., et al. [2002]. *Obstetric and gynecologic dermatology* [2nd ed.]. St. Louis, MO: Mosby.)

Fig. 87.2 Perianal condylomata acuminata. (Adapted from White, G., & Cox, N. [2006]. *Diseases of the skin* [2nd ed]. St. Louis, MO: Mosby.)

✅ Patients should be warned that persistent hypopigmentation or hyperpigmentation is common with ablative modalities. Rarely, treatment can result in disabling chronic pain syndromes (e.g., vulvodynia or hyperesthesia of the treatment site).

Patient-Applied Treatment

✅ **Prescribe imiquimod (Aldara) cream 5%, 12 single-use packets for dry or moist warts. Have the nonpregnant patient apply a thin layer of cream once daily to external genital and perianal warts, rubbed in until the cream is no longer visible, with hand washing before and after cream application.** This should be repeated three times per week, prior to normal sleeping hours, and left on the skin for 6 to 10 hours before being washed off. This should continue until there is total clearing of the warts or for a maximum of 16 weeks. Avoid with warts larger than a 10-cm^2 area. **This cream is very expensive.**

✅ **An alternative for self-treatment is to prescribe podofilox (Condylox) 0.5% solution (3.5 mL) or gel 0.5% (3.5 g) for moist warts. Both are relatively inexpensive. Nonpregnant patients may apply podofilox solution with a cotton swab or podofilox gel with a finger twice daily for 3 days, followed by 4 days of no treatment.** The patient should be careful to avoid the surrounding normal tissue. This cycle may be repeated as necessary for a total of four cycles. Total wart area treated should not exceed 10 cm^2, and the total volume of podofilox should not exceed 0.5 mL/day. If possible, apply the initial treatment to demonstrate the proper application technique and identify which warts should be treated.

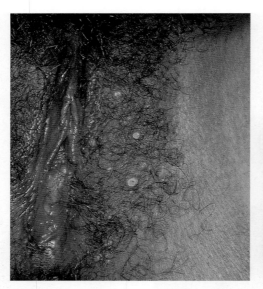

Fig. 87.3 Molluscum contagiosum on the labia majora. (Adapted from Black, M., McKay, M., Braude, P., et al. [2002]. *Obstetric and gynecologic dermatology* [2nd ed.]. St. Louis, MO: Mosby.)

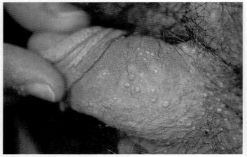

Fig. 87.4 Molluscum on the shaft of the penis. (Adapted from White, G., & Cox, N. [2006]. *Diseases of the skin* [2nd ed]. St. Louis, MO: Mosby.)

⊘ **Another option, sinecatechins (Veregen) 15% ointment for dry warts should be applied tid (do not wash off) for use up to 16 weeks.**

Provider-Administered Treatment

⊘ **Apply 25% podophyllin in tincture of benzoin (Podocon-25, Podofilm) for moist warts. Use applicator provided. A thin layer should be applied to each wart and allowed to air dry. Do not exceed a 10-cm² area. Leave on briefly for the first treatment to assess for sensitivity (approximately 30 minutes). Thereafter the nonpregnant patient may thoroughly wash off the podophyllin in 1 to 4 hours.** Patient may leave on overnight if tolerated. This may be repeated weekly if necessary, but if warts persist after six applications, the patient should be referred for alternative therapy. This is not to be used on mucosal surfaces— never to be applied on cervical or vaginal epithelium.

⊘ **Alternatively, apply a small amount of trichloroacetic acid (TCA) or bichloroacetic acid (BCA), 80% to 90%, only to small, few moist warts and allow it to dry, at which time a white frosting-like film develops.** If an excess amount of acid is applied, the treated area can be powdered with baking soda to neutralize unreacted acid. This treatment can be repeated weekly, if necessary. A barrier of petroleum jelly helps protect unaffected surrounding skin because the solution is highly caustic.

⊘ **The treatment modality should be changed if the patient has not improved substantially after three provider-administered treatments or if warts have not completely cleared after six treatments.**

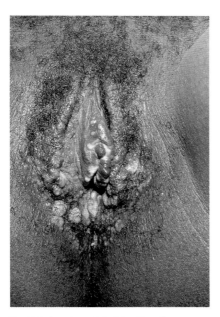

Fig. 87.5   Secondary syphilis. (Adapted from White, G., & Cox, N. [2006]. *Diseases of the skin* [2nd ed]. St. Louis, MO: Mosby.)

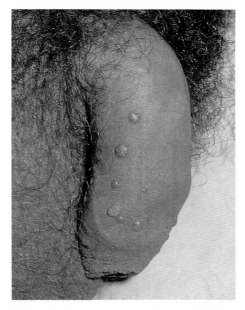

Fig. 87.6   Condylomata acuminata; multiple lesions on the shaft of the penis. (Adapted from White, G., & Cox, N. [2006]. *Diseases of the skin* [2nd ed]. St. Louis, MO: Mosby.)

If the patient is pregnant, has severe involvement, or has profuse anal or rectal warts, she should be referred for cryotherapy, ablation with carbon dioxide laser, electrocautery, or surgical excision.

If the patient's male partner also has visible lesions (Fig. 87.6), he can be treated using the same regimens. Examination of asymptomatic sex partners is not necessary, but they may benefit from counseling about their potential for future disease.

Provide patient education and counseling. Inform the patient of the following:

- Genital human papillomavirus (HPV) is a viral infection that is common among sexually active adults.

- Infection is almost always sexually transmitted, but the incubation period is variable, and it is often difficult to determine the source of infection. Within ongoing relationships, sex partners usually are infected by the time of the patient's diagnosis, although they may have no symptoms or signs of infection.

- The natural history of genital warts is generally benign; the types of HPV that usually cause external genital warts are not associated with cancer.

- Recurrence of genital warts within the first several months after treatment is common and usually indicates recurrence rather than reinfection.

○ The likelihood of transmission to future partners and the duration of infectivity after treatment are unknown. The use of latex condoms may help to prevent the likelihood of further transmission.

○ The value of disclosing a past diagnosis of genital HPV infection to future partners is unclear. Candid discussions about other sexually transmitted diseases (STDs) should be encouraged and attempted whenever possible.

○ After visible genital warts have cleared, a follow-up evaluation is not mandatory but may be helpful. Patients concerned about recurrences should be offered a follow-up evaluation 3 months after treatment.

✓ **Women should be counseled to undergo regular Papanicolaou (Pap) screening, as recommended for women without genital warts. The presence of genital warts is not an indication for a change in the frequency of Pap tests or for cervical colposcopy.**

✓ Counsel both partners about the unpredictable natural history of the disease and the possible increased risk for lower genital tract malignancy (see Discussion box). Infected women should have an annual Pap smear.

What Not to Do

✗ Do not use imiquimod, podofilox, or podophyllin during pregnancy. Safety during pregnancy has not been established for these agents, and there have been a few cases of toxicity reported when large amounts of podophyllin have been used.

✗ Do not mistake pearly penile papules for warts (Fig. 87.7). These dome-shaped or hairlike projections around the corona of the glans penis are normal variants in up to 10% of men.

✗ **Do not mistake condyloma acuminata for other lesions. Other lesions include condylomata lata, micropapillomatosis of vulva, molluscum contagiosum, and squamous cell carcinoma. If lesions are not responding to therapy, consider biopsy.**

✗ **Do not advise patients that clearing is a cure; recurrence is the norm.**

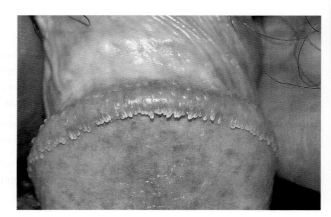

Fig. 87.7 Pearly penile papules. (Adapted from White, G., & Cox, N. [2006]. *Diseases of the skin* [2nd ed]. St. Louis, MO: Mosby.)

Discussion

Genital warts are a result of infection with HPV. Approximately 35 types of HPV can infect the genital tract. Most HPV infections are asymptomatic, unrecognized, or subclinical. The sexual transmission of HPV is well documented, with the highest prevalence in young, sexually active adolescents and adults. **HPV types 6 and 11 are the most prevalent types associated with condylomata acuminata and are not considered to have the malignant potential of types 16, 18, 31, 33, and 35. The types with malignant potential are found occasionally in visible genital warts and have been associated with external genital squamous intraepithelial neoplasia. Patients who have visible genital warts can be infected simultaneously with multiple HPV types. In addition, HPV frequently coexists with other sexually transmitted diseases.** HPV lesions are difficult to eradicate, with a very high recurrence rate, and there is still no definitive therapy. No evidence indicates that either the presence of genital warts or their treatment is associated with the development of cervical cancer.

Despite current infection with genital warts, patients may still be candidates for the new HPV vaccine. They should be encouraged to seek a specialist's advice.

Prevention options include HPV vaccination, abstinence, routine condom use, and limiting sexual partners. Once patients have condyloma, they should be encouraged to use condoms consistently. Educate patients that condoms can decrease transmission but might not completely prevent infection.

Two HPV vaccine series are currently available in the United States. Gardasil is a quadrivalent HPV vaccine indicated for male and female patients aged 9 to 25 years for prevention of cervical cancer and genital warts. Cervarix is the bivalent vaccine indicated for female patients aged 9 to 25 years for prevention of cervical cancer.

Imiquimod is a topically active immune enhancer that stimulates production of interferon and other cytokines. Local inflammatory reactions are common with the use of imiquimod; these reactions are usually mild to moderate.

Podofilox, 0.5% solution or gel, an antimitotic drug that destroys warts, is relatively inexpensive, easy to use, safe, and self-applied by patients.

Most patients experience mild to moderate pain or local irritation after treatment.

Podophyllin resin, which contains several compounds, including antimitotic podophyllin lignans, must be allowed to air dry before the treated area comes into contact with clothing, or local irritation caused by spread of the compound to adjacent areas can result.

Both TCA and BCA are caustic agents that destroy warts by chemical coagulation of proteins. TCA solutions have low viscosity, comparable with that of water, and can spread rapidly if applied excessively; thus they also can damage adjacent tissues if not applied sparingly and allowed to dry before the patient sits or stands.

Surgical therapy is a treatment option that has the advantage of usually eliminating warts at a single visit. However, such therapy requires substantial clinical training, additional equipment, and a longer office visit.

Newer therapies, such as topical cidofovir, are under study and show promise. For the treatment of condylomata acuminata (genital warts), in a placebo-controlled trial, 30 patients were treated with cidofovir 1% gel once daily or placebo. Overall, 16 of 19 patients had a complete or partial response to cidofovir (9 complete responses) versus only 2 patients in the placebo group after a median of 43 days of treatment. The Centers for Disease Control and Prevention (CDC) suggests cidofovir as an alternative regimen but provides no further recommendations.

The goal of present treatments is clearance of visible warts; some evidence exists that treatment reduces infectivity, but there is no evidence that treatment reduces the incidence of genital cancer. Patient-applied therapy, such as imiquimod cream or podofilox, is increasingly recommended. These treatments, used at times in conjunction with surgical excision and/or cryotherapy, are presently the most convenient and effective options.

Biopsy, viral typing, acetowhite staining, and other diagnostic measures are not routinely required.

In patients who fail to respond to therapy or who have extremely large lesions, consider evaluating for an immunosuppressed state, including human immunodeficiency virus (HIV).

Suggested Readings

Kodner, C. M., & Nasraty, S. (2004). Management of genital warts. *American Family Physician*, *70*, 2335–2342.

Long, M. C. (2020). Condylomata acuminata. In *Conn's current therapy 2020* (pp. 955–958). Philadelphia, PA: Elsevier.

Snoeck, R., Bossens, M., Parent, D., et al. (2001). Phase II double-blind, placebo controlled study of the safety and efficacy of cidofovir topical gel for the treatment of patients with human papillomavirus infection. *Clinics in Infectious Diseases*, *33*, 597–602.

Contact Vulvovaginitis

Presentation

A patient presents for evaluation of severe vulvar itching that may be accompanied by edematous swelling. Occasionally there will be tenderness, pain, burning, and dysuria severe enough to cause urinary retention. The vulvovaginal area is variably inflamed, erythematous, and edematous. In more severe cases there may be a microvesicular papular eruption with excoriations. In cases where there is chronic contact dermatitis, there may be an eczematoid appearance with cracks, fissures, scaling, and skin thickening (lichenification).

What to Do

✓ **Try to determine if the condition is exogenous (from contact) or endogenous (atopic). If an offending agent can be identified, have the patient stop using it. Most reactions are caused by agents that the patient unknowingly applies or uses for hygienic or therapeutic purposes.** Chemically scented douches, soaps, bubble baths, deodorants, perfumes, dyed or scented toilet paper, dyed underwear, scented tampons or pads, and additional feminine hygiene products are the most common causative agents. Neomycin-containing topical medication is another frequent source. Less commonly, plant allergens, such as poison oak or poison ivy (see Chapter 184), may trigger the reaction. Use of latex condoms, lubricants, and proteins in seminal fluid may also cause contact dermatitis.

✓ If the diagnosis is unclear, rule out an alternative cause of vulvar pruritus, such as pinworms (see Chapter 70) or *Trichomonas* organisms (see Chapter 94). Superimposed *Candida albicans* may also contribute to pruritus. Atypical herpes simplex virus should also be considered (examine closely for vesicular lesions). Atopic or eczematous changes can be causative as well (examine closely the gluteal and labial folds).

✓ **When the findings are typical for contact vulvovaginitis, instruct the patient in the use of warm to cool sitz baths twice a day for 5 minutes. Cool compresses may provide comfort throughout the day. Have the patient practice vulvar hygiene (avoid synthetic underwear, tight jeans or pants, leotards, swimsuits, panty liners, or other close-contact irritants). Choose fragrance-free, pH-neutral soaps and unscented detergents; avoid wipes or topical powders, sprays, douches.**

✓ **Prescribe liberal amounts of topical corticosteroids, such as fluocinolone (Synalar cream 0.025%) or triamcinolone (Aristocort A 0.025% cream) two to four times a day (dispense 15-g tube).** For mild symptoms, hydrocortisone 1% or 2.5% or triamcinolone 0.1% can be used daily for 2 to 4 weeks, then twice per week. For moderate to severe symptoms, clobetasol propionate or betamethasone dipropionate ointment 0.05% can be used nightly for 30 days. One can also try tapering starting with applications twice daily for 2 weeks; then daily for 2 weeks; then on Mondays, Wednesdays, and Fridays for 2 weeks; finally, the patient should be reevaluated. In the past, there has been concern about atrophy with steroid use. These potent steroids have been used up to 12 weeks on the vulva without adverse effects.

✓ **In more severe cases, or if topical application is increasing the irritation, use triamcinolone intramuscular 60 mg. This may be used every 6 weeks for up to three doses. Alternatively, a steroid taper dose pack, such as prednisone (Sterapred DS or Sterapred DS 12 day) or methylprednisolone (Medrol Dosepack 4-mg tablets) for systemic therapy could be prescribed.**

✓ **A sedating antipruritic agent may help with nighttime itching and scratching. Consider the antihistamine hydroxyzine (Atarax, Vistaril), 25 to 50 mg every night at bedtime.**

What Not to Do

✗ Do not have the patient use hot baths or compresses. This will usually exacerbate the burning and pruritus.

✗ Do not prescribe nonsedating antihistamines. They are relatively ineffective in treating contact vulvovaginitis and may increase discomfort by drying the vaginal mucosa.

Discussion

The major problem with managing contact vulvovaginitis is identifying the primary irritant or allergen. In many cases, more than one substance is involved, or potentially involved, and may be totally unsuspected by the patient (such as the use of scented toilet paper). For this reason, a thorough investigative history is important. Include questions about hygiene practices, clothing, and fabrics.

An allergic reaction can take 12 to 72 hours to develop, is usually very pruritic, and can often last for weeks.

Suggested Readings

Miller, M. (2014). Recurrent vulvovaginitis: Tips for treating a common condition. *Contemporary OB/GYN*, *59*(8), 22–27.

Paladine, H. L., & Urmi, A. D. (2018). Vaginitis: Diagnosis and treatment. *American Family Physician*, *97*(5), 321–329.

Stricker, T. (2010). Vulvovaginitis. *Paediatrics and Child Health*, *20*(3), 143–145.

Dysmenorrhea

(Menstrual Cramps)

Presentation

A young female presents with crampy, laborlike pains that began shortly before or at the onset of the visible bleeding of her menstrual period. The pain is focused in the lower abdomen, low back, suprapubic area, or thighs and may be associated with nausea, vomiting, increased defecation, headache, muscular cramps, or passage of clots. The pain is most severe on the first day of the menses and may last from several hours to days. Often this is a recurrent problem, dating back to early menarche. Rectal, vaginal, and pelvic examinations disclose no abnormalities.

What to Do

⊘ Ask about the duration of symptoms and pattern of similar episodes. Onset of dysmenorrhea after adolescence or pain that is not limited to the time of menses suggests other pelvic disease. Ask about appetite, diarrhea, dysuria, dyspareunia, abnormal vaginal discharge, and other symptoms suggestive of pelvic disease.

⊘ Perform a thorough abdominal, speculum, and bimanual pelvic examination. Look for signs of trauma, infection, or other uterine or adnexal disease. Evaluate for pregnancy and sexually transmitted diseases (STDs) in sexually active patients. **It is appropriate to perform only an abdominal examination and forgo the pelvic examination in young adolescents with a typical history and who truly have never been sexually active; imaging is useful in this situation.**

⊘ **Confirm that the patient is not pregnant, using a urine pregnancy test (or serum β–human chorionic gonadotropin [β-hCG], if available).**

⊘ When the history and physical examination suggest other pelvic disease, the evaluation should follow accordingly, usually with pelvic ultrasonography as the initial diagnostic test to rule out anatomic abnormalities, such as mass lesions.

⊘ **For uncomplicated dysmenorrhea, nonsteroidal anti-inflammatory drugs (NSAIDs) and hormonal therapy are the mainstays of treatment. If one of these agents fails after 2 to 3 months, then consider the other.**

⊘ **Start with NSAIDs, such as ibuprofen (Motrin), 600 mg once every 6 hours or 800 mg once every 8 hours, or naproxen (Naprosyn), 500 mg once every 12 hours. NSAIDs may be most effective when therapy is started before the onset of menstrual pain, and continue for the first 2 to 3 days of bleeding or until the cramping resolves.** Approximately 70% of patients have moderate to complete relief of painful cramps with these drugs. **NSAIDs should not be** offered to women with a history of gastrointestinal bleeding, ulceration, or perforation. Treat with an alternative approach (e.g., oral contraceptives).

✅ **If hormonal contraception is desired, monophasic oral contraceptive pills (OCPs) and depo-medroxyprogesterone acetate (Depo-Provera) may be considered.** OCPs are up to 90% effective. Extended oral contraceptive formulations (i.e., usually taking OCPs for 12 weeks followed by 1 week off) lead to less frequent menstrual periods and is associated with less menstrual pain than do monthly OCP regimens. Both, however, are effective. A disadvantage of the longer regimen is unscheduled spotting that occurs, causing some women to discontinue use; this, however, does decrease over time.

✅ Use of the transdermal contraceptive patch in a randomized trial found dysmenorrhea more common in patch users than in oral users. Vaginal rings and intrauterine devices (IUDs) have shown variable results on dysmenorrhea symptoms. Implanted contraception has not been well studied for this condition. **At this time, oral contraception appears to be the most efficacious hormonal agent for dysmenorrhea.**

✅ **Use of topical heat appears to be as effective as oral analgesics. Systematic reviews found that exercise also appears to reduce menstrual symptoms. Behavior modification with biofeedback, electromyographic training, Lamaze exercises, and relaxation training may also be helpful.**

✅ Limited data demonstrate some promise in the following:

- One study found that 100 mg of thiamine (vitamin B_1) taken daily reduced symptoms in 87% of women tested.
- Diet modifications may help alleviate dysmenorrhea, including a low-fat diet rich in fish (e.g., salmon, tuna, halibut), beans, seeds (e.g., sesame, pumpkin, sunflower), whole grains, fruits, and vegetables.
- Acupuncture, acupressure, and aromatherapy have also been shown to be effective in treating dysmenorrhea.
- Smoking has been associated with prolonged duration of dysmenorrhea, prompting the recommendation to quit smoking to improve dysmenorrhea.

✅ If pain is not controlled with any of these approaches, pelvic ultrasonography should be performed, and gynecologic referral should be arranged for the workup of endometriosis or other secondary causes of dysmenorrhea.

What Not to Do

❌ Do not overlook the possibility of chronic pelvic inflammatory disease (PID), which can present with cyclic lower abdominal pain (associated with menses). In contrast to benign dysmenorrhea, PID would be expected to show abnormal cervical motion tenderness, uterine tenderness, and/or adnexal tenderness on pelvic examination.

❌ Do not recommend spinal manipulation for pain relief. There is reasonable evidence that it is ineffective.

Ⓧ Do not use NSAIDs if the patient wants to get pregnant; NSAIDs have been linked to reduced ovulation. If the patient is trying to get pregnant, use of these agents should be avoided.

Ⓧ Do not delay further gynecologic evaluation if the patient's symptoms persist for more than three cycles.

Discussion

Dysmenorrhea affects more than half of all menstruating women, with 10% to 15% suffering enough pain to interfere with work performance and home activities; it is a leading cause of short-term absenteeism from school in adolescent patients. It is most common during the late teens and 20s. Overproduction of prostaglandins E and F and leukotrienes in menstrual blood appears to stimulate uterine contractions and thus results in many of the symptoms of dysmenorrhea, including cramps, nausea, vomiting, bloating, and headaches. Vasopressin also may play a role by increasing uterine contractility and causing ischemic pain as a result of vasoconstriction. Risk factors for dysmenorrhea include nulliparity, heavy menstrual flow, smoking, and depression.

Most dysmenorrhea in adolescents is primary (or functional), associated with normal ovulatory cycle, with no anatomic pelvic disease. Family history of dysmenorrhea is predictive of dysmenorrhea, especially in a first-degree relative. Secondary dysmenorrhea can occur at any time after menarche, but usually occurs in the 20s through 40s and is more common in patients with first-degree relatives with endometriosis.

Empiric therapy can be initiated based on a typical history of painful menses and a normal physical examination. NSAIDs are the initial therapy of choice in patients with presumptive primary dysmenorrhea. There is no clear-cut advantage of one NSAID versus another in the treatment of dysmenorrhea. Therefore agent selection should be guided by cost, convenience, and patient preference, with ibuprofen or naproxen being good choices for most patients. Treatment with NSAIDs is most effective when initiated 1 to 2 days before the onset of menses. An adolescent who cannot predict the start of her period should be instructed to begin NSAID treatment as soon as menstrual bleeding begins or as soon as she has any menstruation-associated symptoms.

In the nonmenstruating adolescent with cyclic pain, a complete exam should be performed to evaluate for an anatomic abnormality such as transverse vaginal septum, imperforate hymen, or noncommunicating uterine horn.

Dysmenorrhea that does not respond to treatment (NSAIDs, OCPs, or other) administered for at least three ensuing menstrual cycles should raise suspicion of secondary dysmenorrhea. Refer to gynecology for further evaluation. Diagnosis of secondary dysmenorrhea often requires pelvic ultrasonography, hysteroscopy, laparoscopy, and/or endometrial biopsy to identify the underlying cause, including endometriosis (with or without endometrioma formation), uterine fibroids, and adenomyosis (ectopic endometrium within myometrium).

Primary dysmenorrhea often improves after childbirth.

Suggested Readings

Elsevier Point of Care. (2020). *Dysmenorrhea*. Amsterdam, Netherlands: Elsevier BV.

French, L. (2005). Dysmenorrhea. *American Family Physician, 71*, 285–291.

Harel, Z. (2004). Cyclooxygenase-2 specific inhibitors in the treatment of dysmenorrhea. *Journal of Pediatric and Adolescent Gynecology, 17*, 75–79.

Foreign Body, Vaginal

Presentation

Vaginal foreign bodies occur in both children and adults. The patient presents for care with a foul-smelling, bloody or brown purulent discharge, or pain. Children may insert a foreign body and not tell their parents or may be the victims of child abuse. Vaginal foreign bodies in the adult may be a result of a psychiatric disorder or sexual practices. Frequently, patients are reluctant to inform the examiner of the presence of the foreign body. Common vaginal foreign bodies in adults include condoms, contraceptive diaphragms, drug-smuggling devices, and sexual stimulation devices. Occasionally, a retained tampon or pessary is forgotten or lost and causes discomfort and a vaginal discharge. One study in children found the most common vaginal foreign bodies were toilet paper, beads, small parts of toys, cap of watercolor brush, and crayons.

What to Do

✅ **Visualize the vaginal vault to identify a foreign body or signs of vaginal trauma using a vaginal speculum for adults or a pediatric or nasal speculum for the pediatric patient. After performing a gentle speculum examination, if a foreign body is not visualized, consider bimanual or rectovaginal examination. Use procedural sedation (see Appendix E) in a child or frightened adult as necessary.**

✅ Other noninvasive methods used to identify foreign bodies in young patients include transperineal/transabdominal sonography, plain abdominal radiography, computed tomography (CT), and magnetic resonance imaging (MRI), all of which are imperfect and can miss foreign bodies.

✅ **Pediatric patients** may be placed in the knee-chest position. While a rectal examination is being performed, the foreign body may be expelled from the vagina by pushing it with the examining finger in the rectum.

✅ **Friable foreign bodies,** such as wads of toilet paper (one of the most common foreign bodies), may be flushed out using warm water or saline, an infant feeding tube, or a pediatric Foley catheter attached to a 60-mL syringe. The catheter tip is inserted into the vagina past the object, then flushed (using a moderate amount of pressure) with approximately 200 mL of fluid.

✅ **Lost or forgotten tampons can be removed with vaginal forceps that are first pierced through the finger of a polyvinyl glove, so that when the malodorous foreign body is extracted, the glove can immediately be pulled over it to reduce the odor before it is discarded in a sealed plastic bag. The vagina may then be swabbed with a Betadine solution. (See Video 90.1)**

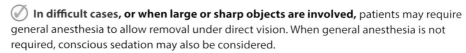

✓ **In difficult cases, or when large or sharp objects are involved,** patients may require general anesthesia to allow removal under direct vision. When general anesthesia is not required, conscious sedation may also be considered.

✓ **With objects that are not likely to cause harm,** the patient should first empty her bladder and then be examined in the lithotomy position. **Most objects can then be grasped with ring forceps, a tenaculum, or using a Foley catheter.** A Foley catheter can be used to break any suction between the foreign body and the vaginal mucosa, or it can be advanced past the object, inflated, and used to pull gentle traction on the object.

✓ In adults, objects in the vagina are usually apparent on examination. Radiographs are rarely indicated but can be considered for suspected radiopaque foreign bodies when ultrasonography is unavailable or nondiagnostic. When deep injury or deep migration of a long-standing foreign body is suspected, a CT scan or MRI might be indicated.

✓ When a foreign body is suspected in a child but cannot be visualized, refer the patient for examination under anesthesia and vaginoscopy, which allows the identification of foreign bodies, aids in the diagnosis of other conditions, and allows for a complete examination. A CT scan and MRI might be indicated as noted earlier.

What Not to Do

✗ Do not ignore a vaginal discharge in a pediatric patient or assume it is the result of benign vaginitis. A gentle rectoabdominal exam may reveal a hard object within the vagina.

✗ Do not forget to consider sexual abuse; therefore consult with protective services as needed.

Discussion

Always consider vaginal foreign body when evaluating a patient with vaginal complaints. Removal of a vaginal foreign body is generally successful, but when large objects make removal more difficult, use the additional techniques described for rectal foreign bodies (see Chapter 72).

Vaginal discharge in children is a common gynecologic complaint. Common sources for vaginal irritation or discharge include fecal contamination from poor perineal hygiene, spread of respiratory bacteria from hand-to-perineal contact, and local irritants such as bubble bath or nylon underwear. Recurrent or persistent vaginal discharge should raise concerns of an undiagnosed bacterial source, possible sexual abuse, and the possibility of a foreign body. Foreign bodies are the cause for 10% of girls presenting with a complaint of bloody discharge.

If a patient presents with vaginal discharge that does not respond to hygiene measures and medical therapy for other causes of vaginitis (see Chapter 94), or if the vaginal discharge is unusual, associated with bleeding, malodorous, and/or not consistent with clinical findings, a thorough investigation to rule out a foreign body must be performed.

Suggested Readings

Simon, D. A., Berry, S., Brannian, J., & Hansen, K. (2003). Recurrent, purulent vaginal discharge associated with longstanding presence of a foreign body and vaginal stenosis. *Journal of Pediatric and Adolescent Gynecology, 16,* 361–363.

Smith, Y. R., Berman, D. R., & Quint, E. H. (2002). Premenarchal vaginal discharge: Findings of procedures to rule out foreign bodies. *Journal of Pediatric and Adolescent Gynecology*, *15*, 227–230.

Yang, X., Sun, L., Ye, J., Li, X., & Tao, R. (2017). Ultrasonography in detection of vaginal foreign bodies in girls: A retrospective study. *Journal of Pediatric and Adolescent Gynecology*, *30*(6), 620–625. https://doi.org/10.1016/j.jpag.2017.06.008

Pelvic Inflammatory Disease (PID)

Presentation

A sexually active female, possibly with a new sex partner or multiple sex partners, presents with lower abdominal pain beginning with or soon after her last menstrual period. There may be associated vaginal discharge, malodor, dysuria, dyspareunia, menorrhagia, or intermenstrual bleeding. In patients with more severe infections, systemic symptoms such as fever, chills, malaise, nausea, and vomiting may also be present.

Women with severe pelvic pain tend to ambulate in a slightly bent-over position, holding their lower abdomen and shuffling their feet. Abdominal examination reveals lower quadrant tenderness, sometimes with rebound, and occasionally right upper quadrant tenderness resulting from perihepatitis (Fitz-Hugh–Curtis syndrome). Pelvic examination typically demonstrates bilateral adnexal tenderness as well as uterine fundal and cervical motion tenderness.

Many women with pelvic inflammatory disease (PID) exhibit subtle or mild symptoms with absence of fever and leukocytosis as well as minimal cervical motion tenderness and adnexal tenderness. Asymptomatic infections or atypical presentations may occur.

What to Do

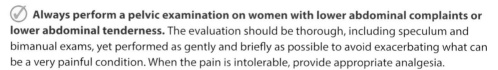 **Always perform a pelvic examination on women with lower abdominal complaints or lower abdominal tenderness.** The evaluation should be thorough, including speculum and bimanual exams, yet performed as gently and briefly as possible to avoid exacerbating what can be a very painful condition. When the pain is intolerable, provide appropriate analgesia.

Obtain urine for urinalysis and pregnancy testing. A catheterized urine specimen may be necessary when vaginal discharge or bleeding is present.

Evaluate for *Neisseria gonorrhoeae* and *Chlamydia trachomatis* with nucleic acid amplification testing if available. If not available, cultures or older nonculture techniques such as direct fluorescent antibody, enzyme immunoassay, and nonamplified nucleic acid hybridization can be used; however, these are less sensitive.

When PID is suspected, strongly consider testing for other sexually transmitted infections (STIs), including syphilis, hepatitis B, hepatitis C, and human immunodeficiency virus (HIV), as these infections may be contracted simultaneously.

Consider obtaining an erythrocyte sedimentation rate and C-reactive protein level. These are indicators of clinical severity, but normal results do not rule out PID.

✅ **Determine the pH of any vaginal discharge, and make wet-mount examinations of endocervical secretions, looking for** *Candida*, *Trichomonas*, **leukocytes, and clue cells** (see Chapter 94).

✅ Perform pelvic ultrasonography if there is a suspected mass, severe pain, or a positive pregnancy test. One of the most specific criteria for diagnosing PID is the finding of thickened, fluid-filled fallopian tubes, with or without free pelvic fluid, on transvaginal sonography.

✅ **Maintain a low threshold for diagnosing PID. No laboratory tests are diagnostic for PID, and the clinical diagnosis is imprecise. In addition, the long-term sequelae of missing PID are significant and include infertility, tubo-ovarian abscess (TOA), perihepatitis, chronic pelvic pain, and ectopic pregnancy.**

✅ **Maintain a low threshold to initiate treatment of PID in sexually active young women (highest rates in women ages 15–19 years) and other women at risk for STIs if no other causes for their illness can be identified and they have cervical motion and uterine or adnexal tenderness.** Risk factors for STIs include new or multiple sex partners, sexual debut at age younger than 18 years, inconsistent use of barrier precautions, sexual intercourse during menses, and previous STI or PID.

✅ These **additional criteria** may be used to enhance the specificity of the minimum criteria already mentioned and further support a diagnosis of PID:

- Oral temperature greater than 101° F (>38.3° C)
- Abnormal cervical or vaginal mucopurulent discharge
- Presence of white blood cells (WBCs) on wet-mount examination of vaginal secretions
- Elevated erythrocyte sedimentation rate
- Elevated C-reactive protein level
- Laboratory documentation of cervical infection with *N. gonorrhoeae* and/or *C. trachomatis*

✅ **Investigate alternative causes for pain if the cervical discharge appears normal and no WBCs are found on the wet-mount examination. Consider transvaginal sonography and spiral computed tomography (CT) scanning to help rule out other potential gynecologic, gastrointestinal (especially appendicitis), or urologic causes.**

✅ **When in doubt, always treat.** Subtle findings may include only a history of abnormal uterine bleeding, dyspareunia, vaginal discharge, or cervical purulence.

✅ **The presence of an intrauterine device (IUD) does not affect management. It is unnecessary to immediately remove an IUD if clinically improving. Consider removing the device if there is no improvement after 3 days from initiation of therapy.**

✅ **The presence of HIV infection alone should not change management of PID.**

✅ **Treat suspected cases while awaiting diagnostic confirmation.** Prevention of long-term sequelae has been linked directly with early administration of appropriate antibiotics. When selecting a treatment regimen, consider availability, cost, medication allergies, and antimicrobial susceptibility.

✓ **Hospitalize all patients with pelvic abscess or TOA, pregnancy, high fever (≥38.5° C), septicemia, nausea and vomiting that preclude oral antibiotics, as well as when surgical emergencies (e.g., appendicitis) cannot be excluded.** Inpatient treatment may be necessary when there are complicating issues such as immune compromise, failure of oral therapy after 48 hours, or inability to complete outpatient treatment or follow-up plan.

✓ Inpatient treatment for PID, with or without TOA, consists of intravenous (IV) antibiotics. Give cefotetan, 2 g intravenously once every 12 hours, or cefoxitin, 2 g intravenously once every 6 hours, plus doxycycline, 100 mg orally once every 12 hours. (Because of pain associated with infusion, doxycycline should be administered orally when possible, even when the patient is hospitalized.) Alternatively, give clindamycin, 900 mg intravenously once every 8 hours, plus gentamicin, 3 to 5 mg/kg intravenously daily. The transition to oral therapy from parenteral can start after 24 to 48 hours, with demonstrated clinical improvement.

✓ **Treat mild to moderate cases on an outpatient basis.** Coverage of *Neisseria gonorrhoeae* and *Chlamydia trachomatis* should be provided even if test results for these organisms are negative. **Give ceftriaxone (Rocephin), 500 mg intramuscularly in a single dose, plus doxycycline, 100 mg orally twice a day for 14 days, with or without metronidazole (Flagyl), 500 mg orally twice a day for 14 days. Coverage of anaerobes may require the addition of metronidazole, which will also effectively treat bacterial vaginosis and trichomoniasis, frequently associated with PID.**

✓ When ceftriaxone cannot be used for treating urogenital or rectal gonorrhea because of cephalosporin allergy, a single 240 mg IM dose of gentamicin plus a single 2 g oral dose of azithromycin is an option. Gastrointestinal symptoms, primarily vomiting within 1 hour of dosing, have been reported among 3%–4% of treated persons (26). If administration of IM ceftriaxone is not available, a single 800 mg oral dose of cefixime is an alternative regimen. However, cefixime does not provide as high, or as sustained, bactericidal blood levels as does ceftriaxone and demonstrates limited treatment efficacy for pharyngeal gonorrhea.

✓ **Because of the changing patterns of antibiotic resistance, always check for the latest CDC antimicrobial guidelines for the treatment of all STIs.**

✓ **Arrange for follow-up examination within 72 hours.** Patients should demonstrate substantial clinical improvement (e.g., defervescence, reduction in direct or rebound abdominal tenderness, and reduction in uterine, adnexal, and cervical motion tenderness) within 3 days of initiation of therapy. Patients who do not improve within this period usually require hospitalization, additional diagnostic tests, and possible surgical intervention.

✓ **Provide analgesics as needed.**

✓ **Instruct the patient to abstain from sexual intercourse for at least 2 weeks.**

✓ **Treat sexual partners for presumptive gonorrhea and chlamydia if they had sexual contact with the patient during the 60 days preceding the patient's onset of symptoms. Use ceftriaxone (Rocephin), 500 mg intramuscularly once, PLUS doxycycline (Vibramycin), 100 mg orally twice a day for 7 days.** In cases where gonococcal expedited partner therapy (provision of prescriptions or medications for the patient to take to a sex partner without the health care provider first examining the partner) is permissible by state law and the partner is unable or unlikely to seek timely treatment, the partner may be treated with a single 800 mg oral dose of cefixime, provided that concurrent chlamydial infection in the patient has been excluded. Otherwise, the partner may be treated with a single oral 800 mg cefixime dose plus oral doxycycline 100 mg twice daily for 7 days.

✓ Male partners of women who have PID caused by *C. trachomatis* and/or *N. gonorrhoeae* often are asymptomatic. Sex partners should be treated empirically with regimens that are effective against both of these infections, regardless of the pathogens isolated from the infected woman. Patient-delivered treatment of sex partners was associated with a reduced risk for recurrent gonorrhea and/or chlamydia in a University of Washington study.

✓ **Counsel the patient about the sexually transmitted nature of PID and its risks** for infertility and ectopic pregnancy. (Three years after treatment for PID, 18% of women reported infertility, and the risk for ectopic pregnancy is increased 6-fold to 10-fold.) Importantly, as many as 29% of women diagnosed with PID will develop chronic pelvic pain, which is associated with a lower quality of physical and mental health. Counsel the patient on the importance of barrier methods of contraception (condoms) to reduce the risk of STI transmission.

✓ **Test-of-cure is recommended to be done in 7-14 days following treatment.**

✓ **Rescreen the patient in 3 to 4 months** because reinfection is common. In one study, 15% to 23% of patients had one or more new infections, and 66% were asymptomatic.

What Not to Do

✗ Do not miss the more unilateral disorders such as ectopic pregnancy, appendicitis, ovarian cyst or torsion, and diverticulitis.

✗ Do not diagnose PID in a patient with a positive pregnancy test without ruling out ectopic pregnancy.

✗ Do not ignore pelvic symptoms if the patient has perihepatic inflammation.

✗ Do not assume sexual activity based on age.

Discussion

The Centers for Disease Control and Prevention (CDC) recommends a low threshold for empiric treatment of PID based on minimal criteria that can be assessed by history and physical examination alone.

The clinical diagnosis of acute PID is imprecise. The positive predictive value (PPV) of a clinical diagnosis of acute PID differs, depending on epidemiologic characteristics and the clinical setting. There is a higher PPV among sexually active young women (particularly adolescents) and among patients attending STI clinics or from settings in which rates of gonorrhea or chlamydia are high. In all settings, however, no single historical, physical, or laboratory finding is both sensitive and specific for the diagnosis of acute PID (i.e., can be used both to detect all cases of PID and to exclude all women without PID).

In spite of this, **prompt diagnosis and early presumptive treatment are crucial to maintaining** fertility and avoiding the other complications of PID. It should be kept in mind that the diagnosis and management of other common causes of lower abdominal pain (e.g., ectopic pregnancy, acute appendicitis, and functional pain) are unlikely to be impaired by initiating empiric antimicrobial therapy for PID.

PID is defined as salpingitis, often accompanied by endometritis or secondary pelvic peritonitis, which results from an ascending genital infection. In the United States there is an increased risk for PID with multiple sex partners, nonbarrier contraceptive use, instrumentation of the cervix, smoking, minority race, use of an IUD, previous history of PID, and vaginal douching. The incubation period for PID varies from 1 to 2 days to weeks or months.

Gonorrheal and chlamydial infections are thought to initiate conditions that allow organisms from

(continued)

Discussion continued

the lower genital tract to ascend into the upper genital tract. The resulting polymicrobial infection includes facultative and anaerobic organisms. A variety of gram-positive and gram-negative aerobic and anaerobic pathogens, such as aerobic streptococci, *Escherichia coli*, *Bacteroides fragilis*, *Proteus* spp., and *Peptostreptococcus* spp. can be recovered from the uterus, fallopian tubes, and peritoneal cavity. Gonococcal and chlamydial PID often occur within a week of the onset of menses. **The absence of a positive test for *N. gonorrhoeae* or *C. trachomatis* does not rule out PID,** because these microbes are only found in 25% to 40% of patients. A mixed aerobic and anaerobic infection is found in 25% to 60% of cases. **PID associated with gonorrhea produces relatively rapid and more severe symptoms than chlamydia, whereas the latter is associated with more severe scarring.**

Tubo-ovarian abscess should be suspected in the setting of PID with persistent fever, despite adequate antibiotics, continued lower abdominal pain, or adnexal mass. Pelvic ultrasonography is

highly sensitive (90–95%) in diagnosing TOA. It is usually amenable to medical therapy but requires surgical intervention in up to 25% of cases. Surgical intervention for TOA should be considered if there is an increase in the size of the abscess, or a size larger than 10 cm, persistent fever spikes, suspected abscess rupture (requiring urgent surgery), or lack of clinical improvement in 48 to 72 hours. Drainage of the abscess can be done percutaneously (by interventional radiology) or laparoscopically.

Although all of the gonorrheal isolates in the United States are susceptible to cephalosporins, resistance to quinolones has developed. Fluoroquinolones are no longer recommended for the treatment of PID. Laparoscopy is indicated in severe cases if diagnosis is uncertain or there is inadequate response to initial antibiotic therapy.

Consult public health authorities or websites for local and national reporting requirements.

A diagnosis of PID in children or young adolescents should prompt an evaluation for possible child abuse.

Suggested Readings

Arrendondo, J. L., Oyarzún, E., Paz, R., et al. (1997). Oral clindamycin and ciprofloxacin versus intramuscular ceftriaxone and oral doxycycline in the treatment of mild-to-moderate pelvic inflammatory disease in outpatients. *Clinical Infectious Diseases*, *24*, 170–178.

Braverman, P. K. (2000). Sexually transmitted diseases in adolescents. *Medical Clinics of North America*, *84*, 869–889.

Campion, E. W., Brunham, R. C., Gottlieb, S. L., & Paavonen, J. (2015). Pelvic inflammatory disease. *New England Journal of Medicine*, *372*(21), 2039–2048.

Elsevier Point of Care. (2018). *Pelvic inflammatory disease*. Amsterdam, Netherlands: Elsevier BV.

Epperly, A. T. A., & Viera, A. J. (2005). Pelvic inflammatory disease. *Clinics in Family Practice*, *7*, 67–78.

Ford, G. W., & Decker, C. F. (2016). Pelvic inflammatory disease. *Disease-a-Month*, *62*(8), 301–305.

Golden, M. R., Whittington, W. L., Handsfield, H. H., et al. (2005). Effect of expedited treatment of sex partners on recurrent or persistent gonorrhea or chlamydial infection. *New England Journal of Medicine*, *35*, 676–685.

Nasraty, S. (2003). Infections of the female genital tract. *Primary Care*, *30*, 193–203. vii.

Ness, R. B., Soper, D. E., Holley, R. L., et al. (2002). Effectiveness of inpatient and outpatient treatment strategies for women with pelvic inflammatory disease: Results from the pelvic inflammatory disease evaluation and clinical health (PEACH) randomized trial. *American Journal of Obstetrics and Gynecology*, *186*, 929–937.

Sancta St. Cyr, MD1; Lindley Barbee, MD1,2; Kimberly A. Workowski, MD1,3; Laura H. Bachmann, MD1; Cau Pham, PhD1; Karen Schlanger, PhD1; Elizabeth Torrone, PhD1; Hillard Weinstock, MD1; Ellen N. Kersh, PhD1; Phoebe Thorpe, MD1; Update to CDC's Treatment Guidelines for Gonococcal Infection, 2020 Weekly / December 18, 2020 / 69(50);1911–1916.

Simms, I., Wharburton, F., & Weström, L. (2003). Diagnosis of pelvic inflammatory disease: Time for a rethink. *Sexually Transmitted Infections*, *79*, 491–494.

Prophylaxis Following Sexual Exposure

Presentation

A female patient presents for evaluation after sexual contact. There was no barrier to prevent sexually transmitted infections (STIs) or pregnancy, or the barrier method being used was suspected to have failed (e.g., a condom broke or contraceptive pills were used imperfectly). Sexual contact may be described as consensual or nonconsensual, such as the result of a sexual assault or sexual abuse. Patients may present asymptomatic or with a variety of symptoms or examination findings.

What to Do

✓ **Try to determine if the sexual contact was consensual,** and if it was not, contact your local antisexual violence resources for further forensic examination of the patient and evidence collection if the patient desires. **Assist the patient in contacting law enforcement if they desire.**

✓ **The type of sexual contact should be discussed,** as anal receptive or insertive intercourse has a significantly higher risk of HIV transmission than oral insertive or receptive, which is quite low.

✓ **A thorough physical exam on any patient reporting assault or abuse is necessary,** looking for signs of trauma such as evidence of strangulation (petechia, subconjunctivial hemorrhage, neck bruising or ligature marks), as well as external genitalia and pelvic speculum examinations. Apply basic first aid if needed, with further testing or consultation as necessary for complex injuries such as strangulation injuries, extensive vaginal lacerations/hemorrhage, etc.

✓ **All female patients who present for evaluation after unprotected intercourse, contraception failure, or sexual assault should be offered emergency contraception.** Patients should be given information on options for STI testing and treatment, including HIV postexposure prophylaxis (PEP). (See CDC Guidelines: https://www.cdc.gov/hiv/pdf/programresources/cdc-hiv-npep-guidelines.pdf.)

✓ **Emergency contraception (EC)** is important to decrease the incidence of undesired pregnancy. A copper intrauterine device (IUD) placed within 5 days of unprotected or underprotected sex is the most effective method of EC, however is not routinely utilized in urgent care centers or emergency departments.

✓ **Common oral EC methods** include ulipristal (Ella) and levonorgestrel (Plan B). Ulipristal 30 mg as a one-time dose can be used up to 5 days after unprotected intercourse and is available by prescription only. Ulipristal is a selective progestin receptor modulator and therefore delays ovulation. There are no contraindications. Levonorgestrel 1.5 mg can be used up to 3 days after unprotected intercourse and is available over the counter. It is ideally taken as a single 1.5-mg dose; however, it can be given in two doses of 0.75 mg separated by 12 hours. Levonorgestrel can thicken the cervical mucus and inhibits or delays ovulation. Both medications are safe in breastfeeding mothers and have not been linked to any adverse pregnancy outcomes. The most common side effects of both oral EC methods include nausea, vomiting, abdominal pain, and irregular menses.

✅ **In addition to EC, patients should also be offered testing or treatment for STIs** including gonorrhea, chlamydia, and trichomoniasis (see Chapter 91) as well as HIV PEP (see Chapter 147).

What Not to Do

❌ Do not forget to consider sexual abuse or assault and examine for additional injuries such as evidence of vaginal or anal lacerations, bruises, or ligature marks to suggest strangulation.

❌ Do not exclude sexual assault based on a normal physical exam. Many survivors of sexual assault will have no visible injuries and may have highly variable emotional responses to trauma.

❌ Do not forget to attempt to interview the patient alone, as they may withhold part of the history if others are in the room.

❌ Do not forget to screen patients for indicators of human trafficking (e.g., suspicious injuries, minors being involved, apparent prostitution, a dependency relationship, signs of punishment or being restrained, being seen with a known suspect, unexplained STIs or perineal injuries, depression, malnourished or unkempt appearance, and as noted below).

❌ Do not forget to arrange follow-up for further evaluation of patients who are at risk for contracting HIV or hepatitis C or are being prescribed HIV PEP.

❌ Do not forget to provide the patient with support from the appropriate local social services and if necessary help ensure that they have a safe plan upon discharge.

Discussion

EC should be routinely offered to patients presenting for evaluation within 5 days after sexual exposure without adequate protection. Copper IUDs are the most effective EC; however, urgent care and emergency departments are often unequipped to insert these. Both Ulipristal and Levonorgestrel can both be taken as a single dose in the first 3 to 5 days after unprotected intercourse. Both oral ECs are safe in breastfeeding mothers, and neither have been linked to adverse pregnancy outcomes. The most common side effects of oral EC methods include nausea, vomiting, abdominal pain, and irregular menses.

Evaluation of patients presenting for evaluation after unprotected or underprotected sexual exposure should include a thorough history and physical examination. Determine if the sexual contact was consensual, and if it was not, contact local forensic nursing and social support or advocacy resources as needed. **Screen patients for indicators of human trafficking, such as delayed presentation of illnesses, domineering or controlling family or visitors, and/or inconsistent histories.** If abuse or assault is reported or suspected, physical exams should include genitourinary exams as well as a more thorough skin and musculoskeletal exam to assess for other injuries. In addition to EC, patients should be counseled on and offered STI testing or treatment as well as HIV PEP when appropriate. Ensure patients have a safe plan upon discharge.

Suggested Reading

Bullock, H., & Salcedo, J. (2015). Emergency contraception. *Obstetrics and Gynecology Clinics, 42*, 699–712.

Vaginal Bleeding

Presentation

A worried menstruating female presents with greater-than-usual bleeding, which is either off of her usual schedule (metrorrhagia), lasts longer than a typical period, or is heavier than usual (menorrhagia), perhaps with crampy pains and passage of clots. Bleeding is considered prolonged when lasting longer than 7 days. Profuse bleeding is generally defined as soaking a large sanitary pad or tampon every 1 to 2 hours and continuing for more than 2 hours. Excessive menstrual bleeding is quantified typically as greater than 80 mL, with normal menstrual losses over an average cycle of 5 to 7 days of 30 to 45 mL.

What to Do

✅ Establish whether there is hemodynamic instability, clearly identify the source of bleeding, and evaluate the volume of blood loss.

✅ **Obtain orthostatic pulse and blood pressure measurements, a complete blood count, type and screen, and pregnancy test** (urine or serum β-human chorionic gonadotropin [β-hCG]). Measurement of β-hCG is required in all menstruating women, except when there are positive fetal heart tones, a known pregnancy, or a definite history of hysterectomy. All others should have β-hCG measured, including those with tubal ligation, implantable contraception, claims of celibate lifestyle, female partners, and those whose doctors have told them they cannot get pregnant. (To avoid unintentionally insulting a patient, inform her that pregnancy testing is routinely required in all cases of vaginal bleeding.) Although less reliable than hemoglobin and hematocrit measurements, try to quantify the amount of bleeding by the presence of clots and the number of saturated pads used. In the United States, regular to super-plus tampons hold 6 to 15 mL of blood.

✅ **If the patient is deemed hemodynamically unstable,** arrange for rapid transport to an acute care setting, such as an emergency department by ambulance. Start an intravenous (IV) infusion of normal saline or lactated Ringer solution and have blood ready to transfuse on short notice if there is significant bleeding—demonstrated by pallor, lightheadedness, tachycardia, orthostatic pressure changes, a pulse increase of more than 20 beats per minute on standing, or a hematocrit below 30%. Consider intrauterine tamponade by packing the uterus with Kerlix. A Foley catheter inflated within the cervical os can also help tamponade uncontrolled hemorrhage. Uterine curettage is first-line therapy for the unstable patient with acute or prolonged uterine bleeding. Uterine artery embolization is first-line therapy for those with uterine arteriovenous malformation. Hysterectomy is recommended when all other treatments have failed.

✓ **If the patient is hemodynamically stable, obtain a thorough history, including a menstrual, sexual, and reproductive history.** Inquire if the patient's menses are usually irregular, occasionally heavy. Ask about oral contraceptive pills (OCPs) and compliance·with these medications as missed doses can initiate a withdrawal bleed. Ask if there is an intrauterine device (IUD) in place, which may be contributing to cramps, bleeding, or a source of infection. It is important to consider the most recent menstrual cycle. If this was missed or light, or if this period is late, that may be suggestive of an anovulatory cycle, a spontaneous abortion, or an ectopic pregnancy. Ask about a family history of bleeding disorders and a personal history of bruising, petechiae, or other signs suggestive of coagulopathy, especially when onset of menorrhagia began at menarche. Ask about use of anticoagulants, such as aspirin or warfarin (Coumadin). Other medications such as antiepileptic agents (especially valproic acid), as well as typical and atypical antipsychotics and steroids, can also cause abnormal uterine bleeding. Ask about any history of thyroid, renal, or hepatic disease; determine if the patient is involved in high-risk sexual activity (e.g., unprotected sexual intercourse, new and/or multiple sexual partners, trauma). Also inquire about any known structural abnormalities, such as a history of fibroid uterus.

✓ **Determine the source of bleeding. Perform a speculum and bimanual vaginal examination, inspecting the vulva, vagina, cervical surface/os, uterus, and anus.** Look for signs of early pregnancy (e.g., a soft blue cervix, enlarged uterus, passage of fetal parts with the blood) and visualize for menstrual flow, lacerations, pathologic lesions, or rectal bleeding. For patients with vaginal bleeding in early pregnancy (before 20 weeks of gestation and prior to fetal viability), the differential diagnosis includes miscarriage, ectopic pregnancy, implantation bleeding, molar pregnancy, and ruptured corpus luteum cyst.

✓ **Recognition and management of second- and third-trimester bleeding are beyond the scope of this book and are not covered in this chapter.**

✓ Ascertain that the blood is coming from the cervical os and not from a laceration, polyp, cervical lesion, or other vaginal or uterine disease or infection. Test for sexually transmitted infections (STIs), including gonorrhea and chlamydia when infection may be a factor, particularly in the young sexually active patient with intermenstrual spotting and/or prolonged menses (see Chapters 83, 91, and 94). Palpate for adnexal masses as well as pelvic tenderness. Spread any questionable products of conception on gauze or suspend in saline to differentiate from organized clot. Gently press sterile ring forceps against the cervix to see whether they enter the uterus, indicating that the internal os is open (a sign of an inevitable, complete, or incomplete abortion) or closed (not pregnant or a threatened abortion, the fetus having roughly even odds of survival, which is generally treated with bed rest alone).

Pregnant Patients:

✓ **Obtain a transvaginal ultrasonogram and quantitative β-hCG level if the urine β-hCG is positive or there is any uterine or adnexal abnormality on pelvic examination.** A sonogram will help assess the age and viability of a fetus in an intrauterine pregnancy. An ectopic gestational sac may be seen. **A sonogram showing an empty uterus, despite a positive pregnancy test, may be indicative of either a very early intrauterine pregnancy, an ectopic pregnancy, or a recent complete abortion.** It should be noted that ectopic pregnancy is the leading cause of first trimester maternal death and is common among patients presenting with pain or bleeding in the first trimester of pregnancy. When an ectopic gestational sac is discovered, urgent gynecologic consultation is required.

✅ **When the β-hCG result is positive, there is no clear evidence of an ectopic or intrauterine pregnancy, and the patient's condition remains stable**, repeat the quantitative measurement in 48 hours. In a healthy pregnancy, the hCG should approximately double in 48 hours. An inappropriate rise in the hCG without a visible intrauterine pregnancy on ultrasound should raise suspicion for an ectopic pregnancy.

✅ **With incomplete spontaneous abortions, deliver any products of conception that protrude from the cervical os using steady gentle traction with sponge forceps while compressing and massaging the uterus. If bleeding continues**, consider starting an IV infusion of oxytocin (Pitocin) 10 U, at 20 milliunits (mU)/min, to diminish the rate of hemorrhage. Alternatively, place 10 IU of oxytocin in 1 L of 0.9% normal saline and run it at 200 to 500 mL/hr, or give methylergonovine (Methergine), 0.2 mg intramuscularly (contraindicated in the hypertensive patient). Obtain gynecologic consultation to consider performing a dilation and curettage (D&C) for emergent termination of the uterine bleeding. **With all bleeding while pregnant, test the mother's Rh status;** if negative, administer Rh immunoglobulin (RhoGAM). A 50-μg IM dose can be given if the uterus is less than 12 weeks in size. If this is not available, or if the gestation is greater than 12 weeks, then a 300-μg IM dose should be administered.

✅ **It is appropriate to discharge the stable patient with a threatened abortion, as determined by an intrauterine pregnancy on ultrasound, unless there is severe pain or hemorrhage.** Bed rest has not been shown to improve the outcome for a threatened abortion but is still usually part of the regimen.

Nonpregnant Patients:

✅ **Treatment of stable nonpregnant patients with menorrhagia includes nonhormonal treatments such as nonsteroidal anti-inflammatory drugs (NSAIDs). Despite their varying degree of platelet activity inhibition, NSAIDs decrease blood loss by reducing endometrial prostaglandin levels and promoting vasoconstriction in the uterus.**

✅ **Treat simple menorrhagia and suspected anovulatory bleeding with standard regimens of OCPs plus NSAIDs given on the first 3 days of the menstrual period.** Anovulatory bleeding is typically not accompanied by breast discomfort, increased vaginal discharge, or premenstrual cramping and bloating. Ovulatory dysfunction encompasses abnormal uterine bleeding as a result of an immature hypothalamic-pituitary axis (in adolescents), endocrinopathy (e.g., polycystic ovary syndrome, hypothyroidism), mental stress, anorexia, weight loss, or extreme exercise.

✅ **In stable patients with suspected moderate anovulatory bleeding, consider the tapering of OCPs for treatment. Prescribe an OCP with at least 35 μg ethinyl estradiol (Necon 10/11 or Ortho Novum 10/11), administered at a dose of one pill four times a day tapered for 3 to 5 days until the bleeding stops, and then decreased to one pill per day until the month's pack is completed. Provide the patient with an antiemetic and discuss the possibility of withdrawal bleeding at the end of this new cycle.** This regimen is contraindicated in women over age 35 years who smoke and in women who have a history of deep vein thrombosis or pulmonary embolism, breast cancer, liver disease, known thromboembolic disorders, pregnancy, ischemic heart disease, cerebrovascular disease, or uncontrolled hypertension.

✅ **When it is necessary to help control vaginal bleeding in the nonpregnant patient who has moderate to heavy bleeding, oral conjugated estrogen (Premarin), 2.5 mg orally four** times a day, can be given until the bleeding subsides. Typically bleeding will stop within 10 to 24 hours. For mild to moderate bleeding, the dose can be twice a day, but is not to be continued for more than 21 to 25 days. After the estrogen, a progestin should be given, medroxyprogesterone acetate, 5 to 10 mg orally, daily for 5 to 10 days, start on day 16 or 21 of cycle. Warn the patient that after the initial reduction of bleeding, there will be an increase in hemorrhage when the uterine lining is sloughed.

✓ For acute severe abnormal uterine bleeding, conjugated estrogen (Premarin), 25 mg, can be given IV (inject slowly to reduce flushing) and repeated every 6 to 12 hours until bleeding stops, up to 24 hours. It will take several hours to have an effect. When available, this treatment should be coordinated with a consulting gynecologist. This drug is contraindicated in patients with active or past thromboembolic disease, breast cancer, or liver disease. Estrogens cause nausea and vomiting in high doses, so an antiemetic should also be prescribed.

✓ Tranexamic acid (TXA), 1300 mg, by mouth, three times a day for 5 days, is a medication that helps prevent clot breakdown and may be used in the event of uncontrolled bleeding associated with heavy menorrhagia. It has an onset of 2 to 3 hours. Use with caution when there is renal impairment or a thromboembolic history. Use is contraindicated in women using combined hormonal contraception or those with active thromboembolic disease.

✓ If the cause of the uterine bleeding was from missed OCPs, advise the patient to resume the pills but use additional contraception for the first cycle to prevent pregnancy.

✓ If the cause is a new IUD, the patient may elect to have it removed and use another contraceptive technique.

✓ In most cases, the patient should be referred for follow-up to a gynecologist for definitive diagnosis, adjustment of medications, or further treatment. Further evaluation may include hysteroscopy, ultrasonography, and endometrial biopsy. Endometrial ablation is an option for those for whom medical therapy has been unsuccessful or is contraindicated because of thrombosis risks. This procedure is also recommended, rather than D&C, for those patients bleeding from polyps or intracavitary leiomyomas.

✓ D&C is recommended for removing retained products of conception and for those women wishing to maintain fertility.

✓ Medical evaluation may reveal liver disease, hypothyroidism (even when there is a minimally high thyroid-stimulating hormone [TSH] level, there may be a response to treatment), or a bleeding disorder (especially thrombocytopenia and von Willebrand disease).

What Not to Do

✗ Do not prescribe estrogen therapy to women at risk for intravascular thrombosis. In these women, use progestins or provide surgical intervention. Be aware that TXA may also increase the risk of thromboembolic events; monitor appropriately.

✗ Do not leap to a diagnosis of anovulatory bleeding or benign menorrhagia without ruling out pregnancy.

✗ Do not forget to rule out pregnancy or STI in patients on the basis of a negative sexual history alone—confirm with physical examination and laboratory tests.

Do not give aspirin for menorrhagia. It is not effective and may increase bleeding.

Do not attempt to use methylergonovine in the nonpregnant patient. It has no effect.

Discussion

Abnormal uterine bleeding occurs in women of all ages and is the most common reason why women seek gynecologic care. Abnormal vaginal bleeding in nonpregnant women is rarely life threatening but may herald serious underlying pathology such as cancer. Bleeding as a complication of pregnancy poses significant risk of morbidity and mortality to the fetus and mother.

The patient's age should direct you to the most likely cause of her vaginal bleeding. Vaginal bleeding in a newborn may be the result of withdrawal of maternal hormones. In **prepubertal girls,** look for anatomic lesions, urethral prolapse, vulvovaginal infections, endocrinopathies, neoplasia, rectal fissures, trauma, or foreign bodies, and consider abuse. Scratching prompted by dermatoses may also cause bleeding. In **postmenarchal adolescents and women of reproductive age,** consider pregnancy first, then bleeding due to ovulatory dysfunction (anovulatory cycles), infection with STIs, anatomic lesions (fibroids, cervical polyps), and systemic illnesses (hypothyroidism, bleeding disorders). In **nonpregnant adolescents,** 50% of severe menorrhagia at the first menses is the result of a coagulopathy (i.e., thrombocytopenia, immune thrombocytopenic purpura, platelet dysfunction, and von Willebrand disease). In **perimenopausal and postmenopausal women,** rule out malignant disease; then evaluate for atrophic vaginitis, fibroids, polyps, anovulatory dysfunctional uterine bleeding, liver disease, anticoagulation therapy, and bleeding disorders. One-third of postmenopausal bleeding is associated with common premalignant or malignant conditions of the endometrium (e.g., hyperplasia and atypia). The most common cause in this age group is endometrial atrophy.

Ovulatory dysfunction and iatrogenic uterine bleeding are diagnoses of exclusion. It is usually hormonal in etiology and can be the result of either abnormal endogenous hormone production or the administration of prescribed synthetic sex hormones, such as OCPs. During an anovulatory cycle, there is no progesterone, which results in a chaotic estrogen-stimulated endometrial proliferation. The uterine lining therefore hypertrophies and sloughs erratically, resulting in excessive or irregular uterine bleeding. This occurs most commonly around the time of menarche in girls and menopause in women. Other causes include a severely restricted diet, including eating disorders, prolonged exercise, and significant emotional stress.

Breakthrough bleeding is a form of estrogen withdrawal while taking low-dose estrogen OCPs. Changing to a higher-dose pill will generally eliminate this problem. Also consider drug interactions with certain anticonvulsants and antibiotics.

The essential steps in the emergency evaluation and management of vaginal bleeding are fluid resuscitation of shock, if present; recognition of any anatomic lesion, infection, or pregnancy; and complications of pregnancy, such as spontaneous abortion or ectopic pregnancy. Treatment of the more chronic and less severe causes of abnormal uterine bleeding usually consists of iron replacement and optional use of OCPs to decrease menstrual irregularity (metrorrhagia) and volume (menorrhagia).

The half-life of β-hCG after the end of pregnancy is 1.5 days, and a sensitive pregnancy test may remain positive for 2 to 4 weeks after a miscarriage or abortion.

There has been an important change in the accepted nomenclature used to describe abnormal bleeding in nonpregnant women. Since 2011, the American College of Obstetricians and Gynecologists (ACOG) has recommended the PALM-COEIN classification system, which uses the all-inclusive term *abnormal uterine bleeding* (AUB) and divides the causes of AUB into structural and nonstructural causes. Structural causes include **p**olyps, **a**denomyosis, **l**eiomyomas, and **m**alignancy (**PALM**). Nonstructural causes include **c**oagulopathy, **o**vulatory dysfunction, **e**ndometrial, **i**atrogenic, and **n**ot yet classified causes (**COEIN**). The use of the term *dysfunctional uterine bleeding* is no longer recommended.

Suggested Readings

Bevan, J. A., Maloney, K. W., Hillery, C. A., et al. (2001). Bleeding disorders: A common cause of menorrhagia in adolescents. *The Journal of Pediatrics, 138*, 856–861.

Borhart, J. (2018). Vaginal bleeding. In *Rosen's emergency medicine: Concepts and clinical practice* (pp. 270–274 e1 [chap 31]). Philadelphia, PA: Elsevier. e1 [chap 31]).

Elsevier Point of Care. (2019). *Abnormal uterine bleeding in women of reproductive age.* Amsterdam, Netherlands: Elsevier BV.

Falcone, T., Desjardins, C., Bourque, J., et al. (1994). Dysfunctional uterine bleeding in adolescents. *Journal of Reproductive Medicine, 39*, 761–764.

Heller, D. S. (2005). Lower genital tract disease in children and adolescents—a review. *Journal of Pediatric and Adolescent Gynecology, 18*, 75–83.

Vaginitis

Presentation

A patient presents for evaluation of vaginal discharge, possibly with itching and/or irritation of the labia and vagina. Odor, dysuria, vague low abdominal discomfort, or dyspareunia may be present.

Abdominal examination is benign, but examination of the introitus may reveal erythema of the vulva and edema of the labia, often with pustulopapular peripheral lesions (especially with *Candida* organisms). Speculum examination may disclose a diffusely red, inflamed vaginal mucosa with an adherent thick, white discharge resembling cottage cheese. These findings are also most likely the result of *Candida* organisms, especially when associated with vulvar pruritus.

A thin, homogeneous, gray-to-white milklike discharge smoothly coating the vaginal wall and having a fishy odor is characteristic of bacterial vaginosis (BV).

Profuse yellow-green or gray, sometimes frothy discharge with an unpleasant malodor and associated vulvar irritation is characteristic of *Trichomonas* organisms. Up to 70% of women infected with trichomonas, however, are asymptomatic. Cervical inspection may reveal a strawberry or punctate appearance.

Bimanual examination should demonstrate a nontender cervix and uterus, without adnexal tenderness or masses or pain on cervical motion (if present, see Chapter 91).

The appearance of the discharge is not pathognomonic, and testing needs to confirm any suspicion.

What to Do

⊘ Take a sexual history. Ask if partners are experiencing related symptoms.

⊘ Perform speculum and bimanual pelvic examination.

⊘ **Collect urine for urinalysis, possible culture, and pregnancy test.**

⊘ **Collect endocervical or vaginal swabs for nucleic acid amplification testing for *Neisseria gonorrhoeae* and *Chlamydia*. Patients may be instructed to self-collect a vaginal swab.**

⊘ **Touch pH indicator paper to the vaginal mucus.** A pH greater than 4.5 suggests BV or *Trichomonas* organisms, but this is only useful if there is no blood or semen to buffer vaginal secretions. A normal pH (4–4.5) is found with *Candida* vulvovaginitis. Normal pH for a premenarchal or postmenopausal woman is 4.7, thus a less reliable test in these patients.

✅ **For wet-mount examination,** dab a drop of vaginal secretions on a slide, add a drop of 0.9% NaCl and a cover slip, and examine under 400× magnification for swimming protozoa (*T. vaginalis*), semen, epithelial cells covered by adherent bacilli (clue cells) of BV, or pseudohyphae and spores (i.e., spaghetti and meatballs) appearance of *C. albicans* (Figs. 94.1 and 94.2).

✅ If epithelial cells obscure the view of yeast, add a drop of 10% potassium hydroxide (KOH) and smell whether this liberates the odor of stale fish (Whiff test), which is characteristic of *Gardnerella* organisms that cause BV. Unfortunately the sensitivity of saline and KOH microscopy for yeast is about 40% to 80%.

✅ Gram stain a second specimen. This is an even more sensitive method for detecting *Candida* organisms (see Fig. 94.2C) and clue cells (see Fig. 94.2B), as well as a means to assess the general vaginal flora, which is normally mixed with occasional predominance of gram-positive rods.

✅ ***T. vaginalis* testing should be performed in symptomatic or high-risk patients. Testing options include saline microscopy (which has a sensitivity of only 51–65%), or if available, nucleic acid amplification, which has a sensitivity and specificity of 95% to 100%, with 100% concordance between urine and vaginal samples. Thus nucleic acid amplification testing is currently the gold standard.**

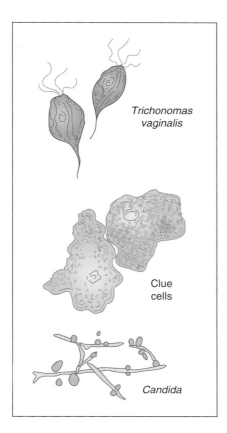

Trichonomas vaginalis

Clue cells

Candida

Fig. 94.1 Test vaginal mucus on a slide with saline.

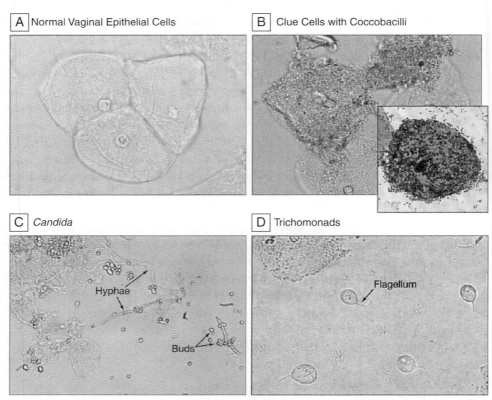

Fig. 94.2 Microscopic examination of vaginal samples. (Adapted from Anderson, M. R., Klink, K., & Cohrssen, A. [2004]. Evaluation of vaginal complaints. *JAMA, 291*, 1368–1379.)

✅ **If *T. vaginalis* is identified** (see Fig. 94.2D), previous recommendations were to treat with metronidazole (Flagyl), 2 g, as one oral dose. A more expensive and slightly more effective alternative treatment was tinidazole (Tindamax), also taken as a single 2-g oral dose. **However, a recent multicenter randomized control trial found the 7-day course of metronidazole to be superior to single-dose metronidazole. Therefore the present recommendation is either oral metronidazole, 500 mg twice daily for 7 days, or oral tinidazole, 2000 mg as one oral dose.** For recurrent infection, prescribe oral metronidazole, 1000 mg twice daily for 7 days

✅ **The patient must abstain from alcohol for 24 hours post metronidazole and 3 days after the last dose of tinidazole because of the disulfiram-like activity of these drugs.**

✅ **Men infected with *T. vaginalis* may be asymptomatic** or have symptoms of urethral irritation and/or discharge, or they may develop prostatitis (see Chapters 82 and 83). **Sex partners must receive the same treatment as the patient.** Advise the patient and partner(s) to refrain from intercourse or to use a condom until therapy has been completed and patient and partner(s) are asymptomatic, at least 7 days. Follow-up is unnecessary for men and women who become asymptomatic after treatment or who are initially asymptomatic.

✓ **Pregnant women who are symptomatic with trichomoniasis** should be treated either with a single 2-g dose of metronidazole or with 500 mg twice a day for 5 to 7 days as this may be better tolerated in patients already prone to nausea. Multiple studies and meta-analyses have not demonstrated a consistent association between metronidazole use during pregnancy and teratogenic or mutagenic effects in infants. However, **one study did note preterm labor increased when treating with metronidazole orally, thus treatment of asymptomatic pregnant patients can be delayed until after delivery.** If symptomatic, consider clotrimazole 1% intravaginally for 7 days. This will relieve symptoms but is unlikely to eradicate the organisms; thus delayed treatment postdelivery will be needed.

✓ **The diagnosis of vulvovaginal candidiasis (VVC) is suggested clinically by a white cottage cheese–like discharge, pruritus and erythema in the vulvovaginal area, and vaginal pH less than or equal to 4.5, and when yeasts or pseudohyphae are demonstrated on either a wet preparation or a Gram stain.** If clinical suspicion is for vulvovaginal candidiasis and microscopy is negative, then culture with speciation should be obtained. Newer, more costly tests are available for diagnosis such as a deoxyribonucleic acid (DNA) homology probe 2728 or a polymerase chain reaction (PCR) test.

✓ **Treat with fluconazole 150 mg PO as a single dose if no contraindications.** Fluconazole is secreted in vaginal secretions for 72 hours postingestion and is at least as effective as intravaginal treatment. Alternatively, miconazole, clotrimazole, or tioconazole intravaginal topical preparations are available over the counter (OTC) without a prescription.

✓ **With severe VVC** (i.e., extensive vulvar erythema, edema, excoriation, and fissure formation), have the patient use a topical prescription intravaginal medication such as terconazole 0.4% cream, 5 g intravaginally for 7 days, or prescribe 150 mg fluconazole in two sequential doses (second dose 72 hours after the initial dose). **In patients with severe discomfort secondary to vulvovaginitis, low-potency steroid creams used for the first 48 hours, in combination with a topical antifungal cream, may be of benefit.** Women **with medical conditions such as uncontrolled diabetes or those receiving corticosteroid treatment** also require more prolonged (i.e., 7–14 days) antimycotic treatment. **During pregnancy,** only topical azole therapies, applied for 7 days, are recommended. Sex partners need not be treated unless they have balanitis. The patient only needs to return for follow-up visits if the symptoms persist or recur within 2 months of the initial treatment.

✓ For recurrent infections, fluconazole may be repeated every 3 days for three doses, and thus taken on days 1, 4, and 7. Gastrointestinal side effects are fairly common, and serious side effects can occur. For recurrent *Candida,* the Infectious Diseases Society of America recommends 10 to 14 days of a topical therapy, such as miconazole or clotrimazole or oral fluconazole, followed by 6 months of weekly doses of oral fluconazole, 150 mg.

✓ **The diagnosis of BV is suggested clinically by profuse, thin homogenous discharge with a fishy odor.** Of women with vaginal complaints, 40% to 50% will be diagnosed with BV. **The presence of three or more of the Amsel diagnostic criteria establishes an accurate diagnosis in 90% of patients. The criteria include thin homogenous discharge, positive whiff test, clue cells present on microscopy, and vaginal pH above 4.5.** Vaginal culture for bacteria is not recommended in the evaluation of BV and should be actively discouraged.

✅ Molecular testing can improve the accuracy of diagnosing BV and trichomoniasis and may be useful in cases that have not responded to therapy or when microscopy is not available. Molecular diagnostic tests include two direct DNA probe assays (BV/vaginitis panel and the Affirm VPIII assay) and four nucleic amplification tests (Nu Swab, Sure Swab, BD Max vaginal panel, and the BV Panel). These testing modalities are substantially more costly than saline microscopy. The benefit of molecular technology over classic diagnostic methods is not yet clear when microscopy is available.

✅ **Treat with metronidazole (Flagyl), 500 mg orally twice a day for 7 days; or tinidazole (Tindamax), given orally at 1 g daily for 5 days or 2 g daily for 2 days (taken with food). Alternatively, metronidazole, 0.75% vaginal gel (MetroGel-Vaginal), one applicator intravaginally once before bedtime for 5 days; or clindamycin, 2% vaginal cream (Cleocin), one 5-g applicator intravaginally once before bedtime for 7 days.**

✅ Alternative therapy includes metronidazole as a single 2-g oral dose (noted to have lower efficacy than the abovementioned regimen); clindamycin, 300 mg orally twice a day for 7 days; or clindamycin vaginal ovules, 100 mg intravaginally once before bedtime for 3 days. **Clindamycin vaginal ovules have been shown to be as effective as the 7-day course of clindamycin.** In 2018, secnidazole granules, 2-g single dose, was approved for the treatment of BV. Secnidazole has a much longer half-life than metronidazole, and the single-dose regimen was found to be at least as effective as the 7-day oral metronidazole regimen.

✅ **Intravaginal treatment for BV is more expensive but carries fewer gastrointestinal side effects than the oral form**, and some patients prefer using intravaginal products for treating this vaginosis. Vaginal therapy is considered more inconvenient by other patients and is associated with a high risk for vaginal candidiasis (10–30%). Metronidazole and tinidazole cannot be used for 3 days after drinking alcohol. Sex partners need not be treated unless they are symptomatic.

✅ **For recurrent BV** (defined as three or more episodes in 1 year), treat as above. Additionally, consider intravaginal metronidazole 0.75% gel twice weekly for 4 to 6 months.

✅ **Treat BV during pregnancy** with metronidazole, 500 mg orally twice a day or 250 mg orally three times a day for 7 days; or clindamycin, 300 mg orally twice a day for 7 days. Some prefer to use oral rather than topical therapy in pregnancy because it may also treat subclinical coinfections. Vaginal treatment is less preferred in pregnancy because of concerns about possible preterm labor.

✅ **To prevent developing *C. albicans* vaginitis after antibiotic treatment** reduces the normal vaginal flora, consider having patients douche with 1% acetic acid (half-strength white vinegar) to maintain a normal low pH vaginal ecology.

✅ **Follow-up visits are unnecessary unless symptoms recur.**

✅ Instruct patients in the prevention of vaginitis. They should avoid routine douching, perfumed soaps and feminine hygiene sprays, and tight/poorly ventilated clothing.

✅ **The differential diagnosis**

  ○ **Remember that a patient may harbor more than one infection.**

  ○ **Seventy percent of all cases of vaginitis are caused by BV, vulvovaginal candidiasis, or trichomonal vaginitis.** However, there are **noninfectious causes** as well. **Physiologic leukorrhea**, a generally nonmalodorous, mucouslike, white or yellowish discharge without other symptoms, is usually estrogen induced. **Atrophic vaginitis,** caused by estrogen deficiency, leads to inflammation of the vagina, and topical estrogen is the treatment of choice. **Desquamative inflammatory vaginitis is rare,** with signs and symptoms of pain, vaginal erythema, profuse discharge, and epithelial cell exfoliation. Intravaginal clindamycin works well for these patients due to its antibacterial and anti-inflammatory effects. **Vaginal erosive disease** consists of multimucosal erosive diseases (e.g., erosive lichen planus, pemphigus vulgaris, and cicatricial [mucous membrane] pemphigoid). The multimucosal erosive diseases are autoimmune disorders that result in erosions or blisters that affect mucosal surfaces such as the mouth, esophagus, eyelid, vagina, and vulva. The treatment of these conditions will not be covered here. **Seminal plasma allergy** is in the differential; **although rare,** it presents with postcoital itching, burning, edema, and erythema and can have systemic symptoms as well. Management of this problem will also not be covered in this chapter.

What Not to Do

(X) Do not blindly prescribe creams or other therapies for nonspecific symptoms of vaginitis. Perform the appropriate physical examination and laboratory tests before initiating one of the treatment regimens recommended.

(X) Do not miss underlying pelvic inflammatory disease (PID), pregnancy, or diabetes, all of which can potentiate vaginitis.

(X) Do not attempt to treat trichomoniasis with metronidazole gel. It is unlikely to achieve therapeutic levels in the urethra and perivaginal glands where infection is also located, and it is considerably less efficacious than oral preparations.

(X) Do not miss candidiasis because the vaginal secretions appear essentially normal in consistency, color, volume, and odor. Nonpregnant patients may not develop thrush patches, curds, or caseous discharge.

(X) Do not treat patients based on self-diagnosis. In one study, only 33.7% of women who self-diagnosed vulvovaginal candidiasis were ultimately confirmed to have the disorder.

(X) Do not treat sex partners of patients with BV or *C. albicans* unless they show signs of infection or have had recurrent infections.

Discussion

Vaginitis is one of the most common causes of patient visits to gynecologists, primary care providers, and urgent care centers. However, many women leave without a clear diagnosis or experience recurrent symptoms despite treatment. The three most common etiologies of vaginitis are trichomonas, BV, and vulvovaginal candidiasis, which account for an estimated 70% of cases. The remaining 30% may be related to other causes of vaginitis, including atrophic

vaginitis, desquamative inflammatory vaginitis, and vaginal erosive disease.

Trichomoniasis and BV are often grouped together, despite major differences in etiology, pathophysiology, and transmission implications. The reason that these two entities are frequently considered together is that they present with elevated vaginal pH, major shifts in vaginal flora, and abnormal vaginal discharge that is characteristically malodorous. They also frequently coexist.

(continued)

Discussion continued

Trichomonas vaginalis is a parasite that is transmitted primarily through sexual activity. In addition to the vaginal discomfort, trichomoniasis facilitates the transmission of human immunodeficiency virus (HIV) and an increased incidence of PID in HIV-infected women. During pregnancy, infection has been associated with delivery of low-birthweight infants and preterm deliveries. Diagnosis is typically made by identification of motile trichomonads on a saline wet preparation. It is important to note that wet-mount examination can be negative in up to 50% of culture-confirmed cases. Therefore, in suspect cases in which the wet-mount examination is negative, it is important to confirm using nucleic acid amplification tests. Other testing options include a 10-minute point-of-care test to detect antigens via dipstick with a sensitivity of 82% to 95% and specificity of 97% to 100%. A 45-minute DNA hybridization probe test evaluates for *T. vaginalis*, *G. vaginalis*, and *C. albicans* with a sensitivity of 63% and specificity of 99.9%. The CDC recommends retesting within 3 months for women diagnosed with a trichomonas infection, regardless of partner treatment status because of high rates of recurrence (17%). Testing can be performed as soon as 28 days after treatment.

It is thought that BV results from a disturbance in the normal vaginal flora, whereby the normal levels of *Lactobacillus* are reduced. *Lactobacillus* is necessary to maintain normal vaginal pH (<4.5) and to prevent proliferation of other organisms. In BV, *Lactobacillus* is replaced by less dominant organisms, such as *G. vaginalis*, *Mycoplasma*, *Mobiluncus*, *Bacteroides* spp., and *Peptostreptococcus*. This polymicrobial mix of facultative anaerobes aids in the transmission and persistence of BV. Bacterial vaginosis is also considered a biofilm infection, which consists of a complex polysaccharide matrix that adheres to epithelial cells in the genital tract of women. The bacterial biofilm provides a biologic explanation for treatment resistance and recurrence because antibiotic therapy alone is unable to disrupt the BV biofilm.

Greater than 50% of women will have a repeat episode of BV within 1 year of treatment with 7 days of metronidazole therapy. With the realization that a bacterial biofilm is implicated in recurrent or persistent BV, disruption of the bacterial biofilm has become the target of in vitro studies. Boric acid combined with nitroimidazole therapy (i.e., metronidazole) has been used to treat recurrent

BV and has been shown to disrupt the biofilms of both BV and *Candida*. While these results are promising, larger, prospective, comparative studies are recommended.

When asked about the ingestion of yogurt, placing yogurt or garlic in the vagina, or oral supplementation with probiotic species, a review and meta-analysis from 2017 found no significant difference in the efficacy of metronidazole combined with probiotics compared with metronidazole alone for the treatment of BV. At this time there is not sufficient evidence to support the use of probiotics for BV, and they are not recommended in the CDC treatment guidelines.

Risk factors associated with BV include the number of sex partners in the previous 12 months, douching, smoking, and low socioeconomic conditions.

Patients with BV usually complain of thin, off-white, fishy-smelling discharge. However, because studies have demonstrated a poor correlation between vaginal symptoms and the final cause of vaginitis, clinicians should not treat vaginal complaints empirically based on patient history alone. BV is often diagnosed on the basis of a typical history in conjunction with clue cells on a wet preparation or an elevated vaginal pH. Although this approach to diagnosis is not unreasonable, accuracy can be improved by using complete Amsel criteria. This includes (1) milky homogeneous adherent discharge, (2) vaginal pH greater than 4.5, (3) more than 20% clue cells in the vaginal fluid on saline light microscopy, and (4) a positive whiff test. If three of the four criteria are present, there is a 90% likelihood of BV; however, some studies have shown that two of the four Amsel criteria may perform just as well as three of four. Cultures are not helpful in diagnosing BV. The Affirm VPIII DNA probe is a highly sensitive and specific test but is expensive, and there is a moderate delay for results. Gram staining is highly reliable and inexpensive, but it is not always available in a doctor's office.

Bacterial vaginosis has been so called because of the absence of inflammatory signs traditionally associated with *G. vaginitis*. As such, in the absence of pain, soreness, burning, and dyspareunia, BV has been considered a noninflammatory condition— hence the term *vaginosis*, not *vaginitis*. The lack of major inflammatory signs has correlated with the lack of polymorphonuclear leukocyte accumulation

(continued)

Discussion continued

in vaginal secretions in BV. If vaginal or vulvar irritation is present, the clinician should have a strong suspicion for mixed infection with *Candida* or other inflammatory processes.

In pregnant women, BV has been associated with an approximately twofold risk for developing preterm delivery, premature rupture of membranes, low birthweight, and postpartum endometritis. Therefore all symptomatic pregnant women should be treated for BV with either the oral or the topical regimen of metronidazole, neither of which has demonstrated teratogenic or mutagenic effects in newborns.

It should also be noted that women who have BV are more likely to have persistence of human papillomavirus (HPV), increased HIV acquisition, PID, and tubo-ovarian abscess formation than those who do not. Multiple studies have also illustrated increased acquisition of *T. vaginalis*, *N. gonorrhea*, and *C. trachomatis* in women with BV.

About 75% of all women will develop symptomatic vulvovaginal candidiasis *at least once in their lifetime. One half of all women will have sporadic recurrences, with about 8% having at least four episodes every year. OTC antifungal medications are in the top 10 of all OTC medications sold in the United States.* **C. albicans** *is usually implicated as the cause of this yeast infection. Vulvovaginal candidiasis may be caused by less common nonalbicans species, such as C. glabrata and C. tropicalis, which tend to be more resistant to standard treatment.*

Established risk factors for VVC include uncontrolled diabetes, steroid-induced immunosuppression, recent antibiotic use, and infection with HIV. *C. albicans* is more common in the summer under tight or nonporous clothing (jeans, synthetic underwear, and wet bathing suits). Vulvar pruritus

is the most common symptom of VVC. Vaginal discharge is often minimal and sometimes absent. Although described as cottage cheese–like in character, the discharge may vary from watery to homogeneously thick.

Symptoms and signs of all forms of vaginitis are extremely nonspecific and can be simulated by a variety of noninfectious causes (e.g., contact and irritant dermatitis). In fact, only 20% of women presenting with pruritus have VVC. A recent assessment of the criteria for wet-preparation–based diagnosis suggests that this approach is neither highly sensitive nor specific when using culture as the gold standard for diagnosis. Although costly, vaginal culture can be helpful in cases of recurrent symptoms or in women with typical symptoms and a negative KOH preparation. A reasonable approach is to reserve culture for cases of treatment failure and to routinely use a wet mount and KOH preparation or a Gram stain of a vaginal discharge in conjunction with physical examination findings. DNA-based diagnostic tools with fairly good degrees of sensitivity and specificity are also useful when available.

To emphasize, symptoms alone do not allow clinicians to distinguish confidently between the causes of vaginitis. However, if there is no itching, candidiasis is less likely, and lack of perceived odor makes BV unlikely. Similarly, physical examination signs are limited in their diagnostic power. The presence of inflammatory signs is associated with candidiasis. Presence of a "high cheese" odor on examination is predictive of bacterial vaginosis, whereas lack of odor is associated with candidiasis.

In conclusion, laboratory tests, particularly the microscopy of a vaginal discharge, are the most useful way of diagnosing the three conditions described in this chapter when taken together with a patient's clinical picture.

Suggested Readings

Abbott, J. (1995). Clinical and microscopic diagnosis of vaginal yeast infection: A prospective analysis. *Annals of Emergency Medicine*, *25*, 587–591.

Anderson, M. R., Klink, K., & Cohrssen, A. (2004). Evaluation of vaginal complaints. *JAMA*, *291*, 1368–1379.

Brown Mills, B. (2017). Vaginitis. *Obstetrics and Gynecology Clinics*, *44*(2), 159–177.

Carr, P. L., Rothberg, M. B., Friedman, R. H., et al. (2005). "Shotgun" versus sequential testing: Cost-effectiveness of diagnostic strategies for vaginitis. *Journal of General Internal Medicine*, *20*, 793–799.

Clenney, T. L., Jorgensen, S. K., & Owen, M. (2005). Vaginitis. *Clinics in Family Practice*, *7*, 57–66.

Ferris, D. G., Litaker, M. S., Woodward, L., et al. (1995). Treatment of bacterial vaginosis: A comparison of oral metronidazole, metronidazole vaginal gel, and clindamycin vaginal cream. *Journal of Family Practice, 41*, 443–449.

Klebandt, M. A., Carey, J. C., Hauth, J. C., et al. (2001). Failure of metronidazole to prevent preterm delivery among pregnant women with asymptomatic *Trichomonas vaginalis* infection. *New England Journal of Medicine, 345*, 487–493.

Martin, D. H., Mroczkowski, T. F., Dalu, Z. A., et al. (1992). A controlled trial of a single dose of azithromycin for the treatment of chlamydial urethritis and cervicitis. *New England Journal of Medicine, 327*, 921–925.

Neal, C. M., Kus, L. H., Eckert, L. O., & Peipert, J. F. (2020). Noncandidal vaginitis: A comprehensive approach to diagnosis and management. *American Journal of Obstetrics and Gynecology, 222*(2), 114–122.

Postenrieder, N. R., Reed, J. L., et al. (2016). Rapid antigen testing for trichomoniasis in an emergency department. *Pediatrics, 137*(6), 2015–2072.

Schwebke, J. R., Hillier, S. L., Sobel, J. D., et al. (1996). Validity of the vaginal Gram stain for the diagnosis of bacterial vaginosis. *Obstetrics & Gynecology, 88*, 573sssss–576.

Sobel, J. D. (2005). What's new in bacterial vaginosis and trichomoniasis? *Infectious Disease Clinics of North America, 19*, 387–406.

Spence, M. R., Hartwell, T. S., Davies, M. C., et al. (1997). The minimum single oral metronidazole dose for treating trichomoniasis: A randomized, blinded study. *Obstetrics & Gynecology, 85*, 699–703.

Swedberg, J., Steiner, J. F., Deiss, F., et al. (1985). Comparison of a single-dose vs one-week course of metronidazole for symptomatic bacterial vaginosis. *JAMA, 254*, 1046–1049.

Trager, J. D. K. (2005). What's your diagnosis? Well-demarcated vulvar erythema in two girls. *Journal of Pediatric and Adolescent Gynecology, 18*, 43–46.

Vazquez, J. A., & Sobel, J. D. (2002). Mucosal candidiasis. *Infectious Disease Clinics of North America, 16*, 793–820.

Watson, M. C., Grimshaw, J. M., Bond, C. M., et al. (2002). Oral versus intravaginal imidazole and triazole antifungal agents for the treatment of uncomplicated vulvovaginal candidiasis (thrush). *British Journal of Obstetrics and Gynecology, 109*, 85–95.

Zeger, W., & Holt, K. (2003). Gynecologic infections. *Emergency Medicine Clinics of North America, 21*, 631–648.

PART 9

Musculoskeletal Emergencies

■ Katherine Dolbec   ■ Joe Ravera

Acromioclavicular (Shoulder) Separation

Presentation

After a direct blow to or a fall onto the lateral shoulder with the arm adducted, the patient complains of shoulder pain increased by motion of the arm (Fig. 95.1A). An indirect mechanism of injury commonly involves a fall onto an outstretched arm or falling back onto an elbow (Fig. 95.1B). Patients are generally able to localize their pain to the acromioclavicular (AC) joint.

Inspection may reveal no deformity (type I), a small step-off between the acromion process of the scapula and the distal end of the clavicle (type II) (Fig. 95.3), or significant superior displacement of the distal end of the clavicle with respect to the acromion process (type III) (Figs. 95.2 and 95.4).

Signs such as swelling, abrasions, or bruising may be evident, either on the superior shoulder, implying a direct mechanism, or on the elbow or forearm, implying an indirect mechanism. The AC joint, which is superficial and easily palpated, is tender to palpation.

Patients with a type I or II AC sprain often present with pain. Patients with a type III injury may present noting a deformity, with or without pain (Fig. 95.4). There is a 5-to-1 male-to-female injury rate.

What to Do

⊘ **Provide analgesia as needed.**

⊘ **Palpate the entire shoulder girdle**, including the sternoclavicular joint, the clavicle, and the proximal humerus, assessing for deformities and tenderness. There should be tenderness only over the AC joint with varying prominence of the distal clavicle, depending on the severity of the injury. Gentle passive rotation of the humerus should not cause more pain, but there should be pain with the cross-body adduction, or scarf, test. This is done by elevating the arm on the affected side to 90 degrees of forward flexion and then adducting it passively as far as possible. Pain localized over the AC joint is a positive test.

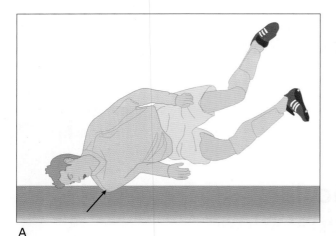

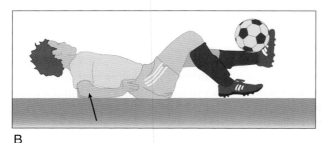

A

B

Fig. 95.1 (A) The most common mechanism of injury to the AC joint results from a direct blow onto the tip of the shoulder. (B) An indirect force, such as a fall onto the elbow, may also disrupt the AC joint. (Adapted from Buss, D. D., & Watts, J. D. [2003]. Acromioclavicular injuries in the throwing athlete. *Clinics in Sports Medicine, 22,* 327–341.)

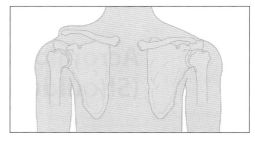

Fig. 95.2 Type III injury with rupture of the AC ligament. (Adapted from Montellese, P., & Dancy, T. [2004]. The acromioclavicular joint. *Primary Care, 31,* 857–866.)

⊘ Strength and range of motion (ROM) may be limited by pain. Perform a complete neurovascular examination of the upper extremity and assess for neurologic injury due to the close proximity of the brachial plexus.

⊘ **Obtain x-ray or bedside ultrasound imaging of the shoulder to be sure that there is no associated fracture of the lateral clavicle or coracoid or fracture or dislocation of the humerus.** Comparison views may be useful to allow measurements of the coracoclavicular distance and distal clavicle position in the unaffected AC joint. **Weight-bearing stress views are uncomfortable and unnecessary.**

⊘ **In a type I injury**, the acromioclavicular ligament and the coracoclavicular ligament are sprained but intact, and the distal clavicle is stable and in normal anatomic alignment. **In a type II injury**, the acromioclavicular ligament is torn, the coracoclavicular ligament is sprained but intact, and the distal clavicle is mobile in the axial plane with less than 50% subluxation.

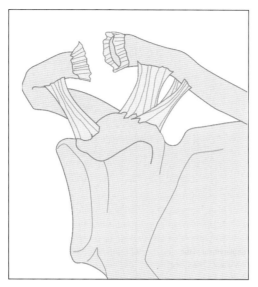

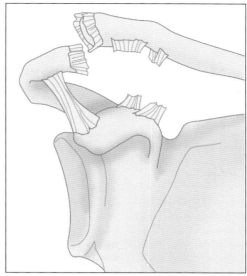

Fig. 95.3 Type II injury with rupture of the AC and coracoclavicular ligaments. (Adapted from Montellese, P., & Dancy, T. [2004]. The acromioclavicular joint. *Primary Care, 31,* 857–866.)

Fig. 95.4 Step-off deformity of type III injury. (Adapted from Knoop, K. J., Stack, L. B., & Storrow, A. B. [1997]. *Atlas of emergency medicine.* New York, NY: McGraw-Hill.) (Courtesy Frank Birinyi, MD.)

✅ **Type I and II injuries are treated the same** and **differ only in the time to recovery. Provide analgesics and a sling, as needed, for comfort. Cold packs can be helpful; ultrasound-guided analgesic injection of bupivacaine has been shown, in one case study, to relieve severe pain when oral pain medications were inadequate.** Pain relief lasted for approximately 8 hours.

✅ **As quickly as tolerated, the patient should come out of the sling and begin active ROM exercises.** Once the range of motion is full and pain free, progressive strengthening and activity-specific exercises will prove that the patient is capable of returning to activity successfully and safely. Recovery from this injury takes 2 to 12 weeks of rest and rehabilitation.

✅ **Type III injuries** involve disruption of both the acromioclavicular and coracoclavicular ligaments, resulting in an unstable joint. There is a 25% to 100% superior displacement of the AC joint. The distal clavicle is mobile in the axial and coronal planes.

✅ **Treatment of type III injuries remains controversial, and there is no good evidence to suggest that surgical repair is routinely superior to nonoperative management. The evidence suggests that conservative therapy is the initial treatment of choice and that surgery should be reserved for patients who have chronic pain and weakness. Conservative treatment is performed exactly as outlined for type I and type II injuries, but the resumption of full activity and return to play will likely be slower.**

✅ Type IV injuries (Fig. 95.5) include the previous findings, plus the distal clavicle tears the deltotrapezius fascia, which remains fixed posteriorly. In type V injuries, there is a 100% to 300%

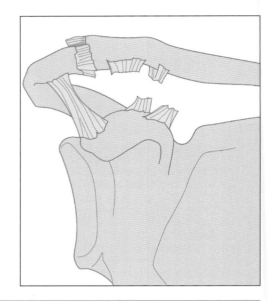

Fig. 95.5 Type IV injury with posterior displacement of the distal clavicle. (Adapted from Montellese, P., & Dancy, T. [2004]. The acromioclavicular joint. *Primary Care, 31,* 857–866.)

joint displacement and tearing of the deltotrapezius fascia. In rare type VI injuries, the clavicle is fixed beneath the acromion or coracoid; this injury is usually accompanied by a neurologic deficit.

✓ **Type IV, V, and VI injuries require urgent orthopedic consultation and** are often operative.

✓ **For type I, II, and III injuries, arrange for follow-up with an orthopedic surgeon or sports medicine physician within 7 to 10 days. Physical therapy may begin around 1 week postinjury, but the patient should engage in ROM exercises as soon as possible.**

What Not to Do

✗ Do not confuse the deformity of a displaced AC ligament tear with a dislocated shoulder, which is accompanied by loss of the normal deltoid convexity and inability to rotate the shoulder internally and externally at the side.

✗ Do not bother with weight-bearing radiographs to differentiate separations based on the widening of the distance between the clavicle and scapula. These views are painful and inaccurate.

✗ Do not try to tape or strap the clavicle and scapula back into position. Patients have suffered ischemic necrosis of the skin from overzealous strapping. This includes the use of a Kenny-Howard sling.

✗ Do not allow the patient to wear a sling and immobilize the shoulder for more than 1 week without at least beginning pendulum exercises. Adhesive capsulitis may result, causing decreased ROM, increased pain, and delayed recovery.

Discussion

The AC joint is a diarthrodial synovial joint of the acromion and the distal clavicle with an intraarticular disk. This disk degenerates rapidly, resulting in narrowing of the joint space by age 40 years. The clavicle is the last bone in the body to ossify the physes; therefore Salter-Harris injuries can occur up to the age of 25 years.

The static stabilizers are the ligaments, but significant functional stability arises from the muscles attached to the shoulder girdle as well. The AC ligaments, which are incorporated into the AC joint capsule, provide most of the resistance to anteroposterior displacement and rotation of the clavicle. The two coracoclavicular ligaments, the conoid and trapezoid, prevent superior displacement of the distal clavicle. The dynamic stabilizers are the deltoid and trapezius muscles.

In patients with open physes, the physis is the weak link in the AC joint. When injured, the physis fractures and the metaphysis tears through the superior aspect of the periosteum. Because the AC joint remains in its anatomic position, but the metaphysis is displaced, these injuries are called pseudodislocations. Because the inferior slip of periosteum remains in its original position, the bone it lays down is in the original orientation. Once the fracture gap is bridged, remodeling occurs, which usually brings the clavicle to its original position. These injuries are treated conservatively in the same manner as described for AC joint separations.

A partial tear of the ligaments between acromion and clavicle produces pain but no widening of the joint (type I separation). A type II AC separation is visualized on radiographs as a widened joint but is otherwise the same with regard to examination and treatment. In a type III or complete separation, the coracoclavicular ligament is also torn, allowing the clavicle to be pulled superiorly by the sternocleidomastoid muscle.

Nearly all patients with type I and 90% of those with type II injuries recover fully after 10 to 14 days of simple sling immobilization and early ROM exercise. The patient should avoid heavy lifting for 8 to 12 weeks and be referred to an orthopedic surgeon for any problems with pain or diminished ROM.

Long-term shoulder joint stability and strength after a type III tear remain nearly normal in most patients, but the visible deformity persists. Patients may desire surgical repair to regain normal shoulder appearance or to regain maximal function in the case of elite athletes. These patients should be counseled regarding the risks of surgery. Some of the literature on the treatment of AC separations listed visual prominence as a possible indication for surgery. This may be a consideration for thin patients who may have compromise of the skin or in patients who put excessive direct pressure on the AC joint, such as soldiers carrying backpacks. Caution is advised prior to surgical intervention for a cosmetic deformity, however. The surgical risks have been documented in the literature and include infection, hardware migration, failure to maintain a reduction, and scarring from the procedure.

A review of the current state-of-the-art management of AC joint injuries summarized that the evidence would seem to broadly support the consensus that low-grade (types I and II) injuries be treated conservatively, with initial rest, but early mobilization as pain allows. Equally, acute surgical repair, ideally within 10 days but at least within 30 days of injury, should be considered for types IV to VI. For type III injuries, though still the subject of much debate, the literature would seem to suggest that it is reasonable to treat conservatively initially, opting for delayed reconstruction for those who remain symptomatic following full rehabilitation. Based on some military studies, however, in young, high-physical-demand patients, acute surgical intervention may also be a reasonable consideration given the high (>70%) incidence of delayed surgical intervention, and so prolonged morbidity, in this population.

Suggested Readings

Buss, D. D., & Watts, J. D. (2003). Acromioclavicular injuries in the throwing athlete. *Clinics in Sports Medicine, 22,* 327–341, vii.

Mickell, C., Gelber, J., & Nagdev, A. (2020). Ultrasound-guided analgesic injection for acromioclavicular joint separation in the emergency department. *American Journal of Emergency Medicine, 38*(1), 162.e3–e5

Montellese, P., & Dancy, T. (2004). The acromioclavicular joint. *Primary Care, 31,* 857–866.

Radhakrishnan, G., & Henderson, D. (2019). Injuries of the acromioclavicular joint. *Orthopaedics and Trauma, 33*(5), 276–282.

Tamaoki, M. J. S., Belloti, J. C., Lenza, M., Matsumoto, M. H., Gomes dos Santos, J. B., & Faloppa, F. (2010). Surgical versus conservative interventions for treating acromioclavicular dislocation of the shoulder in adults. *Cochrane Database of Systematic Reviews, 8,* CD007429. https://doi.org/10.1002/14651858.CD007429.pub2.

Ankle Sprain

(Twisted Ankle)

Presentation

Most patients with ankle sprains describe an inversion injury; eversion injuries are less common. Inversion injuries constitute 85% of ankle sprains. Patients may report having stepped off a curb or into a hole. Sports-related injuries often occur after jumping and landing on another player's foot, which causes an inversion or supination of the ankle. There may be a sensation of a "pop" or "snap" at the time of injury with immediate loss of function suggesting disruption of a ligament. Severe swelling in the first hour suggests bleeding from the torn ligament ends. The body will rapidly respond with an inflammatory response, producing swelling, warmth, pain, and stiffness that build during the first few days postinjury.

Patients may present immediately after the injury or in the days following the injury complaining of pain, swelling, and partial or complete inability to walk. Patients are usually tender around the lateral malleolus, particularly anteriorly, because the anterior talofibular ligament is the first to tear when the ankle is inverted. Although the pain during the first hours after injury is often localized to the injured area, it becomes diffuse during the first few days. Once the initial inflammatory response has dissipated, careful palpation will confirm which ligaments were most likely injured.

What to Do

✅ **Obtain a detailed description of the mechanism of injury; ask if the patient could bear weight immediately after the injury. Ask if there have been previous injuries of the ankle.** Patients with a previous ankle injury have an increased risk for recurrence due to persistently impaired proprioception through the injured ligaments.

✅ **Document the degree and location of swelling and discoloration.** Check the sensation and circulation distal to the injury. (A slight decrease relative to the uninjured foot might be attributed to the swelling.)

✅ **Palpate sites of potential injury: the fibula up to the knee, the base of the fifth metatarsal on the lateral foot, the tarsal navicular bone anteriorly, the anterior tibiotalar joint line, the deltoid ligament medially, and (finally) the anterior talofibular ligament (ATFL) in front of the lateral malleolus. Note if there is tenderness along the posterior distal 6 cm of the lateral malleolus, the posterior medial malleolus, or the tip of either malleolus.** Start palpating gently and away from the injury, saving the most likely site of injury for last, as pain may inhibit the reliability of any further examination.

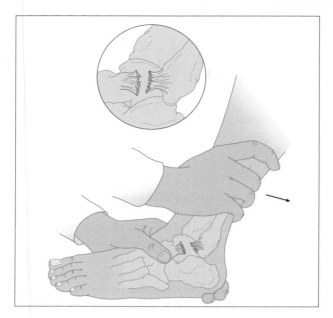

Fig. 96.1 Anterior drawer test.

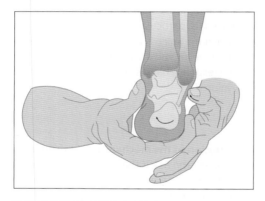

Fig. 96.2 Talar tilt test.

⊘ **If there is not too much pain, check joint stability with the anterior drawer test (Fig. 96.1) and the talar tilt test (Fig. 96.2).** Perform these tests gently. For the anterior drawer test, grasp the tibia with one hand and the heel with the other hand; with the ankle in slight plantar flexion, stabilize the distal leg while gently translating the foot anteriorly at the ankle. Anterior displacement of the talus can be felt or seen as a dimple over the anterolateral ankle compared with the uninjured side. A positive anterior drawer indicates a significantly torn anterior talofibular ligament. The talar tilt test is also performed with the foot in the neutral position. Gently invert the ankle and compare the range of movement (ROM) and the softness of the end point with the uninjured side. An intact calcaneofibular ligament should prevent inversion. **Often these tests cannot be accomplished because the ankle is too painful, in which case the tests may be deferred for up to 1 week.** A delayed physical examination (4–5 days) has been shown to give better diagnostic results and is considered the gold standard in the diagnosis of acute lateral ligament injury, with a sensitivity of 96% and a specificity of 84%.

✓ **If there is significant medial ankle injury or severe lateral injury, perform a squeeze test to determine if there is a tear of the syndesmosis between the distal tibia and fibula.** With the knee flexed at 90 degrees, place a hand over the midportion of the lower leg, with the thumb on the fibula and fingers on the medial tibia. Squeeze the fibula and tibia together. Pain radiating toward the ankle during this test signifies syndesmotic injury, or **high ankle sprain**. This diagnosis generally portends a more prolonged recovery than that from a low ankle sprain. These patients will require orthopedic or sports medicine referral to ensure that healing is progressing. **High-energy high-ankle sprains may have an associated fracture of the fibular head**; this pattern is called a Maisonneuve fracture when there is an associated deltoid ligament tear or medial malleolus fracture. Magnetic resonance imaging (MRI) has been considered the investigation of choice for suspected syndesmotic ligament injury.

✓ **With low-ankle sprains, radiographs or bedside ultrasound scans of the ankle or foot may be ordered to rule out a fracture. However, radiographs are not necessary (and likely to be negative) if none of the following are present: (1) inability to bear weight both immediately and at the initial physical examination or (2) bony tenderness to palpation of the ankle in the posterior distal 6 cm of the lateral malleolus or the posterior distal medial malleolus, or bony tenderness of the foot at the tarsal navicular or the base of the fifth metatarsal bone. These constitute the Ottawa ankle rules.** If any of these are present, imaging should be ordered. The use of this decision rule must remain secondary to the judgment and common sense of the clinician. Patient satisfaction can be maintained by informing patients, "Studies show that your type of ankle sprain does not need an x-ray, and I would prefer not to expose you to unnecessary radiation." You can still give the autonomy of decision making to the patient by stating, "I'd be glad to order an x-ray if you still want it."

✓ Be liberal in imaging patients with other distracting painful injuries, altered sensorium, intoxication, paraplegia, or bone disease. Weight bearing is defined as the ability to transfer weight twice onto each leg for a total of four steps, regardless of limping. Assess ability to bear weight after determining bony tenderness, and do not coerce the patient.

✓ Both ultrasonography and MRI can be valuable in diagnosing any concomitant chondral or tendon injury. Recently a study compared ultrasonography in the emergency room with MR images for injuries of the ATFL and found no differences in diagnostic accuracy. The sensitivity and specificity of MRI in diagnosing ATFL injuries are 92% to 100% and 100%, respectively.

✓ **When there is no suspected or demonstrated ankle fracture:**

○ **Initial management for low-ankle sprains is symptomatic and may include elevation of the foot to limit pain and swelling, application of an ice pack to the ankle (over a protective barrier) for pain management, and compression of the ankle with a splint or elastic bandage to limit swelling for the first 4 to 5 days.** The RICE principle (rest, ice [cryotherapy], compression, and elevation) is the classic approach to ankle sprains, although a recent systematic review found no conclusive value for the application of that principle. Therefore, if patients find any of these modalities bothersome, they may discontinue them, as they are unlikely to change the course of injury. **After the initial inflammatory phase has resolved, generally after 3 days, early mobilization with weight bearing as tolerated and ROM exercises should be encouraged.**

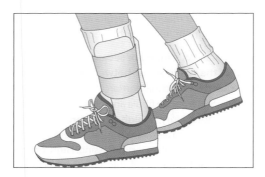

Fig. 96.3 Grade I and II sprains should be fitted with a stirrup splint.

○ **Nonsteroidal anti-inflammatory drugs (NSAIDs) may be used for pain management if there are no contraindications** (gastrointestinal [GI] bleed, hypertension, kidney disease, allergy, cardiac disease) to their use. **Acetaminophen may also be effective without the risk for GI, renal, and cardiac side effects.**

○ **The patient should begin active and passive ROM exercises as soon as possible. The patient may use an exercise band or a rolled-up towel to stretch the ankle in plantar flexion, dorsiflexion, inversion, and eversion.**

○ **Patients with mild to moderate sprains (grades I and II) should be fitted with a stirrup-type, lace-up, or compression sleeve splint** (Fig. 96.3) **that provides external proprioception and helps limit recurrent inversion and eversion injuries of the ankle. Patients who are unable to bear weight** or **who have a substantially antalgic gait should be given crutches and instructions on their use.**

○ **Upon discharge, instruct the patient to begin weight bearing with the crutches as soon as it is tolerable. The crutches may be discarded when the patient is able to walk without a limp. ROM exercises should be aggressively undertaken as soon as possible after injury. Once normal weight bearing and pain-free range of motion are achieved, muscle strengthening can begin.** Early phases of treatment should begin with low-resistance exercises, such as stationary cycling or swimming. Further strengthening can be accomplished using resistance bands while performing resisted plantar flexion, dorsiflexion, inversion, and eversion exercises. Patients with these sprains can be referred to their primary care provider or a primary care sports medicine specialist for follow-up in 2 weeks. They will frequently require physical therapy to recover full proprioception, which will help prevent recurrent injuries and chronic ankle instability.

○ **Patients with severe low-ankle sprains (grade III), high-ankle sprains, recurrent sprains, sprains with instability or syndesmotic injury, and most injuries with associated fractures will require a walking boot or a short leg splint** (Figs. 96.4 and 96.5) **and crutches. They should generally be non–weight bearing initially. These patients will require follow-up with an orthopedic surgeon or primary care sports medicine physician in approximately 1 week, and reassessment at that time will help guide the rehabilitation plan.**

○ Obtain urgent or emergent orthopedic consultation in cases of delayed recovery, diagnostic uncertainty, neurovascular compromise, pain out of proportion to the injury (think compartment syndrome), and treatment involving competitive athletes.

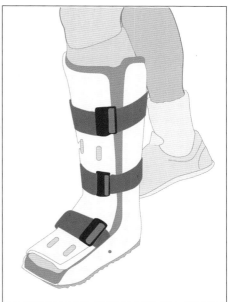

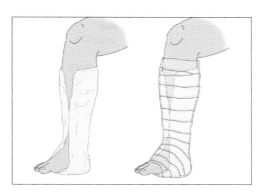

Fig. 96.4 Severe sprains and fractures should be treated with a sugar-tong splint or Jones dressing.

Fig. 96.5 Walking boot for grade III sprains.

○ **Tender or swollen ankle sprains in children** with open growth plates should incite consideration of a nondisplaced physeal (Salter I) fracture, even with negative radiographs. Consider more aggressive immobilization for these injuries with plaster or fiberglass splinting preferred. Orthopedic or sports medicine follow-up should be arranged in 1 to 2 weeks. Bony structures and growth plates are often weaker than the contiguous ligaments and tendons. Care should be taken to palpate both malleoli and their respective physes, the proximal fifth metatarsal (a site of peroneus brevis avulsion), and the tarsal navicular, which may reveal an occult fracture.

⊘ **Patients not receiving radiographs at the initial visit** should be instructed to seek follow-up if their symptoms have not improved after 1 week. Persistent ankle pain beyond 6 to 8 weeks could indicate a complication or overlooked injury. MRI, which is seldom needed at the initial presentation, may be very useful if symptoms have persisted this long.

What Not to Do

✗ Do not have the patient apply heat during the recovery phase. It is unnecessary and increases swelling.

✗ Do not recommend ointments or creams. They offer no benefit for ankle sprains.

✗ Do not overlook fractures of the anterior process of the calcaneus, the tarsal navicular, the talar dome or the rest of the talus, or the os trigonum, all visible on the ankle radiographs.

✗ Do not completely rule out a fracture based on a negative radiograph.

Discussion

Blunt ankle trauma is one of the most common injuries seen in emergency departments, and ankle sprains are the most common sports-related orthopedic injuries, but less than 15% have associated clinically significant fractures. The old tradition of radiographic examination of all ankle injuries is no longer required. The Ottawa decision rules described here have led to reductions in the number of negative radiographs, decreases in the use of unnecessary radiation, with shorter waiting times and lower costs—all without an increase in missed fractures or patient dissatisfaction.

The ankle ligaments can be divided into three groups: lateral ligaments, medial ligaments, and the ligaments of the syndesmosis. The most common injuries involve the lateral ligaments. These three groups of ligaments function as the static stabilizers of the ankle joint. The dynamic stabilizers consist of the muscles of the anterior, lateral, and posterior compartments of the leg. Mild or grade I sprains usually involve partial tearing of ligament fibers and minimal swelling, with no joint instability. Moderate or grade II sprains are characterized by some pain, edema, ecchymosis, and point tenderness over the involved structures, resulting in partial loss of joint motion. Some ligament fibers may be completely torn, but overall stability of the joint remains intact. Severe or grade III sprains exhibit gross instability with complete tearing of all ligament fibers, marked swelling, and severe pain. In general, the more extensive the ligament injury, the more difficult it is to bear weight, the more swelling noted acutely, and the more ecchymosis that develops over a few days.

Medial ligament injuries usually result from an eversion stress. Because the deltoid ligament is so strong, it is rarely injured in isolation and is often associated with a lateral malleolus fracture.

Current research recommends early weight bearing and mobilization for lateral ligament injuries. Four stages characterize the biology behind functional treatment of acute lateral ankle ligament tears. Immediately after the injury, hemorrhage, swelling, inflammation, and pain develop. Rest, ice, compression, elevation (RICE), NSAIDs, and acetaminophen may provide some pain relief during this phase. During the following 1 to 3 weeks, called the healing or proliferation phase, fibroblasts invade the injured area and proliferate to form collagen fibers. During this phase a brace, wrap, or sleeve will provide some additional support and external proprioception, which may be beneficial in preventing recurrent injury. Three weeks after the injury, the maturation phase begins, during which the collagen fibers mature and become scar tissue. Controlled stretching of muscles and movement of the joint as well as focused balance exercises encourage the orientation of the collagen fibers along the stress lines and the recreation of proprioceptive connections, creating a stronger ligamentous repair and a more stable complex. After 6 to 8 weeks, the new collagen fibers can withstand almost normal stress, and full return to activity is the goal. The entire maturation and remodeling of the injured ligaments lasts 6 to 12 months. Reports indicate that up to 73% of people who sustain a lateral ankle sprain have recurrent sprains, but it is unknown how many of these participants partake in rehabilitation.

A minor sprain usually keeps an athlete out of competition for several days to 2 weeks, and a moderate sprain usually keeps an athlete out of competition for 2 to 4 weeks. Time to return to play for severe sprains will be greater than 4 weeks. Taping, lace-up braces, and air stirrup orthoses can all be helpful in the rehabilitation of ankle injuries and the prevention of recurrence.

When the patient reports a snapping sensation and states that it felt like something "slipped out of place," accompanied by pain in the posterolateral aspect of the ankle, consider the diagnosis of a peroneal tendon dislocation. This is seen more frequently in skiers but does occur to a lesser extent in other sport activities. Swelling and tenderness are found posteriorly and extending 6 inches proximally from the lateral malleolus. Circumduction of the ankle with palpation over the peroneal tendons may elicit a dislocation or subluxation of the peroneal tendons. These injuries require orthopedic consultation and may require acute surgical repair to prevent recurrence.

Typically, a patient with a Maisonneuve fracture will not complain of pain in the region of the proximal fibula but rather only of ankle pain in the region of the medial malleolus. Morbidity associated with proximal fibular fractures includes contusion or laceration of the common peroneal nerve (resulting in footdrop), injury to the anterior tibial artery, damage to the lateral collateral ligament of the knee, and even compartment syndrome.

The application of ice (cryotherapy) for the prevention of swelling and inflammation has

(continued)

Discussion continued

traditionally been accepted as a standard of care for the treatment of sprains. Although it is theorized that cryotherapy can be beneficial both immediately after injury and in the rehabilitation phase, the available scientific evidence does not provide much support for this belief. There is also some limited evidence that ice may delay healing and impair proprioception. **Ice may be used as an adjunct for pain management but is not necessary for healing or recovery.** Additionally, no benefit was found for the usage of laser therapy, ultrasound therapy, or electrotherapy.

On the positive side, compression and elevation may help reduce swelling after an ankle sprain, and **early mobilization seems to be the most beneficial approach to encourage rapid and full recovery.**

A Thompson test should be performed if inspection and examination of the Achilles tendon suggests a full or partial tear there (see Fig. 126.1).

Suggested Readings

Anis, A. H., Steill, I. G., Stewart, D. G., et al. (1995). Cost-effectiveness analysis of the Ottawa ankle rules. *Annals of Emergency Medicine, 26*, 422–428.

Arnold, B. L., & Docherty, C. L. (2004). Bracing and rehabilitation—what's new? *Clinics in Sports Medicine, 23*, 83–95.

Auleley, G. R., Kerboull, L., Durieux, P., et al. (1998). Validation of the Ottawa ankle rules in France: A study in the surgical emergency department of a teaching hospital. *Annals of Emergency Medicine, 32*, 14–18.

Auleley, G. R., Ravaud, P., Giraudeau, B., et al. (1997). Implementation of the Ottawa ankle rules in France: A multicenter randomized controlled trial. *Journal of the American Medical Association, 277*, 1935–1939.

Bachmann, L. M., Kolb, E., Koller, M. T., et al. (2003). Accuracy of Ottawa ankle rules to exclude fractures of the ankle and midfoot. *BMJ, 326*, 417–419.

Baumhauer, J. F., Nawoczenski, D. A., DiGiovanni, B. F., et al. (2004). Ankle pain and peroneal tendon pathology. *Clinics in Sports Medicine, 23*, 21–34.

Bleakley, C., McDonough, S., & MacAuley, D. (2004). The use of ice in the treatment of acute soft tissue injury. *The American Journal of Sports Medicine, 32*, 251–261.

Braun, B. L. (1999). Effects of ankle sprain in a general clinic population 6 to 18 months after medical evaluation. *Archives of Family Medicine, 8*, 143–148.

Chande, V. T. (1995). Decision rules for roentgenography of children with acute ankle injuries. *Archives of Pediatric and Adolescent Medicine, 149*, 255–258.

Cydulka, R. K. (2004). Accuracy of Ottawa ankle rules to exclude fractures of the ankle and midfoot. *Annals of Emergency Medicine, 43*, 675–676.

Deal, D. N., Tipton, J., Rosencrance, E., et al. (2002). Ice reduces edema: A study of microvascular permeability in rat. *Journal of Bone and Joint Surgery, 84*, 1573–1578.

D'Hooghe, P., Alkhelaifi, K., Abdelatif, N., & Kaux, J. F. (2018). From "low" to "high" athletic ankle sprains: A comprehensive review. *Operative Techniques in Orthopaedics, 28*(2), 54–60.

DiGiovanni, B. F., Partal, G., & Baumhauer, J. F. (2004). Acute ankle injury and chronic lateral instability in the athlete. *Clinics in Sports Medicine, 23*, 1–19 v.

Doherty, C., Bleakley, C., Delahunt, E., & Holden, S. (2017). Treatment and prevention of acute and recurrent ankle sprain: An overview of systematic reviews with meta-analysis. *British Journal of Sports Medicine, 51*, 113–125.

Eggli, S., Sclabas, G. M., Eggli, S., et al. (2005). The bernese ankle rules: A fast, reliable test after low-energy, supination-type malleolar and midfoot trauma. *The Journal of Trauma, 59*, 1268–1271.

Eiff, M. P., Smith, A. T., & Smith, G. E. (1994). Early mobilization versus immobilization in the treatment of lateral ankle sprains. *The American Journal of Sports Medicine, 22*, 83–88.

Graham, I. D., Stiell, I. G., & Laupacis, A. (2001). Awareness and use of the Ottawa ankle and knee rules in 5 countries: Can publication alone be enough to change practice? *Annals of Emergency Medicine, 37*, 259–266.

Halvorson, G., & Iserson, K. V. (1987). Comparison of four ankle splint designs. *Annals of Emergency Medicine, 16,* 1249–1252.

LeBlanc, K. E. (2004). Ankle problems masquerading as sprains. *PrimaryCare, 31,* 1055–1067.

Lucchesi, G. M., Jackson, R. E., Peacock, W. F., et al. (1995). Sensitivity of the Ottawa rules. *Annals of Emergency Medicine, 26,* 1–5.

MacAuley, D. (2001). Do textbooks agree on their advice on ice? *Clinical Journal of Sports Medicine, 11,* 67–72.

Markert, R. J., Walley, M. E., Guttman, T. G., et al. (1998). A pooled analysis of the Ottawa ankle rules used on adults in the. *American Journal of Emergency Medicine, 16,* 564–567.

Pommering, T. L., Kluchurosky, L., & Hall, S. L. (2005). Ankle and foot injuries in pediatric and adult athletes. *PrimaryCare, 32,* 133–161.

Stiell, I. G., Greenberg, G. H., McKnight, R. D., et al. (1993). Decision rules for the use of radiography in acute ankle injuries: Refinement and prospective validation. *Journal of the American Medical Association, 269,* 1127–1132.

Stiell, I. G., McKnight, R. D., Greenberg, G. H., et al. (1994). Implementation of the Ottawa ankle rules. *Journal of the American Medical Association, 271,* 827–832.

van Dijk, C. N., Lim, L. S., Bossuyt, P. M., et al. (1996). Physical examination is sufficient for the diagnosis of sprained ankles. *Journal of Bone and Joint Surgery, 78,* 958–962.

Wilson, D. E., Noseworthy, T. W., Rowe, B. H., et al. (2002). Evaluation of patient satisfaction and outcomes after assessment for acute ankle injuries. *American Journal of Emergency Medicine, 20,* 18–20.

Annular Ligament Displacement, Radial Head Subluxation

(Nursemaid's Elbow)

Presentation

A toddler who is between 1 and 4 years of age presents with upper extremity pain and reluctance to use that extremity following a sudden jerk on the arm. Circumstances surrounding the injury may be obvious (such as a parent pulling the child up by the arm to avoid stepping into a puddle, pulling a child back by the arm who is trying to run out into the street, or a child having been swung by forearms during play). On the other hand, the mechanism of injury may be obscure (the untruthful babysitter who reports that the child "just fell down"). The patient and family may not be accurate about localizing the injury and think that the child has injured the shoulder or wrist. The patient is comfortable at rest, splinting the arm limply at the side (pseudoparalysis) with mild flexion at the elbow and pronation of the forearm. There should be no deformity, crepitation, swelling, or discoloration of the arm. There is also no palpable tenderness, except possibly over the radiohumeral joint. However, the child will start to cry with any movement of the elbow, especially attempted supination. The left arm is affected more frequently than the right, as most caregivers are right-handed and hold the child's left hand.

What to Do

✅ **Ask about a history of any significant trauma,** such as a fall from a height.

✅ **Thoroughly examine the entire extremity,** including inspection and palpation of the shoulder girdle, hand, and wrist. To avoid obtaining a false-positive examination, special effort should be made to keep the elbow joint perfectly immobile while evaluating for tenderness throughout the rest of the upper extremity.

✅ **If the diagnosis is unclear or there is a history of trauma** (i.e., injury caused by a fall), point tenderness, swelling, ecchymosis, or any other reason to suspect a fracture, obtain a radiograph or bedside ultrasound.

✅ **When nursemaid's elbow is confidently suspected,** place the patient in the parent's lap and inform the mother or father that it appears that a ligament in the child's elbow is slightly out of place and that you are going to put it back in place. Warn the parent that this is going to hurt the child for a few moments.

✅ **The traditional reduction technique is to put a thumb over the head of the radius with the fingers supporting the elbow and press down with the thumb while smoothly and fully**

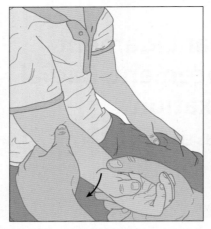
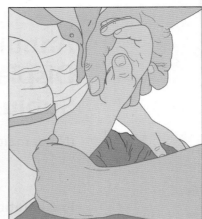

Fig. 97.1
Supination
technique for
annular ligament
displacement
(ALD) reduction.

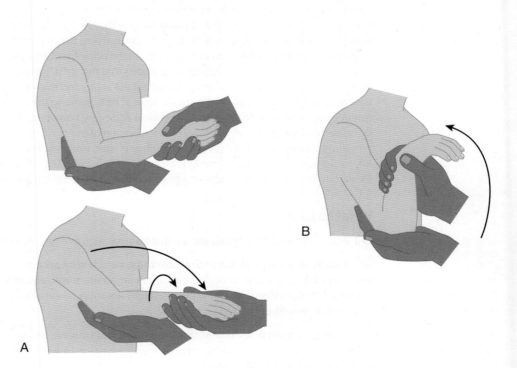

A

B

Fig. 97.2 "Handshake" or hyperpronation maneuver. Simultaneous pronation of the wrist and extension of the elbow (A), followed by flexion of the elbow with the forearm maintained in pronation (B).

supinating the forearm and extending the elbow. Complete the procedure by fully flexing the elbow while keeping the thumb pressing against the radial head and the forearm supinated (Fig. 97.1). At some point, you should feel a click beneath your thumb. The patient will usually scream at this point. **Leave the bedside for about 10 minutes, then return and**

reexamine the elbow to see that the child has fully recovered as if nothing had happened. This recovery may take as long as 30 minutes. Postreduction immobilization is unnecessary.

✅ **An alternative maneuver that some believe is more successful and less painful and should be the preferred first reduction technique is the "handshake" or hyperpronation maneuver.** Following the preparation as noted earlier, **grasp the hand of the patient's affected arm as if to shake it, place your other hand under the affected elbow with your thumb over the radial head, and slowly pronate the wrist so the hand is facing down. This can be done alone or while simultaneously extending the elbow, followed by fully flexing the elbow while still maintaining pronation of the forearm** (Fig. 97.2). A palpable or audible click may be appreciated as subluxation is reduced. While the child cries, leave the bedside for about 10 minutes as noted earlier.

✅ **Initial attempts at reduction using either technique are usually successful.** The majority of children need only a single manipulation, and soon afterward the patient should be able to use the arm normally. Failure is more likely to occur if reduction is attempted 12 or more hours after the injury has occurred.

✅ **If there is not full recovery after 30 minutes, a repeated attempt using the alternative maneuver may be warranted. If this is also unsuccessful, imaging should be obtained to evaluate for occult fracture.** Examine again for possible injury to the clavicle or humerus (particularly the lateral condyle and supracondylar region), and consider other bone and joint disorders. Differential diagnosis includes fracture, soft tissue injury, infection, arthritis, tumor, neurologic injury, and vaso-occlusive crisis in sickle cell.

✅ **In the event that an alternative diagnosis is ruled out and nursemaid's elbow is still the leading diagnosis even without a full recovery** (most likely due to a treatment delay), **place the child in a sling**, with or without posterior splinting. (The elbow should be kept at 90-degree flexion with as much supination of the forearm as comfort will allow.) Provide pediatric or orthopedic follow-up within 24 to 48 hours. Self-reduction almost always occurs during this period of immobilization.

✅ **When full recovery has been obtained, reassure the parents, explain the mechanism involved in the injury, and teach them how to prevent and treat recurrences.**

What Not to Do

❌ Do not attempt to reduce an elbow where the possibility exists of fracture or dislocation such as humerus (e.g., supracondylar), radial head, or Monteggia fracture.

❌ Do not attempt further reduction maneuvers when previous attempts have failed.

❌ Do not get unnecessary radiographs when all the findings are consistent with nursemaid's elbow. The radiographs will appear normal.

❌ Do not confuse nursemaid's elbow with the more serious brachial plexus injury, which occurs after much greater stress and results in a flaccid paralysis of the arm.

Discussion

Nursemaid's elbow or annular ligament displacement (ALD), formerly called radial head subluxation (RHS), is a common pediatric orthopedic problem. It is most often seen in children who are between 1 and 4 years of age and is extremely rare in children who are older than 5 years of age. Injury frequency has been reported to peak twice for both boys and girls at 6 months and 2 years of age. This displacement usually occurs as the result of a sudden forceful longitudinal traction on the hand while the forearm is pronated and the elbow is extended, as when one pulls the forearm of a resisting child.

This condition is actually a displacement of the annular ligament between the capitulum of the distal humerus and the radial head. The annular ligament is displaced from its normal position, covering the radial head, into the radiohumeral joint (Fig. 97.3). Radiographs of an untreated nursemaid's elbow are normal without any evidence of abnormal positioning of the radial head. Although there is a transient subluxation of the radial head, prolonged subluxation does not occur. ALD is more common in girls and in the left arm. About one-third have had a previous episode.

The assessment of the young child is especially challenging because the child cannot relate a coherent history, has difficulty localizing pain, and is often frightened and uncooperative, hindering physical examination. The classic history of a child being pulled up by the arm while falling or lifted by the arm is obtained in only 50% of patients. **The diagnosis is nonetheless made by history and physical examination and confirmed by prompt reuse of the affected arm following reduction.**

Supination or pronation of the forearm usually causes reduction of the annular ligament back into its normal position. The reported recurrence rate involving either the same or contralateral arm is extremely variable, ranging from 5% to 39%.

ALD should be considered in any toddler presenting with arm injury without obvious evidence of trauma. The key to diagnosis is the observation that the child is not in pain; has no swelling, ecchymosis, or deformity; holds the elbow in a slightly flexed position with wrist pronated; refuses to use the arm; and resists supination. When history and physical examination suggest ALD, it is appropriate to attempt reduction without obtaining radiographs. Successful reduction is more likely when a click is felt. On occasion, if the injury has been present for several hours, edema, pain, and natural splinting will continue even after reduction or may prevent reduction.

Although not fully proven safe, parents or caretakers can be instructed by telephone to treat ALD, especially in those cases in which there is a previous history and in which the history is typical of recurrent ALD. Instruct the caregiver to restrain the child by placing him or her in a second adult's lap and then grasp the child's hand. With the treating adult's other hand under the child's affected elbow, straighten out the arm with the palm of the child's hand facing upward. Then have the child bend the elbow up, touching the palm of his or her hand to the same shoulder. After 20 minutes, the child should be moving the arm normally.

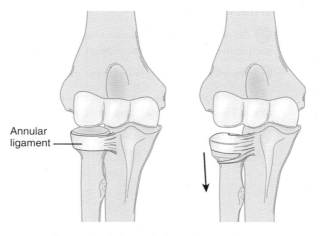

Annular ligament —

Fig. 97.3 Annular ligament displacement (nursemaid's elbow).

Suggested Readings

Elsevier Point of Care. (2020). *Radial head subluxation (nursemaid's elbow)*. Amsterdam, Netherlands: Elsevier BV.

Frumkin, K. (1985). Nursemaid's elbow: A radiographic demonstration. *Annals of Emergency Medicine, 14*, 690–693.

Meiner, E. M., Sama, A. E., & Lee, D. C. (2004). Bilateral nursemaid's elbow. *American Journal of Emergency Medicine, 22*, 502–503.

Quan, L., & Marcuse, E. K. (1985). The epidemiology and treatment of radial head subluxation. *American Journal of Diseases of Children, 139*, 1194–1197.

Schunk, J. E. (1990). Radial head subluxation: Epidemiology and treatment of 87 episodes. *Annals of Emergency Medicine, 19*, 1019–1023.

Schutzman, S. A., & Teach, S. (1995). Upper-extremity impairment in young children. *Annals of Emergency Medicine, 26*, 474–479.

Boutonnière Finger

Presentation

After jamming the tip of a partially or fully extended finger (resulting in hyperflexion of the proximal interphalangeal [PIP] joint) or with direct trauma over the joint, the patient develops a painful, swollen PIP joint. These injuries are seen in basketball players and martial artists, who use open-hand blocking techniques, as well as when an athlete's hand is stepped on or after a volar dislocation at the PIP joint.

Tenderness is greatest over the dorsum of the base of the middle phalanx, and there is diminished extensor tendon strength with pain when the middle phalanx is extended against resistance. **The classic boutonnière deformity is rarely present immediately after injury**; therefore early recognition and intervention are key to preventing this deformity from developing. Radiographs are usually normal.

What to Do

✅ **Obtain a detailed history of the mechanism of injury.**

✅ **Perform a complete examination,** palpating for point tenderness of the dorsum of the PIP joint, the collateral ligaments, and the volar plate. Test for joint stability in all directions, test sensation, and check for injuries proximal and distal to the PIP joint.

✅ **Check for a possible tear of the central slip of the extensor digitorum communis tendon. With the patient's PIP joint flexed at 90 degrees over a straight edge (such as a countertop), apply resistance to active extension over the middle phalanx. If the central slip is ruptured, the patient will not be able to easily extend the middle phalanx at the PIP joint** against resistance (Fig. 98.1A), *as opposed to maintaining strength when the central slip is intact* (see Fig. 98.1B). **In the presence of central slip rupture, the DIP joint can be extended when the PIP joint is flexed because of the recruitment of the lateral bands** (see Fig. 98.1C). **The distal interphalangeal (DIP) joint is in slight hyperextension at rest.**

✅ **Therefore if the patient is unable to extend the finger at the PIP joint against resistance or shows marked weakness, a central-slip extensor injury should be suspected. To make a more definitive diagnosis, the affected finger should be compared with the noninjured finger of the other hand using the modified Elson test (Fig. 98.2).** The injured finger is flexed at about 90 degrees in the PIP joint and pushed against the dorsal side of the midphalanx of the same finger of the noninjured hand. Once in this position, the patient is asked to extend the DIP joints. The finger with a central slip lesion will be able to extend the distal phalanx more than the noninjured distal phalanx.

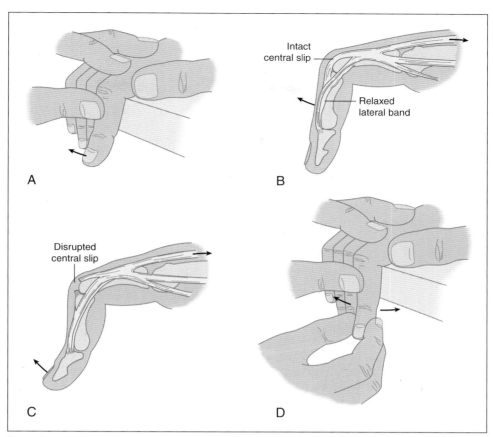

Fig. 98.1 Extension against resistance tests for a central slip avulsion (A–C). Varus and valgus stress at the PIP joint tests for collateral ligament instability (D).

✅ **The difference between the extension at the DIP joint of the injured and noninjured hand is easily observed. Asymmetric position of the two distal phalanges in an effort to extend the distal phalanges suggests that the central slip is avulsed from its insertion on the base of the middle phalanx. If the two fingers remain in a symmetric position when trying to extend the distal phalanges, a central slip lesion is highly unlikely.**

✅ Bedside or formal ultrasonography is a very accurate noninvasive study that can also help to identify central slip injuries in the extensor mechanism of the finger. This can confirm the diagnosis and either allow early initiation of splinting or eliminate the need for prolonged splinting.

✅ Test for collateral ligament stability at the PIP joint with varus and valgus stress (see Fig. 98.1D).

✅ **If avulsion of the central slip of the extensor tendon is suspected or confirmed, splint the PIP joint in extension. The splint should leave the DIP and metacarpophalangeal (MCP) joints completely mobile, or the collateral ligaments will contract.** Active DIP flexion should be encouraged. This action pulls the PIP extensor hood mechanism distally, thereby further approximating the two ends of the ruptured central slip. The PIP joint should remain constantly splinted for 6 weeks followed by another 6 weeks of night splinting (Fig. 98.3). The finger should be splinted for an additional 8 to 10 weeks during contact activity that places the finger at risk of reinjury.

(Modified) Elson Test

- Injured and contralateral fingers knuckle to knuckle in 90° PIP flexion, pt extends DIPs

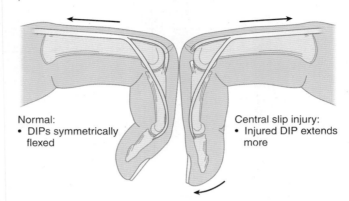

Normal:
- DIPs symmetrically flexed

Central slip injury:
- Injured DIP extends more

Fig. 98.2 Modified Elson test.

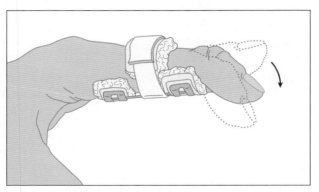

Fig. 98.3 Suspected avulsion of the central slip of the extensor tendon necessitates splinting of the PIP joint in extension, while allowing the DIP joint to go through a full range of motion. (Adapted from Ruiz, E., & Cicero, J. J. [1995]. *Emergency management of skeletal injuries.* St. Louis, MO: Mosby.)

⊘ Prompt referral should be made to a hand surgeon to evaluate for potential acute operative repair and to follow along to ensure complete healing.

⊘ Provide standard acetaminophen or nonsteroidal anti-inflammatory drugs (NSAIDs) along with initial cold compresses and elevation for pain management.

What Not to Do

✗ Do not assume that posttraumatic swelling of a PIP joint represents a simple sprain until testing for extension against resistance and performing the modified Elson test.

✗ Do not overlook associated injuries that may cause joint instability. Such injuries may require immediate orthopedic consultation.

✗ Do not be fooled by the patient's ability to actively extend the PIP joint without resistance. In the acute setting, the patient may be able to fully extend through the action of the lateral bands, despite a complete rupture of the central slip.

Discussion

Thin, soft tissue covering extensor tendons make them prone to injury. The boutonnière (buttonhole) injury or deformity refers to a rupture of the central slip of the extensor tendon at the PIP joint. Early diagnosis and treatment are essential to optimal outcome. Similar to the mechanism of injury in mallet finger, there is forced PIP flexion at the same time the PIP joint is held rigidly in extension. Volar dislocation of the PIP joint is another mechanism that can result in a boutonnière deformity if a central slip injury is unrecognized and left untreated.

Although the acute manifestations of a disrupted central slip may be limited to swelling and tenderness over the PIP joint, with time the central slip retracts. The lateral bands will slip and displace volarly, becoming flexors of the PIP joint and allowing the joint to herniate dorsally through the defect in the tendon (like a button through a buttonhole), thereby creating a flexed PIP joint. Eventually, a position of flexion at the PIP joint and hyperextension at the DIP joint become fixed, producing the classic buttonhole or boutonnière deformity (Fig. 98.4). This clinical presentation may only occur 10 to 14 days after the initial injury.

Early diagnosis is clearly the key to prevention. Because the acute injury may suggest nothing more than a contusion or sprain, any injury around the PIP joint should be viewed with suspicion.

A boutonnière finger, like a mallet finger, requires complete and prolonged immobilization. Unfortunately, many people do not seek help for a central slip avulsion until a deformity has developed; at that point, surgery may be required to correct the retinacular structures and the subluxed lateral bands. Once a deformity becomes chronic or fixed, it presents a difficult surgical challenge with potentially permanent functional deficits.

A hyperextension injury at the PIP joint that disrupts the volar plate and tears the accessory collateral ligaments may lead to chronic pseudoboutonnière deformity if there is a delay in diagnosis. This pseudoboutonnière is generally less severe than a true boutonnière deformity. Treatment of a pseudoboutonnière deformity consists of progressive stretching of the contracture with dynamic splinting before considering surgical release.

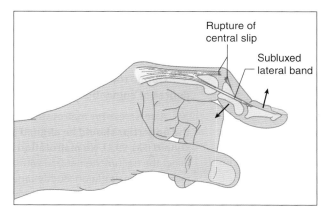

Rupture of central slip

Subluxed lateral band

Fig. 98.4 Boutonnière deformity.

Suggested Readings

Hong, E. (2005). Hand injuries in sports medicine. *PrimaryCare*, *32*, 91–103.

Netscher, D. T., Pham, D. T., & Staines, K. G. (2017). Finger injuries in ball sports. *Hand Clinics*, *33*(1), 119–139.

Patel, D., Dean, C., & Baker, R. J. (2005). The hand in sports: An update on the clinical anatomy and physical examination. *PrimaryCare*, *32*, 71–89.

Perron, A. D., & Brady, W. J. (2003). Evaluation and management of the high-risk orthopedic emergency. *Emergency Medicine Clinics of North America*, *21*, 159–204.

Westerheide, E., Failla, J. M., van Holsbeeck, M., et al. (2003). Ultrasound visualization of central slip injuries of the finger extensor mechanism. *Journal of Hand Surgery*, *28*, 1009–1013.

Boxer's Fifth Metacarpal Fracture

Presentation

The patient seeks help for painful swelling of the hand over the distal fifth metacarpal (MC) after punching an object or another person with a closed fist. It occurs commonly during fistfights or from punching a hard object, such as a wall or a filing cabinet, and may be an act of deliberate self-harm or a compulsive action while enraged.

What to Do

✓ **Obtain a clear history regarding the mechanism of injury** and the circumstances that led up to the punching incident.

✓ **Examine the patient's hand, with attention to inspection and palpation of the fifth MC.** The normal prominence of the fifth knuckle may be lost, and most often there will be tenderness at the neck of the fifth MC, where the shaft meets the head. **Any overlying laceration obtained in a fistfight should be considered a human bite and needs to be treated aggressively (see Chapter 140).**

✓ **Obtain routine radiographs of the injured hand to determine the exact nature and degree of angulation of any fracture.**

✓ **Also assess for malrotation by examining the direction of the fingers in flexion. All of the fingertips should be aligned parallel to one another and pointing toward the radial styloid** (Fig. 99.1). **No malrotation is acceptable. If any malalignment is present** (Fig. 99.2), inject the fracture hematoma with a local anesthetic and, with traction and counterrotation, reduce the malrotation. Buddy-tape the fifth finger to the fourth finger while padding between the fingers to maintain normal alignment and place the hand and wrist in an ulnar gutter splint.

✓ **Most fractures occur just below the metacarpal head without rotation but are usually displaced in a volar direction. Up to 40 to 70 degrees of volar angulation is acceptable in the nonoperative management of a boxer's fracture.**

✓ **Traditionally, patients with a boxer's fracture were all placed in an ulnar gutter splint** with the fourth and fifth metacarpophalangeal (MCP) joints in a 90-degree flexed position and given orthopedic follow-up within 1 week. **This gutter splinting may not be necessary; buddy-taping of the fourth and fifth fingers alone, with padding between them, should be adequate management. A randomized controlled Australian study**, designed and endorsed by emergency and orthopedic specialists, demonstrated that buddy-taping resulted

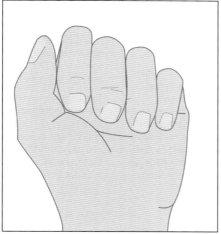

Fig. 99.1   Normal alignment.

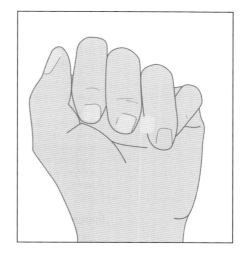

Fig. 99.2   Rotational deformity.

in outcomes similar to those of plaster casting. Patients in both the buddy-taping and plaster groups had the same good functional outcomes, and the buddy-taping group returned to work earlier than those randomized to the plaster group. Pain and satisfaction scores were similar for both groups at 1 and 12 weeks. There were no radiographic complications in either group, and healed fracture angles were similar. In addition, patients randomized to the buddy-taping group spent, on average, 36 minutes less time in the emergency department than those randomized to the plaster group.

✅ **Pain management is with acetaminophen alone or in addition to nonsteroidal anti-inflammatory drugs (NSAIDs), where there is no contraindication.**

✅ Self-harmers and patients who are having problems controlling their anger should be considered for psychiatric assessment and referral.

What Not to Do

❌ Do not overlook a so-called fight bite injury. All open wounds over the MCP joints should be considered fist-to-mouth human bite wounds, which have the highest incidence of infectious complications of any closed-fist injury and of any type of bite wound (see Chapter 142). These should be treated with antibiotics prophylactically, even if there is no current evidence of infection.

Discussion

An isolated fracture of the distal fifth metacarpal bone, known as a boxer's fracture, is the most common type of metacarpal fracture. Boxer's fractures are named for one of their most common causes—punching an object with a closed fist. This is somewhat of a misnomer because boxers learn not to punch this way,

and the injury is seen more commonly in laypeople striking a hard object with a closed fist.

Detailed physical examination is crucial, as open fractures with tendinous involvement can be very

(continued)

Discussion continued

subtle. If missed, however, these injuries can lead to devastating infections and permanent disability.

There is no good evidence to guide conservative treatment of boxer's fractures, and a Cochrane review on the topic was unable to make any definitive recommendations. Although some studies have reported no loss of function in patients with fractures that are volarly angulated up to 70 degrees, common practice is to reduce angulated fractures of the fifth metacarpal neck of greater than 40 degrees. Without reduction, pseudoclawing of the hand may result in a functional deficit. Any rotational deformity needs to be reduced to preserve maximal hand function. All boxer's fractures should be given an orthopedic or sports medicine follow-up.

This injury has been described as "a tolerable fracture in an intolerable patient." Anxiety symptoms and maladaptive personality traits are very common in patients with boxer's fractures. Psychiatric assessment and counseling should be strongly considered in these patients, who actually have a high risk for recurrence of self-harm or aggressive acts.

Suggested Readings

Hong, E. (2005). Hand injuries in sports medicine. *Primary Care, 32*, 91–103.

Mercan, S., Uzun, M., Ertugrul, A., et al. (2005). Psychopathology and personality features in orthopedic patients with boxer's fractures. *General Hospital Psychiatry, 27*, 13–17.

Muller, M. G. (2003). Immediate mobilization gives good results in boxer's fractures with volar angulation up to 70 degrees: A prospective randomized trial comparing immediate mobilization with cast immobilization. *Archives of Orthopedic Trauma Surgery, 123*, 537.

Patel, D., Dean, C., & Baker, R. J. (2005). The hand in sports: An update on the clinical anatomy and physical examination. *Primary Care, 32*, 71–89.

Pellatt, R., Fomin, I., Pienaar, C., Bindra, R., Thomas, M., Tan, E., et al. (2019). Is buddy taping as effective as plaster immobilization for adults with an uncomplicated neck of fifth metacarpal fracture? A randomized controlled trial. *Annals of Emergency Medicine, 74*(1), 88–97.

Perron, A. D., & Brady, W. J. (2003). Evaluation and management of the high-risk orthopedic emergency. *Emergency Medicine Clinics of North America, 21*, 159–204.

Poolman, R. W., Goslings, J. C., Lee, J., Statius Muller, M., Steller, E. P., & Struijs, P. A. A. (2005). Conservative treatment for closed fifth (small finger) metacarpal neck fractures. *Cochrane Database of Systematic Reviews, 3*, CD003210.

Sanderson, M., Mohr, B., & Abraham, M. K. (2020). The emergent evaluation and treatment of hand and wrist injuries. *Emergency Medicine Clinics of North America, 38*(1), 61–79.

Bursitis

Presentation

Following minimal trauma or repetitive motion, a nonarticular synovial sac or bursa protecting a tendon or prominent bone becomes swollen and possibly painful, inflamed, and fluctuant. It may be nontender or tender. The elbow, hip, knee, and shoulder are most commonly involved unilaterally.

Olecranon bursitis of the elbow can be caused by trauma from a direct blow (often only causing acute hemorrhage into the bursa), chronic crushing friction from prolonged leaning on the elbows, crystal deposition (gout), systemic diseases (rheumatoid arthritis, diabetes, systemic lupus erythematosus [SLE], alcoholism, uremia), or infection (usually from an overlying skin lesion or wound).

Trochanteric bursitis causes pain and tenderness that is greatest over the lateral hip. Active resistance to abduction of the hip may increase the pain.

Ischial bursitis can result from trauma or prolonged sitting on a hard surface. This causes buttock pain that may radiate down the back of the thigh. Palpation will reveal point tenderness over the ischial tuberosity.

Prepatellar bursitis, also known as housemaid's knee, is caused by frequent or prolonged kneeling on hard surfaces. There may be marked swelling and tenderness over the anterior surface of the patella.

Pes anserine bursitis is located on the medial inferior aspect of the knee on the anterior medial aspect of the knee about 4 to 5 cm below the joint margin and just superior to the pes anserinus tendon. Inflammation of this bursa is common in overweight middle-aged and elderly women with knee pain. It is also seen in those people beginning an exercise program, distance runners, and individuals with osteoarthritis of the knee. The knee pain is worsened when climbing stairs, and there is tenderness to direct palpation over the area of the bursa.

Subdeltoid (or subacromial) bursitis can be the result of traumatic injury or chronic overuse of the shoulder, and it frequently accompanies other shoulder problems. A history of pain in the lateral shoulder, which can be severe with acute onset, and tenderness to palpation along the acromial border help make the diagnosis. Shoulder strength should be intact, although active strength testing may be limited due to pain.

Because there is no joint involved, there is usually little decreased range of motion, except in the shoulder, where bursitis can produce dramatic limitation. If the tendon sheath is involved, there may be some stiffness and pain with motion. Swelling is less evident when the bursa is deep, such as in the case of ischial bursitis.

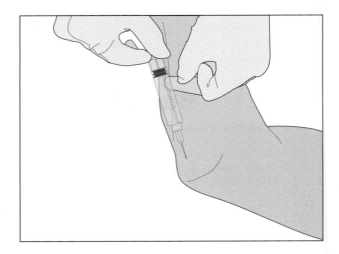

Fig. 100.1 Technique for draining olecranon bursitis.

What to Do

✓ **Obtain a detailed history of the injury or precipitating activity, document a thorough physical examination, and rule out a joint effusion** (see Chapter 118).

✓ Obtain a radiograph or ultrasound study, especially if the possibility of a foreign body exists.

✓ **Bursae can become infected, and when there is swelling and fluctuance of a bursa accompanied by overlying erythema, warmth, tenderness, and fever, the possibility of septic bursitis should be explored. Prepare the skin with alcohol and povidone-iodine antiseptic solution, and either anesthetize the skin with 1% lidocaine using a 30-gauge needle or spray with ethyl chloride. Puncture the swollen bursa with a needle (18 or 20 gauge) using aseptic technique, withdraw some fluid to drain the effusion, and have the fluid analyzed to rule out a bacterial infection.** Attempt to penetrate the skin tangentially in an area without overlying erythema and cellulitis, if possible (Fig. 100.1).

✓ **Relatively clear yellow or serosanguineous fluid** drained from a minimally inflamed or noninflamed bursa **needs to be sent only for culture**, because clear fluid indicates a nonseptic bursitis. Crystal analysis can be considered, as well, if the history suggests gout or pseudogout as the etiology of the bursitis. **If there is no concern for infection, corticosteroid can be injected into the bursa after aspiration to help resolve inflammation.** Using a hemostat to grasp the needle hub to twist off and remove the syringe, the needle can be left within the bursa, and the syringe containing the corticosteroid can then be connected to it. **When the fluid appears purulent or cloudy, or if the clinical picture is unclear, the needle should be removed and no corticosteroid should be instilled. The aspirated fluid should be sent for leukocyte count, Gram stain, culture, and sensitivity; it should also be analyzed for crystals when there is suspicion of gout or pseudogout.**

✓ **Examine a Gram stain of the effusion.** This may be negative in about 30% of patients with septic bursitis. **Leukocyte counts greater than 2000/mm³ have a high sensitivity and specificity for bursal infections.** The white blood cell (WBC) count for the nonseptic bursitis will usually be only a few hundred/mm³. <u>With or without fluid to examine, it is often difficult to clinically distinguish an inflamed bursa from an infected one.</u> Therefore, if there is any

suggestion or sign of a bacterial infection, hold any steroids and prescribe appropriate oral antibiotics. Bacterial bursal infections tend to result from gram-positive cocci, specifically *Staphylococcus aureus*, and respond well to appropriate coverage. Consider covering for methicillin-resistant *S. aureus* (MRSA) when indicated. Serial aspirations of purulent fluid or surgical drainage may be indicated.

✅ Initially, reaspirate any recurrent infected effusion on a daily basis. **Severe infections will require parenteral antibiotics and hospitalization.**

✅ When there is no indication of a bacterial infection, **inflammatory bursitis may respond to injection of local anesthetics such as lidocaine 1% (Xylocaine) or bupivacaine 0.25% (Marcaine), 5 to 9 mL, mixed with corticosteroids, such as methylprednisolone (Depo-Medrol), 40 mg, triamcinolone (Kenalog), 15 to 40 mg, or betamethasone (Celestone Soluspan), 1 mL. When available, use the aspiration needle (18 or 20 gauge) left in place. Alternatively, use a 25-gauge, 1.25-inch needle** and review the anatomy so that the needle can be carefully pushed through the lowest-density tissue and the shortest pathway, causing the least amount of pain while probing for the bursa sac. For olecranon bursitis, perform the injection with the arm in extension, and penetrate the sac parallel to the ulna on the lateral side, away from the ulnar nerve. Approach the greater trochanteric bursae from the lateral and posterior side. For the subacromial bursa, insert the needle just inferior to the posterolateral edge of the acromion and then direct the needle toward the opposite nipple. **The anesthetic and steroid should flow freely into the space without any resistance or significant discomfort to the patient. Ultrasound-guided corticosteroid injections potentially offer a significantly greater clinical improvement over blind subacromial bursitis injections in adults with shoulder pain.** After injection of local anesthetic and steroid, it may take several minutes or longer for patients to perceive pain relief and regain lost range of motion. The literature suggests that the instillation of a long-acting corticosteroid in a noninfected bursitis is associated with a significantly better cure rate than aspiration or nonsteroidal anti-inflammatory drugs (NSAIDs) alone or in combination.

✅ **For knee and elbow, apply a bulky compressive dressing after aspiration and/or injection for protection and comfort. A sling should suffice for the shoulder.**

✅ Awaiting effect of the steroid injection, acetaminophen can be used for pain management. NSAIDs can be used if there is no contraindication (gastrointestinal bleeding, hypertension, kidney disease, coronary artery disease). Follow-up with primary care, orthopedics, or sports medicine should be arranged.

✅ Fluid may reaccumulate and require additional aspiration.

✅ When symptoms have subsided, prior to returning to any previous activity, have the patient take measures (padding bony prominences [i.e., knee pads], correcting any muscle imbalances, slowly ramping up a new exercise regimen) to prevent further bursal irritation.

✅ Septic bursitis resolves slowly over weeks; 2 to 3 weeks of antibiotics are required, and close follow-up is mandatory.

What Not to Do

❌ Do not inject corticosteroids into a potentially infected bursa. The infection is likely to worsen and spread.

(X) Do not puncture an area of olecranon bursitis by needling perpendicular to the ulna. Flexion and trauma may produce a chronic sinus. Use a tangential approach (Fig. 100.1).

(X) Do not routinely obtain radiographs when there is minimal trauma involved and the nature of the bursitis is obvious. They are generally not helpful or necessary in these circumstances. Ultrasound imaging may be more helpful when location and size of fluid accumulation is unclear.

Discussion

Common sites for bursitis include the subacromial bursa of the shoulder, the prepatellar bursa of the knee, the olecranon bursa of the elbow, and the trochanteric bursa of the hip. **In shoulder bursitis, radiographs may reveal calcific bursitis. There may be bony spurs in olecranon bursitis, but these images are not needed for routine emergency department or urgent care management.**

Burning pain and sometimes numbness in the anterolateral thigh, which may be worsened by prolonged standing or walking, may be caused by compression of the lateral femoral cutaneous nerve in the area of the anterior superior iliac spine **(meralgia paresthetica). This should not be confused with bursitis.** There is no tenderness over the greater trochanter of the hip. Obese, pregnant, or diabetic patients or workers who carry a heavy tool belt are commonly affected. Tightly fitting garments that also crush the cutaneous nerves against the hard underlying ileum may also precipitate the syndrome. Meralgia paresthetica usually resolves after conservative treatment, such as weight loss and the wearing of loose-fitting clothes.

Patients with septic bursitis, unlike those with septic arthritis, can often be safely discharged on oral antibiotics because the risk for permanent damage is much less when there is no joint involvement. Severe cases with extensive cellulitis or lymphangitis, however, may require hospitalization and intravenous (IV) antibiotics. Immunocompromised patients may require longer courses of antibiotics. Grossly purulent fluid that reaccumulates must be repeatedly aspirated.

Some long-acting corticosteroid preparations can produce rebound bursitis several hours after injection, after the local anesthetic wears off but before the corticosteroid crystals dissolve and take therapeutic effect. Patients should be so informed. **Patients should prevent recurrence** by wearing knee or elbow pads at work, avoiding pressure and trauma to vulnerable areas, limiting repetitive motion that exacerbates activities, correcting muscle imbalances, and incorporating new physical activity gradually.

Suggested Readings

Deu, R. S., & Carek, P. J. (2005). Common sports injuries: Upper extremity injuries. *Clinics in Family Practice, 7,* 249–265.

McFarland, E. G., Gill, H. S., Laporte, D. M., et al. (2004). Miscellaneous conditions about the elbow in athletes. *Clinics in Sports Medicine, 23,* 743–763, xi-xii.

Pien, F. D., Ching, D., & Kim, E. (1991). Septic bursitis: Experience in a community practice. *Orthopedics, 14,* 981–984.

Smith, D. L., McAfee, J. H., Lucas, L. M., et al. (1989). Treatment of nonseptic olecranon bursitis. *Archives of Internal Medicine, 149,* 2527–2530.

Tallia, A. F., & Cardone, D. A. (2003). Diagnostic and therapeutic injection of the shoulder region. *American Family Physician, 67,* 2147–2152.

Wu, T., Song, H. X., Dong, Y., & Li, J. H. (2015). Ultrasound-guided versus blind subacromial—subdeltoid bursa injection in adults with shoulder pain: A systematic review and meta-analysis. *Seminars in Arthritis and Rheumatism, 45*(3), 374–378.

Carpal Tunnel Syndrome

Presentation

The patient complains of pain, tingling, or a "pins and needles" sensation in the hand(s) or fingers. There may be the sensation of swelling or tightness in the absence of edema in the affected hand(s) as well as the sensation of extreme temperature. Onset may have been abrupt or gradual, but the problem is most noticeable after extended use of the hand or when driving or holding up reading material. There may be decreased grip strength, resulting in loss of dexterity, and patients may complain of dropping things and having difficulty with opening jars. Symptoms are usually worse at night and commonly awaken the patient. Sports such as racquetball and handball or activities such as assembly-line work and use of vibratory tools (e.g., jackhammers) are frequently associated with carpal tunnel syndrome (CTS). CTS has also been associated with a number of systemic conditions, including rheumatoid arthritis, sarcoidosis, multiple myeloma, leukemia, diabetes, hypothyroidism, acromegaly, gout, renal failure, obesity, pregnancy, and menopause. The dominant hand can be affected initially but the uncomfortable sensation is often bilateral, may include pain in the wrist or forearm, and, is usually ascribed to the entire hand until specific physical examination localizes it to the median nerve distribution (thumb, index, and middle finger on the palmar side). Strenuous use of the hand almost always aggravates the symptoms. To relieve the symptoms, patients often flick the wrist as if shaking down a thermometer (flick sign). More established cases may include weakness of the thumb and atrophy of the thenar eminence. Although one hand typically has more severe symptoms, as previously mentioned, both hands are often affected.

Physical examination localizes paresthesia and decreased sensation to the median nerve distribution (which may vary) (Fig. 101.1). Motor weakness, if present, is localized to intrinsic muscles with median innervation. Innervation varies widely, but the muscles most reliably innervated by the median nerve are the abductors and opponens of the thumb (Fig. 101.2). CTS typically occurs after 30 years of age and is three times more common in women than in men.

What to Do

⊘ Perform and document a complete examination, illustrating the area of decreased sensation and grading (on a scale of 1–5) the strength of the muscles of the hand. **One clinical finding that best identifies patients** with electrodiagnostic studies that are positive for CTS is hypalgesia (diminished perception of painful stimuli) along the palmar aspect of the index finger, compared with the ipsilateral little finger. Another typical finding is weakness of resistance to downward pressure applied to the distal phalanx of the thumb, while the patient rests the dorsal surface of the hand on a hard surface with the thumb raised perpendicular to the palm** (see Fig. 101.2).

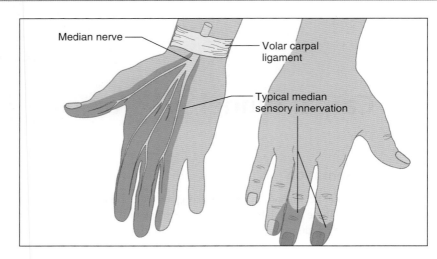

Median nerve

Volar carpal ligament

Typical median sensory innervation

Fig. 101.1 Sensory abnormalities are found along the median nerve distribution.

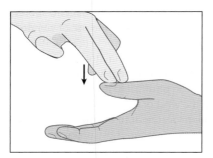

Fig. 101.2 Testing thumb abduction.

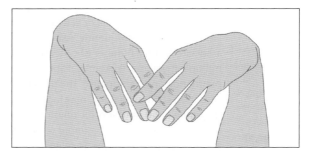

Fig. 101.3 The Phalen test.

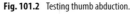

(✓) **Although the Tinel sign and a positive Phalen maneuver are classic clinical signs of CTS, their actual utility in the diagnosis is not clear.** With the Phalen test (Fig. 101.3), the patient passively drops both wrists to 90 degrees of flexion for 60 seconds to see if this reproduces symptoms. It is more sensitive than the reverse (hyperextending the wrist) and more specific than tapping over the volar carpal ligament to elicit paresthesia in the distribution of the median nerve (Tinel sign).

(✓) **The hand elevation test is comparable in accuracy to the Phalen test and only requires the patient to hold the arm over the head as high as comfortably possible.** Reproduction of CTS symptoms within 1 minute is considered a positive test.

(✓) **Patients should be told to avoid repetitive wrist and hand motions that may exacerbate symptoms or make symptom relief difficult to achieve.** If possible, they should not use vibratory tools (e.g., jackhammers, floor sanders).

(✓) **Wrist splints that maintain the wrist in a neutral position may be helpful for patients who engage in repetitive wrist motion often. These may also be beneficial for use at nighttime to prevent the natural wrist flexion position that most assume while sleeping.**

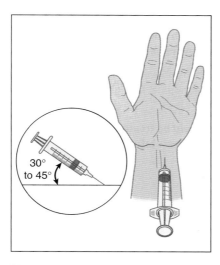

Fig. 101.4 Location for needle insertion.

☑️ **A 4-week course of oral prednisone (e.g., 20 mg daily for 2 weeks, then 10 mg daily for another 2 weeks) may offer short-term relief in mild to moderate cases.**

☑️ **When a patient is not on anticoagulation therapy and does not have a coagulopathy,** injections of corticosteroids directly into the carpal tunnel **can often dramatically alleviate symptoms and may improve symptoms for a longer period with fewer systemic symptoms. When combined with a local anesthetic, such injections can be diagnostic as well as therapeutic.** Using a 1-inch, 25-gauge needle with 40 mg of methylprednisolone (Depo-Medrol) or 0.5 mL of betamethasone (Celestone Soluspan) along with 5 mL of bupivacaine (Marcaine), 0.25%, or 5 mL of lidocaine 1% with the hand facing toward the ceiling and a rolled towel positioned under the dorsal wrist to create moderate wrist extension, inject on the ulnar side of the palmaris longus tendon, which is midway between the flexor carpi radialis and the flexor carpi ulnaris tendons, just proximal (1 cm) to the flexor crease of the wrist, distally into the central portion of the flexor tendon mass (Fig. 101.4). The palmaris longus tendon can be identified by having the patient pinch the thumb and fifth fingers together while slightly flexing the wrist. Avoid injecting either the median or ulnar nerve or radial or ulnar artery. If injection produces paresthesia in the distribution of the median or ulnar nerve, withdraw the needle and redirect it to avoid intraneural injection. If the patient gets immediate relief of the symptoms, the diagnosis of CTS is very likely. When the local anesthetic wears off and after 1 day of wrist splinting, the patient can expect symptomatic relief, but the maximum effect may not come until up to 1 week later. Warn the patient that the hand will feel somewhat numb for a few hours and that a rebound phenomenon or flare may develop within 12 hours after the injection. Nonsteroidal anti-inflammatory drugs (NSAIDs), elevation, and ice packs will help if this rebound pain occurs.

☑️ **If the first injection is successful, a repeat injection can be considered after a few months.** Surgery should be considered if a patient needs more than two injections. An orthopedic referral can be made for these patients.

☑️ **A diagnosis may be established in borderline cases with electrodiagnostic studies (nerve conduction and electromyography [EMG]),** but they have significant false-positive and false-negative results. **These studies may also be considered when surgical management is being considered, in patients with thenar atrophy and/or when there is persistent numbness (to document more severe nerve injury).**

✅ If symptoms are refractory to the above-mentioned conservative measures or if nerve conduction studies show severe entrapment, surgical referral for open or endoscopic carpal tunnel release may be necessary.

✅ **Carpal tunnel syndrome should be treated conservatively** in pregnant women because spontaneous postpartum resolution is common.

What Not to Do

❌ Do not rule out thumb weakness just because the thumb can touch the little finger. Thumb flexors may be innervated by the ulnar nerve.

❌ Do not diagnose carpal tunnel syndrome solely on the basis of a positive Tinel sign. Paresthesia can be produced in the distribution of any nerve if one taps hard enough.

❌ Do not perform the Phalen test for more than 60 seconds; maintaining a flexed wrist for longer may produce paresthesia in a normal hand.

❌ Do not persist with prolonged, nonoperative treatment in patients with more severe or prolonged carpal tunnel syndrome. These patients may only benefit from surgical intervention.

❌ Do not prescribe or recommend NSAIDs, pyridoxine (vitamin B_6), diuretics, or chiropractic therapy for CTS symptoms. They have been shown to be no more effective than a placebo in relieving these symptoms.

Discussion

Carpal tunnel syndrome is one of the most common causes of hand pain, particularly in middle-aged women. There is little space to spare where the median nerve and digit flexors pass beneath the volar carpal ligament, and very little swelling may produce this specific neuropathy. There is no single reference standard for the diagnosis of CTS. Whether CTS is a clinical or electrophysiologic diagnosis remains somewhat controversial. Professional consensus committees have recognized nerve conduction studies as the diagnostic standard for CTS. It must still be appreciated that although electrodiagnostic studies may assist in confirming the diagnosis, they unfortunately have significant false-positive and false-negative results.

Although most cases are idiopathic or the result of nonspecific flexor tenosynovitis, CTS is also associated with trauma and a number of systemic conditions previously mentioned. There is also

strong evidence of a positive association of CTS with exposure to forceful work and repetition (e.g., in meat packers, poultry processors, and automobile assembly workers).

Although the incidence of diagnosed CTS has increased over time, and public attention has focused on excessive keyboard use, frequent computer use has not yet been established as a cause of CTS. Although 30% of frequent computer users complain of hand paresthesias, only 10% meet clinical criteria for CTS, and nerve conduction studies are abnormal in only 3.5% of these persons.

Usually the initial diagnosis of CTS is made on clinical grounds. Because about 50% will resolve spontaneously, not all need to be referred for nerve conduction studies or surgical assessment.

Patients with mild symptoms should be offered conservative treatment such as activity modification and splinting. In those cases clearly related to

(Continued)

Discussion continued

occupational job tasks, such as highly repetitive forceful work or work involving hand and wrist vibration, the patient should be advised to modify the activities or movements that caused the CTS. Splinting is a low-cost option that may provide benefit and certainly warrants a trial. Compared with nighttime-only splint use, full-time use has been shown to provide greater improvement of symptoms and electrophysiologic measures; however, compliance with full-time use is more difficult.

With moderate symptoms, steroid injection and, to a lesser extent, oral corticosteroids provide the most effective nonsurgical treatment.

After conservative measures have been performed, **surgical referral** should be considered in patients **with symptoms that are causing persistent sleep disturbance, interfering with their ability to work, causing weakness and/or atrophy, or otherwise adversely affecting their lifestyle.** In general, surgical management is indicated for persistent symptoms (not resolving after 1 year) or deteriorating symptoms (worsening clinical plus or minus deterioration on nerve conduction studies). Indications for surgery also include severe symptoms, persistent dysesthesia, thenar weakness or atrophy, and acute median neurapraxia caused by the closed compartment compression. One study showed that patients who had surgery within 3 years of the initial diagnosis were twice as likely to have symptom relief than were those whose surgery was delayed more than 3 years. **Endoscopic carpal tunnel release** is a newer procedure that allows division of the transverse carpal ligament, with the overlying structures left intact. Use of this procedure purportedly lessens scar formation and allows an earlier return to work and activities of daily living. Neither open nor endoscopic technique has been conclusively proven superior. The wrist is generally splinted for 3 to 4 weeks after surgery.

Less often, the median nerve can be entrapped more proximally, where it enters the medial antecubital fossa through the pronator teres (pronator teres syndrome). Symptoms of this type of entrapment syndrome may be reproduced with resisted pronation of the forearm and wrist flexion. The differential diagnosis of CTS also includes cervical radiculopathy (neck pain with associated radiation to upper extremity in a specific dermatomal distribution), osteoarthritis (results in severe pain and restricted movement of wrist), and diabetic neuropathy (frequently bilateral; causes tingling and numbness in a stocking-and-glove distribution).

Suggested Readings

Atroshi, I., Gummesson, C., Johnsson, R., et al. (1999). Prevalence of carpal tunnel syndrome in a general population. *Journal of the American Medical Association, 282,* 153–158.

Burke, D. T., Burke, M. M., Stewart, G. W., et al. (1994). Splinting for carpal tunnel syndrome: In search of the optimal angle. *Archives of Physical Medicine and Rehabilitation, 75,* 1241–1244.

Chang, M. H., Chiang, H. T., Lee, S. S., et al. (1998). Oral drug of choice in carpal tunnel syndrome. *Neurology, 51,* 390–393.

D'Arcy, C., & McGee, S. (2000). Does this patient have carpal tunnel syndrome? *Journal of the American Medical Association, 283,* 3110–3117.

De Smet, L. (2003). Value of some clinical provocative tests in carpal tunnel syndrome: Do we need electrophysiology and can we predict the outcome? *Hand Clinics, 19,* 387–391.

Deu, R. S., & Carek, P. J. (2005). Common sports injuries: Upper extremity injuries. *Clinics in Family Practice, 7,* 249–265.

Dias, J. J., Burke, F. D., Wildin, C. J., et al. (2004). Carpal tunnel syndrome. *Journal of Hand Surgery (Britain), 29,* 329–333.

Elsevier Point of Care. (2018). *Carpal tunnel syndrome.* Amsterdam, Netherlands: Elsevier BV.

Goodyear-Smith, F., & Arroll, B. (2004). What can family physicians offer patients with carpal tunnel syndrome other than surgery? A systematic review of nonsurgical management. *The Annals of Family Medicine, 2,* 267–273.

Hui, A. C. F., Wong, S., Leung, C. H., et al. (2005). A randomized controlled trial of surgery vs steroid injection for carpal tunnel syndrome. *Neurology, 64,* 2074–2078.

Kamath, V., & Stothard, J. (2003). A clinical questionnaire for the diagnosis of carpal tunnel syndrome. *Journal of Hand Surgery (Britain)*, *28*, 455–459.

Kele, H., Verheggen, R., Bitterman, H., et al. (2003). The potential value of ultrasonography in the evaluation of carpal tunnel syndrome. *Neurology*, *61*, 389–391.

Kuhlman, K. A., & Hennessey, W. J. (1997). Sensitivity and specificity of carpal tunnel syndrome signs. *American Journal of Physical Medicine and Rehabilitation*, *76*, 451–457.

Tallia, A. F., & Cardone, D. A. (2003). Diagnostic and therapeutic injection of the wrist and hand region. *American Family Physician*, *67*, 1356–1362.

Viera, A. J. (2003). Management of carpal tunnel syndrome. *American Family Physician*, *68*, 265–272.

Cervical Strain

(Whiplash)

Presentation

The patient will complain of neck pain after any mechanism that caused forceful neck hyperextension followed by hyperflexion. This is most commonly seen after a motor vehicle collision when the vehicle is struck from behind, but sports injuries and falls may also cause this injury. Patients may present directly after sustaining the injury complaining of acute neck pain, may arrive the following day complaining of increased neck stiffness and pain, or may seek medical attention any time afterward to have the injuries documented. The injury was incurred when the neck was subjected to sudden extension and flexion, possibly injuring intervertebral joints, disks, and ligaments; cervical muscles; or even nerve roots. As is common with other strains and sprains, the stiffness and pain tend to peak 1 to 3 days after the injury.

What to Do

✅ **Obtain a detailed history** to determine the exact mechanism and severity of the injury. Was the patient wearing a seat belt? Was the headrest up? Were eyeglasses thrown into the rear seat? Was the seat broken? Was the car damaged? Was the car drivable afterward? Was the windshield shattered? Was there intrusion into the passenger compartment?

✅ **Did a sports injury include a worrisome mechanism of injury,** such as axial loading with the neck flexed or hyperextended, or did it involve spear tackling (using the helmet as the point of impact when tackling)?

✅ **Historical red flags that suggest a serious spinal injury include any dangerous mechanism of injury (e.g., a fall from a height >1 m; an axial loading injury, as described earlier or a diving injury; high-speed [>60 m/hr or >100 km/hr] motor vehicle collision, rollover, or ejection; motorized recreational vehicle or bicycle collision) or the presence of paresthesias in the extremities, severe neck pain, or persistent patient apprehension.**

✅ **To evaluate the possibility of head trauma**, ask about loss of consciousness or amnesia, headache, and nausea or vomiting (see Chapter 10).

✅ **Examine the patient for involuntary splinting, point tenderness over the spinous processes of the cervical vertebrae, cervical muscle spasm or tenderness, and strength, sensation, and reflexes in the arms to evaluate the cervical nerve roots.**

✅ **Objective red flags that suggest a serious spinal injury include age of 65 years or older, inability of the patient to actively rotate the neck 45 degrees to the left and to the right, any focal neurologic findings, or midline cervical tenderness.**

✓ **If there is any question of an unstable neck injury based on historical or objective red flags** mentioned previously or if there is altered mentation, intoxication, or painful distracting injuries, **immobilize the cervical spine. Traditionally this is done with a rigid collar, manual in-line stabilization, and often a rigid backboard/spineboard. Although this approach initially appears to provide the safest framework, in practice, research suggests it may be causing more harm than good, and a more flexible stabilization protocol may lead to better overall outcomes.** (See discussion.)

✓ **After the neck is satisfactorily secured, proceed to imaging of the cervical spine. Although a cross-table radiograph of the cervical spine may be useful, computed tomography (CT) scanning is far more sensitive for diagnosing cervical spinal injuries and is generally preferred if there is more than a minimal index of suspicion** or if there are reasons why plain radiograph will be technically limited, such as obesity, demineralization, or significant degenerative disease.

✓ **Most minor neck injuries can be safely cleared without obtaining any radiologic studies.** Using the **Canadian C-spine rule** if there are no historical or physical high-risk factors (red flags noted previously), and the patient has low-risk factors that allow a safe assessment of neck range of motion (ROM; e.g., simple rear-end motor vehicle collision, ability to sit at the time of the examination, ability to ambulate at any time after the injury, or delayed onset of neck pain) and is able to actively rotate the neck 45 degrees to the left and to the right, without midline C-spine tenderness, imaging is not necessary.

✓ Alternatively, the **National Emergency X-ray Use Study (NEXUS)** can be applied to safely clear the cervical spine without any imaging studies in patients who have normal alertness, are not intoxicated, have no painful distracting injuries, and, on examination, have no midline cervical tenderness or focal neurologic deficits.

✓ **Initially, if the neck cannot be cleared**, routine cervical spine immobilization in a hard cervical collar may provide more harm than benefit in neck injuries, and a more individualized approach may be more reasonable.

✓ **If the C-spine has been cleared clinically or radiographically and history and physical examination are consistent with a stable, mild to moderate joint, ligament, and/or muscle injury, the patient can be safely discharged home. Explain to the patient that the stiffness and pain are often worse after 24 hours but usually begin to resolve over the next 3 to 5 days.** Most patients are back to normal in 1 week, although some have persistent pain.

✓ **When there is significant discomfort, provide 1 or 2 days of intermittent immobilization by fitting a soft cervical collar to wear when out of bed.** Place the wide side of the cervical collar either anterior or posterior, based on the position of maximum comfort. When worn in reverse, the collar allows neck flexion and may be valuable, particularly when carrying out certain activities of daily living, such as driving. **If neither position improves comfort, omit the collar entirely. Under any circumstances, a collar should be used for as brief a time as possible because early mobilization has been shown to speed recovery,** and a soft cervical collar has not been shown to provide any benefit in outcome and may actually lead to stiffness and delayed recovery.

✓ **Instruct the patient to apply heat or cold if either is found to be beneficial and to take over-the-counter (OTC) acetaminophen or anti-inflammatory analgesics such as ibuprofen or naproxen, unless there are any contraindications to the use of NSAIDs.**

✓ **Have the patient begin gentle ROM exercises as soon as possible.** One exercise and mobilization protocol consists of small-range and amplitude rotational movements of the neck, first in one direction, then the other, to be repeated 10 times in each direction every waking hour. The movements should be performed up to a maximum comfortable range. These home exercises can be done in the sitting position if symptoms are not too severe or in the unloaded supine position when the sitting position is too painful.

✓ **The athlete** must regain full ROM and strength without pain before return to play can be advised.

✓ Arrange for follow-up for patients, as necessary.

What Not to Do

✗ Do not forget to tell the patient that symptoms may well be worse the day after the injury.

✗ Do not refer the patient for chiropractic manipulation of the cervical spine. There is risk for cervical myelopathy, cervical radiculopathy, and vertebral basilar artery strokes, with little chance of any improvement.

✗ Do not forget to be thorough in recording the history and physical examination. This sort of injury may end up in litigation, and a detailed record can obviate the physician being subpoenaed to testify in person.

✗ Do not check neck movement by using passive ROM testing. This has the potential for causing serious neurologic injury.

✗ Do not obtain a radiograph of every neck. A thousand negative cervical spine radiographs are cost effective if they prevent one paraplegic from an occult unstable fracture, but with the Canadian C-spine rules and NEXUS establishing a standard of care for the evaluation of neck injuries, not all patients need radiography just because they were in a motor vehicle collision, fell, or hit their head.

✗ Do not remove shoulder pads and helmets in football and hockey players until the cervical spine has been cleared, unless there is airway compromise or the helmet prevents cervical immobilization. To safely remove this equipment, the patient's torso, head, and neck are elevated about 30 to 40 degrees by a four-person team. With manual stabilization of the neck, the helmet and shoulder pads are removed simultaneously, and the patient is lowered to the supine position.

Discussion

In general, patients with suspected neck injuries can be thought of as falling into one of four categories: uninjured or minor injury, stable cervical spine fractures, unstable cervical spine fractures with completed neurologic deficits, and unstable cervical spine fractures without or with incomplete neurologic deficits. An overwhelming majority of patients (96%) fall into the first category, whereas stable fractures make up approximately 3% of the total. Fewer than 1%, then, have unstable fractures that may potentially benefit from immobilization. Even among patients who have unstable fractures,

(Continued)

Discussion continued

neurologic deficits are rare, and most of those happen immediately at the time of injury. Deficits that develop only later are extremely rare, with one review finding only 41 such case reports in the literature. Of those, 30 had no identifiable trigger, and only 1 developed deficits after the removal of a cervical collar. In multiple cases, neurologic deficits actually developed after the application of a cervical collar, which can be especially dangerous in patients with preexisting cervical spine abnormalities, such as ankylosing spondylitis.

A more commonsense, individualized approach has been proposed, aimed at limiting spinal motion and protecting the patient in transport without attempts at full immobilization. This approach calls for special attention and a more conservative management plan for patients with altered mental status or existing neurologic symptoms, but would allow for awake, alert patients with no neurologic deficits to be transported in a position of comfort.

The most commonly encountered injuries are soft tissue trauma and include ligament sprains, muscle strains, and soft tissue contusions. Fortunately, these injuries generally heal without producing long-term problems.

The cervical spine is made up of seven specialized vertebrae, which together provide a wide ROM to the head. As with other joints, the large ROM afforded by the cervical spine comes at the cost of stability because the cervical region has relatively little intrinsic bony stability and relies on ligament restraints to avoid excessive or pathologic mobility.

The primary static stabilizers of the neck include the anterior longitudinal ligament, intervertebral disks, posterior longitudinal ligament, ligamentum flavum, facet capsules, and interspinous and supraspinous ligaments. Important dynamic stabilizers consist of the sternocleidomastoid, trapezius, strap, and paraspinal muscles. This muscular envelope functions as a dynamic splint and protects the cervical spine during the full ROM, whereas the ligamentous structures act as a check rein, limiting motion at the end points.

Strains are defined as stretch injuries occurring at the musculotendinous junction or within the muscle substance. **Sprains** involve stretch injuries to ligamentous structures. Cervical **contusions** involve a blunt-force injury to the soft tissues. Sprains occur with a spectrum of ligamentous disruptions, ranging from

mild pain without instability to gross ligamentous disruption. Injuries to the facet joints and capsular ligaments have been blamed for chronic neck pain following forced flexion injuries such as whiplash.

Typically patients who have sustained a cervical sprain, strain, or contusion present with painful, limited cervical motion and tenderness over the involved structure. The management of cervical sprains, strains, and contusions is similar, although ligament injuries usually take more time to heal.

Cervical spine imaging should begin with radiographs or CT. When indicated, magnetic resonance imaging (MRI) should be used to evaluate for ligamentous, muscle, and spinal cord involvement.

Whiplash, in contrast with most other injuries, has a female preponderance of 2:1. Some have speculated that this gender difference reflects a woman's smaller, less muscular neck. Most patients presenting for evaluation in a delayed fashion have less specific symptoms and few hard signs on examination. Localized neck pain, neck stiffness, occipital headache, dizziness in all of its forms, malaise, and fatigue are common whiplash symptoms and may be associated with comorbid concussion (see Chapter 10). Localized paracervical tenderness to palpation, reduced range of neck motion, and weakness of the upper extremities secondary to guarding are common findings.

Although most patients with myofascial symptoms recover in several months, 20% to 40% complain of debilitating symptoms for extended periods, sometimes years.

When litigation is involved, some patients exaggerate or lie about persisting symptoms to help make their legal case. Most plaintiffs who have persistent symptoms at the time of settlement of their litigation, however, are not cured by a verdict. The clinician should evaluate the merits of each case individually. The available evidence does not support bias against patients just because they have pending litigation.

The **term** *whiplash* is probably best reserved for describing the mechanism of injury and is of little value as a diagnosis. Because of the many undesirable legal connotations that surround this term, it may be advisable to substitute the term *flexion/extension injury.*

(Continued)

Discussion continued

Brachial plexus injuries, which are commonly referred to as stingers or burners, are a common occurrence in athletics, especially in football. Either traction on the brachial plexus or compression of the dorsal nerve roots can cause these injuries. When the neck is flexed laterally and the contralateral shoulder is depressed, a traction force is created on the brachial plexus. Conversely, extreme lateral flexion of the neck can cause cervical nerve root compression by narrowing the neural foramen. Both types of stingers usually result in transient neuropraxia, manifested in the injured athlete as a burning sensation down the affected arm and weakness of C5-6–innervated muscles (deltoid, biceps, supraspinatus, infraspinatus). The athlete is usually seen coming off the field or mat shaking the arm, which may be hanging limply at the side, and leaning toward the side of injury.

Usually a stinger is a self-limited injury that does not require anything more than keeping the athlete out of the game until the neurologic symptoms have resolved. Pain usually resolves in less than 15 minutes; strength returns in 24 to 48 hours.

The athlete should not return to play if there is any cervical pain, limited cervical ROM, bilateral limb involvement, or persistent neurologic deficits.

Suggested Readings

Bandiera, G., Stiell, I. G., Wells, G. A., et al. (2003). The Canadian C-spine rule performs better than unstructured physician judgment. *Annals of Emergency Medicine*, *42*, 395–402.

Borchgrevink, G. E., Kaasa, A., McDonagh, D., et al. (1998). Acute treatment of whiplash neck sprain injuries: A randomized trial of treatment during the first 14 days after a car accident. *Spine*, *23*, 25–31.

Daffner, R. H. (2001). Identifying patients at low risk for cervical spine injury: The Canadian C-spine rule for radiography. *Journal of the American Medical Association*, *286*, 1893–1894.

Demetriades, D., Charalambides, K., Chahwan, S., et al. (2000). Nonskeletal cervical spine injuries: Epidemiology and diagnostic pitfalls. *The Journal of Trauma*, *48*, 724–727.

Devereaux, M. W. (2004). Neck pain. *Primary Care*, *31*, 19–31.

Dickinson, G., Stiell, I. G., Schull, M., et al. (2004). Retrospective application of the NEXUS low-risk criteria for cervical spine radiography in Canadian emergency departments. *Annals of Emergency Medicine*, *43*, 507–514.

Dorshimer, G. W., & Kelly, M. (2005). Cervical pain in the athlete: Common conditions and treatment. *Primary Care*, *32*, 231–243.

Evans, R. W. (2004). The postconcussion syndrome and whiplash injuries; a question-and-answer review for primary care physicians. *Primary Care*, *31*, 1–17.

Gennis, P., Miller, L., Gallagher, J., et al. (1996). The effect of soft cervical collars on persistent neck pain in patients with whiplash injury. *Academic Emergency Medicine*, *3*, 568–573.

Griffen, M. M., Fryberg, E. R., Kerwin, A. J., et al. (2003). Radiographic clearance of blunt cervical spine injury: Plain radiograph or computed tomography scan? *The Journal of Trauma*, *55*, 222–227.

Hoffman, J. R., Mower, W. R., Wolfson, A. B., et al. (2000). Validity of a set of clinical criteria to rule out injury to the cervical spine in patients with blunt trauma. *New England Journal of Medicine*, *343*, 94–99.

Kerr, D., Bradshaw, L., & Kelly, A. (2005). Implementation of the Canadian C-spine rule reduces cervical spine x-ray rate for alert patients with potential neck injury. *Journal of Emergency Medicine*, *28*, 127–131.

Mower, W. R., Hoffman, J. R., Pollack, C. V., et al. (2001). Use of plain radiography to screen for cervical spine injuries. *Annals of Emergency Medicine*, *38*, 1–7.

Oshlag, B., Ray, T., & Boswell, B. (2020). Neck injuries. *Primary Care: Clinics in Office Practice*, *47*(1), 165–176.

Richell-Herren, K. (1999). Mobilization of neck sprains. *Journal of Accident and Emergency Medicine*, *16*, 363.

Rosenfeld, M., Gunnarsson, R., & Borenstein, P. (2000). Early intervention in whiplash-associated disorders. *Spine, 25,* 1782–1787.

Stiell, I. G., Clement, C. M., McKnight, R. D., et al. (2003). The Canadian C-spine rule versus the NEXUS low-risk criteria in patients with trauma. *New England Journal of Medicine, 349,* 2510–2518.

Stiell, I. G., Wells, G. A., Vandemheen, K. L., et al. (2001). The Canadian C-spine rule for radiography in alert and stable trauma patients. *Journal of the American Medical Association, 286,* 1841–1848.

Viccellio, P., Simon, H., & Pressman, B. D. (2001). A prospective multicenter study of cervical spine injury in children. *Pediatrics, 108:* Article e20.

Zmurko, M. G., Tannoury, T. Y., Tannoury, C. A., & Anderson, D. G. (2003). Cervical sprains, disc herniations, minor fractures, and other cervical injuries in the athlete. *Clinics in Sports Medicine, 22,* 513–521.

Clavicle (Collarbone) Fracture

Presentation

A patient presents with anterior shoulder pain after falling onto the lateral shoulder or, less commonly, an outstretched arm, or has received a direct blow to the clavicle. With distal clavicle fractures, patients may complain of pain on the top of the shoulder. There may be deformity of the bone with swelling, abrasion, and/or ecchymosis. This is usually seen in the midclavicle and is exquisitely tender if palpated. The deformity may appear similar to an acromioclavicular (AC) joint separation with distal clavicle fractures, but the tenderness is usually more medial along the clavicle than with AC injuries (see Chapter 95). The affected shoulder may appear slumped inward and downward compared with the contralateral shoulder, and the patient is usually supporting the injured side by holding the arm adducted. Paresthesias in the distribution of the supraclavicular nerves can occur.

An infant or small child might present not moving the arm after a fall, but examination of the arm will be normal, and only further examination of the clavicle will reveal the actual site of the injury.

What to Do

✓ **Perform a detailed history and physical examination.** A high-energy mechanism of injury should raise the suspicion for associated injuries. A motorcycle collision or fall from a great height should lead to suspicion of ipsilateral rib fractures and/or pulmonary injury. All patients with suspected clavicle fractures should be questioned with respect to any neck pain, numbness or paresthesias, chest pain, or shortness of breath. Palpation of the ribs and assessment of chest excursion are essential. Cervical motion should be full and pain free.

✓ **After completing a musculoskeletal examination, including gentle palpation along the entire length of the clavicle and proximal humerus, evaluate the neurovascular status of the arm.**

✓ **Obtain radiographs or bedside ultrasound to rule out or accurately define a suspected clavicle fracture. A simple anteroposterior (AP) view of the clavicle will demonstrate most midclavicle fractures. An acromioclavicular (Zanca) view, which is a 20-degree cephalad view, is normally included.** If there is suspicion of glenohumeral joint injury, shoulder imaging should be added. If there is any shortness of breath, chest imaging should be performed. Occasionally, a **computed tomography (CT) scan can be useful for evaluation of comminution, position of fracture fragments, and (most importantly when there is tenderness at the medial end of the clavicle) evaluation of a suspected sternoclavicular (SC) joint injury.** Fractures or dislocations at the sternal end of the clavicle are often difficult to see on plain radiographs but are well visualized on CT scans.

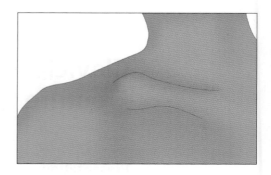

Fig. 103.1 Clinical appearance of a type II distal clavicle fracture.

✅ **Obtain orthopedic consultation if there is any evidence of neurovascular compromise. Consultation should also be obtained with open fractures or if there is significant displacement (>2 cm) between fracture fragments or if the overlying skin is tented and appears to be under tension. Fractures of the distal third of the clavicle medial to the acromioclavicular joint, where the proximal fragment is detached from the coracoclavicular ligaments and is unstable (type II)** (Fig. 103.1)**, also require orthopedic consultation to consider surgical reduction. Additionally, fractures with complete displacement (displacement greater than one bone width) also need orthopedic consultation.**

✅ **The majority of lateral clavicle fractures are nondisplaced and can be managed conservatively.**

✅ **All uncomplicated fractures can simply be treated with a cold pack and sling to provide comfort and appropriate immobilization. Rotation exercises at the glenohumeral joint should be encouraged. The cold pack is optional, and the sling can be discontinued when the pain has resolved.** Passive and active range-of-motion (ROM) exercises can begin as soon as the patient's comfort allows.

✅ **Analgesics,** usually acetaminophen or nonsteroidal anti-inflammatories, can be recommended.

✅ **Inform that the patient may be more comfortable sleeping in a semi-upright position, with a sling.**

✅ **Arrange for orthopedic follow-up in 1 week to evaluate healing.** Pendulum exercises, or passive shoulder ROM exercises, should begin within the first week. Resistive strengthening can commence when the fracture site is nontender and full ROM exists.

✅ Contact sports are to be avoided until the fracture appears clinically and radiographically healed.

✅ Inform the patient that the bone will likely heal with a noticeable callus (visible lump).

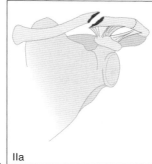
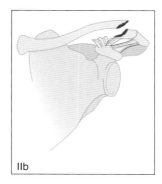

Fig. 103.2 Types IIa and IIb clavicle fractures.

What Not to Do

🚫 Do not apply a figure-of-eight dressing or a Kenny-Howard–type splint. They are not necessary and often cause greater patient discomfort and have been associated with brachial plexus injuries.

🚫 Do not leave an arm fully immobilized in a sling for more than 7 to 10 days. This can result in loss of ROM or adhesive capsulitis (frozen shoulder).

Discussion

The clavicle is the first bone to ossify, a process that starts in the fifth to sixth week of intrauterine life and is the only long bone of the body to form by intramembranous ossification.

The clavicle connects the shoulder girdle to the axial skeleton and articulates with the acromion laterally and the sternum medially. Clavicle fractures are classified by the location of the fracture, with the clavicle divided into thirds. Most fractures involve the middle third of the clavicle (approximately 69%). The distal third of the clavicle is fractured roughly 28% of the time, and the proximal third is the least common site of fracture (about 5%, but in some studies, up to 22%).

Distal clavicle fractures are classified into five categories. A type I distal clavicle fracture is minimally displaced and occurs lateral to the coracoclavicular (CC) ligaments. Type II fractures may be medial to the CC ligaments (IIa) or lateral to the CC ligaments with CC ligament disruption from the proximal fragment (IIb) (Fig. 103.2) which in both cases results in the proximal segment being detached from the CC ligaments and therefore more prone to distraction of the fracture fragments. Type III distal clavicle fractures extend into the AC joint,

type IV involves periosteal sleeve disruption (seen in younger patients), and type V involves an avulsion fracture that leaves only an inferior cortical fragment attached to the CC ligaments and is functionally similar to type II. **Only the type II and type V distal clavicle fractures are considered unstable and warrant early orthopedic consultation.**

The management of type II distal clavicle fractures is controversial. Although many authors advocate a surgical approach, because of the relatively high risk of nonunion (approximately 11%), only a small minority of those nonunions have significant functional limitation.

One approach to surgical intervention in both midclavicular and distal clavicular fractures is to treat marked displacement, high-energy injuries, and potential skin compromise with acute surgical fixation. In addition, advanced age, female sex, displacement, and comminution of the fracture have been found to be independent predictors of nonunion.

Significant overlap of bony fragments (>1.5 cm) causing substantial clavicular shortening with increased risk of nonunion, decreased shoulder

(continued)

Discussion continued

strength, and patient dissatisfaction is also sometimes cited as a reason to pursue surgical repair. On the other hand, there is not currently robust evidence to suggest improved functional outcome for this indication.

Proximal clavicle fractures are the least common but are associated with subluxation or dislocation of the corresponding SC joint. CT scans are far superior to plain radiographs in determining the extent of these injuries. **In general, most isolated, minimally displaced, proximal fractures are treated in the same manner as midclavicular fractures. Significant displacement and SC dislocation require rapid orthopedic consultation, as they place posterior mediastinal structures at risk. Fractures of the proximal clavicle should always prompt a thorough examination to look for other injuries because approximately 90% have an associated injury.**

In children, fracture of the clavicle requires very little force and usually heals rapidly and without complication. In adults, however, this fracture usually results from a greater force and is associated with other injuries and complications. In the elderly population, these fractures can be sustained by a simple fall from a standing height. **Nonaccidental injuries should be suspected in high-risk patients (vulnerable adults and children).**

Clavicle fractures are sometimes associated with a hematoma from the subclavian vein. However, other nearby structures, including the carotid artery, brachial plexus, and lung, are usually protected by the underlying anterior scalene muscle as well as the tendency of the sternocleidomastoid muscle to pull the medial fragment of bone upward.

A great deal of angulation deformity and distraction on radiographs of midshaft fractures are usually acceptable because the clavicle mends and remodels itself so well. In addition, the clavicle does not have a significant skeletal support role. As with rib fractures, respiration prevents full immobilization, and therefore the relief that comes with callus formation may be delayed.

Suggested Readings

Anderson, K., Jensen, P. O., & Lauritzen, J. (1987). Treatment of clavicular fractures: Figure-of-eight bandage versus a simple sling. *Acta Orthopaedica Scandinavica*, *58*, 71–74.

Eskola, A., Vainionpaa, S., Myllynen, P., et al. (1986). Outcome of clavicular fracture in 89 patients. *Archives of Orthopedic and Trauma Surgery*, *105*, 337–338.

Shuster, M., Abu-Laban, R. B., Boyd, J., et al. (2003). Prospective evaluation of clinical assessment in the diagnosis and treatment of clavicle fracture: Are radiographs really necessary? *Canadian Journal of Emergency Medicine*, *5*, 309–313.

Stanley, D., & Norris, S. H. (1988). Recovery following fractures of the clavicle treated conservatively. *Injury*, *19*, 162–164.

Stelter, S., Malik, S., & Chiampas, G. (2020). The emergent evaluation and treatment of shoulder, clavicle, and humerus injuries. *Emergency Medicine Clinics of North America*, *38*(1), 103–124.

Woltz, S., Sengab, A., Krijnen, P., & Schipper, I. B. (2017). Does clavicular shortening after nonoperative treatment of midshaft fractures affect shoulder function? A systematic review. *Archives of Orthopedic and Trauma Surgery*, *137*(8), 1047–1053.

Coccyx Fracture

(Tailbone Fracture)

Presentation

The patient presents after falling onto the buttocks or getting kicked in the sacrococcygeal synchondrosis during an athletic activity, complaining of pain at the tip of the spine that is worse with sitting and perhaps with defecation owing to the use of the levator ani and the anococcygeal muscles. There is little or no pain with standing, but walking may be uncomfortable. Because part of the gluteus maximus inserts on the coccyx, pain can also occur when rising from a seated position.

On physical examination, there is point tenderness and perhaps deformity of the coccyx that may be best palpated by examining through the rectum with a gloved finger (Fig. 104.1).

What to Do

✅ **Verify the history** (Was this actually a straddle injury?) **and examine thoroughly,** including the lumbar spine, pelvis, and legs. **Palpate the coccyx** from inside and out, feeling primarily for point tenderness and/or pain with motion. **Often, with gentle examination with a gloved hand, the entire coccyx can be examined and tested for stability without the discomfort of a rectal examination.**

✅ **Radiographs should generally be avoided.** Any noticed variation can be an old fracture or an anatomic variant, and a fractured coccyx can appear within normal limits. There is no specific change in management that will come about as a result of radiographic findings.

✅ **The diagnosis can usually be made clinically. If there is a tender deformity, especially if accompanied by movement or crepitus of the distal segment, a fracture of the coccyx is most probable.** Exquisite tenderness alone is an indication of contusion or a stable nondisplaced fracture. **The therapy is the same for both contusion and fracture.**

✅ **Reassurance and an explanation of the examination findings and presumed diagnosis will satisfy most patients even in the absence of radiographs.**

✅ **Instruct the patient in how to sit forward, resting on the ischial tuberosities and thighs using a hard chair, instead of resting on the coccyx. As an alternative approach, a foam-rubber doughnut cushion or gel cushion may also be helpful. Limit the patient's activity. If necessary, prescribe or recommend acetaminophen or anti-inflammatory pain medications and stool softeners. Cold packs or hot sitz-type baths may provide further comfort. Avoid narcotics when possible because constipation may aggravate coccygeal pain.**

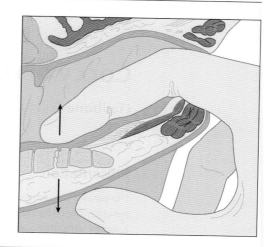

Fig. 104.1 Finger palpating the coccyx by rectal examination.

✅ Inform the patient that the pain will gradually improve over 1 to 4 weeks as bony callus forms and motion decreases. Arrange for follow-up as needed.

✅ **If pain persists** for greater than 2 months, consider injection of corticosteroid (i.e., methylprednisolone [Depo-Medrol], 20 mg) or therapeutic ultrasound. Chronic pain is rare but can be treated by surgically removing the coccyx or by coccygeoplasty, injection of polymethylmethacrylate cement, which can result in immediate relief of symptoms.

What Not to Do

❌ Do NOT routinely order radiographs, as the diagnosis can be made clinically.

❌ Do NOT routinely prescribes opiates, as constipation can exacerbate the pain.

Discussion

The term *coccyx* actually comes from the Greek term *kokkoux* (for "cuckoo") because it resembles the shape of a cuckoo's beak.

A fracture, contusion, or partial dislocation of the sacrococcygeal junction can cause painful, abnormal movement of the coccyx, especially when sitting pressure is applied to this region. Resulting pain can involve use of the levator ani muscle and the anococcygeal, sacrotuberal, and sacrospinal ligaments, as well as the gluteus maximus muscles.

Suggested Reading

Wang, H., Coppola, P. T., & Coppola, M. Orthopedic emergencies. *Emergency Medicine Clinics of North America*, 33(2), 451–473.

De Quervain Paratenonitis

(Thumb Tenosynovitis)

Presentation

The patient experiences an insidious onset of difficulty with tasks such as opening jars because of pain localized to the dorsoradial aspect of the wrist that is exacerbated with thumb and wrist motion, and which may also be present on awakening.

On examination, the first dorsal compartment over the radial styloid is thickened and tender to palpation. Crepitus of the tendon may be felt on active and passive thumb motion. Tenderness will be elicited on palpating or stretching the extensor pollicis brevis and abductor pollicis longus tendons bordering the palmar side or, less commonly, the extensor pollicis longus tendon bordering the dorsal side of the anatomic snuff box (Fig. 105.1).

What to Do

✅ **Obtain a careful history** to reveal the underlying causative activity as well as to inquire into the patient's general health. An alternate source of this paratendinopathy may be uncovered, such as gonococcal tenosynovitis or fluoroquinolone-induced tendinopathy.

✅ **Perform a physical examination** to determine the exact source of pain and tenderness.

✅ Document circulatory and sensation examination findings. Compress the thumb metacarpal onto the scaphoid (axial loading of the carpometacarpal joint) to rule out arthritis at the joint as an alternative cause of symptoms.

✅ **Have the patient fold the thumb into the palm, close the fingers over it into a fist, then passively ulnar deviate the wrist. This is known as the Finkelstein test** (Fig. 105.2) **and reproduces the pain of de Quervain tenosynovitis of the extensor pollicis brevis and abductor pollicis longus tendons.** A positive test causes sharp pain over the first dorsal compartment.

✅ **Acute de Quervain paratenonitis responds best to corticosteroid injection into the tendon sheath** (Fig. 105.3). Results of a meta-analysis of treatments for de Quervain tenosynovitis showed that there was an 83% cure rate with injection alone. This rate was much higher than any other therapeutic modality (61% for injection and splint, 14% for splint alone, and 0% for rest or nonsteroidal anti-inflammatory drugs [NSAIDs]). **Tendon-sheath injection is a technique that can be used by the more experienced clinician.** This can be done using ultrasound guidance. Alternatively, a landmark-based approach can be used. Using a 27-gauge, 0.5-inch to 1-inch needle and sterile technique, slowly penetrate the skin and soft tissue, aiming for the middle of the tendon. When the tendon is hit, it may produce a muscle reflex, increased

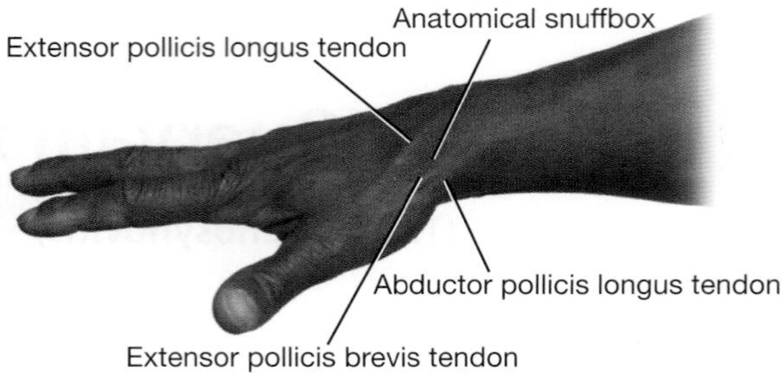

Fig. 105.1 First dorsal wrist compartment and extensors of the thumb. (Modified from Drake RA, Vogl W, Mitchell A: *Gray's Anatomy for Students*. 4e, Philadelphia, 2021, Elsevier.)

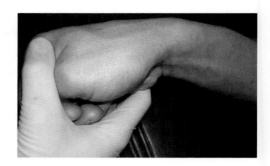

Anatomical snuffbox

Extensor pollicis longus tendon

Abductor pollicis longus tendon

Extensor pollicis brevis tendon

Fig. 105.2 Demonstration of the Finkelstein test. (Adapted from Parmelee-Peters, K., & Eathorne, S. W. [2005]. The wrist: Common injuries and management. *Primary Care, 32,* 35–70.)

Fig. 105.3 Inject site for de Quervain tenosynovitis. (Adapted from Parmelee-Peters, K., & Eathorne, S. W. [2005]. The wrist: Common injuries and management. *Primary Care, 32,* 35–70.)

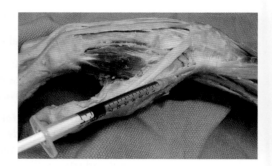

resistance to advancement of the needle, and pain, which are signals to withdraw the needle slightly. Move the muscle-tendon unit so it slides back and forth, and readvance the needle until the tendon is felt slightly scraping the point. Back off 1 mm, steady the syringe and needle, and slowly inject a steroid and anesthetic mixture. While injecting, palpate the tendon, feeling for a "sausaging" effect as the mixture inflates the sheath. Warn the patient that there may be a transient flare in pain when the anesthetic wears off, which may last 24 to 48 hours. The corticosteroid should begin to have a noticeable therapeutic effect within a few days.

What Not to Do

⊗ Do not allow NSAIDs to be used. They have been shown to be of no value in this condition and have potentially hazardous side effects.

⊗ Do not inject steroid directly into the tendon. This may weaken the tendon and lead to future rupture.

⊗ Do not inject steroids into the very superficial layer of the subcutaneous tissue. This may cause skin depigmentation, which is particularly noticeable in dark-skinned individuals.

⊗ Do not splint the wrist and thumb after steroid injection. This reduces the cure rate over injection alone.

Discussion

Symptoms of de Quervain syndrome are related to overuse. The involved tendons course under the extensor retinaculum in a groove along the radial styloid process. Repetitive wrist motion causes shear stress on the tendons in their small compartment, which results in inflammation of the tenosynovium. This is more accurately called paratenonitis. The term includes what was previously called peritendinitis, tenosynovitis (single layer of areolar tissue covering the tendon), and tenovaginitis (double-layer tendon sheath). Clinically, paratenonitis presents with acute edema and hyperemia of the paratenon with infiltration of inflammatory cells. After a few hours to a few days, a fibrinous exudate fills the tendon sheath and causes the crepitus that can be felt on clinical examination. **This condition is often seen in supermarket cashiers and piecework factory workers and after intensive computer keyboarding. Mothers of infants aged 6 to 12 months and day care workers are frequently affected because of repetitive lifting of infants. De Quervain disease is also common in racquet sports, fishing, and golf. It is approximately six times more common in women than in men. Patients should avoid the activity that brought on the condition.**

Tendon sheath injections are well tolerated and can be repeated safely at least three times, spaced several months apart. Most often, one injection is effective. **One small study suggested that postpartum women with de Quervain disease respond well to conservative management without steroid injection.**

Suggested Readings

Carek, P. J., & Hunter, M. H. (2005). Joint and soft tissue injections in primary care. *Rheumatology*, *7*, 359–378.

Maffulli, N., Wong, J., & Almekinders, L. C. (2003). Types and epidemiology of tendinopathy. *Clinics in Sports Medicine*, *22*, 675–692.

Rajwinder, S. D., & Carek, P. J. (2005). Common sports injuries: Upper extremity injuries. *Clinics in Family Practice*, *7*, 2.

Richie, C. A. (2003). Corticosteroid injection for treatment of de Quervain's tenosynovitis: A pooled quantitative literature evaluation. *Journal of the American Board of Family Practice*, *16*, 102–106.

Weiss, A. P. C., Akelman, E., Tabatabai, M., et al. (1994). Treatment of de Quervain's disease. *Journal of Hand Surgery*, *19*, 595–598.

Extensor Tendon Avulsion—Distal Phalanx

(Baseball or Mallet Finger)

Presentation

A patient arrives with a tender fingertip injury with a noticeable deformity. There is a history of a sudden resisted flexion of the distal interphalangeal (DIP) joint, such as when the fingertip is struck by a ball or jammed against a stationary object, resulting in pain and tenderness over the dorsum of the base of the distal phalanx. This injury can occur with relatively minor trauma (such as jamming a finger while reaching for a light switch in the dark) or even as a result of a direct blow to the dorsum of the finger. It may or may not be accompanied by swelling and ecchymosis over the DIP joint. When the finger is at rest or held in extension, the injured DIP joint remains in slight or moderate flexion (Fig. 106.1).

What to Do

✅ **Obtain imaging.** A radiograph with anteroposterior and lateral views should be obtained to evaluate for an avulsion fracture, which, if present, will be best seen on the lateral view at the dorsal base of the distal phalanx (Fig. 106.2). Bedside ultrasound may reveal bony injury or ligament rupture.

✅ **Test for stability of the collateral ligaments** of the DIP joint with varus and valgus stress.

✅ While stabilizing the metacarpophalangeal (MCP) and the proximal interphalangeal joint (PIP) in extension, **ask the patient to extend the DIP joint. When the extensor tendon is avulsed, there should be a loss of full active extension while active flexion and passive range of motion remain intact.**

✅ **If the avulsion fragment is small or there is no bone involvement, nonoperative treatment is preferred. Apply a finger splint that will hold the DIP joint in neutral position or slight hyperextension and gently secure it in place with tape.** Either a dorsal or a volar splint of aluminum and foam may be used. Plastic fingertip splints are manufactured in various sizes (e.g., Stax extension splints) (Figs. 106.3, 106.4, and 106.5).

✅ **Instruct the patient to keep the DIP joint in full extension continuously and seek hand specialist, orthopedic, or sports medicine follow-up care within 1 week.**

✅ **Closed mallet fingers should be immobilized in extension full time for 8 weeks. Patients must understand that if they take the finger out of the splint, they cannot let the DIP joint fall into flexion. Each time the DIP joint flexes, the treatment clock starts over again at time zero.**

✅ **Skin breakdown can be a significant problem,** and patients should be instructed to remove the splint daily while holding the joint in extension, resting the joint on a flat surface to

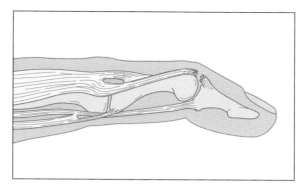

Fig. 106.1 Injured distal interphalangeal joint in slight flexion.

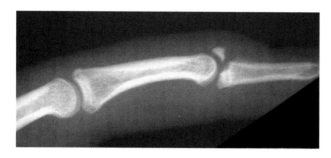

Fig. 106.2 Radiograph showing avulsion fracture. (Adapted from Raby, N., Berman, L., & de Lacey, G. [2005]. *Accident and emergency radiology.* Philadelphia, PA: WB Saunders.)

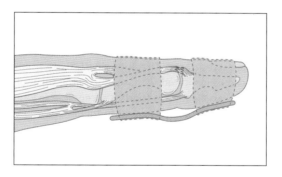

Fig. 106.3 Commercial concave aluminum splint.

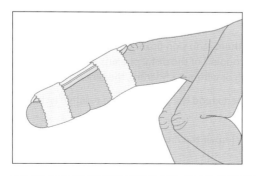

Fig. 106.4 Dorsal aluminum splint.

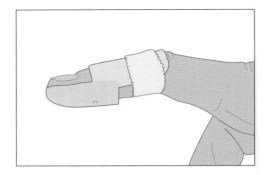

Fig. 106.5 Commercial Stax extension splint.

allow the skin to dry and reduce the chance of maceration. **One splint that is well tolerated and can be left on continuously (but is moderately expensive and somewhat difficult to learn how to mold) is the MEALS splint** (George Tiemann & Co., 25 Plant Ave., Hauppauge, NY, 11788; phone: 800-843-6266).

✓ In addition to the verbal instructions, patients can be provided with an online video link specific for the type of orthotic:

- ○ Stack splint: https://www.youtube.com/watch?v=8b_9Fz2edw0
- ○ Trough splint: https://www.youtube.com/watch?v=e7aHOTHx-8o
- ○ Thermoplastic splinting: https://www.medscape.com/answers/1242305-99723/where-can-video-demonstration-of-thermoplastic-splinting-for-mallet-finger-be-accessed

✓ An additional 6 weeks of splinting can follow the initial 8 weeks of treatment if there is not a full ability to extend against resistance. After full active DIP extension is achieved, a gradual withdrawal of the splint can be instituted, with wearing of the splint only at night and with sports for another 6 weeks. Participation in sports is acceptable so long as the DIP joint is firmly immobilized in extension and is protected against further injury.

✓ **Surgery is recommended for displaced avulsion fractures with a large articular component** (>50% of the articular surface), volar subluxation of the distal phalanx, or failure of splinting.

What Not to Do

✗ Do not assume that there is no significant injury if the radiograph is negative. The clue to this injury is persistent drooping of the distal phalanx and tenderness over the bony insertion of the extensor tendon. With or without a fracture, the tendon avulsion requires splinting.

✗ Do not forcefully hyperextend the joint. This can result in ischemia and dorsal skin necrosis over the joint.

✗ Do not unnecessarily impair the movement of the PIP joint.

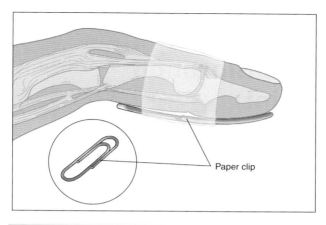

Paper clip

Fig. 106.6 Paper-clip splint.

Discussion

Mallet finger, also known as baseball finger or drop finger, involves disruption of the extensor tendon or an avulsion fracture of the distal phalanx. The classic mechanism involves a direct blow to the tip of the finger while the DIP joint is held in extension. Although this injury is commonly caused during participation in athletic activities (e.g., by contact with a baseball, volleyball, or basketball), mallet finger may occur with household activities, such as pushing off a sock or tucking in bed sheets. Given the mechanism, it makes sense that the middle finger, the longest one, is most commonly involved, although a mallet finger may involve any of the digits, including the thumb.

Swelling and tenderness may be found on the dorsum of the DIP joint, but commonly the injury is painless, and the loss of extension may not appear for several days to weeks.

Patients may wait weeks to months before being seen and may present with a subsequent swan neck deformity. This is caused by the unopposed extensor mechanism on the middle phalanx leading to hyperextension of the PIP joint.

Patients presenting with chronic mallet finger injuries without significant bone involvement should still be treated with splinting in extension, but treatment duration is anticipated to be longer.

There are many commercially available splint options for treatment of this injury (e.g., Stax hyperextension splints, padded aluminum, and frog splints), but, in a pinch, a paper clip will do (Fig. 106.6). A dorsal splint allows more use of the finger but requires more padding and may contribute to ischemia of the skin overlying the DIP joint. Figure-of-eight taping can also provide some limitation of flexion. A Cochrane review looking at interventions for treating mallet finger injuries found insufficient evidence to establish the effectiveness of different finger splints in determining when surgery is indicated. The MEAL splint noted earlier must be heated in hot water in a nonstick container before it can be molded and stretched to fit the finger. It is very comfortable for the patient, has no absorbent surfaces, and can be worn after washing without having to remove it to prevent skin maceration. Patients have to be warned that the MEAL splint may slide off when showering.

Mallet thumb can be treated similarly to mallet finger, with a trial of splinting in extension; however, because larger forces are required to cause mallet thumb and because full function of the thumb is critical, consider earlier surgical intervention than with the same injury in a triphalangeal digit.

Suggested Reading

Hong, E. (2005). Hand injuries in sports medicine. *Primary Care, 32*, 91–103.

Finger Dislocation (PIP Joint)

CHAPTER

107

Presentation

The patient will have jammed a finger, causing a hyperextension injury that forces the middle phalanx dorsally and proximally out of articulation with the distal end of the proximal phalanx. A swollen, painful deformity of the proximal interphalangeal (PIP) joint will be present, unless the patient or a bystander has reduced the dislocation prior to presentation.

There should be no sensory or vascular compromise.

What to Do

✓ **When a deformity is present**, unless there is crepitus or bony instability and a shaft fracture is suspected, **radiographs may be deferred, and joint reduction can be carried out first. If the nature of the injury is at all unclear, obtain radiographs before attempting a reduction.**

✓ **If there has been significant delay in seeking help or if the patient is suffering considerable discomfort,** a digital block over the proximal phalanx or, most effectively, **1% lidocaine or 0.25% bupivacaine injected directly into the joint will allow for a more comfortable reduction. The patient may be given the choice of receiving anesthesia prior to reduction.**

✓ To reduce a dorsal dislocation, **do not just pull on the fingertip; instead, with the joint mildly extended, push the base of the middle phalanx distally using your thumb while holding the patient's middle and distal phalanx with your other thumb and index finger. Then, apply traction and gently flex the middle phalanx until it slides smoothly into its natural anatomic position** (Fig. 107.1).

✓ **Lateral PIP dislocations** are dramatic in appearance (pointing laterally at a very unnatural angle), and often they have been self-reduced. When this type of dislocation requires reduction, grasp the end of the affected finger between your thumb and index finger and apply steady traction along the long axis with ulnar or radial directed force, based on the direction of dislocation. The joint will often reduce with longitudinal traction alone. Bring the middle phalanx into line with the proximal phalanx and squeeze the sides of the PIP joint to correct any residual lateral displacement. A collateral ligament rupture from its proximal attachment, with resultant ulnar or radial joint instability, generally accompanies these dislocations.

✓ **Volar PIP dislocations** are uncommon but are almost always accompanied by an injury to the central slip of the extensor tendon, which can lead to a disabling boutonnière deformity if not properly treated (see Chapter 98). These dislocations can be reduced by applying the same principles used for the dorsal dislocation but in reverse. With mild flexion, push the proximal end

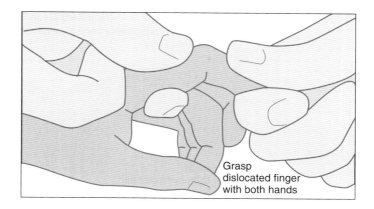

Grasp
dislocated finger
with both hands

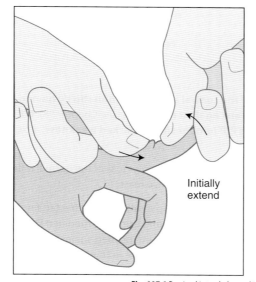

Initially
extend

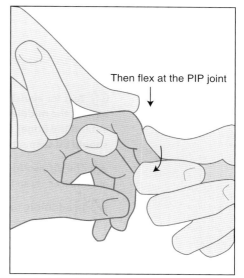

Then flex at the PIP joint

Fig. 107.1 Proximal interphalangeal joint reduction for dorsal dislocation.

of the middle phalanx distally with one thumb, while applying traction on the **middle and** distal phalanx held between your other thumb and index finger, until finally pushing and pulling the middle phalanx dorsally into its normal position.

✅ **Irreducible dislocations** may be caused by avulsion and entrapment of the volar plate in the joint, entrapment of the long flexor tendon in the joint, or entrapment of an osteochondral fragment. **These and all open dislocations necessitate immediate consultation with an orthopedist or hand surgeon. Surgical repair will also be required if there is an avulsion fracture of more than 33% of the articular surface area.**

✅ **When the joint is reduced, test the PIP joint for collateral ligament instability by applying varus and valgus stress in full extension and 20 degrees of flexion.** A partial ligament tear allows no laxity, but there is little or no resistance to stress if the collateral ligament tear is complete.

(Modified) Elson Test

- Injured and contralateral fingers knuckle to knuckle in 90° PIP flexion, pt extends DIPs

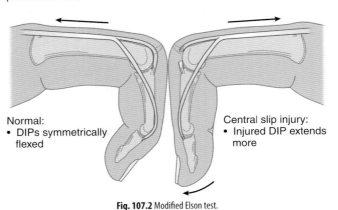

Normal:
- DIPs symmetrically flexed

Central slip injury:
- Injured DIP extends more

Fig. 107.2 Modified Elson test.

✓ **Test for avulsion of the central anterior tendon slip by having the patient attempt to extend the middle phalanx against resistance** (see Chapter 98). **If the patient is unable to extend the finger at the PIP joint or shows marked weakness, a central-slip extensor injury should be suspected.**

✓ The **ultrasound** of a central slip tear shows loss of the normal reflective tendon fibrils that are replaced by an ill-defined, low-reflective mass.

✓ **In addition, to test for a central slip avulsion,** the affected finger should be compared with the noninjured finger of the other hand using the modified Elson test. The injured finger is flexed at about 90 degrees in the PIP joint and pushed against the dorsal side of the midphalanx of the same finger of the noninjured hand. Once in this position, the patient is asked to extend the distal interphalangeal (DIP) joints. The finger with a central slip lesion will be able to extend the distal phalanx more than the noninjured distal phalanx (Fig. 107.2).

✓ When using the modified Elson test, the difference between the extension at the DIP joint of the injured and noninjured hand is easily observed. Asymmetric position of the two distal phalanges in an effort to extend the distal phalanges suggests that the central slip is avulsed from its insertion on the base of the middle phalanx. If the two fingers remain in a symmetric position when trying to extend the distal phalanges, a central slip lesion is highly unlikely (see Chapter 98).

✓ **Testing for avulsion of the volar carpal plate, you will be able to hyperextend the PIP joint more than that of the same finger on the uninjured hand if a disruption is present.**

✓ **If any of these associated injuries exist, orthopedic or surgical hand consultation should be sought, and prolonged splinting and rehabilitation may be required.**

✓ **Postreduction radiographs should be taken.** Chip fractures may represent tendon or ligament avulsions. Radiographs will also allow you to detect an incomplete reduction. The true lateral view is most helpful in detecting subtle subluxation and small avulsion fractures on the volar surface. In an unsatisfactory reduction, the joint's surfaces will be misaligned.

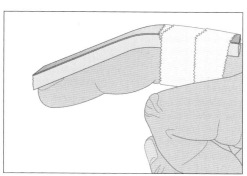

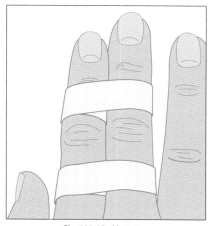

Fig. 107.3 Dorsal extension block splint for proximal interphalangeal dislocation.

Fig. 107.4 Buddy-taping.

✅ **If the joint feels unstable with a tendency to dislocate when extended, or there are minor fractures present, then splint the finger 20 to 30 degrees short of full extension with a padded dorsal splint for 3 to 4 weeks** (Fig. 107.3). Follow up the splinting with buddy-taping (Fig. 107.4) to the adjacent finger for another 2 to 4 weeks and provide follow-up for active range of motion (ROM) exercises to restore normal joint mobility. **When collateral ligament instability is present**, **buddy-tape the affected finger to the finger adjacent to the ruptured ligament. In both situations, early specialty consultation should be obtained.**

✅ **When a central extensor tendon slip injury is suspected**, splint the PIP joint in full extension without immobilizing the DIP or metacarpophalangeal (MCP) joints (see Chapter 98).

✅ **If the joint feels stable, buddy-taping to adjacent digits for 2 weeks is an acceptable immobilization technique** (see Fig. 107.4). **The tape should be removed at night or if the skin becomes wet (to prevent skin maceration). Have the patient dry the skin thoroughly prior to retaping.** Cotton padding placed between fingers can also be used to prevent skin breakdown.

✅ Inform the patient that joint swelling and stiffness with loss of motion may persist for several months after the initial injury. Prophylactic nighttime PIP extension splinting can be used to prevent the mild PIP joint flexion contractures that are common consequences of these injuries. Active ROM exercises performed by squeezing a soft foam ball can be helpful.

✅ Remind the patient to keep the injured finger elevated when possible to limit swelling and resultant pain. If it provides comfort, you can recommend ice application for 20 minutes three to four times over the next 24 hours and acetaminophen or nonsteroidal anti-inflammatory drugs (NSAIDs) for pain.

What Not to Do

❌ Do not immobilize the PIP joints by taping over them when buddy-taping. Early mobilization of this joint is beneficial.

Discussion

Proximal interphalangeal joint dislocations are a common hand injury, especially in the athlete, and have good outcomes if treated properly. PIP dislocations are often simple and easily reduced; however, they may also lead to severely restricted hand function. Most are dorsal dislocations, with the middle phalanx dislocating dorsally from forced hyperextension, axial load, and radial or ulnar deviation. They may involve disruption of the volar plate at its distal attachment. These dorsal dislocations have good outcomes when hyperextension with immobilization is limited (allowing the volar plate to heal back to its distal attachment). However, delayed diagnosis or splinting the patient in too much flexion or for too long a period of time puts the patient at risk for flexion contracture and a pseudo-boutonniere deformity (see Chapter 98).

Often, an athlete reduces the finger alone, or a coach does it (hence the term *coach's finger*).

Early recognition of instability—either dorsal, volar, or lateral—offers the best possibility of closed treatment leading to satisfactory functional healing. The main goals are to enable volar plate, collateral ligament, or central slip healing and to restore normal joint function.

Fracture dislocation is the most disabling PIP joint injury and can result in both dorsal and volar instability (Fig. 107.5).

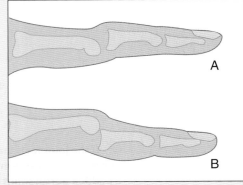

Fig. 107.5 (A) Dorsal dislocation. (B) Volar dislocation.

Suggested Readings

Hong, E. (2005). Hand injuries in sports medicine. *Primary Care, 32,* 91–103.

Patel, D., Dean, C., & Baker, R. J. (2005). The hand in sports: An update on the clinical anatomy and physical examination. *Primary Care, 32,* 71–89.

Saitta, B. H., & Wolf, J. M. (2018). Treating proximal interphalangeal joint dislocations. *Hand Clinics, 34*(2), 139–148.

Singer, A. J. (1999). Comparison of patient and practitioner assessments of pain from commonly performed emergency department procedures. *Annals of Emergency Medicine, 33,* 652–658.

Finger Sprain

(PIP Joint)

108

Presentation

During a sports activity or a fall, the patient's finger is jammed or hyperextended, resulting in a painful, swollen, possibly ecchymotic proximal interphalangeal (PIP) joint. The patient is most often worried that the finger is broken. There may have been an initial dislocation, which was reduced by the patient or a bystander (see Chapter 107).

What to Do

✓ **Get a detailed history** of the exact mechanism of injury.

✓ **Palpate to locate precise areas of tenderness.** Pay particular attention to the collateral ligaments, the volar plate, and the dorsal insertion of the central slip of the extensor tendon at the base of the middle phalanx. Note any associated injuries above and below the PIP joint.

✓ **Obtain anteroposterior and lateral radiograph views of the finger.** "Chip fractures" may represent tendon or ligament avulsions. Surgical **repair and orthopedic consultation are required if there is an avulsion fracture of more than 33% of the articular surface.**

✓ **If pain precludes active motion testing or passive stressing of the joint ligaments,** consider using a 1% lidocaine digital block or, more effectively, direct joint injection. The patient may decide if this anesthesia is used or not, as the pain of the examination may be preferred over the pain of the injection.

✓ **Assess collateral ligament stability by stress testing the injured joint both radially and ulnarly—performed with the joint at about 20 degrees of flexion. A partial ligament tear allows no laxity, but there is little or no resistance to stress if the collateral ligament tear is complete.**

✓ **Test for avulsion of the central anterior tendon slip by having the patient attempt to extend the middle phalanx against resistance** (see Chapter 98). **If the patient is unable to extend the finger at the PIP joint or shows marked weakness, a central-slip extensor injury should be suspected.**

✓ **The ultrasound of a central slip tear** shows loss of the normal reflective tendon fibrils that are replaced by an ill-defined, low-reflective mass.

✓ **In addition, the affected finger should be compared with the noninjured finger of the other hand using the modified Elson test (see Chapter 98).** The injured finger is flexed at about 90 degrees in the PIP joint and pushed against the dorsal side of the midphalanx of the same finger of the noninjured hand. Once in this position, the patient is asked to extend the distal interphalangeal (DIP) joints. The finger with a central slip lesion will be able to extend the distal phalanx more than the noninjured distal phalanx.

✅ **The difference between the extension at the DIP joint of the injured and noninjured hand is easily observed using the modified Elson test.** Asymmetric position of the two distal phalanges in an effort to extend the distal phalanges suggests that the central slip is avulsed from its insertion on the base of the middle phalanx. If the two fingers remain in a symmetric position when trying to extend the distal phalanges, a central slip lesion is highly unlikely.

✅ **Test for an avulsion of the volar carpal plate by passively attempting to hyperextend the PIP joint.** If hyperextension is greater than that of the same finger on the uninjured hand, a disruption of the volar plate must be considered, because delay in making this diagnosis may lead to chronic pseudoboutonnière deformity (see Chapter 98).

✅ **If any of these associated injuries exist,** orthopedic or surgical hand consultation should be sought, and prolonged splinting and rehabilitation may be required.

✅ **When there is no loss of function and no significant joint instability or fracture, immobilize the joint by buddy-taping adjacent digits.** Have the patient remove the tape while sleeping or if the hand becomes wet (to prevent maceration of the skin) and dry the skin thoroughly prior to retaping. **Prophylactic nighttime PIP extension splinting can be used with the more serious sprains to prevent the mild PIP joint flexion contractures that are common consequences of these injuries.** Very minor sprains may not require any special splinting.

✅ **When a central extensor tendon slip injury is suspected,** splint the PIP joint in full extension without immobilizing the DIP or metacarpophalangeal (MCP) joint (see Chapter 98).

✅ **Disruption of the volar plate with abnormal hyperextension at the PIP joint and injuries with minor associated fractures require splinting with a padded dorsal splint in 20 to 30 degrees of flexion for 3 to 4 weeks with buddy-taping to the adjacent finger for another 2 to 4 weeks.** Provide follow-up for active range-of-motion (ROM) exercises to restore normal joint mobility.

✅ **When collateral ligament instability is present, splint the affected finger to the finger adjacent to the ruptured ligament.**

✅ Instruct the patient to use elevation for swelling and acetaminophen or nonsteroidal anti-inflammatory drugs (NSAIDs) for pain. Ice may be used if it provides comfort.

✅ Inform the patient that swelling, stiffness, and discomfort may persist for several months, and provide follow-up for continued care or physical therapy. Active ROM exercises performed by squeezing a soft foam ball can be helpful for regaining strength and function.

What Not to Do

❌ Do not miss joint instability or tendon avulsion—these injuries require special splinting and orthopedic or hand referral.

❌ Do not immobilize the PIP joints when buddy-taping by taping over the PIP joints. Early mobilization is an important benefit.

Discussion

Most PIP joint sprains are stable and heal well with minimal splinting and early mobilization.

The major complications of the more severe PIP joint injuries are stiffness, joint enlargement, ligamentous laxity, and boutonnière deformity. Temporary stiffness and joint enlargement are to be expected for most PIP joint sprains. Boutonnière deformity (see Chapter 98) can be prevented by adequate examination and diagnosis of volar-plate disruption and central-slip injuries. Ligamentous laxity is not common, but if there is significant laxity, which usually affects the index or small finger, the ligament may need to be surgically reattached or reconstructed.

Early recognition of instability—either dorsal, volar, or lateral—as well as discovering weakness to extension against resistance, offers the best possibility of closed treatment leading to satisfactory functional healing. The main goals are to enable volar plate, collateral ligament, or central slip healing and to restore normal joint function.

Fingertip (Tuft) Fractures

Presentation

The patient seeks help after a crushing injury to the fingertip, such as closing it in a car door. The fingertip will be swollen and painful, with ecchymosis. There may or may not be a subungual hematoma, open nail bed injury, or finger pad laceration.

What to Do

✓ Assess for associated injuries and distal interphalangeal (DIP) joint instability.

✓ **Finger radiographs with anteroposterior** (Fig. 109.1) **and lateral views**.

✓ **If there are open wounds, perform a digital block** (see Appendix B), **thoroughly cleanse and débride any open wounds, and repair any nail bed lacerations** (see Chapter 144).

✓ **For open tuft fractures with clean wounds, prophylactic antibiotic coverage is not indicated. Early aggressive local wound care has been found to be the best prevention against infection in open fingertip fractures. When there is gross contamination with marginally viable tissue,** prophylactic antibiotics such as cephalexin, 500 mg orally four times a day for 5 days, may be appropriate. If there is a contraindication to oral antibiotics, cefazolin, 1000 mg intravenously (IV), may be used.

✓ **Provide tetanus prophylaxis** for open fractures.

✓ **Treat painful subungual hematomas** (see Chapter 156).

✓ **Apply a sterile, nonadhesive protective dressing to open wounds** (see Appendix C), **and with or without an open wound, provide an aluminum fingertip splint** (Fig. 109.2) **to prevent further injury and pain.**

✓ **If necessary, provide oral analgesics and advise the patient to elevate the injury above the heart to minimize swelling and reduce pain.**

✓ Ensure follow-up to monitor the patient's recovery, and in the case of open fracture to intervene in the event of infection.

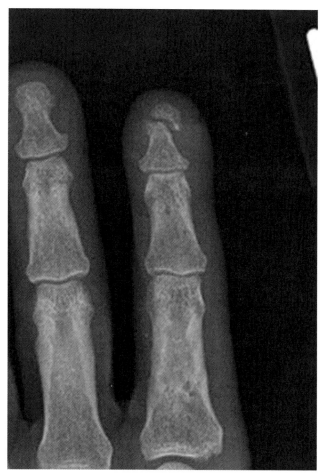

Fig. 109.1 X-ray of tuft fracture. (From Kee C, Massey P: Phalanx Fracture. StatPearls. Treasure Island, 2020, StatPearls Publishing. Figure from Dalton McDaniel, DO. Available under the terms of the Creative Commons Attribution 4.0 International License (http://creativecommons. org/licenses/by/4.0/), which permits use, duplication, adaptation, distribution, and reproduction in any medium or format, as long as you give appropriate credit to the original author(s) and the source, a link is provided to the Creative Commons license, and any changes made are indicated.)

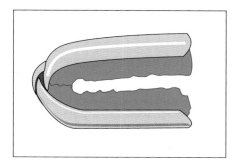

Fig. 109.2 Aluminum fingertip splint.

What Not to Do

🚫 Do not splint the proximal interphalangeal joint.

🚫 Do not prescribe prophylactic antibiotics for clean and uncomplicated open fractures of the distal tuft. Prophylactic antibiotics have been shown to be of no benefit when aggressive irrigation and débridement have been provided.

🚫 Do not obtain cultures from acute open tuft fractures. They have not been shown to be helpful in making therapeutic decisions.

Discussion

Distal phalanx fractures are the most frequently seen fractures of the hand, with the tuft being the most common site. Tuft fractures are inherently stable due to the nail plate dorsally and the dense fibrous septa volarly in the pulp. Generally these can be simply treated with protective splinting, allowing prompt return to their normal activities.

Fractures at the base of the distal phalanx may lead to chronic pain and degenerative changes in the DIP joint if there is significant intraarticular involvement, and these may require referral to an orthopedic or hand surgeon.

Suggested Readings

Sloan, J. P., Dove, A. F., Maheson, M., et al. (1987). Antibiotics in open fracture of the distal phalanx? *Journal of Hand Surgery (British)*, *12*, 123–124.

Stevenson, J., McNaughton, G., & Riley, J. (1990). The use of prophylactic flucloxacillin in treatment of open fractures of the distal phalanx within an accident and emergency department: A double-blind randomized placebo-controlled trial. *Journal of Hand Surgery (British)*, *28*, 388–394.

Suprock, M. D., Hood, J. M., & Lubahn, J. D. (1990). Role of antibiotics in open fractures of the finger. *Journal of Hand Surgery (American)*, *15*, 761–764.

Flexor Digitorum Profundus Tendon Avulsion—Distal Phalanx

(Splay Finger, Jersey Finger)

Presentation

The patient injures the fingertip by falling backward and striking it on the floor or hitting it in some other way, causing sudden and forceful hyperextension at the distal interphalangeal (DIP) joint against resistance. Alternatively, this injury can befall a football player trying to tackle the ball carrier but only catching the jersey or belt with the distal phalanx of one finger (Fig. 110.1). The ring finger is especially susceptible to this injury. Both mechanisms can avulse the insertion of the flexor tendon on the distal phalanx. The patient may feel a pop, followed by immediate pain and swelling. The distal fingerpad becomes markedly swollen, often with ecchymosis. The patient is often unaware that the DIP joint cannot be actively flexed.

What to Do

✓ **Have the patient try to close the fingers against the palm in a loose fist.** All the fingers will readily flex into the palm, but the DIP joint of the injured digit is unable to bend, and the patient cannot bring the fingertip into the palm. The patient will have full range of motion of the proximal interphalangeal (PIP) joint (Fig. 110.2).

✓ Neurovascular examination reveals intact function.

✓ **Obtain radiographs of the finger with anteroposterior and lateral views.** The radiograph is usually normal, although occasionally a small avulsion fracture may be visible on the proximal volar aspect of the distal phalanx.

✓ **When the exam reveals a Flexor Digitorum Tendon Avusion, request consultation from a hand surgeon for early surgical repair.** If this injury is not treated within 3 weeks, the tendon will shorten and retract into the palm.

✓ **A protective dorsal splint (positioned for greatest comfort) incorporating the adjacent finger and extending to the midforearm can be applied to reduce pain and help prevent further injury.**

✓ Provide necessary analgesia with nonsteroidal anti-inflammatory drugs (NSAIDs) or acetaminophen.

What Not to Do

✗ Do not assume a simple sprain exists because of negative radiographs. When there is marked swelling of the distal finger pad following a grabbing injury, be mindful of the possibility of a flexor digitorum profundus avulsion.

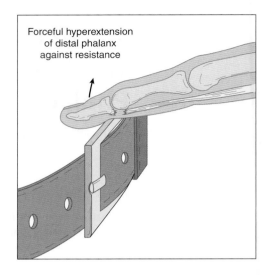

Forceful hyperextension
of distal phalanx
against resistance

Fig. 110.1 Avulsion of the flexor digitorum profundus tendon.

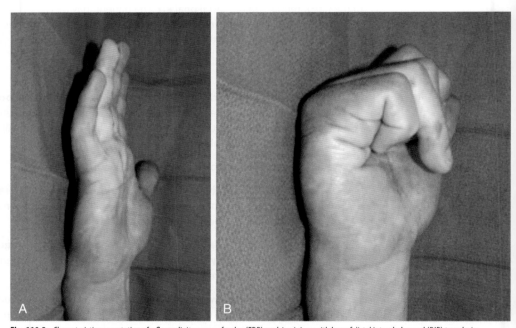

A

B

Fig. 110.2 Characteristic presentation of a flexor digitorum profundus (FDP) avulsion injury with loss of distal interphalangeal (DIP) tenodesis. (A) Fingers extended. (B) Fingers flexed demonstrate a lack of DIP joint flexion indicative of an FDP avulsion injury. (With permission from Polfer, E. M., Sabino, J. M., & Katz, R. D. [2019]. Zone I flexor digitorum profundus repair: A surgical technique. *Journal of Hand Surgery (American), 44,* e1–e5.)

Discussion

Avulsion of the insertion of the flexor digitorum profundus tendon results from the sudden forced extension of a finger during resisted flexion of the digit with the metacarpophalangeal (MCP) joint in extension. Jersey finger injuries should be promptly diagnosed to allow timely surgical repair and prevention of complications.

Unless the clinician specifically examines for active flexion of the DIP joint, the opportunity to repair the tendinous insertion may be lost.

Suggested Readings

Grant, I., Berger, A. C., & Ireland, D. C. (2005). Rupture of the flexor digitorum profundus tendon to the small finger within carpal tunnel. *Hand Surgery, 10,* 109–114.

Polfer, E. M., Sabino, J. M., & Katz, R. D. (2019). Zone I flexor digitorum profundus repair: A surgical technique. *Journal of Hand Surgery (American), 44,* e1–e5.

Shapiro, L. M., & Kamal, R. (2020). Evaluation and treatment of flexor tendon and pulley injuries in athletes. *Clinics in Sports Medicine, 39*(2), 279–297.

Ganglion Cysts

Presentation

The patient is concerned about a rubbery, rounded swelling most commonly emerging from the dorsal or volar aspect of the wrist or the flexor tendon sheath of the hand. It may have appeared abruptly, been present for years, or fluctuated, suddenly resolving and gradually returning in much the same place (Fig. 111.1). The patient often first notices it when a minor injury brings it to attention. People may be troubled with these cysts at any age, but they tend to be most common in midlife.

There is usually little tenderness, inflammation, or interference with function, but ganglion cysts may be bothersome with symptoms that include pain, paresthesias, limitation of motion, or weakness. Often the patient is only disturbed by the presence of a lump.

What to Do

✓ Take a thorough history and perform a complete physical examination of the hand to ascertain that everything else is normal. These cysts are usually self-evident and generally no larger than 2 cm in diameter. They are soft and ballotable and appear on the dorsal or volar aspect of the wrist. Gentle percussion over the mass should not elicit electric shocks as seen with digital nerve abnormalities. Also, a ganglion should not be pulsatile or compressible as seen with an aneurysm.

✓ **It is unnecessary to obtain a radiograph of a classic, asymptomatic ganglion cyst.** Standard radiographs will not demonstrate the cyst and need only be obtained when the cyst is symptomatic and there is a question of underlying bony disease or injury.

✓ **Although most ganglions can be diagnosed easily on physical examination, ultrasonography may be helpful in diagnosing a small or questionable lesion. Transillumination with an otoscope light will demonstrate its clear cystic nature, in contrast to a lipoma, sarcoma, or other solid soft tissue mass.**

✓ **Explain to the patient that this is a benign, fluid-filled cyst, spontaneously arising from a bursa, ligament, tendon sheath, meniscus, or joint capsule.**

✓ **Treatment options include the following: (1) doing nothing; (2) draining the contents of the cyst with a needle (18 or 20 gauge) to reduce its size, with or without injecting it afterward with a corticosteroid; or (3) arranging for a surgical excision.**

✓ Conservative management is an option for asymptomatic patients; it consists of reassurance that the lesion is benign, and that spontaneous resolution often occurs (about 40–60% of cysts).

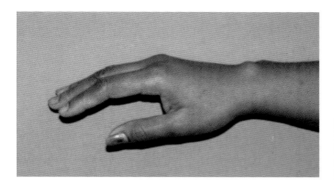

Fig. 111.1 Typical dorsal wrist ganglion cyst. (From Waldman, S. D. [2019]. Ganglion cysts of the wrist. In: S. D. Waldman (Ed.), *Atlas of common pain syndromes* [4th ed., fig. 54.2]. Philadelphia, PA: Elsevier.)

✅ If the patient has symptoms, including pain or paresthesias, or is disturbed by the cosmetic appearance, aspiration with or without injection of a corticosteroid is effective, without recurrence in 27% to 67% of patients. Surgical treatment involves total ganglionectomy, with removal of a modest portion of the attached capsule. Recurrence after surgical treatment is between 5% and 15%.

✅ Follow the wishes of the patient regarding treatment and arrange for the appropriate corresponding follow-up.

✅ **If the patient requests immediate decompression, prepare the skin and anesthetize the skin and cyst wall using a small-gauge needle and a small amount of injectable local anesthetic. With a needle (18 or 20 gauge) on a 10-mL syringe, aspirate the mucinous contents. Following aspiration, you can consider instilling a long-acting corticosteroid mixed with a local anesthetic through the same needle used to aspirate.** When injecting a corticosteroid after aspiration, a hemostat is used to stabilize the needle while the syringe is changed.

✅ Provide appropriate follow-up care. Refer patients who desire surgical resection to an orthopedic surgeon; for hand or wrist ganglion cysts, referral to a hand surgeon is appropriate if one is available.

What Not to Do

❌ Do not ignore a cyst that drains spontaneously. With external drainage, there is the risk for developing a serious joint or soft tissue infection.

❌ Do not forget to allay any concerns about possible malignancy. Reassure the patient that this lesion is benign and poses no potential for malignant transformation.

Discussion

Ganglion cysts are outpouchings of joint capsules, menisci, bursae, ligaments, or tendon sheaths, with no clear cause and no relation to nerve ganglia. Perhaps ganglion cysts got their name because their contents are like glue.

Ganglion cysts may be caused by trauma or tissue irritation when modified synovial cells lining the synovial-capsular interface are stimulated to produce mucin. This mucin dissects along the attached joint ligament and capsule to form capsular ducts and dilatations (lakes) of mucin. The ducts and lakes of mucin coalesce to form a solitary ganglion cyst. Their viscous mucin consists of hyaluronic acid, albumin, globulin, and glucosamine.

Dorsal wrist ganglia represent 60% to 70% of all ganglia. Twenty percent of all ganglia occur in the volar wrist. The flexor tendon sheath of the fingers is involved in 10% to 12% of ganglia. A dorsally located ganglion of the distal interphalangeal joint is also known as a mucous cyst. Reassurance about their insignificance is often the best we can offer patients.

Suggested Readings

Elsevier Point of Care. (2020). *Ganglion cyst*. Amsterdam, Netherlands: Elsevier BV.

Tallia, A. F. (2003). Diagnostic and therapeutic injection of the wrist and hand region. *American Family Physician, 67,* 745–750.

Zubowicz, V. N., & Ishii, C. H. (1987). Management of ganglion cysts of the hand by simple aspiration. *Journal of Hand Surgery American, 12,* 618–620.

Gouty Arthritis, Acute

Presentation

A patient rapidly develops an intensely painful monoarticular arthritis, often in the middle of the night, but sometimes a few hours following a minor trauma. The first attack of acute gouty arthritis usually occurs between the ages of 40 and 60 years in men and after the age of 60 years in women.

Any joint may be affected, but the most common is the metatarsophalangeal joint of the great toe (podagra). Other lower limb joints, including the ankle, knee, and tarsal joints, are commonly involved. The joint is red, warm, swollen, and intensely tender to touch or movement. There is increased sensitivity of the overlying skin, and pain can be precipitated with little stimulation, such as a bed sheet touching the area. There is usually no fever, rash, or other sign of systemic illness, although low-grade fever, leukocytosis, and an elevation of the erythrocyte sedimentation rate may occur.

The patient may have predisposing factors that increase the risk for developing gout, such as obesity, moderate to heavy alcohol intake (especially beer), high blood pressure, diabetes, a family history of gout, and abnormal kidney function. Certain medications, including thiazide diuretics, low-dose aspirin, and tuberculosis medications (pyrazinamide and ethambutol), can also precipitate gout.

What to Do

✅ **If the patient has not been previously diagnosed by arthrocentesis that showed crystals, tap the involved joint as described for acute monoarticular arthritis** (see Chapter 118). In addition to ruling out infection with Gram stain and culture of the synovial fluid, laboratory analysis should include microscopy to look for crystals in the joint fluid. Urate crystals of gout look like needles; calcium pyrophosphate dihydrate crystals of pseudogout are rhomboid shaped. Polarizing filters above and below the sample help distinguish the strongly negative birefringent crystals of sodium urate (Fig. 112.1) from the weakly positive birefringent calcium pyrophosphate dehydrate. Cell counts should be performed on the synovial fluid. Gout produces an inflammatory arthritis, and synovial white blood cell (WBC) counts will range from 5000 to 50,000/mL with a neutrophilic predominance. Higher counts with more than 75% polymorphonuclear cells should always raise the question of an infection. **If septic arthritis is suspected, urgent initiation of antibiotics along with orthopedic and infectious disease referral should be provided.**

✅ Radiographs may be obtained but are only likely to be helpful in the late stages of the disease (Fig. 112.2) or if other underlying disease is in question (e.g., pseudogout, tumor).

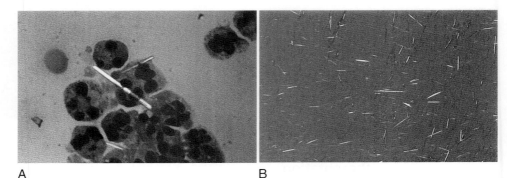

Fig. 112.1 Microscopic examples of monosodium urate monohydrate microcrystals under (A) polarized light and (B) light microscopy. (Adapted from Knoop, K. J., Stack, L. B., & Storrow, A. B. [2002]. *Atlas of emergency medicine* [2nd ed.]. New York, NY: McGraw-Hill.)

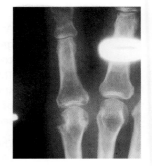

Fig. 112.2 The fifth metacarpophalangeal joint in this radiograph is fairly characteristic of the late stages of gout. Marginal erosions of the metacarpal head result in prominent overhanging edges. (Adapted from Yu, J. [2001]. *Musculoskeletal imaging.* St. Louis, MO: Mosby.)

✅ **For most otherwise healthy patients with acute gout, nonsteroidal anti-inflammatory drugs (NSAIDs) are the treatment of choice.** Treatment of an acute attack is most effective when started within the first 24 hours.

✅ **Provide rapid pain relief with loading doses of NSAIDs. All NSAIDs have been shown to be equally effective. The choice of NSAID is not as important as initiating therapy early in an attack. One potential example is** naproxen oral tablets (750 mg, then 250 mg once every 8 hours as needed; treat with the lowest effective dose and for the shortest duration; consider lower doses in geriatric patients). All NSAIDs should be used with caution or not at all in patients with any of the following: significant renal impairment (creatinine >2), poorly controlled congestive heart failure, history of or active peptic ulcer disease, anticoagulation therapy, or hepatic dysfunction.

✅ **Corticosteroids are effective in the treatment of gout. When used appropriately for a short duration, they are a safe alternative for patients in whom NSAIDs are contraindicated.** Care must be used in patients with diabetes, but in recent years corticosteroids have been used more often in older patients with multiple comorbid conditions because of their low-toxicity profile.

✅ **For a monoarticular flare-up, an intraarticular injection of a long-acting corticosteroid is often the safest treatment.** Delay injecting corticosteroids into the joint until the possibility of infection is eliminated (see Chapter 118). After draining as much fluid as possible from the joint, using aseptic techniques, inject a mixture of corticosteroid and local anesthetic into the affected joint. Methylprednisolone acetate suspension for injection (Depo-Medrol) can be used in a dose range from 10 to 80 mg at the appropriate site, depending on degree of inflammation and size and location of the affected joint. Repeat doses are usually not required for 1 to 5 weeks. Dose ranges for large joints: 20 to 80 mg; medium joints: 10 to 40 mg; small joints: 4 to 10 mg.

✅ **Oral corticosteroids may also be used.** Start with a loading dose of oral steroid such as 20 to 40 mg of prednisone and then provide a tapering course over 8 days. If tapered too rapidly, a rebound flare-up of gout may occur.

✅ **A single dose of intramuscular (IM) steroid** is an alternative in patients who cannot take oral medications. Triamcinolone acetonide (Aristocort, Kenalog), 60 mg IM once, is an acceptable option.

✅ **Adrenocorticotropic hormone (ACTH), 80 units IM, is also effective and can be used in patients with multiple medical problems, including congestive heart failure, chronic renal insufficiency, and peptic ulcer disease.** Its use is limited by patient comfort (IM administration), cost, and availability.

✅ **Another alternative treatment** for acute gouty arthritis within the first 12 to 24 hours of an attack is colchicine, 1.2 mg orally, at onset of flare-up, followed by 0.6 mg 1 hour later (max total dose 1.8 mg orally over a 1-hour period). Higher doses are not more effective. IV administration can cause anaphylaxis, and extravasation can cause tissue necrosis. At high doses, colchicine is bone marrow suppressive; in patients with renal insufficiency or who are taking cyclosporine or statins, colchicine can cause neuromyopathy. **Because of its small benefit-to-toxicity ratio, colchicine should only be considered if there is no alternative therapy.**

✅ Colchicine is usually used at low doses, 0.6 mg once or twice daily, to prevent attacks or rebound flare-ups in patients in whom steroids are being tapered or urate-lowering therapy is being started. It should still be used with caution in older patients with reduced renal function. All patients should be informed that the dose required for gout control is often associated with diarrhea.

✅ **It should be remembered that gout is a self-limited disease. At times, the risks of certain treatments may outweigh the benefits, especially in elderly patients.**

✅ **Instruct the patient** to elevate and rest the painful extremity, apply ice packs, and **arrange for follow-up.** In gouty arthritis, the application of ice may be therapeutic and can help discriminate gout from other forms of inflammatory arthritis. **In other words, topical ice has been shown to help relieve joint pain in patients with gouty arthritis but not in patients with other inflammatory arthritides.**

✅ Patients should be informed about the factors contributing to their hyperuricemia, such as obesity, a high-purine diet, regular alcohol consumption, and diuretic therapy, which may all be modifiable.

✅ After the acute attack has subsided, urate-lowering therapy with probenecid or allopurinol is considered cost effective for patients who have two or more attacks of gout per year.

✅ Most patients will note improvement within the first 12 to 24 hours, with resolution of symptoms in the next 7 to 10 days.

What Not to Do

(X) Do not depend on serum uric acid to diagnose acute gouty arthritis—it may or may not be elevated (>8 mg/dL) at the time of an acute attack. Hyperuricemia will be found in 70% of patients with their first attack of gout.

(X) Do not use NSAIDs when a patient has a history of active peptic ulcer disease with bleeding. Relative contraindications include renal insufficiency, volume depletion, gastritis, inflammatory bowel disease, asthma, and congestive heart disease.

(X) Do not insist on reconfirming an established diagnosis of gout by ordering serum uric acid levels (which are often normal during the acute attack) or tapping an exquisitely painful joint at every attack in a patient with known gout and a typical presentation.

(X) Do not, on the other hand, miss a septic arthritis in a patient with gout who is toxic with shaking chills and has a high fever, an elevated WBC count, an identified source of infection, or comorbidities such as diabetes, alcohol abuse, and advanced age. Septic arthritis carries the potential for a high morbidity and mortality.

(X) Do not attempt to reduce the serum uric acid level with probenecid or allopurinol during an acute attack of gouty arthritis. This will not help the arthritis and may even be counterproductive. Leave it for follow-up. Because of the high frequency of comorbid conditions and decreased life expectancy in elderly patients, it may be less important to institute urate-lowering therapy in these patients than in younger patients with many years of cumulative attacks and joint damage in their future.

(X) Do not stop urate-lowering maintenance therapy during an acute attack. In these cases, therapy should be continued, and the acute gouty flare treated in the usual manner.

Discussion

Among mammals, only humans and other primate species excrete uric acid as the end product of purine metabolism. This is because humans and primates lack the enzyme uricase, which converts uric acid to allantoin, a more soluble excretory product.

When overproduction or underexcretion of uric acid occurs, the serum urate concentration may exceed the solubility of urate (a concentration of approximately >6.8 mg/dL), and supersaturation of urate in the serum and other extracellular spaces results. This state (called hyperuricemia), increases the risk for crystal deposition of urate, from the supersaturated fluids, in tissues. Hyperuricemia is defined as a serum uric acid level of more than 7.0 mg/dL in men or more than 6.0 mg/dL in women. **Acute gouty arthritis results from an inflammatory response to deposition of monosodium urate crystals in the joints, creating intense inflammation in the joints or other soft tissues.**

Hyperuricemia is clearly associated with an increased risk for the development of gout, although most patients with hyperuricemia are asymptomatic and never develop gout. In the general population, 80% to 90% of gout patients are underexcreters, although renal function is otherwise normal. The risk for the development of gout increases with increasing serum uric acid level.

In younger patients, hyperuricemia and gout are overwhelmingly observed in men. The initial attack of gout is monoarticular in 85% to 90% of patients. Lower extremity joints are usually affected, with approximately 60% of first attacks involving the first metatarsophalangeal joints. Attacks may last from a few days to 2 to 3 weeks without treatment, with a gradual resolution of all inflammatory signs and a return to apparent normalcy. A so-called intercritical period, lasting weeks to months, may elapse before a new attack occurs in the same or another joint. Without specific therapy, a second attack will

(continued)

Discussion continued

occur in 78% of patients within 2 years, and in 93% within 10 years. Over subsequent years, attacks occur more frequently and may be polyarticular and associated with fever and constitutional symptoms. Tophaceous deposits become apparent over the elbows, fingers, or other areas over the years (tophaceous gout); chronic polyarticular arthritis may develop, which is often less severe, sometimes resembling rheumatoid arthritis or degenerative joint disease. Distal interphalangeal (DIP) joint involvement is a little more common than proximal interphalangeal (PIP) involvement, and tophaceous deposits on Heberden nodes can often be confused with osteoarthritis.

In patients older than 60 years with newly diagnosed gout, approximately 50% are women. Elderly women may have more finger involvement than men; 25% of women present with hand involvement and polyarticular disease.

Obesity, genetic predisposition, high intake of meat and seafood, hyperlipidemia, hypertension, and heavy alcohol use are associated with younger gout patients, whereas renal insufficiency, low-dose salicylates, and thiazide diuretic use are more often associated with elderly onset gout.

Transplant patients and patients on cyclosporine therapy are also at increased risk for developing gout, as are patients with myeloproliferative disorders, polycythemia vera, myeloid metaplasia, and chronic myelogenous leukemia.

Trauma, surgery, infection, and starvation as well as alcoholic or dietary indiscretions may provoke acute attacks. Acute attacks have been known to follow a game of golf, a long walk, or a hunting trip, leading to the name "pheasant hunter's toe." The solubility of uric acid decreases with a lower body temperature and in a lowering pH. These properties may provide an explanation for the increase in gouty attacks in the peripheral joints in cold weather.

Radiographs in gout characteristically demonstrate normal bone mineral density until the late stages of the disease. Well-marginated paraarticular erosion with overhanging edges or margins is the characteristic lesion of chronic gouty arthritis.

The gold standard for establishing a definite diagnosis of gout is the presence of monosodium urate crystals in aspirated joint fluid or tophus.

Caution should be used when trying to reach a diagnosis based on clinical features and a lab finding of hyperuricemia. No studies have been published on the usefulness or validity of any diagnostic clinical criteria. Additionally, the serum uric acid level is commonly elevated in patients without gout and normal or even low in patients with gout. It is therefore not particularly useful in ruling in or out the diagnosis.

When it is impractical or not possible to obtain joint fluid, supportive data that can be used to make a diagnosis of gout include a history of gout; a typical clinical history of sudden onset of an exquisitely painful joint, classically the first metatarsophalangeal joint; a history of underlying renal disease or use of medications that cause hyperuricemia; an elevated serum urate level; radiologic evidence suggestive of gouty arthritis; and a favorable response to topical cold applications.

Suggested Readings

Elsevier Point of Care. (2020). *Gout*. Amsterdam, Netherlands: Elsevier BV.

Monu, J. U., & Pope, T. L. (2004). Gout: A clinical and radiologic review. *Radiology Clinics of North America, 42*, 169–184.

Rott, K. T., & Agudelo, C. A. Gout. *JAMA, 289,* 2857–2860.

Wise, C. M. (2005). Crystal-associated arthritis in the elderly. *Clinics in Geriatric Medicine, 21*, 491–511. v-vi.

Knee Sprain

Presentation

After twisting the knee during a fall or sports injury, the patient complains of knee pain, possible swelling, and variable ability to bear weight. There may be a joint effusion or spasm of the quadriceps, forcing the patient to hold the knee at 10 to 20 degrees of flexion. See Fig. 113.1 for normal anatomy.

With an **anterior cruciate ligament (ACL) tear,** there will most likely be a noncontact injury involving a sudden deceleration (landing from a jump, cutting, or sidestepping), hyperextension, or twisting, as is common in basketball, football, and soccer. This may be accompanied by the sensation of a "pop," immediately followed by significant nonlocalizing pain and rapid development of swelling and effusion. Significant injuries will have a positive Lachman test on examination.

The **medial collateral ligament (MCL)** is another frequently injured knee ligament. This may be torn with a direct blow to the lateral aspect of a partially flexed knee, such as being tackled from the side in football, or by an external rotational force on the tibia, which can occur in snow skiing when the tip of the skin is forced out laterally. There may also be an awareness of a "pop" during the injury, but unlike the ACL tear, it is localized to the medial knee, along with more focal pain and swelling. Significant injuries cause laxity of the MCL with valgus stress testing at 30 degrees of flexion.

The **medial or lateral meniscus** can be torn acutely with a sudden twisting injury of the knee while the knee is partially flexed, such as may occur when a runner suddenly changes direction or when the foot is firmly planted, the tibia is rotated, and the knee is forcefully extended, as when a football lineman turns and springs up at the beginning of a play. Pain along the joint line is felt immediately, and there is often a mild effusion with tenderness to palpation along the corresponding medial or lateral joint line. There may be a positive McMurray test.

Posterior cruciate ligament (PCL) injuries occur with forced hyperflexion, as can occur in high-contact sports, such as football and rugby. Tears of the PCL can also occur with a posterior blow to the proximal tibia of a flexed knee, as occurs with dashboard injuries to the knee during motor vehicle collisions. Hyperextension, most often with an associated varus or valgus force, can also cause PCL injury. There is no report of a tear or pop, only vague symptoms, such as unsteadiness or discomfort. There is commonly a mild to moderate knee effusion, and a significant injury will have a positive posterior drawer test, and a posterior sag sign will be present (Fig. 113.2).

Injury of the **lateral collateral ligament (LCL)** is much less common than injury of the MCL. This usually results from varus stress to the knee, as occurs when a runner plants the foot and then

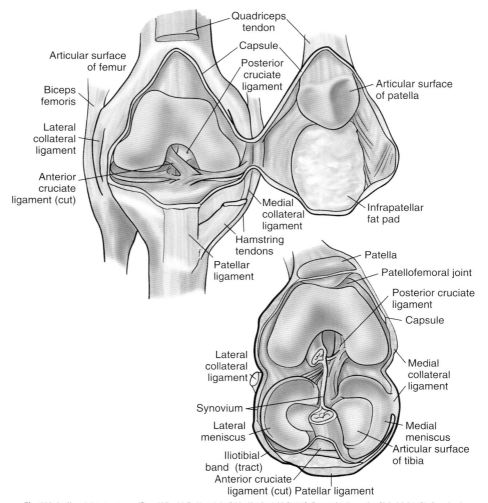

Fig. 113.1 Knee joint structures. (From Miller, M. D., Hart, J. A., & MacKnight, J. M. [2010]. *Essential orthopaedics.* Philadelphia, PA: Saunders.)

turns toward the ipsilateral knee or when there is a direct blow to the anteromedial knee. The patient reports acute onset of lateral knee pain that requires prompt cessation of activity.

What to Do

⊘ If there is any delay in examining the knee, provide ice, a compression dressing, and elevation above the level of the heart to try to minimize pain and swelling. **For severe pain, provide immediate analgesia.**

⊘ **Ask about the mechanism of injury, which is often the key to diagnosis.** The position of the joint and direction of traumatic force dictates which anatomic structures are at greatest risk for injury. The patient can usually recreate exactly what happened by using the uninjured knee to demonstrate.

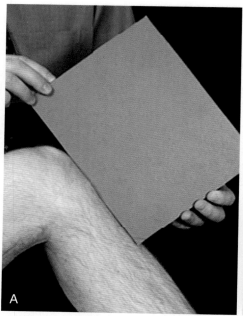
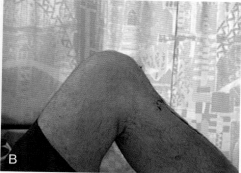

Fig. 113.2 Posterior sag sign (left knee viewed from the side). (A) Normal. (B) Posterior sagging as a result of a posterior cruciate ligament injury. (From Ghosh, K. M., et al. [2010]. Soft tissue knee injuries. *Surgery (Oxford), 28*[10], 494–501.)

Obtain information about associated symptoms. Knee buckling/instability with pivoting or walking is associated with ACL tear. A knee-joint effusion within 4 to 6 hours of injury suggests an intraarticular injury, such as ACL, meniscus, or osteochondral fracture. Sensations of locking or catching inside the knee may be associated with meniscal tears.

During inspection and examination of the injured knee, comparison with the normal knee is important. Initiate the examination by focusing first on the leg that is healthy. This helps to create trust and allows the patient to relax for a more accurate examination. Inspect the knee for swelling, ecchymosis, malalignment, or disruption of skin. Palpate the bony and ligamentous structure on the medial and lateral aspect of the knee and palpate along both joint lines to elicit any point tenderness. With the patient supine, feel for an effusion and discomfort with patellar motion. Determine if there is any crepitus or limitation in range of motion (ROM) by gently attempting to fully flex and extend the knee. Look for injuries of the back and pelvis. Check hip flexion, extension, and rotation. Thump the sole of the foot as an axial loading clue to a tibia or fibula fracture.

Document any effusion, discoloration, heat, deformity, or loss of function, circulation, sensation, or movement.

Stress the four major knee ligaments, comparing the injured with the uninjured knee to determine if there is any instability. A complete knee examination will help to detect isolated ligamentous injuries but will also help the examiner find coexisting injuries.

Perform a Lachman test to diagnose injury of the ACL (Fig. 113.3). With the knee flexed 20 to 30 degrees, place one hand on the proximal tibia and the other on the distal femur,

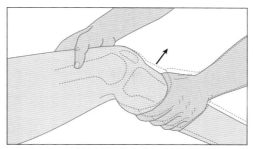

Fig. 113.3 The Lachman test.

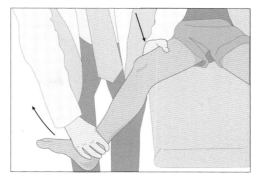

Fig. 113.4 Valgus stress test.

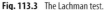

with the patient's heel on the examination table. Stabilize the femur, grasp the tibia, and pull it anteriorly with a brisk tug. ACL tears will have increased anterior translation, at least 3 mm greater than the noninjured side, and a soft or nonexistent end point.

✅ **Test MCL stability with the valgus stress test** (Fig. 113.4). With the knee still flexed 20 to 30 degrees, grasp the tibia distally to stabilize the lower leg, then apply direct, firm pressure in a medial direction from the lateral femoral condyle. Pain in the location of the MCL during valgus stressing, but no laxity, is called a grade I sprain. Grade II sprains have some laxity during valgus load; however, there is still a solid end point. When there is a soft or nonexistent end point, this constitutes a grade III MCL sprain, which represents a complete tear of the ligament. **Repeat valgus stress testing in full extension.** If there is joint laxity when the knee is locked in full extension, there is a strong possibility of an accompanying **ACL, posterior oblique ligament, or posteromedial capsular tear.**

✅ **Test the integrity of the PCL and posterior capsule with the posterior drawer test** (Fig. 113.5). The test is performed with the patient supine and the hip flexed to 45 degrees. Flex the knee to 90 degrees and apply firm, direct pressure in a posterior direction to the anteroproximal tibia with the thumbs located on the medial and lateral joint lines. If the force displaces the anterior superior tibial border beyond the medial femoral condyle, this suggests a complete PCL injury; posterior displacement of the tibia more than 5 mm posterior to the femur suggests a **combined PCL and posterolateral corner injury.** Look for increased posterior displacement of the tibia and a soft or mushy end point. When the knee is in 90 degrees of flexion, the proximal tibia normally sits about 10 mm anterior to the femoral condyles. If no step-off is present, a posterior sag sign exists and is also associated with PCL injury. **These tests may be difficult to perform if there is a large effusion.** Fifteen percent of patients with **posterolateral corner knee injuries** have a common **peroneal nerve injury.** It is important to ask patients about sensory changes or muscle weakness and to examine ankle dorsiflexion and great-toe extension.

✅ **Test LCL stability with the varus stress test** (Fig. 113.6), pressing laterally on the medial femoral condyle with the knee flexed to 20 to 30 degrees and in full extension. Grading is the same as for MCL sprains. **Lateral joint line opening in full extension typically indicates a multiligament injury.** Grade III tears are indicative of complete LCL tear and have a high association with **posterolateral corner injury** or **cruciate tears.** If there is varus laxity, also check the function of the **peroneal nerve** by asking the patient to dorsiflex the big toe.

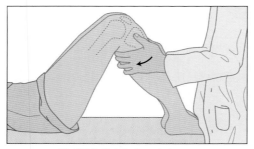

Fig. 113.5 Posterior drawer test.

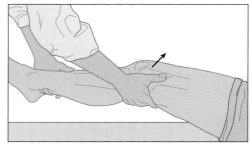

Fig. 113.6 Varus stress test. (The valgus stress test is the opposite of this test.)

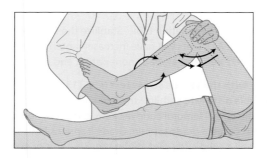

Fig. 113.7 The McMurray test.

✓ **Examine for an injury to the medial or lateral meniscal cartilage with the McMurray test** (Fig. 113.7). With the patient supine, hold the knee anteriorly at the femoral condyle with one hand, fingers positioned along the joint line, and while applying a valgus force to the knee, hold the foot with the other hand. Then, while externally rotating the lower leg, fully flex the knee and hip, slowly extend, and then repeat with the lower leg internally rotated. Keep repeating this maneuver several times. Pain associated with audible sounds or palpable crepitus suggests a tear of the meniscus. **This test may be difficult to complete if there is acute pain and muscle spasm.**

✓ **A negative McMurray test does not rule out a meniscal tear.** Tenderness from meniscal tears is localized along the joint line, most prominently at or posterior to the collateral ligament. The medial meniscus is more susceptible to injury than the lateral meniscus is.

✓ **Palpate the patella and head of the fibula, looking for tenderness associated with fracture.**

✓ **Assess for effusion** by placing a finger lightly on the patella with the knee relaxed and fully extended and, with the other hand, gently pinching the soft tissue on both sides of the patella, feeling for a fluid wave. In the presence of an intraarticular effusion, the patella can also be bounced or balloted against the underlying femoral condyle. Alternatively the knee joint can be milked, gently pushing on the medial side of the joint with a flat palm in a superior to inferior motion and then repeating the same motion on the lateral side of the joint, and then again on the medial side, back and forth. While doing this, look for fluid to flow away from the hand providing pressure and toward the opposite side of the joint.

✓ **Radiographs to rule out fracture may be deferred or avoided if the patient does not meet one of the following Ottawa knee rules:**

- ○ Age 55 years or older
- ○ Tenderness at the head of the fibula
- ○ Isolated tenderness of the patella
- ○ Inability to flex the knee to 90 degrees
- ○ Inability to bear weight (four steps) both immediately after injury and at initial physical assessment

✓ **These criteria do not apply to patients younger than 5 years of age or patients with an altered level of consciousness, multiple painful injuries, paraplegia, or diminished limb sensation.**

✓ **Treatment:**

- ○ **Minor (grade I) sprains that do not exhibit any joint instability or intraarticular effusion can be treated with rest, elevation, and, if comfort is improved, ice (20-minute periods three or four times a day for 3 days), and acetaminophen or nonsteroidal anti-inflammatory drugs (NSAIDs) (ibuprofen, naproxen).** The patient can usually return to previous activities as rapidly as pain allows. Provide follow-up if symptoms do not improve in 5 to 7 days.

- ○ **Moderate (grade II) and severe (grade III) ACL, MCL, and PCL sprains with partial or complete ligament tears, meniscal tears, joint effusion, or instability should be treated with rest, elevation, and ice, as mentioned, but can also be provided with crutches for additional stability and pain management with ambulation. In the absence of associated fractures, patients may bear weight as tolerated. A sleeve brace or wrap may provide external proprioception and compression, which may improve symptoms. A knee immobilizer is only indicated for quadriceps and patellar tendon ruptures, displaced tibial plateau fractures, tibial spine avulsion fractures, patellar fractures or dislocations, and knee dislocations. In pediatric patients and those with severe pain, knee immobilizer use can be considered.** They should be encouraged to work actively on regaining full ROM through active and passive knee flexion and extension exercises several times a day. They should also work to preserve quadriceps and hamstrings strength by performing active quadriceps and hamstrings flexion exercises while seated with the knee extended at least three times daily.

- ○ **Patients with grade II and grade III LCL injuries, which are frequently accompanied by disruptions in the posterolateral corner of the knee, should be treated with knee immobilization and remain non-weightbearing until seen by orthopedics in follow-up and cleared to mobilize the joint and bear weight.**

- ○ **All patients with grade II and III knee ligament sprains should be referred for orthopedic assessment within 5 to 7 days.**

- ○ Instruct the patient that additional injuries may become apparent as the spasm and effusion abate.

- ○ **If vascular injury is strongly suspected (e.g., multiligamentous disruption),** urgently consult with a vascular surgeon. Ultrasonography may be used to evaluate the popliteal artery for suspected injury.

○ **Thromboprophylaxis is not recommended for most patients with lower leg injuries** requiring short-term leg immobilization. However, consider using low-molecular-weight heparin for adult outpatients at high risk for deep vein thrombosis who are expected to be immobilized for at least 1 week. Examples of high-risk conditions include active malignancy, pregnancy, and inherited thrombophilia.

What Not to Do

Ⓧ Do not assume that a negative radiograph means a major injury does not exist.

Ⓧ Do not rely on magnetic resonance imaging (MRI) to assess all injured knees. MRI is not cost effective or superior to clinical assessment in accuracy. MRI is a useful surgical planning tool for assessing a knee before operative intervention, especially with posterolateral corner injuries, which may require the reconstruction of multiple ligaments and the lateral meniscus.

Ⓧ Do not inject or prescribe corticosteroids for acute knee injuries. These drugs may delay soft tissue healing.

Ⓧ **Do not miss vascular injuries with bicruciate ligament injuries. These injuries are equivalent to knee dislocations with regard to mechanism of injury, severity of ligamentous injury, and frequency of major arterial injuries.**

Discussion

The ACL, PCL, MCL, and LCL make up the main static stabilizers of the knee. Together the four ligaments enable the knee to function as a complex hinge joint, with rotational capabilities that allow the tibia to rotate internally and glide posteriorly on the femoral condyles during flexion and to rotate externally 15 to 30 degrees during extension.

The menisci are crescent-shaped cartilaginous structures that provide a cushioning congruous surface for the transmission of 50% of the axial forces across the knee joint. The menisci increase joint stability, facilitate nutrition, and provide lubrication and shock absorption for the articular cartilage.

Most patients with a knee injury suffer soft tissue damage, including ligament, tendon, meniscal cartilage, and muscle tears. In most cases, plain radiographs do little to aid diagnosis of soft tissue injury. Plain radiographs can show findings suggestive of ACL injury, such as an avulsion of the lateral capsule, known as a Segond fracture or a tibial spine avulsion. They can also show subtle fractures of the posterior tibial plateau or associated fibular head avulsion fractures. However, **clinicians must rely on physical examination to identify patients with serious knee injuries that require splinting and/or orthopedic referral.**

Joint aspiration of hemarthrosis to reduce severe pain should be reserved for patients with very large or tense effusions and should be performed with sterile technique. Fat globules in bloody joint fluid suggest occult fracture.

Conservative treatment versus surgical reconstruction is the main treatment decision when managing an ACL tear. ACL reconstruction is the preferred treatment for adolescents and most young adults who are unwilling to modify their physical activity levels. In older patients, there is support for both conservative and operative treatment. Patients with a sedentary or low-impact lifestyle are ideal candidates for conservative or nonoperative management. Patients who compete in jumping or cutting sports are likely to benefit from ACL reconstruction.

Hinged knee braces can be prescribed for grade II and III ACL and MCL injuries in patients who feel unstable without them. If used, patients should come out of the brace multiple times daily to work on ROM and strength exercises to prevent joint stiffness and muscle atrophy. Surgical repair of a grade III MCL tear is generally reserved for the patient who has associated damage to the ACL or meniscus.

(continued)

Discussion continued

A long-leg knee brace can be prescribed for grade I and II LCL sprains, which are generally managed nonoperatively. The brace should be removed multiple times daily to allow for performance of ROM and strength exercises to prevent joint stiffness and muscle atrophy. **Grade III LCL and posterolateral corner injuries with or without PCL involvement are generally treated with surgical repair, and more often reconstruction, which should be completed within the first 1 to 2 weeks following the injury.**

In general, a patient who has had a knee injury can be given the go-ahead to resume sports activities **when examination demonstrates that the cruciate and collateral ligaments are intact, the knee is capable of moving from full extension to flexion of 120 degrees, and there is no effusion. The patient's pain should be markedly diminished, and there should be no locking, instability, or limp.**

Suggested Readings

Bauer, S. J., Hollander, J. E., Fuchs, S. H., et al. (1995). A clinical decision rule in the evaluation of acute knee injuries. *Journal of Emergency Medicine, 13*, 611–615.

Brown, J. R., & Trojian, T. H. (2004). Anterior and posterior cruciate ligament injuries. *PrimaryCare, 31*, 925–956.

Bulloch, B., Neto, G., Plint, A., et al. (2003). Validation of the Ottawa knee rule in children: A multicenter study. *Annals of Emergency Medicine, 42*, 48–55.

Elsevier Point of Care. (2018). *Knee injury (other than dislocation or fracture).* Amsterdam, Netherlands: Elsevier BV.

Emparanza, J. I., & Aginaga, J. R. (2001). Validation of the Ottawa knee rules. *Annals of Emergency Medicine, 38*, 364–368.

Gelb, H. J., Glasgow, S. G., Sapega, A. A., et al. (1996). Magnetic resonance imaging of knee disorders: Clinical value and cost-effectiveness in a sports medicine practice. *The American Journal of Sports Medicine, 24*, 99–103.

Johnson, L. L., Johnson, A. L., Colquitt, J. A., et al. (1996). Is it possible to make an accurate diagnosis based only on a medical history? A pilot study on women's knee joints. *Arthroscopy, 12*, 709–714.

Muellner, T., Weinstabl, R., Schabus, R., et al. (1997). The diagnosis of meniscal tears in athletes: A comparison of clinical and magnetic resonance imaging investigations. *The American Journal of Sports Medicine, 25*, 7–12.

Nichol, G., Stiell, I. G., Wells, G. A., et al. (1999). An economic analysis of the Ottawa knee rule. *Annals of Emergency Medicine, 34*, 438–447.

O'Shea, K. J., Murphy, K. P., Heekin, R. D., & Herzwurm, P. J. (1996). The diagnostic accuracy of history, physical examination and radiographs in the evaluation of traumatic knee disorders. *The American Journal of Sports Medicine, 24*, 164–167.

Quarles, J. D., & Hosey, R. G. (2004). Medial and lateral collateral injuries: Prognosis and treatment. *PrimaryCare, 31*, 957–975 ix.

Scholten, R. J., Devillé, Opstelten, W., et al. (2001). The accuracy of physical diagnostic tests for assessing meniscal lesions of the knee: A meta-analysis. *Journal of Family Practice, 50*, 938–944.

Seaberg, D. C., Yealy, D. M., Lukens, T., et al. (1998). Multicenter comparison of two clinical decision rules for the use of radiography in acute, high-risk knee injuries. *Annals of Emergency Medicine, 32*, 8–13.

Solomon, D. H., Simel, D. L., Bates, D. W., et al. (2001). Does this patient have a torn meniscus or ligament of the knee? *Journal of the American Medical Association, 286*, 1610–1620.

Stiell, I. G., Greeberg, G. H., Wells, G. A., et al. (1995). Derivation of a decision rule for the use of radiography in acute knee injuries. *Annals of Emergency Medicine, 26*, 405–414.

Stiell, I. G., Greeberg, G. H., Wells, G. A., et al. (1996). Prospective validation of a decision rule for the use of radiography in acute knee injuries. *Journal of the American Medical Association, 275*, 611–615.

Stiell, I. G., Wells, G. A., Hoag, R. H., et al. (1997). Implementation of the Ottawa knee rule for the use of radiography in acute knee injuries. *Journal of the American Medical Association, 278*, 2071–2079.

Strayer, R. J., & Lang, E. S. (2006). Does this patient have a torn meniscus or ligament of the knee? *Annals of Emergency Medicine, 47*, 499–501.

Wascher, D. C., Dvirnak, P. C., & DeCoster, T. A. (1997). Knee dislocation: Initial assessment and implications for treatment. *Journal of Orthopedic Trauma, 11*, 525–529.

Weber, J. E., Jackson, R. E., Peacock, W. F., et al. (1995). Clinical decision rules discriminate between fractures and nonfractures in acute isolated knee trauma. *Annals of Emergency Medicine, 26*, 429–433.

Lateral Epicondylitis and Medial Epicondylitis

(Tennis Elbow, Golfer's Elbow)

Presentation

In lateral epicondylitis, the patient complains of pain in the lateral elbow that frequently radiates down the lateral aspect of the forearm. Because the lateral epicondyle is the bony origin of wrist extensors, patients are usually involved in an activity that requires repetitive wrist extension, such as tennis or mechanical work. Occasionally, the patient can recall a specific injury to the area, but more often the pain is of gradual, insidious onset. Most patients relate symptoms to activities that stress the wrist extensor and supinator muscles, and especially to activities that involve forceful gripping or lifting of heavy objects. Even holding lightweight objects such as a cup may be difficult. There is tenderness to palpation over the origin of the extensor carpi radialis brevis tendon immediately anterior, medial, and distal to the lateral epicondyle. This tenderness is more pronounced with resisted wrist extension while the elbow is in extension or when the forearm is pronated.

Patients **with medial epicondylitis** complain of pain over the medial epicondyle and the proximal forearm. The pain may radiate down the medial aspect of the forearm. Medial epicondylitis has been associated with activities involving repetitive forearm pronation and wrist flexion, as this is the insertion point for wrist flexors. It occurs frequently in baseball pitchers and is also related to golf, tennis, bowling, racquetball, archery, weightlifting, and javelin throwing. It is also associated with occupations such as carpentry, plumbing, and meat cutting. Onset is usually insidious, but there may be an inciting event. The patient may also complain of a weak grasp and pain with repetitive wrist flexion and pronation. There will be tenderness to palpation just anterior to the medial epicondyle at the origin of the pronator teres and flexor carpi radialis muscles. Resisted wrist flexion and forearm pronation while the patient's elbow is in extension will reproduce symptoms.

What to Do

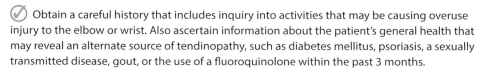 Obtain a careful history that includes inquiry into activities that may be causing overuse injury to the elbow or wrist. Also ascertain information about the patient's general health that may reveal an alternate source of tendinopathy, such as diabetes mellitus, psoriasis, a sexually transmitted disease, gout, or the use of a fluoroquinolone within the past 3 months.

Physical examination should concentrate on localizing the precise site of musculotendinous tenderness but should also include neck examination to help rule out cervical spinal disease as the cause of symptoms.

✅ **Initial treatment begins with the immediate, temporary cessation of offending activities. Complete immobilization or inactivity is not recommended.**

✅ **There are no specific treatment modalities that have been shown to substantially improve symptoms long term, and patients should be advised that regardless of the therapies attempted, the vast majority of these tendinopathies will resolve spontaneously within 1 year.**

✅ If a patient would like to try home treatments, ice massage for 5 to 15 minutes may be trialed, two to four times per day, for its local vasoconstrictive and analgesic effects. When comfort allows, deep friction massage, muscle stretching, and grip strengthening may help with early rehabilitation.

✅ Consider prescribing a nonsteroidal anti-inflammatory drug (NSAID) if it is not contraindicated by allergy, bleeding, gastritis, cardiac disease, or renal insufficiency. One trial suggests that a 7-day treatment course with a once-daily, 100-mg ketoprofen topical patch can provide pain relief without the adverse events associated with systemic delivery of an NSAID. Topical therapies tend to be substantially more expensive than oral NSAIDs, however. Always advise patients taking oral NSAIDS to do so with food and plenty of clear fluids to help alleviate stomach discomfort and to protect kidney function. Prescribing a histamine blocker or proton pump inhibitor can also be helpful.

✅ Steroid injection at the site of tendon origin at the epicondyle may improve pain 4 weeks postinjection, but does not appear to improve pain at 3 months and 1 year. There is evidence to suggest that steroid injections for lateral epicondylitis may lead to a lower rate of complete recovery and a greater 1-year recurrence versus placebo injection. **Steroid injections for this condition are therefore not recommended unless a patient requires pain relief in the short term and is willing to accept the risk of a worse long-term outcome.**

✅ **The counterforce brace has been found to be helpful for symptom reduction and is thought to reduce the load at the lateral or medial epicondyle by preventing the forearm muscles from fully expanding. Braces placed just distal to the epicondyles reduce loads greater than pads placed over the epicondyles** (Fig. 114.1).

✅ Patients should be informed that recovery often takes several months to 1 year but that most patients treated with conservative therapy respond successfully without recurrent symptoms. Physical therapy may be considered, but keep in mind that there are no published data proving its efficacy.

What Not to Do

❌ Do not order radiographs for a classic presentation. Reserve them for questions of bony disease.

❌ Do not inject corticosteroids repeatedly into the tendon. They cause it to weaken or possibly rupture. Additionally, corticosteroid injections may decrease cure rate and increase recurrence rate.

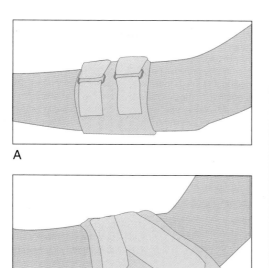

A

B

Fig. 114.1 (A) Lateral elbow brace. (B) Medial elbow brace.

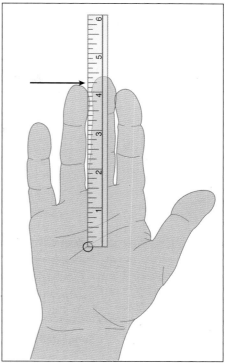

Fig. 114.2 Hand-size measurement to determine proper grip handle size—Nirschl technique. (Adapted from Nirschl, R. P. [1992]. Elbow tendinosis/tennis elbow. *Clinics in Sports Medicine, 11,* 851–870.)

Discussion

The characteristics most likely to result in elbow tendon overuse are age older than 35 years, high activity level (sports or occupational), and demanding activity technique. Lateral epicondylitis, also known as tennis elbow, occurs 7 to 10 times more frequently than medial epicondylitis, commonly referred to as golfer's elbow.

Although the precise universal pathophysiology of epicondylitis has yet to be established, it is now generally accepted that the injury results from microtearing of the tendon origin at the epicondyle. This progresses to a failed reparative response and subsequent tendon degeneration that ultimately alters the typical musculotendinous biomechanics of the elbow. Because of its relationship to other overuse tendinopathies (see Chapter 129), the more appropriate descriptive terms for lateral and medial

epicondylitis are lateral elbow tendinosis and medial elbow tendinosis.

Both tennis elbow and golfer's elbow usually affect patients who are between 30 and 60 years of age, with a peak incidence in the 40s. An acute onset of symptoms occurs more often in young athletes; chronic, recalcitrant symptoms typically occur in older patients.

Poor form for the backhand stroke, extending the wrist when striking the ball instead of holding the wrist and elbow immobile, and swinging from the shoulder increase one's risk for lateral elbow tendinosis. There is some evidence to support that a two-handed backstroke may decrease risk because of improved stroke mechanics. Patients with medial

(continued)

Discussion continued

elbow tendinosis who regularly play tennis often exhibit an improper serve and forehand stroke.

Equipment that is properly sized to the athlete is essential, especially in racquet sports, to prevent subsequent bouts of epicondylitis. Correct grip size is calculated by measuring from the proximal palm crease to the tip of the ring finger along its radial border (Fig. 114.2). Lighter graphite frames, racquets less tightly strung (manufacturer's low-range recommendations), racquets with higher string counts per unit area, and a larger racquet head (90–100 in^2 of hitting zone) will help to minimize injurious vibration and help prevent stressful off-center contact. In golf, clubs of proper weight, length, and grip are similarly important and can significantly reduce the injurious forces generated within the elbow.

Continued conditioning of the entire body along with the affected extremity is vital to a patient's successful recovery. Conditioning, including flexibility, strength, and endurance, is best performed with a slow, structured interval program.

Under investigation are novel therapies to regenerate tendon and regain function in patients with epicondylitis. These treatments include platelet-rich plasma (PRP) injection, bone marrow aspirate concentrate (BMAC), collagen-producing cell injection, and stem cell treatments. While these treatments are in early stages of investigation, they may warrant further consideration based on prospects of pain alleviation, function enhancement, and improved healing. Voids in the literature prohibit the recommendation that these treatments are safe and effective at this time. However, the preliminary results of initial clinical trials both in humans and in animals suggest that collagen-producing cell treatments and stem cell treatments have the potential to be more effective for tendon healing, pain management, and restoration of use than surgical techniques or conservative therapies alone.

Suggested Readings

Ciccotti, M. C., Schwartz, M. A., & Ciccotti, M. G. (2004). Diagnosis and treatment of medical epicondylitis of the elbow. *Clinics in Sports Medicine, 23*, 693–705, xi.

Coombes, B. K., Bisset, L., Brooks, P., Khan, A., & Vicenzino, B. (2013). Effect of corticosteroid injection, physiotherapy, or both on clinical outcomes in patients with unilateral lateral epicondylalgia: A randomized controlled trial. *JAMA, 309*(5), 461–469. https://doi.org/10.1001/jama.2013.129

Giangarra, C. E., Conroy, B., Jobe, F. W., et al. (1993). Electromyographic and cinematographic analysis of elbow function in tennis players using single- and double- backhand strokes. *American Journal of Sports Medicine, 21*, 394–399.

Hay, E. M., Paterson, S. M., Lewis, M., et al. (1999). Pragmatic randomised controlled trial of local corticosteroid injection and naproxen for treatment of lateral epicondylitis elbow in primary care. *BMJ, 319*, 964–968.

Mazières, B., Rouanet, S., Guillon, Y., et al. (2005). Topical ketoprofen patch in the treatment of tendinitis: A randomized, double blind, placebo controlled study. *Journal of Rheumatology, 32*, 1563–1570.

Mellor, S. (2003). Treatment of tennis elbow: The evidence. *BMJ, 327*, 330.

Nirschl, R. P., & Ashman, E. S. (2003). Elbow tendinopathy: Tennis elbow. *Clinics in Sports Medicine, 22*, 587–598.

Ranger, T. A., Wong, A. M. Y., Cook, J. L., et al. (2016). Is there an association between tendinopathy and diabetes mellitus? A systematic review with meta-analysis. *British Journal of Sports Medicine, 50*, 982–989.

Sandip, P., Tarpada, M., Morris, T., Lian, J., & Rashidi, S. (2018). Current advances in the treatment of medial and lateral epicondylitis. *Journal of Orthopaedics, 15*(1), 107–110.

Sellards, R., & Kuebrich, C. (2005). The elbow: Diagnosis and treatment of common injuries. *Primary Care, 32*, 1–16.

Smidt, N., van der Windt, D. A., Assendelft, W. J., et al. (2002). Corticosteroid injections, physiotherapy, or a wait-and-see policy for lateral epicondylitis. *Lancet, 359*, 657–662.

Whaley, A. L., & Baker, C. L. (2004). Lateral epicondylitis. *Clinics in Sports Medicine, 23*, 677–691, x.

Ligament Sprains

(Including Joint Capsule Injuries)

Presentation

Ligament sprains occur when a joint is distorted beyond its normal anatomic limits (as when an ankle is inverted, or a shoulder is dislocated and reduced). The patient may complain of a snapping or popping noise at the time of injury, immediate swelling, and loss of function (suggestive of grade II or III sprain or a fracture). Alternatively, the patient may come to the office within hours to days after the injury reporting gradually increasing swelling resulting in pain and stiffness after a less dramatic injury (suggestive of a grade I or II sprain and possibly the development of a traumatic effusion).

What to Do

✓ Obtain a detailed history of the mechanism of injury, and examine the joint for structural integrity, function, and point tenderness. Inability to fully extend an elbow is a strong indicator of significant injury. Use the uninjured limb as a control. **Ligamentous injuries are classified as grade I sprains (minimal stretching causing pain without swelling or laxity); grade II sprains (a partial tear with pain, functional loss and bleeding with swelling and slight laxity), which can be managed conservatively; and grade III sprains (complete tear with significant pain, marked swelling, and gross instability), often requiring a rigid splint and possible surgical intervention.**

✓ A tense joint effusion will limit the physical examination (and is one reason to require reevaluation after the swelling has decreased) but also suggests less than a third-degree ligamentous injury, which is normally accompanied by a tear of the joint capsule, and release of any tense effusion.

✓ **Obtain radiographs (these can be deferred if findings are minimal with full range of motion without bony tenderness or if specific criteria are not met, as for ankle and knee sprains)** (e.g., Ottawa Ankle and Knee Rules—see Chapters 96 and 113).

✓ **Ultrasound evaluation** can be helpful in determining whether a joint effusion is present.

✓ **Treatment:**

○ **For grades I and II sprains, gently immobilize the joint using an elastic bandage alone or in combination with a cotton roll or plaster splint, as discomfort demands. For ankle sprains specifically, soft bracing has been demonstrated to be superior to rigid bracing in stable sprains (grade I). Most upper extremity injuries can be immobilized by a sling alone or in combination with a soft or rigid splint.**

○ Consider prescribing acetaminophen or anti-inflammatory pain medication when the patient complains of pain at rest and provide crutches when discomfort will not allow weight bearing.

○ **If there is a fracture or ligament tear with instability (third-degree sprain), the limb is usually best immobilized in a splint or cast—splint ankles at 90 degrees, wrists in extension, and fingers at slight flexion.**

○ Although opioids should be avoided, provide a short course of narcotic analgesics when necessary to control severe pain.

○ Instruct the patient in rest, elevation above the level of the heart, and, when it provides comfort, application of ice 10 to 20 minutes each hour for the first few hours then three or four times a day for 3 days. Minor injuries may need only 1 day of treatment.

○ Explain to the patient that swelling in acute musculoskeletal injuries usually increases for the first 24 hours, and then decreases over the next 2 to 4 days (longer if the previous treatment is not employed). Also inform the patient that some swelling and discomfort may persist for several weeks and at times for several months.

○ Explain the possibility of occult injuries, the necessity for follow-up, and the slow healing of injured ligaments (usually 6 months until full strength is regained).

○ **Advocate for early mobilization and early return to normal functions for first-degree and second-degree sprains.**

What Not to Do

Ⓧ Do not obtain radiographs before the history or physical examination. Films of the wrong spot can be very misleading. For example, physicians have been steered away from the diagnosis of an avulsion fracture of the base of the fifth metatarsal by the presence of normal ankle films.

Ⓧ Do not base the diagnosis on radiographs. They should be used as confirmatory evidence.

Ⓧ Do not obtain routine comparison views on pediatric patients. They usually do not improve diagnostic accuracy.

Discussion

A tense joint effusion will limit the physical examination (and is one reason to require reevaluation after the swelling has decreased) but also suggests less than a third-degree ligamentous injury, which is normally accompanied by a tear of the joint capsule, and release of any tense effusion.

The benefit of cryotherapy for acute ligamentous injuries is controversial. For this reason, the use of ice should not be mandatory but should be used only when it is comforting to the patient.

Suggested Readings

Bleakley, C., McDonough, S., MacAuley, D., et al. (2004). The use of ice in the treatment of acute soft tissue injury. *American Journal of Sports Medicine*, *32*, 251–261.

Carr, K. E. (2003). Musculoskeletal injuries in young athletes. *Clinics in Family Practice*, *5*, 385–415.

Hocutt, J. E., Jr., Jaffe, R., Rylander, C. R., & Beebe, J. K. (1982). Cryotherapy in ankle sprains. *American Journal of Sports Medicine*, *10*, 316–319.

MacAuley, D. (2001). Do textbooks agree on their advice on ice? *Clinical Journal of Sports Medicine*, *11*, 67–72.

Seah, R., & Mani-Babu, S. (2011). Managing ankle sprains in primary care: What is best practice? A systematic review of the last 10 years of evidence. *British Medical Bulletin*, *97–105*.

Locked Knee

Presentation

The patient, usually with a history of a previous knee injury, and often with previous knee locking, suddenly develops a mechanical inability to extend the knee fully. The knee may flex but not extend and may be causing mild to moderate pain.

What to Do

✓ **Perform a complete knee examination, checking for point tenderness, effusion, meniscal tear, and joint stability.** A comprehensive physical examination should include an assessment of range of motion of both knees, with the unaffected knee examined first to establish a baseline. While supine, both knees are extended passively to assess for hyperextension and alignment, with one hand underneath each heel. The exact location of discomfort should be elicited, with anterior pain often implying an intraarticular block. To assess flexion, the patient is asked to actively flex the knee as far as possible, which is then tested passively, as is extension (Fig. 116.1).

✓ **If the patient feels the knee lock, do not to try to push through; this may cause further, possibly irreparable, damage.** The joint lines should also be palpated, with focal pain suspicious for a meniscal tear. In addition to strength, alignment, and neurovascular assessments, the examination should include a careful analysis of the knee ligaments (see Chapter 113).

✓ **If comfort allows, gently and repeatedly perform the maneuvers of the McMurray test** (see Chapter 113). This alone may release the locked knee. If not, continue as described next.

✓ **Obtain knee radiographs, including anteroposterior, lateral, sunrise, and notch views, looking for an osteocartilaginous loose body or other disease.**

✓ **With pain and persistent locking,** prepare the knee with povidone-iodine solution and, at a point just superior and lateral or medial to the patella, using a 25-gauge, 1-inch needle, inject 10 mL of 0.5% bupivacaine (Marcaine) into the joint space (see Fig. 118.1A).

✓ **With the knee thus anesthetized, place a roll of towels under the heel and ankle to serve as a fulcrum. Leave the patient supine so that gravity will aid in extension and have the patient gently rock and rotate the knee for approximately 20 minutes or until the locked knee has released. Repeated McMurray maneuvers may again be gently performed if joint reduction has not occurred. Alternatively, longitudinal traction can be applied with gentle rotation of the knee internally and externally.**

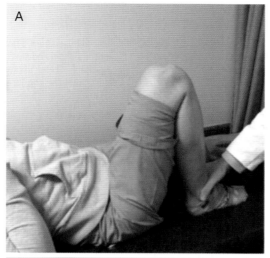

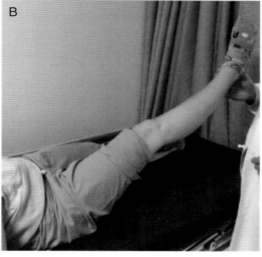

Fig. 116.1 Range of motion assessment. (With permission from Goodman, A. D., Chase, A., & Owens, B. B. [2017]. Locked knee in a 15-year-old girl: The knee examination. *Journal of Pediatrics, 185*, 245,e1.)

✅ **When the mechanical block is dislodged and the knee extended,** place the patient in a knee immobilizer, keep the patient non–weight bearing with crutches, and promptly refer the patient to an orthopedic surgeon for early arthroscopic examination and definitive treatment.

✅ **If full extension cannot be obtained,** the patient can be placed in a soft, bulky, partially immobilizing dressing (thick cotton roll covered with an elastic wrap) and placed on crutches until orthopedic follow-up can be obtained.

What Not to Do

❌ Do not forcefully manipulate or extend the knee. This may produce further intraarticular injury.

Discussion

Knee locking is usually caused by previous injuries that include meniscal tears, partial or complete anterior cruciate ligament tears, osteocartilaginous loose bodies, pathologic medial plicae, and foreign bodies. Less commonly, locking can occur without a history of trauma. In such cases, the cause may be torsion of the infrapatellar fat pad, lateral meniscal dislocation, or an intraarticular tumor such as a ganglion. Locking of the knee occurs when one of these structures has become entrapped between the tibial plateau and the femoral condyles, mechanically blocking extension of the joint. This may happen suddenly and may resolve suddenly.

A locked knee, especially after a past traumatic incident, is most suggestive of medial meniscus pathology, specifically a so-called bucket handle tear. In this pattern, a portion of the meniscus becomes torn and flips up and over, causing a mechanical block to motion. Many of these injuries occur after twisting, jumping, or pivoting, frequently during sports.

An evaluation by an experienced physician will identify meniscus tears with equal or better reliability than magnetic resonance imaging (MRI). However, MRI will often help to narrow the differential diagnosis—meniscus tear (including flipped bucket handle), discoid meniscus, osteochondral fracture, tear of the anterior cruciate ligament, or loose body—and is most useful when ordered as an adjunct to a thorough examination. Based on the examination and imaging, patients will often require prompt arthroscopic surgery.

Suggested Readings

Goodman, A. D., Chase, A., & Owens, B. D. (2017). Locked knee in a 15-year-old girl: The knee examination. *Journal of Pediatrics*, *185*, 245 e1.

Haider, Z., Syed, M. A., & Saran, D. (2017). Atraumatic sequential bilateral locking of the knee joints secondary to dislocation of non-discoid lateral menisci without radiological abnormality. *Journal of Clinical Orthopaedics and Trauma*, *8*, S26–S28.

Lumbar Strain ("Mechanical" Low Back Pain, Sacroiliac Dysfunction), Acute

Presentation

Suddenly or gradually, after lifting, sneezing, bending, or other movement, the patient develops a steady pain in one or both sides of the lower back. At times, this pain can be severe and incapacitating. It is usually better when lying down, worse with movement, and will perhaps radiate around the abdomen or down the thigh but no farther. There is insufficient trauma to suspect bony injury (e.g., a fall or direct blow) and no evidence of systemic disease that would make bony disease likely (e.g., osteoporosis, metastatic carcinoma, multiple myeloma). On physical examination, there may be spasm in the paraspinous muscles (i.e., contraction that does not relax, even when the patient is supine or when the opposing muscle groups contract, as with walking in place), but there is no point tenderness over the spinous processes of lumbar vertebrae and no nerve root signs, such as pain or paresthesia in dermatomes below the knee (especially with straight-leg raising), no foot weakness, and no loss of the ankle jerk. There may be point tenderness to firm palpation or percussion over the sacroiliac joint (SIJ), especially if the patient complains of pain toward that side of the lower back.

What to Do

⊘ **Perform a complete history and physical examination of the abdomen, back, and legs, looking for alternative causes for the back pain.** Pay special attention to **red flags,** such as a history of significant trauma, cancer, weight loss, fever, night sweats, injection drug use, compromised immunity, recumbent night pain, severe and unremitting pain, urinary retention or incontinence, saddle anesthesia, and severe or rapidly progressing neurologic deficit. **Red flags** on physical examination include elderly patients, fever, spinous point tenderness to percussion, abdominal tenderness or mass, and lower extremity motor weakness.

⊘ **Radiographs are generally not required but** consider obtaining plain radiographs of the lumbosacral spine on patients who have suffered injury that is sufficient to cause bony injury. Mild trauma in patients who are older than 50 years, patients younger than 20 years of age with nontraumatic pain, or patients older than 50 years of age who have had pain for more than 1 month warrant radiographs. Radiographs should also be ordered for patients who are on long-term corticosteroid medication, patients with a history of osteoporosis or cancer, and patients who are older than 70 years of age. **A negative radiograph does not rule out disease.**

⊘ **Laboratory investigation is generally not indicated,** but order a complete blood count (CBC) and an erythrocyte sedimentation rate (ESR) on patients with a history of immune deficiency, cancer or intravenous (IV) drug abuse, or signs or symptoms of underlying systemic disease (e.g., unexplained weight loss, fatigue, night sweats, fever, lymphadenopathy, and back pain at night or that is unrelieved by bed rest) or children who are limping, refuse to walk, or bend forward.

✓ **Bone scans, computed tomography (CT) scans, or magnetic resonance imaging (MRI)** may be better than plain radiographs in these patients. Consider diagnoses such as multiple myeloma, vertebral osteomyelitis, spinal tumor, discitis, or spinal subdural abscess.

✓ **Consider abdominal or retroperitoneal pathology** such as renal colic or abdominal aortic aneurysm in **sudden onset severe pain.** If these are suspected a trained provider can utilize **rapid bedside ultrasound** to help evaluate for an abdominal aneurysm or hydronephrosis. An abnormal ultrasound or high index of clinical suspicion may prompt further imaging with a CT scan.

✓ **Consider disc herniation when leg pain overshadows the back pain.** Back pain may subside as leg pain worsens. This pain tends to worsen with coughing, Valsalva maneuver, trunk flexion, and prolonged sitting or standing. Look for weakness of ankle or great-toe dorsiflexion **(drooping of the big toe and inability to heel walk).** Also look for decreased sensation to pinprick over the medial dorsal foot when there is **compression of the fifth lumbar nerve root. Alternatively,** look for weak plantar flexion **(inability to toe walk),** diminished ankle reflex, and paresthesias or decreased sensation to pinprick of the lateral or plantar aspect of the foot when there is **first sacral root compression (L_5 and S_1 radiculopathy account for about 90–95% of all lumbar radiculopathies).** Raise each leg 30 to 60 degrees of elevation from the horizontal (straight leg raise [SLR] test) and consider the test positive for nerve root compression if it produces pain down the leg below the knee along a nerve root distribution, rather than pain in the back. This leg pain is increased by dorsiflexion of the foot and relieved by plantar flexion. Pain generated at less than 30 degrees and greater than 70 degrees is nonspecific. Ipsilateral straight leg raising is a moderately sensitive (but not specific) test. A herniated intervertebral disc is more strongly indicated when **contralateral radicular pain** is reproduced in one leg by raising the opposite leg.

✓ **If nerve root compression is suspected, prescribe short-term bed rest and nonsteroidal anti-inflammatory drugs (NSAIDs) if tolerated. Arrange for general medical, orthopedic, or neurosurgical referral.** Although controversial, some consultants recommend short-term corticosteroid treatment, such as prednisone, 50 mg once a day for 5 days. It should be noted that the 2007 joint guidelines of the American College of Physicians and the American Pain Society recommend against using systemic steroids because of a lack of proven benefit.

✓ The patient should try at least 4 to 6 weeks of conservative treatment before submitting to an operation on the herniated disc. **Surgical treatment should be routinely avoided for patients with disc herniation and radiating pain in the absence of neurologic findings. Eighty percent of patients with sciatica recover with or without surgery. The presence of significant weakness in a myotome is perhaps the most important factor in the decision to perform a relatively early surgical procedure. If the weakness is profound or rapidly progressive, delaying surgery increases the risk for permanent deficit. The rare cauda equina syndrome is the only complication of lumbar disc herniation that calls for emergent surgical referral.** It occurs when a massive extrusion of disc nucleus compresses the caudal sac containing lumbar and sacral nerve roots. Bilateral radicular leg pain or weakness, bladder or bowel dysfunction, perineal or perianal anesthesia, decreased rectal sphincter tone in 60% to 80% of cases, and urinary retention in 90% of cases are common findings. An emergent MRI is the study of choice for confirming this diagnosis.

☑ **For patients who have nonspecific pain that can be treated in an outpatient setting, prescribe a short course of anti-inflammatory analgesics (ibuprofen, naproxen) for patients who do not have any contraindications for using them.** Because gastric bleeding and renal insufficiency are common with long-term use of NSAIDs, consider substituting acetaminophen (Tylenol), 1000 mg every 4–6 hours (maximum four doses daily), especially in the older patient. (Give half this dose if the patient takes greater than or equal to three alcoholic drinks per day). Although their efficacy is questionable, there is little downside to placing a lidocaine patch on the patient's low back for increased analgesia. Furthermore, given the side effects, the addition of a muscle relaxant such as cyclobenzaprine or an opiate pain medication such as oxycodone is not routinely recommended. In addition, recent clinical trials have demonstrated little or no benefit of these drugs when added to the NSAIDs.

☑ **Recommend hot or cold packs** (whichever the patient chooses) or alternate both hot and cold. Although not scientifically supported, these packs can often be comforting.

☑ At times sacroiliac dysfunction **can cause incapacitating spasms of pain that are precipitated by minor movements or attempts to sit up. The patient will usually be able to localize the pain to the right or left side of the sacrum. Firmly palpating the dimple (sacral sulcus) with your thumb and eliciting pain may be the most reliable indication of SIJ pain.** When the pain is significant **and there are no neurologic findings to suggest nerve root compression or any red flags of underlying systemic disease, it can be quite rewarding to provide an intraarticular injection of a local anesthetic mixed with a corticosteroid. When there is improvement of pain, it is both diagnostic and therapeutic. Draw up 10 mL of 0.25% bupivacaine (Marcaine) mixed with 1 mL (40 mg) of methylprednisolone (Depo-Medrol) or 1 to 2 mL (6–12 mg) of betamethasone (Celestone Soluspan). Using a 1.25-inch needle (22 gauge) and sterile technique, inject deeply into the sacroiliac joint at the point of maximal tenderness or into the sacral sulcus immediately lateral to the sacrum** (Fig. 117.1) (See Video 117.1). When the needle is in the joint, the needle should advance freely up to its hub without meeting resistance or bony obstruction. There should be a free flow of medication from the syringe without causing soft tissue swelling. If the needle meets any obstruction, reposition it with slight angulation of the needle tip out laterally until the needle advances easily. During the injection, fan upward into the superior

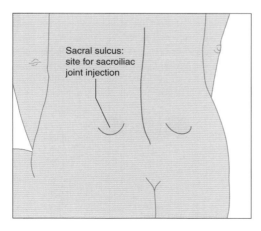

Fig. 117.1 The dimple on either side of the sacrum (sacral sulcus) can serve as a landmark for injecting a painful sacroiliac joint.

501

fibrous tissue of the SIJ. The patient may feel a brief increase of pain, followed by dramatic relief in 5 to 20 minutes that is usually persistent. Pain is often relieved by 50% to 80%. Warn the patient that there may be a flare in pain when the anesthetic component wears off. This could last for 24 to 48 hours. If the patient gets relief initially, any persistent symptoms should subside over the next 5 to 10 days. This should be performed in instances of acute pain or an acute flare-up of chronic recurrent sacroiliac pain. **Sacroiliac or SIJ belts can be used to provide compression and, in some patients, stabilization and pain relief for SIJ dysfunction (samples can be found on the Internet). The belt should be secured posteriorly across the sacral base and anteriorly, inferior to the anterior superior iliac spines** (Fig. 117.2). This belt may be most helpful during walking and standing activities, but for some patients with significant pain and weakness, wearing it during sedentary activities may also be helpful in reducing symptoms.

✅ **For point tenderness of the lumbosacral muscles, substantial pain relief may also be obtained by injecting 10 to 20 mL of 0.25% to 0.5% bupivacaine (Marcaine) deeply into the points of maximal tenderness** of the erector spinae and quadratus lumborum muscles, using a 1.25-inch needle (25–27 gauge). Quickly puncture the skin, drive the needle into the muscle belly, and inject the anesthetic, slowly advancing and withdrawing the needle and fanning out the medication in all directions. Often one fan block can reduce symptoms by 95% after injection and yield a 75% permanent reduction of painful spasms. Following injection, teach stretching exercises.

✅ **For severe pain that cannot be relieved by injections of local anesthetic,** it may be necessary to provide the patient with 1 to 2 days of bed rest, although most patients with acute low back pain recover more rapidly by continuing ordinary activities (within the limits permitted

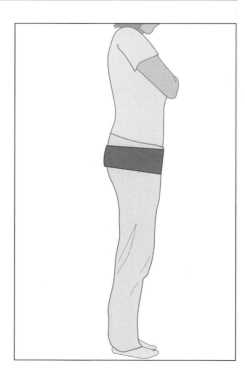

Fig. 117.2 Sacroiliac joint (SIJ) belt.

by their pain) than with bed rest or back-mobilizing exercises. Some patients with intractable excruciating pain (especially the elderly) require hospitalization.

✅ **Refer patients with uncomplicated back pain to their primary care provider for follow-up care in 3 to 7 days.** Reassure patients that back pain is seldom disabling and that it usually resolves rapidly with return to normal activity. Tell patients that the pain may be recurrent, and that cigarette smoking, sedentary activity, and obesity are risk factors for back pain. Teach them to avoid twisting and bending when lifting and show them how to lift with the back vertical, using thigh muscles while holding heavy objects close to the chest to avoid reinjury. **Encourage them to return to work or resume normal activities as soon as possible, with neither bed rest nor exercise in the acute phase, and to participate in an aerobic exercise program when the pain has subsided.** Heavy lifting, trunk twisting, and bodily vibration should be avoided in the acute phase.

What Not to Do

❌ Do not be too eager to use antispasm (muscle relaxant) medicines. Many have sedative or anticholinergic side effects.

❌ Do not apply lumbar traction. It has not been proven to be any better than a placebo for relieving back pain. Do not provide lumbar orthotics, back braces, or lumbar cushions. They have no proven benefit. Lumbar supports have not been proven to reduce the incidence of low back pain in industrial workers and should not be routinely recommended for the prevention of low back pain.

❌ Do not recommend bed rest for more than 2 days and only recommend it when the pain is severe. Bed rest does not increase the speed of recovery from acute low back pain and sometimes delays recovery.

Discussion

Low back pain affects men and women equally, with onset most often between the ages of 30 and 50 years. It is the most common and expensive cause of work-related disability in people who are younger than 45 years of age. A definitive diagnosis for **nonradiating low back pain** cannot be established in 85% of patients because of the weak associations between symptoms, pathologic changes, and imaging results. It can be generally assumed that much of this pain is secondary to musculoligamentous injury, degenerative changes in the spine, or a combination of the two. The approach discussed here is geared only to the management of acute injuries and flare-ups, from which most people recover on their own, which leaves only about 10% developing chronic problems. **With acute pain,** reassurance plus limited medication may be the most useful intervention. The 90% of back pain patients that become pain free are pain free within 3

months, and more than 90% of those patients recover spontaneously within 4 weeks. Even with discogenic back pain or disc herniation with **radicular pain,** there are convincing data to support the nonoperative treatment of these patients in the absence of cauda equine syndrome or progressive neurologic deficit.

History and physical examination are essential to rule out serious pathologic conditions that can present as low back pain but require quite different treatment—aortic aneurysm, pyelonephritis, pancreatitis, abdominal tumors, pelvic inflammatory disease, ectopic pregnancy, and retroperitoneal or epidural abscess.

Older patients who experience radicular symptoms may have **spinal stenosis,** which may be accompanied by **neurogenic claudication,** a

(continued)

Discussion continued

syndrome in which pain radiates down the legs, particularly when walking, and is often relieved by rest. This can be distinguished from vascular claudication because the pain of neurogenic claudication starts even while the patient stands still. The pain is worsened by extension of the spine, which occurs with standing or walking, and improves with flexion, such as sitting or leaning forward.

The standard five-view radiograph study of the lumbosacral spine may entail 500 mrem of radiation, and yet only 1 in 2500 lumbar spine plain films of adults below 50 years of age shows an unexpected abnormality. In fact, many radiographic anomalies, such as spina bifida occulta, single-disc narrowing, spondylosis, facet joint abnormalities, and several congenital anomalies, are equally common in symptomatic and asymptomatic individuals. **It is estimated that the gonadal dose of radiation absorbed from a five-view lumbosacral series is equivalent to that from 6 years of daily anteroposterior (AP) and lateral chest films.** The World Health Organization now recommends that oblique views be reserved for problems remaining after review of AP and lateral films. For simple cases of low back pain, even with radicular findings, both CT scans and MRI are overly sensitive and often reveal anatomic abnormalities that have no clinical significance. In one study of MRI scans, only 36% of asymptomatic patients had normal discs at all levels, whereas 64% had demonstrable disease (52% with at least one bulging disc, 27% with disc protrusion, and 1% with frank herniation). CT and MRI should be reserved for patients for whom there is a strong clinical suggestion of underlying infection, cancer, or persistent neurologic deficit. Both of these tests have similar accuracy in detecting herniated discs and spinal stenosis, but MRI is more sensitive for infections, metastatic cancer, and rare neural tumors.

Although adults are more apt to have disc abnormalities, muscle strain, and degenerative changes associated with low back pain, **athletically active adolescents** are more likely to have **posterior element derangements,** such as stress fractures of the pars interarticularis. Early recognition of this spondylolysis and treatment by bracing and

limitation of activity may prevent nonunion, persistent pain, and disability.

Although the true prevalence of posterior pelvic pain is unknown, researchers estimate that 15% to 30% of patients with low back pain have **SIJ dysfunction.** Radiation of pain down one or both legs may occur, but usually not below the knee or accompanied by positive straight-leg raising or neurologic deficit. Imaging is often not helpful. Radiographs, MRI, bone scan, and CT scans do not differentiate symptomatic from asymptomatic patients. Often SIJ pain presents as a progressive problem with fluctuations in symptoms. There is no gold standard for treatment. The recommendations noted earlier are dependent on the clinician's experience and skills.

Malingering and drug seeking are major psychological components to consider in patients who have frequent visits for back pain and whose responses seem overly dramatic or otherwise inappropriate. These patients may move around with little difficulty when they do not know they are being observed. They may complain of generalized superficial tenderness when you lightly pinch the skin over the affected lumbar area. When straight-leg raising is equivocally positive after testing the patient in a supine position, use distraction and reexamine the patient in the sitting position to see if the initial findings are reproduced. If there is suspicion that the patient's pain is psychosomatic or nonorganic, use the axial loading test, in which the head of the standing person is gently pressed down on. This should not cause significant musculoskeletal back pain. The rotation test can also be performed, in which the patient stands with arms at the sides. Hold the patient's wrists next to the hips and turn the patient's body from side to side, passively rotating the shoulders, trunk, and pelvis as a unit. This maneuver creates the illusion that the spinal rotation is being tested, but in fact the spinal axis has not been altered, and any complaint of back pain should be suspect.

Another technique that is easier to perform is the heel tap test. With the patient supine and with the hips and knees flexed to 90 degrees, suggest to the patient that the next test may cause low back pain, and then lightly tap the patient's heel with the base of your hand. A complaint of sudden low back pain is most likely an indication of malingering.

Suggested Readings

Anderson, G. B. J., Lucente, T., Davis, A. M., et al. (1999). A comparison of osteopathic spinal manipulation with standard care for patients with low back pain. *New England Journal of Medicine*, *341*, 1426–1431.

Baker, R. J., & Patel, D. (2005). Lower back pain in the athlete: Common conditions and treatment. *Primary Care*, *32*, 201–229.

Carey, T. S., Garrett, J., Jackman, A., et al. (1995). The outcomes and costs of care for acute low back pain among patients seen by primary care practitioners, chiropractors and orthopedic surgeons. *New England Journal of Medicine*, *333*, 913–917.

Devereaux, M. W. (2004). Low back pain. *Primary Care*, *31*, 33–51.

Deyo, R. A., Diehl, A. K., & Rosenthal, M. (1986). How many days of bed rest for acute low back pain? *New England Journal of Medicine*, *315*, 1064–1070.

Deyo, R. A., Rainville, J., & Kent, D. L. (1992). What can the history and physical examination tell us about low back pain? *Journal of the American Medical Association*, *268*, 760–765.

Deyo, R. A., & Weinstein, J. N. (2001). Low back pain. *New England Journal of Medicine*, *344*, 363–370.

Elam, K. C., Cherkin, D. C., & Deyo, R. A. (1995). How emergency physicians approach low back pain: Choosing costly options. *Journal of Emergency Medicine*, *13*, 143–150.

Friedman, B. W., Dym, A. A., Davitt, M., et al. (2015). Naproxen with cyclobenzaprine, oxycodone/acetaminophen, or placebo for treating acute low back pain: A randomized clinical trial. *Journal of the American Medical Association*, *314*, 1572–1580.

Frost, H., et al. (2004). Randomised controlled trial of physiotherapy compared with advice for low back pain. *BMJ*, *329*, 708.

Gross, L. (1998). Metaxalone. *Journal of Neurological and Orthopedic Medicine and Surgery*, *18*, 76–79.

Harwood, M. I., & Smith, B. J. (2005). Low back pain: A primary care approach. *Clinics in Family Practice*, *7*, 279–303.

Hurwitz, E. L., Morgenstern, H., Harber, P., et al. (2002). The effectiveness of physical modalities among patients with low back pain randomized to chiropractic care. *Journal of Manipulative and Physiological Therapeutics*, *25*, 10–20.

Jarvik, J. G., Hollingworth, W., Martin, B., et al. (2003). Rapid magnetic resonance imaging vs radiographs for patients with low back pain. *Journal of the American Medical Association*, *289*, 2810–2818.

Malmivaara, A., Hakkinen, U., Aro, T., et al. (1995). The treatment of acute low back pain: Bed rest, exercise, or ordinary activity? *New England Journal of Medicine*, *332*, 351–355.

Miller, P., Kendrick, D., Bentley, E., et al. (2002). Cost-effectiveness of lumbar spine radiography in primary care patients with low back pain. *Spine*, *27*, 2291–2297.

Prather, H., & Hunt, D. (2004). Sacroiliac joint pain. *Disease-a-Month*, *50*, 670–683.

Small, S. A., Perron, A. D., & Brady, W. J. (2005). Orthopedic pitfalls: Cauda equina syndrome. *American Journal of Emergency Medicine*, *23*, 159–163.

Smeal, W. L., Tyburski, M., & Alleva, J. (2004). Discogenic/radicular pain. *Disease-a-Month*, *50*, 636–669.

Suarez-Almazor, M. E., Belseck, E., Russell, A. S., et al. (1997). Use of lumbar radiographs for the early diagnosis of low back pain: Proposed guidelines would increase utilization. *Journal of the American Medical Association*, *277*, 1782–1786.

van Poppel, M. N., Koes, B. W., van der Ploeg, T., et al. (1998). Lumbar supports and education for the prevention of low back pain in industry: A randomized controlled trial. *Journal of the American Medical Association*, *279*, 1789–1794 editorial 1826–1827.

van Tulder, M. W., Assendelft, W. J., Koes, B. W., et al. (1997). Spinal radiographic findings and nonspecific low back pain. A systematic review of observational studies. *Spine*, *22*, 427–434.

van Tulder, M. W., Koes, B. W., & Bouter, L. M. (1997). Conservative treatment of acute and chronic nonspecific low back pain. A systematic review of randomized controlled trials of the most common interventions. *Spine, 22,* 2128–2156.

van Tulder, M. W., Koes, B. W., Bouter, L. M., et al. (1997). Management of chronic nonspecific low back pain in primary care: A descriptive study. *Spine, 22,* 76–82.

Wassell, J. T., Gardner, L. I., Landsittel, D. P., et al. (2000). A prospective study of back belts for prevention of back pain and injury. *Journal of the American Medical Association, 284,* 2727–2732.

Monoarticular Arthritis, Acute

Presentation

The patient complains of one joint that has become acutely red, swollen, hot, painful, and stiff, with pain on minimal range of motion (ROM). Rapid onset with fever and local warmth suggests the possibility of septic arthritis. A prominent monarticular synovitis with comparatively little pain, but where the joint is warm with a large effusion, especially of the knee, is typical of Lyme disease. A migratory tendonitis or arthritis often precedes gonococcal monarthritis. A history of similar attacks, especially of the first metatarsophalangeal joint, suggests the possibility of gouty arthritis. A history of recurrent knee swelling with minimal erythema and gradual onset after overuse or minor trauma is more likely associated with osteoarthritis and pseudogout.

A child between the ages of 3 and 10 years who presents with a limp or inability to walk may have a transient synovitis of the hip or a more serious septic arthritis.

What to Do

✅ **Ask about previous, similar episodes in this or other joints, as well as trauma, systemic illness, fever, tick bites (Lyme arthritis), sexual risk factors, intravenous (IV) drug use, skin infections, or rashes, and ask about any history of gout** (see Chapter 112). Additional clues that might point toward an infectious etiology would be immunosuppression (e.g., human immunodeficiency virus, diabetes, chemotherapy or radiation) and an exotic travel history.

✅ **Determine the rapidity of onset and the duration of symptoms.** Remember that although **a high-grade fever is especially concerning,** the elderly or immunocompromised patient may fail to mount a fever in the face of infection. General malaise and rash can be associated with infection.

✅ **Perform a thorough and complete physical exam** that may reveal findings that are consistent with a specific etiology of the joint pathology as listed above. Obtain cervical, anal, oral, or urethral swabs for culture and Gram stain or deoxyribonucleic acid (DNA) probe when you suspect gonococcal arthritis. Cultures of synovial fluid are positive in no more than 50% of these patients. Mucosal cultures are positive in 80% of cases.

✅ **Examine the affected joint and document the extent of effusion, involvement of adjacent structures, and degree of erythema, tenderness, heat, and limitation of ROM.** True intraarticular problems cause restriction of active and passive ROM, whereas periarticular problems (e.g., prepatellar bursitis, olecranon bursitis), which may mimic joint inflammation, restrict active ROM more than passive ROM. **Maximum pain at the limit of joint motion is characteristic of true arthritis.**

✅ **Intraarticular fluid accumulation** can often be detected by pressing on one side of the affected joint and, at the same time, palpating a wavelike fluctuance on the opposite side of the joint. In the knee, when the medial or lateral compartment is stroked, the fluid moves into the opposite compartment, resulting in a visible bulge. To detect effusion in the elbow joint, the triangular recess in the lateral aspect of the elbow, between the lateral epicondyle, radial head, and the olecranon process, should be palpated. To detect effusion in the ankle, the joint should be palpated anteriorly. **Diagnostic ultrasound will usually be the most accurate method of determining whether a joint effusion is present.**

✅ **Although not always necessary, send a blood sample for complete blood count (CBC), erythrocyte sedimentation rate (ESR), and C-reactive protein (CRP), which may support a suspicion of an inflammatory or infectious process. When sepsis is suspected, obtain blood cultures.** Blood cultures are positive in about 50% of nongonococcal infections but are rarely positive (about 10%) in gonococcal infection. Serum uric acid measurement is not always helpful and may be misleading when considering the diagnosis of gout. **Lyme antibodies** may be appropriate if there are epidemiologic risk factors. The majority of patients with confirmed Lyme in Lyme-endemic areas do not recall a tick bite, as such Lyme studies should be sent in endemic regions. Lyme arthritis has positive two-tier serologic tests for *Borrelia burgdorferi* infection.

✅ **Consider obtaining radiographs of the affected joint** to detect possible unsuspected fractures or evidence of chronic disease, such as rheumatoid arthritis. The finding of crystal-induced chondrocalcinosis could support but not confirm the diagnosis of pseudogout arthritis or osteoarthritis. Occasionally, osteomyelitis or malignancy may be detected. **In most cases, radiographs are not helpful** in the diagnosis of the acute, nontraumatic, swollen, and painful joint, and they are not always a requirement during the initial evaluation.

✅ **Often, the first and most important step in diagnosing a patient with monarticular arthritis is arthrocentesis.** It is a safe and simple procedure that may be indicated in the presence of a joint effusion for either diagnostic or therapeutic purposes.

✅ **Perform an arthrocentesis to remove joint fluid for analysis, to relieve pain, and, in the case of septic or crystal-induced arthritis, to reduce the bacterial and crystal load within the joint.** Identify the joint line to be entered, and make a pressure mark on the overlying skin with the closed end of a retractable pen to serve as a target. Then, using sterile technique throughout, cleanse the skin over the most superficial area of the joint effusion with alcohol and povidone-iodine (Betadine); anesthetize the skin with 1-3 mL of 1% plain buffered lidocaine; and aspirate as much joint fluid as possible through a needle (16 to 18 gauge; smaller needle in small joints). **The joint space of the knee** (Fig. 118.1A) may be entered medially or laterally with the leg fully extended and the patient lying supine. Hold the needle parallel to the bed surface, then direct it just posterior to the patella into the subpatellar space. **The elbow joint** (see Fig. 118.1B) is best entered at about 30 degrees of flexion, with the needle introduced proximal to the olecranon process of the ulna and just below the lateral epicondyle. Advance the needle medially into the joint space. The best site for needle entry of **the wrist** is on the dorsal radial aspect at the proximal end of the anatomic snuff box and the distal articulation of the radius. Place the wrist in about 20 degrees of flexion and introduce the needle perpendicular to the skin, advancing it toward the ulna into the joint space (see Fig. 118.1C). **The ankle joint** (see Fig. 118.1D) may be entered with the patient supine, the knee extended, and the foot plantarflexed. Find the small depression

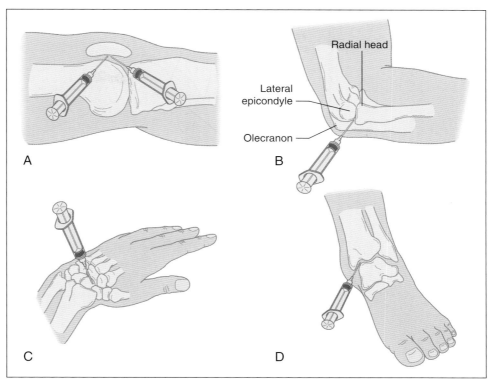

Fig. 118.1 Entry sites for arthrocentesis. **(A, D)** Illustrations provided by Dr. D. H. Neustadt. **(B, C)** (Adapted from Akins, C. M. [1988]. Aspiration and injection of joints, bursae and tendons. In T. J. Vander Salm, B. S. Cutler, & H. Brownell Wheeler [Eds.], *Atlas of bedside procedures* [2nd ed.]. Boston, MA: Little Brown & Co.)

that is just medial to the extensor hallucis longus and tibialis anterior tendons, inferior to the distal tibia, then direct your needle into the tibiotalar articulation. **For small joints,** enter the midline on the dorsolateral aspect and advance a small needle into the joint space. **Joints of the digits** may have to be distracted by pulling on the end to enlarge the joint space.

If the provider is trained, point of care ultrasound can be a useful tool in identifying landmarks for arthrocentesis. In addition, fluoroscopy may be valuable in guiding needle placement **for hip or shoulder joint aspiration. For the lateral approach to the shoulder joint,** the patient should be seated upright with the affected arm hanging by the side. Identify the acromion process of the scapula, then locate the groove just inferior to the lateral aspect of the acromion process. This groove lies between the acromion process and the greater tubercle of the humerus. Insert the needle into the midpoint of the groove, directing it medially and slightly posteriorly. The needle must be inserted at least 2.5 to 3 cm to ensure insertion into the joint capsule (Fig. 118.2).

⊘ **Grossly examine the joint aspirate.** Clear, light-yellow fluid is characteristic of osteoarthritis or mild inflammatory or traumatic effusions. Grossly cloudy fluid is characteristic of more severe inflammation or bacterial infection. Blood in the joint is characteristic of trauma (a fracture or tear inside the synovial capsule) or bleeding from hemophilia or anticoagulants.

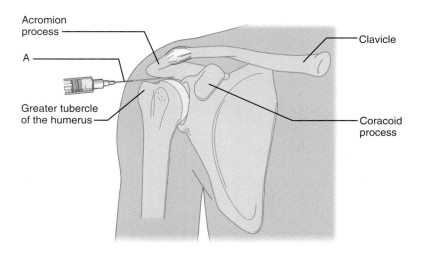

Fig. 118.2 Shoulder joint arthrocentesis. (A) Lateral approach.

A traumatic tap may cause the serous joint fluid to become bloody during aspiration and is not indicative of a previous hemarthrosis. This procedure can be performed safely in patients who are taking warfarin (Coumadin) or an equivalent blood-thinning medication.

✅ **One drop of joint fluid may be used for a crude string or mucin clot test.** Wet the tips of two gloved fingers with joint fluid, repeatedly touch them together, and slowly draw them apart. As this maneuver is repeated 10 or 20 times, and the joint fluid dries, normal synovial fluid will form longer and longer strings, usually to 5 to 10 cm in length. Inflammation inhibits this string formation. This is a nonspecific test but may aid decision making at the bedside.

✅ **If microscopic examinations are delayed,** a tube with ethylenediaminetetraacetic acid should be used for anticoagulation, because anticoagulants (e.g., oxalate, lithium heparin) used in other tubes can confound crystal analysis.

✅ **The most important laboratory tests on joint fluid consist of a Gram stain and culture for possible septic arthritis.** Gram-positive bacteria can be seen in 80% of culture-positive synovial fluid, but gram-negative bacteria are seen less often; gram-negative diplococci are seen rarely. Polymerase chain reaction techniques can detect gonococcal DNA in the synovial fluid of some culture-negative cases of suspected gonococcal arthritis, but this test is not presently considered a standard evaluation.

✅ **A joint fluid total and differential leukocyte count is the next most useful test to order.**

✅ It is important to note that patients may have septic arthritis with any synovial white blood cell (WBC) count; however, the likelihood of septic arthritis increases as the synovial WBC count increases. A comprehensive review from 2007 demonstrated that a synovial WBC count >25,000 had a positive likelihood ratio of 3, a synovial WBC count >50,000 had a positive likelihood ratio of 7, and a synovial WBC count >100,000 had a positive likelihood ratio of 28. Conversely, a synovial WBC count <25,000 had a negative likelihood ratio of 0.3.

✓ **Send a wet preparation to look for crystals.** Identification of crystals can establish a diagnosis of gout or pseudogout and avoid unnecessary hospitalization for suspected infectious arthritis.

✓ **If there is any suspicion of a bacterial infection (based on predisposing factors, fever, elevated ESR, cellulitis, lymphangitis, or the joint fluid results), always treat empirically and start the patient on appropriate IV antibiotics based on results of the Gram stain or the presumptive organism. If the patient does not have a causative organism identified and will be going to the operating room for an operative washout, delaying antibiotics to obtain an intraoperative culture is a reasonable approach if the patient is clinically stable. In older patients,** who are not at risk for sexually transmitted diseases (STDs), antibiotic coverage should be aimed at *Staphylococcus aureus*. Use vancomycin, along with cefotaxime, for uncomplicated infections, or alternatively, use vancomycin with either ceftriaxone, ciprofloxacin, or levofloxacin. **For patients with suspected gonococcus,** use ceftriaxone or cefotaxime. If Gram stain shows gram-positive cocci in clusters, add vancomycin. Provide *Chlamydia* treatment with azithromycin or doxycycline. **For children older than 5 years of age,** prescribe nafcillin or oxacillin, plus ceftriaxone. Consider vancomycin in children with risk factors for methicillin-resistant *S. aureus* (MRSA). **For all patients receiving antibiotics for septic arthritis, the choice of drug and dosage should be coordinated with an Infectious Disease specialist, orthopedist, and/or a clinical pharmacist.**

✓ **Inflammatory arthritis may be treated with nonsteroidal anti-inflammatory drugs (NSAIDs) (unless contraindicated), beginning with a loading dose, such as indomethacin or ibuprofen, tapered to usual maintenance doses.**

✓ **If infection can be confidently excluded from the diagnosis, intraarticular injections of corticosteroids can be a useful adjunctive or alternative therapy.** Using aseptic technique, prepare the skin with povidone-iodine and alcohol. Using the techniques described earlier, with a syringe (3–5 mL) and a needle (1.25 inch, 27 gauge), inject 1 to 2 mL of 40 mg/mL methylprednisolone with 2 to 8 mL of bupivacaine, 0.25% to 0.5%, into the affected joint. For finger or toe joints, use a smaller volume (0.2–0.5 mL) of the more concentrated (80 mg/mL) methylprednisolone, along with a lesser volume of bupivacaine. Alternatively, triamcinolone hexacetonide, 20 to 40 mg/injection, may be used. Warn patients of the 10% to 15% risk for postinjection flare or recurrent pain for
24 to 48 hours after the local anesthetic wears off.

✓ **When joint fluid cannot be obtained to rule out infection, it may be a good tactic to treat simultaneously for infectious and inflammatory arthritis (excluding steroid use).**

✓ **Splint and elevate the affected joint and arrange for admission or follow-up.**

✓ **Children complaining of acute hip pain** must be evaluated for the possibility of a septic arthritis versus a transient synovitis. Similar symptoms are present in these two diseases at the early stages, and differential diagnosis is difficult. To help differentiate between these two diseases, **obtain a CBC, ESR, CRP, and hip radiograph.**

✓ **Five reportedly independent predictors of septic arthritis are a temperature >37° C (>98.6° F), an ESR >20 mm/h, a CRP >1.0 mg/dL, a WBC count >11,000/mm^3, and a radiographic joint space difference between the affected and unaffected hips >2 mm.** The likelihood of septic arthritis is 0.1% if none of the predictors is present, between 3% and 23% with two variables present, 24% to 77% with three, 82% to 97% with four, and 99.1% if all five predictors are present.

✓ **An ultrasound of the hip, either comprehensive or performed at the bedside, can help identify if an effusion is present, which can help guide further management. It should be noted that both transient synovitis and septic arthritis can produce a joint effusion.**

✓ **It may be reasonable to obtain a magnetic resonance image (MRI) or fluoroscopically directed joint aspiration in those children with three or four of these predictors.**

✓ **When there is a low index of suspicion for a septic hip** and there are no contraindications to NSAID use, place the child on ibuprofen, 10 mg/kg three times a day for 5 days. In a small study, this was shown to shorten the duration of symptoms of transient synovitis by 2 days.

What Not to Do

✗ Do not tap a joint through an area of obvious contamination, such as subcutaneous cellulitis. Synovial fluid may consequently be inoculated with bacteria. This is considered a relative contraindication to arthrocentesis.

✗ Do not send synovial fluid for chemistries, proteins, rheumatoid factor, or uric acid because the results may be misleading. Synovial fluid glucose is not discriminatory for joint sepsis.

✗ Do not be misled by bursitis, tenosynovitis, or myositis without joint involvement. An infected or inflamed joint will have a reactive effusion, which may be evident as fullness, fluctuance, reduced ROM, or joint fluid that can be drawn off with a needle. It is usually difficult to tap a joint in the absence of a joint effusion.

✗ Do not treat hyperuricemia with drugs that lower uric acid levels, such as allopurinol or probenecid, during an acute attack of gout (see Chapter 112).

✗ Do not inject corticosteroids into a joint until infection has been ruled out.

✗ Do not use NSAIDs when a patient has a history of active peptic ulcer disease with bleeding. Relative contraindications include renal insufficiency, volume depletion, gastritis, inflammatory bowel disease, asthma, hypertension, and congestive heart disease.

✗ Do not start maintenance NSAID doses for an acute inflammation. It will take 1 day or more to reach therapeutic levels and pain relief. When tolerated, always start with a loading dose.

Discussion

Monoarticular joint disease (especially monoarthritis) should be regarded as infectious until proven otherwise. Infectious arthritis requires prompt treatment to prevent joint destruction and spread of infection.

It should be kept in mind, however, that any polyarticular disease, such as rheumatoid arthritis or systemic lupus erythematosus, can initially present in a single joint and later be revealed to occur in other joints.

The acute, swollen/painful joint is most commonly caused by trauma, infection, or crystal-related disease. Trauma is the most common cause, followed by infection. Gout is the most common crystal-associated arthropathy.

Most acute bacterial arthritis is monoarthritis, but polyarticular infectious arthritis occurs in approximately 12% to 20% of cases. The infectious cause varies according to patient factors, particularly age and sexual activity. *Staphylococcus aureus* is cited as the most common cause of infectious monoarthritis in adults. *Neisseria gonorrhoeae* is the most common cause of acute monoarthritis in young, sexually active adults. It is three to four times more common in women than in men. Neonates and children are at higher risk for group B streptococcus, *S. aureus, Escherichia coli,* and other gram-negative organisms. A few other unique but unusual causes of septic arthritis include infection with *Mycobacterium marinum* in people who clean fish tanks, *Pasteurella multocida* with a cat bite, ingestions of unpasteurized dairy products with *Brucella* species, and *Pseudomonas aeruginosa* or *S. aureus* with IV drug use.

Risk factors for septic joint include skin infection, prosthetic joint, joint surgery, rheumatoid arthritis, age older than 80 years, and diabetes. Also, IV drug abuse allows organisms to access joints, such as the sternoclavicular joint, which is uncommonly thought of in infectious arthritis.

Gout and pseudogout can present with abrupt onset of pain and effusion, raising suspicion of infection. When the history reveals long-standing symptoms in a joint, with exacerbations of preexisting disease (e.g., gout, worsening of osteoarthritis with excessive use), this still should be differentiated from a new superimposed infection.

In patients with rheumatoid arthritis, pain in one joint out of proportion to pain in other joints always suggests infection.

Intraarticular trauma is more likely than extraarticular trauma to present as acute monarthritis; fracture,

meniscal tears, and other internal derangements (e.g., ligament tears) are common forms of intraarticular trauma.

The history of trauma is a potential pitfall in the approach to the patient with acute monoarthritis. Although some patients with a traumatic cause may be unable to recall the event, others falsely and inadvertently attribute their joint pain to a relatively minor injury. Clinically, the physical examination of a patient with traumatic acute monoarthritis may be indistinguishable from crystal deposition and infectious disease. In fact, trauma can be the precipitant of crystal deposition and infection.

Lyme disease presents early with arthralgias and myalgias; however, Lyme arthritis is recognized later in the course of the infection (weeks to months after the initial infection) and typically presents with monoarticular (or occasionally oligoarticular) inflammatory arthritis, most commonly of the knee.

Plant thorn synovitis can be seen in gardeners who inadvertently impale a plant thorn into a joint, which can become inflamed with erythema and warmth. Plain radiographs are often normal, but MRI may help identify the foreign material. Surgical removal of the foreign material is recommended.

Synovial fluid aspiration is universally recommended in the patient with acute monarthritis. The urgent reason for tapping a joint effusion is to rule out a bacterial infection, which could destroy the joint cartilage in as little as 1 or 2 days. Beyond identifying an infection (with the Gram stain, culture, and WBC count), further diagnosis of the cause of arthritis is not particularly accurate, nor is early definitive diagnosis necessary to decide on specific acute treatment.

Reducing the volume of the effusion may alleviate pain and stiffness, but this effect may be short lived because the effusion may reaccumulate within hours.

Identification of crystals is essential for the diagnosis of gout or pseudogout, but one acute attack may be treated in the same manner as any other inflammatory arthritis. The workup for an exact diagnosis may therefore be deferred to follow-up after acute infection has been ruled out.

Infants and young children may present with fever and reluctance to walk from septic arthritis of the hip or knee, and arthrocentesis may require sedation or general anesthesia.

Acute arthritis in prosthetic joints is always of concern. Infections in prostheses are disastrous and require urgent consultation.

Suggested Readings

Arroll, B., & Goodyear-Smith, F. (2004). Corticosteroid injections for osteoarthritis of the knee. *BMJ*, *328*, 869.

Baker, D. G., & Schumacher, H. R. (1993). Acute monoarthritis. *New England Journal of Medicine*, *329*, 1013–1020.

Boss, S. E., Mehta, A., Maddow, C., & Luber, S. D. (2013). Critical orthopedic skills and procedures. *Emergency Medicine Clinics of North America*, *31*(1), 261–290.

Fagan, H. B. (2005). Approach to the patient with acute swollen/painful joint. *Clinics in Family Practice*, *7*, 305.

Jung, S. T., Rowe, S. M., Moon, E. S., et al. (2003). Significance of laboratory and radiologic findings for differentiating between septic arthritis and transient synovitis of the hip. *Journal of Pediatric Orthopedics*, *23*, 368–372.

Kermond, S., Fink, M., Graham, K., et al. (2002). A randomized clinical trial: Should the child with transient synovitis of the hip be treated with nonsteroidal anti-inflammatory drugs. *Annals of Emergency Medicine*, *40*, 294–299.

Li, S. F., Henderson, J., Dickman, E., et al. (2004). Laboratory tests in adults with monoarticular arthritis: Can they rule out a septic joint? *Academy of Emergency Medicine*, *11*, 276–280.

Margaretten, M. E., Kohlwes, J., Moore, D., & Bent, S. (2007). Does this adult patient have septic arthritis? *Journal of the American Medical Association*, *297*(13), 1478–1488.

Singh, N., & Vogelgesang, S. A. (2017). Monoarticular arthritis. *Medical Clinics of North America*, *101*(3), 607–613.

Siva, C., Velazquez, C., Mody, A., et al. (2003). Diagnosing acute monoarthritis in adults: A practical approach for the family physician. *American Family Physician*, *68*, 83–90.

Umberhandt, R., & Isaacs, J. (2012). Diagnostic considerations for monoarticular arthritis of the hand and wrist. *Journal of Hand Surgery*, *37*(7), 1480–1485.

Muscle Cramps

(Charley Horse)

Presentation

The patient complains of painful, visible, palpable muscle contractions, often affecting the gastrocnemius muscle or small muscles of the foot or hand. Ordinary cramps occur chiefly at rest during the night or after trivial movement but also can occur after forceful muscle contraction. Other muscle cramps are associated with exercise in the heat, occupations that cause overuse, pregnancy, hemodialysis, electrolyte disturbances, dehydration, and drug or alcohol use. Most cramps are transient in nature, but they are likely to recur after a severe episode. Following this, the muscles may be tender and painful for some time.

What to Do

⊘ **Look for a specific underlying cause.** Unaccustomed exercise and salt depletion from sweating are common precipitating causes (see Chapter 2). Drug-induced cramps can include those from alcohol, lithium, cimetidine, nifedipine, antipsychotic medications (see Chapter 1), clofibrate, and others. Hypothyroidism, hyperthyroidism, hyponatremia, hypokalemia, hyperkalemia, hypocalcemia, hypomagnesemia, and respiratory alkalosis (see Chapter 3) can all cause muscle cramping.

⊘ **Consider rhabdomyolysis if there are risk factors such as extreme exertion, severe dehydration, concomitant stimulant use such as cocaine or methamphetamine, or other signs, such as dark-colored urine. Consider sending a serum creatine kinase (CK).**

⊘ **Address any specific cause. Intravenous (IV) fluids with electrolyte replacement may help with heat cramps and alcohol-induced cramps.**

⊘ **Ordinary muscle cramps can be treated immediately with passive or active stretching or massage of the cramped muscle (dorsiflexing the foot for calf cramps).**

⊘ **Nocturnal leg cramps have historically been treated with quinine sulfate tablets.** Most studies show that quinine and its derivatives decrease the incidence, severity, and duration of night cramps. However, not all report favorable results, and their use has fallen out of favor. The US Food and Drug Administration (FDA) has warned against using quinine for non–FDA-approved symptoms of leg cramps and restless leg syndrome because of reports of serious hematologic reactions. **A glass of tonic water (a source of quinine) before bed is a less toxic alternative worth trying, although** there is little evidence to suggest that this is effective.

⊘ A small trial using **gabapentin (Neurontin)** showed it was effective in reducing the frequency and severity of muscle cramps and associated sleep disturbances (clinical outcome measures) within the first 2 weeks of medication at 600 mg/day. After 3 months of therapy (mean dosage, 892 ± 180 mg), cramps disappeared in 100% of patients; this benefit persisted as long as 6 months.

The authors concluded that **a gabapentin dose of 600 to 1200 mg/day** would be helpful in the treatment of muscular cramps. Another small study evaluating hemodialysis (HD) patients showed that gabapentin, at a dose of 300 mg orally 5 min before starting HD, could significantly reduce the frequency and the intensity of muscle cramps during HD without any major side effects.

✓ **Oral magnesium (Slo-Mag, Mag 64), four or two times a day, can be used to reduce leg cramps in pregnant women, without increasing serum concentrations.** Although one study failed to find a difference between magnesium and placebo in patients with nocturnal leg cramps, magnesium salts are commonly used to relieve nocturnal leg pain in Europe and Latin America.

✓ Provide appropriate follow-up to patients who have more than benign self-limited cramps.

What Not to Do

✗ Do not ignore muscle weakness, fasciculations, and wasting, which are signs of lower motor neuron disorders, including amyotrophic lateral sclerosis, polyneuropathy, peripheral nerve injury, and nerve root compression. Fasciculation and cramps without weakness or muscle atrophy are recognized as a benign syndrome. If there is any uncertainty, a normal electromyogram will rule out any serious disease processes.

Discussion

A muscle cramp is a sudden, severe, and involuntary muscle contraction or overshortening. It can cause mild to severe pain and a paralysis-like immobility. Usually it resolves on its own over several seconds, minutes, or, in the worst scenario, several hours.

The etiology of this disabling phenomena is multifactorial and can be summarized in three groups of muscle cramps: (1) those caused by pathologic factors (such as metabolic disorders, diabetes, neuropathy), (2) idiopathic nocturnal cramps (painful episodes of muscle spasm that occur during sleep without a clear etiology), and (3) exercise-associated muscle cramps (EAMC; muscle spasm that occurs during or after an exercise).

Most muscle cramps are thought to be caused by hyperactivity of the peripheral or central nervous system rather than the muscle itself. From the latest investigations there seems to be a spinal involvement rather than a peripheral excitation of the motoneurons. The origin and development of muscle cramps can be considered a vicious circle, in which motoneurons receive afferent inputs that result in hyperexcitability.

The pain results from a combination of ischemia, accumulation of metabolites, and possible damage to the muscle fibers. Electromyographic studies indicate that during ordinary muscle cramps, motor units fire at about 300 per second, far more rapidly than any voluntary contraction. This rapid firing rate causes the muscle tightness and pain.

The cramps occur when a muscle already in its most shortened natural position contracts further. True cramps, which by definition occur in the absence of fluid or electrolyte imbalance, are more prevalent in patients with well-developed muscles, in the latter stages of pregnancy, and in patients with cirrhosis. They are typically asymmetric, explosive in onset, and most frequently affect the gastrocnemius muscle and small muscles of the foot. The contraction, which is often visible, may leave soreness and even swelling. The most common type of true muscle cramp occurs at rest, usually during the night. **A small study showed that in elderly patients with nocturnal leg cramps that are unresponsive to quinine sulfate, verapamil provided relief to most.** There are reports that nitroglycerin paste applied to the overlying skin may relieve a muscle cramp rapidly, but the dose must be small to avoid hypotension, headache, and flushing.

Muscle cramps can also be a considerable source of discomfort in patients undergoing hemodialysis. There is limited evidence that nifedipine can also provide significant pain relief to this group of patients. In another study of hemodialysis muscle cramps, the combination of vitamin C and E supplements produced a 97% decrease in cramps.

Suggested Readings

Cohen, S. P., Mullings, R., & Abdi, S. (2004). The pharmacologic treatment of muscle pain. *Anesthesiology*, *101*, 495–526.

De Carvalho, M., & Swash, M. (2004). Cramps, muscle pain, and fasciculations: Not always benign? *Neurology*, *63*, 721–723.

Giuriato, G., Pedrinolla, A., Schena, F., & Venturelli, M. (2018). Muscle cramps: A comparison of the two-leading hypothesis. *Journal of Electromyography and Kinesiology*, *41*, 89–95.

Mousavi, S. S. B., Zeraati, A., Moradi, S., & Mousavi, M. B. (2015). The effect of gabapentin on muscle cramps during hemodialysis: A double-blind clinical trial. *Saudi Journal of Kidney Disease and Transplantation*, *26*(6), 1142–1148. https://doi.org/10.4103/1319-2442.168588

Schaefer, T. J., & Wolford, R. W. (2005). Disorders of potassium. *Emergency Medicine Clinics of North America*, *23* 723–477,viii–ix.

Serrao, M., Rossi, P., Cardinali, P., Valente, G., Parisi, L., & Pierelli, F. (2000). Gabapentin treatment for muscle cramps: An open-label trial. *Clinical Neuropharmacology*, *23*(1), 45–49.

Tews, M. C., Shah, S. M., & Gossain, V. V. (2005). Hypothyroidism: Mimicker of common complaints. *Emergency Medicine Clinics of North America*, *23*, 649–667 vii.

Muscle Strains and Tears

Presentation

Strains are acute injuries to muscle-tendon units that result from overstretching or overexerting. Strains may occur in the trapezius or paravertebral muscles during a motor vehicle collision, with a whiplash-type injury to the neck. A strain can also occur in the anterior thigh, posterior hamstring group, groin, or gastrocnemius muscle while a person is accelerating, running, or playing in a sport such as tennis. There may be an insidious development of pain and tightness, which is worse with use and better with rest. With more severe injury, such as a bicep-tendon rupture, the pain may be immediate and disabling. Tears of the muscle belly tend to be partial, with sudden onset of pain and partial loss of function. Often a tear occurs with considerable bleeding, which can lead to remarkable hematomas, causing swelling at the site and dissecting along tissue planes to create ecchymoses at distant, uninvolved sites. Complete tears are more likely in the tendinous part of the muscle. They can produce immediate loss of function and retraction of the torn end, creating a deformity and bulge.

What to Do

⊘ **Obtain a detailed history** of the mechanism of injury. Elucidating an inciting event, determining the relieving and exacerbating factors, and timing of the pain can be the most important aspects of making an accurate diagnosis.

⊘ **For cervical strains,** see Chapter 102.

⊘ **The anterior thigh (quadriceps)** may be injured while the person is kicking, jumping, and sprinting. **The hamstrings of the posterior thigh (biceps femoris, semitendinosus, semimembranosus, and adductor magnus)** may tear during a powerful acceleration while a person is sprinting. **Adductor strains of the groin** occur during various sports activities, such as playing soccer or hockey. **Calf muscle (gastrocnemius and soleus)** strains are often seen with sudden accelerations from a dorsiflexed position. **Upper arm (biceps)** injury occurs with forceful lifting against resistance and with rupture of the long head of the biceps, usually presenting with anterior shoulder pain, possibly after hearing a "pop."

⊘ Muscle strains may be classified as grade I (mild), grade II (moderate), or grade III (severe, in which the muscle is completely torn). **Grade I strains** are limited to local spasm and tenderness, and the patient may not notice the pain until the day after the injury. **Grade II strains** have a palpable area of tenderness and possible swelling. Passive stretching is usually painful. **Grade III strains** include tendinous rupture or midbelly tears that are usually accompanied by a visible and/or palpable defect or deformity.

✓ **Perform a physical examination** that defines the muscle that is involved and rules out bony involvement and other possible disease or injury.

✓ **Palpate the injured muscle**, attempt active and passive range of motion (ROM), check for bony tenderness, and put proximal and distal joints through ROM in an attempt to elicit any joint pain (see Chapter 124 for specific evaluation of calf muscle strain).

✓ **Most strains can be easily diagnosed on physical examination, with pain on palpation of the involved muscle and pain on muscle contraction against resistance.**

✓ **Without signs of bony injury, plain radiographs are of little value. Ultrasonography can be useful for diagnosing muscle and tendon tears if the diagnosis is in question.**

✓ **When there is a need to know the extent of injury for treatment and prognostic purposes**, magnetic resonance imaging (MRI) can be used to confirm and delineate muscle strain or tears, and partial and complete tendon tears.

✓ **Acute treatment of grades I and II strains should include relative rest and possibly short-term use of acetaminophen or nonsteroidal anti-inflammatory drugs (NSAIDs). Cold packs with compressive soft splinting may be helpful when hemorrhage or swelling is present.** Short-term use of opiates may be required for particularly painful injuries.

✓ **Even without hemorrhage or swelling, ice massage may be preferable to heat for providing comfort in the first 1 to 3 days.** Freeze water in a small paper or foam cup, tear off the upper rim to expose the ice, and then massage the injured muscle with the ice, using slow, circular strokes for 5 to 20 minutes, using the cup as an insulator. It may be helpful to alternate heat and cold treatments and allow the patient to choose which is better for relieving pain or improving ROM.

✓ **Severe grade II or III strains may require maximum immobilization with a rigid splint and/or with a sling or crutches. Midbelly muscular tears** are often treated conservatively, but **complete tears of the tendon's insertion** from the bone may require surgical repair.

✓ Some grade II and most grade III strains require orthopedic consultation and follow-up for treatment and rehabilitation.

✓ **Most minor grade I strains will resolve within 2 to 4 weeks. Healing time for all strains can be extremely variable and prone to exacerbations** (especially hamstring injuries).

✓ **The second stage of therapy** for most strains begins when the patient's pain has subsided and should consist of gentle ROM exercises, followed by progressive strengthening.

✓ **Warn the patient** that potentially alarming ecchymosis may develop in the days following the injury. They will change color and percolate to the skin at distant sites that are dependent to the injury. Let the patient know that these are normal benign occurrences during healing.

What Not to Do

✗ Do not order radiographs when the injury is clearly isolated to a muscle or tendon and there is no bony involvement.

✗ Do not prescribe muscle relaxants for acute muscular strain. One double-blind study demonstrated that adding cyclobenzaprine (Flexeril) to treatment with ibuprofen (Motrin) did not enhance pain relief but was associated with a higher rate of central nervous system side effects.

Discussion

Groin injuries may result from a variety of causes. The most common groin injury in athletes is the abductor strain. Iliopsoas strain usually occurs during resisted hip flexion or hyperextension. Tenderness may be felt on deep palpation over the lateral aspect of the femoral triangle (adjacent to the femoral artery). This may be accentuated by having the patient raise the heel off the examining table to about 15 degrees.

Athletes who participate in sports that require repetitive twisting and turning at speed, such as soccer or ice hockey, may be at risk of developing a **sports hernia**—disruption of the inguinal canal without a clinically detectable hernia. The sports hernia presents as an insidious-onset, gradually worsening, deep groin pain that is diffuse in nature. It may radiate along the inguinal ligament, perineum, and rectus muscles. Coughing may increase the pain. Radiation of pain to the testicles is present in approximately 30% of afflicted men. On physical examination, no true hernia is palpable because only the deep fascia is violated. MRI and bone scan might be helpful in ruling out other conditions (e.g., stress fractures) but not in making a definitive diagnosis of sports hernia. If symptoms persist after several weeks of conservative treatment, an athlete should undergo surgical exploration and repair.

Other potential causes of groin pain include the more common indirect and direct hernias; testicular disease, including torsion; hip disease, including avascular necrosis; and lumbar radiculopathy. Osteitis pubis, or pubic symphysitis, is a painful inflammatory condition involving the pubic symphysis and surrounding structures that is another possible cause for groin pain and is generally thought of as a self-limiting condition.

Potentially more serious intraabdominal disease, including gastrointestinal (e.g., appendicitis), urologic (e.g., renal colic), and vascular (e.g., abdominal aortic aneurysm), can refer pain to the groin and should be considered when clinically compelling.

Quadriceps tendon rupture is often found in younger athletes involved in a high-energy mechanism such as football, hockey, or rugby. However, it is important to note that older athletes can have a less trivial mechanism leading to a partial or complete tear of the quadriceps tendon. Careful physical examination, including documentation of the extensor mechanism, is critical in all lower extremity injuries. If there is a concern for partial or complete tear of the quadriceps tendon, prompt orthopedic referral is preferred, as early surgery is recommended for better functional outcome.

High hamstring strains (partial avulsion of the muscle from its origin on the ischial tuberosity) occur when excessive stress is placed on the stretched hamstrings. Patients usually present with posterior thigh pain and can have radiation to the groin as well. The diagnosis is easily made when the examiner notes pain on palpation directly over the muscle insertion on the ischial tuberosity.

Sartorius strains lead to palpable tenderness over the anterior superior iliac spine.

Avulsion fractures and apophysitis should be considered in the skeletally immature pediatric age group.

Rupture of the long head of the biceps is one of the most common musculotendinous tears. Proximal long-head tendon ruptures account for 96% of all biceps tendon ruptures. Rupture occurs more frequently in an aging population, specifically in patients who are older than 40 years, and generally occurs in tendinopathic tendons. Risk factors for biceps tendon ruptures include recurrent tendinitis, a history of rotator cuff tear, a history of contralateral biceps tendon rupture, age, poor conditioning, and rheumatoid arthritis.

The literature shows no clear consensus on the treatment of biceps tendon rupture. Surgical repair tends to be favored in the younger and more athletic patient, whereas conservative, nonsurgical management is considered to be more appropriate in the middle-aged and older patient.

Overuse injuries affecting the medial aspect of the lower legs have traditionally been referred to as **shin splints.** This catchall diagnosis is gradually being replaced by that of **medial tibial stress syndrome (MTSS).** This condition predominantly affects running athletes. Patients who have MTSS typically present with shin pain that is related to running or jumping. Pain may be unilateral or bilateral. Examination of patients suffering from MTSS frequently reveals pain confined to the medial border of the tibia, although it can also be located laterally. Toe standing or resisted plantarflexion can exacerbate pain.

Rest is crucial for the treatment of MTSS. Ice, stretching, heel cups, NSAIDs, corticosteroid injection, and even crutches have been studied, but none has benefits greater than rest alone. Five to 7 days of rest are often enough to allow return to activity at a reduced intensity, gradually increasing loads to premorbid levels.

Suggested Readings

Glazer, J. L., & Hosey, R. G. (2004). Soft-tissue injuries of the lower extremity. *Primary Care, 31*, 1005–1024.

Harwood, M. I., & Smith, C. T. (2004). Superior labrum, anterior–posterior lesions and biceps injuries: Diagnostic and treatment considerations. *Primary Care, 31*, 831–855.

Ilan, D. I., Tejwani, N., Keschner, M., & Leibman, M. (2003). Quadriceps tendon rupture. *Journal of the American Academy of Orthopedic Surgeons, 11*(3), 192–200.

Kemp, S., & Batt, M. E. (1998/2015). The "sports hernia." A common cause of groin pain. *The Physician and Sports Medicine, 26*(1), 36–44.

Morelli, V., & Espinoza, L. (2005). Groin injuries and groin pain in athletes: Part 2. *Primary Care, 32*, 185–200.

Morelli, V., & Weaver, V. (2005). Groin injuries and groin pain in athletes: Part 1. *Primary Care, 32*, 163–183.

Naticchia, J., & Kapur, E. (2005). New technology, new injuries in the hip/groin. *Clinics in Family Practice, 7*, 267–278.

Turturro, M. A., Frater, C. R., & D'Amico, F. J. (2003). Cyclobenzaprine with ibuprofen versus ibuprofen alone in acute myofascial strain: A randomized, double-blind clinical trial. *Annals of Emergency Medicine, 41*, 818–826.

Myofascial Pain Syndrome

(Trigger-Points)

Presentation

In myofascial pain syndrome, the patient, who is generally 25 to 50 years of age, will be troubled by the gradual onset of localized or regional unilateral fibromuscular pain that at times can be immobilizing. There may be a history of either acute strain or predisposing activities such as holding a telephone receiver between the ear and shoulder to free the arms, prolonged bending, poor postural habits, repetitive motions, and heavy lifting using poor body mechanics. The areas most commonly affected are the axial muscles, used to maintain posture, which include the posterior muscles of the neck and scapula and the soft tissues lateral to the thoracic and lumbar spine.

Careful examination of the painful region will reveal one or more trigger points, which, when firmly pressed with an examining finger, will cause the patient to wince, cry out, or jump with pain. The underlying muscle may contain a small (2–5 mm) firm knot, nodule, or taut band of muscle fibers that produces the exquisitely tender trigger point and reproduces the pain of the patient's chief complaint. Pain is often referred in a radicular pattern that may mimic the pain of cervical or lumbar disc herniation.

The patient with fibromyalgia, on the other hand, has widespread bilateral, symmetric musculoskeletal pain, which is associated with multiple tender points on palpation that do not cause any radiation of pain. This patient is often depressed or under emotional or physical stress and may have associated chronic fatigue with disturbed sleep, irritable bowel syndrome, cognitive difficulties, headache, morning stiffness, and sensations of numbness or swelling in the hands and feet. Other comorbid conditions might include irritable bladder symptoms, temporomandibular joint syndrome, myofascial pain syndrome, restless leg syndrome, and affective disorders. Cold or hot weather may be one of the precipitating causes of pain.

In both syndromes, most affected patients are women. Also, the pain is nonarticular, and there are no abnormal vital signs and no swelling, erythema, or heat over the painful areas.

What to Do

✔ **Obtain a careful history and perform a general physical examination** with special attention to the painful area. **Myofascial pain is focal** or referred regional muscular pain of short (several days) or prolonged (several months) duration, often causing head, neck, shoulder, upper and lower back, buttock, and leg pain and associated with trigger points, as described earlier. The patient can usually point to the pain with one finger (Fig. 121.1).

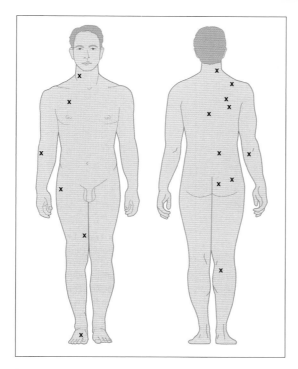

Fig. 121.1 Most frequent locations of myofascial trigger points. (Adapted from Rachlin, E., & Rachlin, I. [2002]. *Myofascial pain and fibromyalgia: Trigger point management* [2nd ed.]. St. Louis, MO: Mosby.)

✓ **The pain of fibromyalgia** is widespread (bilateral, above and below the waist), prolonged (>3 months), and associated with approximately 11 of 18 possible tender points (Fig. 121.2). These tender points are predictable and, unlike trigger points, do not cause radiation of pain or have an underlying small tender muscular knot. The associated coexisting conditions mentioned earlier help to support this diagnosis.

✓ Other conditions should be considered, such as medication-induced myalgias (e.g., statins, colchicines, corticosteroids, fluoroquinolones, antimalarial drugs), connective tissue diseases (e.g., dermatomyositis, polymyalgia rheumatica, systemic lupus erythematosus, rheumatoid arthritis), hypothyroidism and other endocrine disorders, and cancer. In addition, evaluate for true radicular pain with a neurologic examination, and, if indicated, straight-leg raising.

✓ With any suspicion that an underlying systemic illness exists, obtain appropriate radiographs and laboratory tests, such as an erythrocyte sedimentation rate, creatine phosphokinase (CPK), and thyroid-stimulating hormone. These and all other studies should be normal in both myofascial and fibromyalgia pain syndromes.

✓ **With myofascial pain, when a trigger point is found, have the patient maintain a comfortable, relaxed position. Map out its exact location (point of maximum tenderness) and place an X over the site with a marker or ballpoint pen.** If the trigger point is diffuse, there is no need to outline its location.

✓ **When myofascial pain is suspected but trigger points are diffuse**, unless contraindicated, prescribe a nonsteroidal anti-inflammatory drug (NSAID), such as naproxen

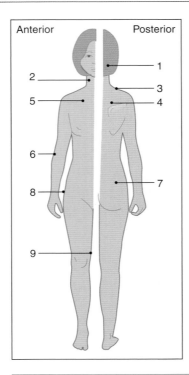

Fig. 121.2 Location of nine bilateral (18) tender point sites for the American College of Rheumatology criteria for the classification of fibromyalgia. *1,* Suboccipital muscle insertions; *2,* cervical, at the anterior aspects of the intertransverse spaces at C5 to C7; *3,* trapezius, at the midpoint of the upper border; *4,* supraspinatus, at the origin, above the scapular spine near the medial border; *5,* second rib, at the costochondral junction; *6,* lateral epicondyle, 2 cm distal to the epicondyle; *7,* gluteal, in the upper outer quadrant of the buttock; *8,* greater trochanter, just posterior to the trochanteric prominence; *9,* knee, at the medial fat pad proximal to the joint line. (Adapted from Rachlin, E., & Rachlin, I. [2002]. *Myofascial pain and fibromyalgia: Trigger point management* [2nd ed.]. St. Louis, MO: Mosby.)

sodium (Naprosyn), 250 mg, two tablets immediately then one four times a day, or ibuprofen (Motrin), 800 mg immediately then 600 mg four times a day for 5 days. A benzodiazepine such as lorazepam (Ativan), 1 mg four times a day, may also be helpful.

⊘ **When a focal trigger point is present, suggest that the patient may get immediate relief with an injection. If the patient is willing, using proper aseptic technique and a needle of 25 or 27 gauge, 1.25 to 1.5 inches, inject through the mark you placed on the skin, directly into the painful site** (Figs. 121.3 to 121.13) (See Video 121.1). **Use 5 to 10 mL of 1% lidocaine (Xylocaine) or longer-acting 0.25% bupivacaine (Marcaine) with or without 20 to 40 mg of methylprednisolone (Depo-Medrol) or 2 to 5 mg of triamcinolone (Aristospan).** Attempt aspiration to be sure you are not in a blood vessel or pleural cavity and then "fan" the needle (while moving it in and out) in all directions while injecting the trigger point. **Advise the patient before the procedure that there may be intensification of the pain before relief.** Intensification of the pain with or without radiation, while injecting slowly, is a good indicator that the needle is in the precise trigger point location. Inject most of the anesthetic into this most painful portion of the site. In addition, massage the area after the injection is complete, to ensure total coverage. Within a few minutes the patient will often get complete or near-complete pain relief, which helps to confirm the diagnosis of myofascial pain syndrome. Inform the patient that there will be approximately 1 day of muscular soreness after the anesthetic wears off. The beneficial effect of this injection may last for weeks or months. A supplementary 5-day course of NSAIDs and/or acetaminophen is optional.

⊘ **Secondary trigger points** may develop in neighboring muscles as a result of stress and muscle spasm. It is common for patients to experience the pain of a secondary trigger point after a primary trigger point is eliminated. These trigger points can be treated in the same manner, either

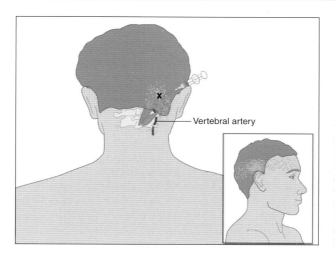

Fig. 121.3 Suboccipital muscle. Injection of trigger point (*x*) in the obliquus capitis superior muscle with the patient in the prone position. Injection is localized directly over the trigger point and the superior portion of the occipital area to avoid the vertebral artery. The occipital triangle and vertebral artery are noted. The pain pattern is shown by stippling. (Adapted from Rachlin, E., & Rachlin, I. [2002]. *Myofascial pain and fibromyalgia: Trigger point management* [2nd ed.]. St. Louis, MO: Mosby.)

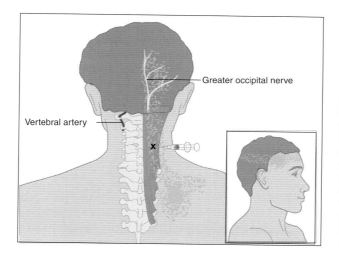

Fig. 121.4 Posterior cervical muscles (semispinalis and multifidi). Injection of trigger point in the right posterior cervical muscles (*x*). The greater occipital nerve is visualized. Anatomic landmarks are noted in addition to visualization of the left vertebral artery. Avoid the vertebral artery by injecting above or below the vertebral artery area. Aspirate prior to injection. The pain pattern is shown by stippling. (Adapted from Rachlin, E., & Rachlin, I. [2002]. *Myofascial pain and fibromyalgia: Trigger point management* [2nd ed.]. St. Louis, MO: Mosby.)

at the same visit or at an early follow-up visit if the symptoms persist. Successful treatment has also been reported with the use of the central α_2-adrenergic receptor agonist tizanidine (Zanaflex) starting with 2 mg every 6 to 8 hours as needed and titrating the dose upward if needed.

✓ **Moist, hot compresses and massage with stretching exercises, as well as the use of a vibrator, may also be comforting to the patient after discharge.**

✓ **Patients with the diffuse symptoms of fibromyalgia usually will not benefit from trigger point injection or NSAIDs. When other causes of such pain have been adequately ruled out, antidepressants, most commonly amitriptyline (Elavil), 5 to 10 mg once before bedtime, titrating up by 5 mg every 2 weeks, improve symptoms for up to several months. The muscle relaxant cyclobenzaprine (Flexeril), which is structurally similar to the tricyclic antidepressants, has also been found to be beneficial in doses of 15 to 45 mg/day divided into three doses.**

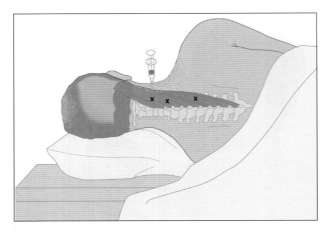

Fig. 121.5 Splenius capitis and splenius cervicis. Injection of trigger points (*xs*) in the right splenius capitis and cervicis with the patient lying on the uninvolved side. Avoid the vertebral artery. Aspirate prior to injection. Anatomic landmarks are noted. The trigger point pattern is shown by stippling. (Adapted from Rachlin, E., & Rachlin, I. [2002]. *Myofascial pain and fibromyalgia: Trigger point management* [2nd ed.]. St. Louis, MO: Mosby.)

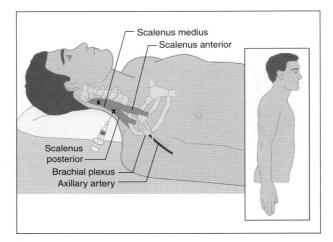

Fig. 121.6 Scalene muscles. Injection of the scalenus medius muscle trigger points (*xs*). The patient is supine, the head turned away from the area of pain. Anatomic landmarks are noted, including axillary artery and lateral chord. The referred pain pattern is shown by stippling. (Adapted from Rachlin, E., & Rachlin, I. [2002]. *Myofascial pain and fibromyalgia: Trigger point management* [2nd ed.]. St. Louis, MO: Mosby.)

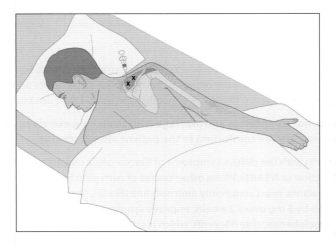

Fig. 121.7 Supraspinatus. Injection of trigger points (*xs*) in the right supraspinatus with the patient prone. The needle is placed directly over the supraspinous fossa of the scapula to avoid penetrating the rib cage. Anatomic landmarks are noted. The pain pattern is shown by stippling. (Adapted from Rachlin, E., & Rachlin, I. [2002]. *Myofascial pain and fibromyalgia: Trigger point management* [2nd ed.]. St. Louis, MO: Mosby.)

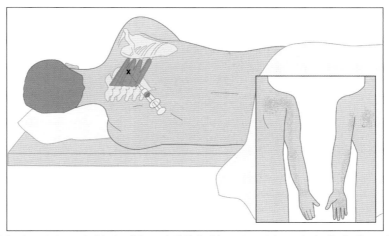

Fig. 121.8 Serratus posterior superior. Injection of trigger point (*x*) in the right serratus posterior superior. Localize the trigger point by palpation and direct the needle in the direction of a rib and tangentially in relation to the chest wall to avoid entering the intercostal space. Aspirate before injection. Trigger points in the region of muscle insertion are more easily palpated with abduction of the right scapula. Observe precautions to prevent pneumothorax. *Inset,* Trigger point pain pattern is shown by stippling. (Adapted from Rachlin, E., & Rachlin, I. [2002]. *Myofascial pain and fibromyalgia: Trigger point management* [2nd ed.]. St. Louis, MO: Mosby.)

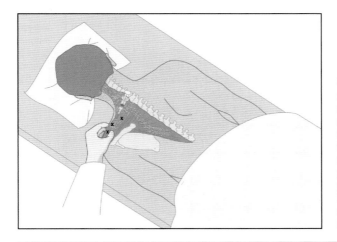

Fig. 121.9 Trapezius. Injection for trigger points (*xs*) in the left trapezius with the patient prone. The upper portion of the left trapezius is grasped between the thumb, index, and middle fingers and is elevated to avoid penetrating the apex of the lung. Several entries are usually necessary to treat all trigger points that are present. Aspirate prior to injection. The pain pattern is shown by stippling. (Adapted from Rachlin, E., & Rachlin, I. [2002]. *Myofascial pain and fibromyalgia: Trigger point management* [2nd ed.]. St. Louis, MO: Mosby.)

⊘ **Aerobic exercise and warm compresses improve function and reduce pain in persons with fibromyalgia.**

⊘ Provide follow-up care for all patients in the event that their symptoms do not clear and thus require further diagnostic evaluation and therapy.

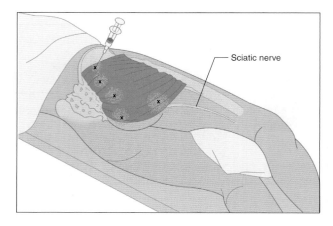

Fig. 121.10 Gluteus maximus. Injection of trigger points (xs) in the gluteus maximus. Anatomic landmarks are noted. Avoid the sciatic nerve. The pain pattern is shown by stippling. Injection may be performed with the patient in the prone or side-lying position. (Adapted from Rachlin, E., & Rachlin, I. [2002]. *Myofascial pain and fibromyalgia: Trigger point management* [2nd ed.]. St. Louis, MO: Mosby.)

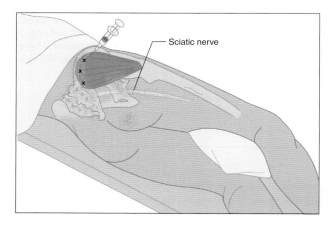

Fig. 121.11 Gluteus medius. Injection of trigger points in the right gluteus medius. Multiple trigger points (xs) are noted. Anatomic skeletal landmarks are shown together with the sciatic nerve. The patient is positioned lying on the uninvolved side. Injection may also be performed with the patient prone. The pain pattern is noted by stippled area. (Adapted from Rachlin, E., & Rachlin, I. [2002]. *Myofascial pain and fibromyalgia: Trigger point management* [2nd ed.]. St. Louis, MO: Mosby.)

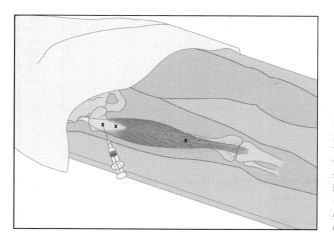

Fig. 121.12 Rectus femoris. Injection of trigger points (xs) in the right rectus femoris. Note trigger points in the area of origin and distally toward the area of insertion. The patient is supine. The trigger point pain pattern is shown by stippling. Anatomic landmarks are noted. (Adapted from Rachlin, E., & Rachlin, I. [2002]. *Myofascial pain and fibromyalgia: Trigger point management* [2nd ed.]. St. Louis, MO: Mosby.)

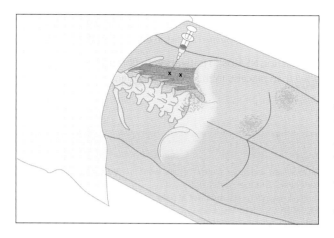

Fig. 121.13 Quadratus lumborum. Injection of trigger points (*xs*) in the right quadratus lumborum with the patient in the prone position. Injection may also be performed with the patient lying on the uninvolved side. The trigger point pain pattern is shown by stippling. Direct the needle tangentially or parallel to the frontal plane of the patient. (Adapted from Rachlin, E., & Rachlin, I. [2002]. *Myofascial pain and fibromyalgia: Trigger point management* [2nd ed.]. St. Louis, MO: Mosby.)

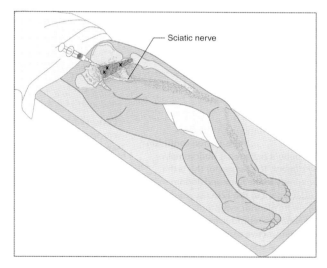

Sciatic nerve

Fig. 121.14 Piriformis. Injection of trigger points in the right piriformis muscle (*xs*). The sciatic nerve is shown in addition to anatomic details. Injection is performed with the patient lying on the uninvolved side. A pillow is placed between the knees. The hip is flexed. The pain pattern is shown by stippling. (Adapted from Rachlin, E., & Rachlin, I. [2002]. *Myofascial pain and fibromyalgia: Trigger point management* [2nd ed.]. St. Louis, MO: Mosby.)

What Not to Do

(X) Do not inject a trigger point while a patient is sitting or standing and is unprotected from a fall caused by vasovagal syncope.

(X) Do not order radiographs or laboratory tests for myofascial pain that is localized and relieved by trigger point injection.

(X) Do not attempt to inject a very diffuse trigger point (>2 cm²) or multiple scattered tender points as found in true fibromyalgia syndrome. Results are generally unsatisfactory.

(X) Do not inject trigger points in the presence of systemic or local infection, in patients with bleeding disorders, in patients on anticoagulants (a relative contraindication), or in patients who appear to be or feel ill.

(X) Do not prescribe narcotic analgesics or systemic steroids. They are no more effective than the abovementioned therapy and add side effects and the risk for dependence.

(X) Do not prescribe NSAIDs to patients with fibromyalgia. They have been found to be no more effective than placebo in this group of patients.

Discussion

Emergency physicians and other acute care clinicians often see patients with trigger points associated with simple self-limiting regional **myofascial pain syndromes,** which appear to arise from muscles, muscle–tendon junctions, or tendon–bone junctions. Myofascial disease can result in severe pain, but it is typically in a limited distribution, without the systemic feature of fatigue and without the multiple somatic complaints of fibromyalgia. Trigger point injection therapy, the treatment of choice for trigger points according to many, has gained widening acceptance in mainstream medicine. When symptoms recur or persist after this basic therapy or are accompanied by generalized complaints, acute care clinicians should refer these patients to a rheumatologist or primary care physician for follow-up and continued management.

When the quadratus lumborum muscle is involved (see Fig. 121.13), **there is often confusion whether the patient has a renal, abdominal, or pulmonary ailment. The reason for this is the muscle's proximity to the flank and abdomen, as well as its attachment to the 12th rib, which, when tender, can create pleuritic symptoms. A careful physical examination reproducing symptoms through palpation, active contraction, and passive stretching of this muscle can save this patient from a multitude of laboratory, ultrasound, and radiographic studies.**

Another affected muscle that often confuses and misleads clinicians is the piriformis (Fig. 121.14). **Piriformis syndrome is an uncommon and often undiagnosed cause of buttock and leg pain. It may be caused by anatomic abnormalities of the piriformis muscle and the sciatic nerve resulting in irritation of the sciatic nerve by the piriformis.**

The typical patient with piriformis syndrome complains of buttock pain with or without radiation to the posterior thigh that sometimes extends below the knee to the calf, resembling typical sciatica and causes difficulty with walking. The cardinal characteristic of the syndrome is sitting intolerance secondary to intense buttock pain. Gluteal atrophy may occur.

Buttock tenderness in the region of the greater sciatic foramen is present in almost all patients, and buttock pain is elicited when the patient lifts and holds the knee several inches off the examination table. There may be moderate relief of pain by applying traction on the affected extremity with the patient in the supine position. A tender sausage-shaped mass may be palpated over the piriformis muscle.

A complete neurologic examination should be performed to test motor power, sensory function, and reflexes of the lower extremities to help rule out spinal causes of sciatic pain. One should also consider intrapelvic diseases, such as tumors and endometriosis, as a possible cause of sciatic pain.

Conservative treatment of piriformis syndrome consists of prescribing NSAIDs, analgesics, and muscle relaxants and providing physical therapy, which includes stretching the piriformis muscle with internal rotation and hip adduction and flexion.

More aggressive therapy includes local injection of anesthetic and corticosteroids that may reconfirm the diagnosis through therapeutic success (see Fig. 121.14). This may be repeated twice with recurrent pain. If this fails, surgery can be considered.

The most likely cause of chronic diffuse myalgia is fibromyalgia. Among adults who seek medical attention for fibromyalgia, less than one-third recover within 10 years of onset. Symptoms tend to remain stable or improve over time.

Although fibromyalgia was long believed to be primarily a muscle disease, research has not found any significant pathologic or biochemical abnormalities in muscle tissue. Many researchers now believe that the disease is caused by abnormalities in central nervous system (CNS) function. This would suggest that the pain of fibromyalgia is in part because of a decrease in the threshold for pain perception and tolerance

(continued)

Discussion continued

experienced by these patients. Fibromyalgia patients also appear to experience pain amplification because of abnormal sensory processing in the CNS.

The diagnosis of fibromyalgia is made by meeting the criteria of having widespread musculoskeletal pain for 3 months or longer and having 11 or more tender points among 18 potential sites defined by the American College of Rheumatology (see Fig. 121.2). **Some patients may not have an adequate number of tender points to make the diagnosis, but when typically associated symptoms are present, these patients should be treated for fibromyalgia.**

Education, reassurance, psychological support, and reminders to exercise regularly are important in all follow-up visits.

Suggested Readings

Abram, S. E. (2005). Does botulinum toxin have a role in the management of myofascial pain? *Anesthesiology, 103,* 223–224.

Benzon, H. T., Katz, J. A., Benzon, H. A., et al. (2003). Piriformis syndrome. *Anesthesiology, 98,* 1442–1448.

Malanga, G., Gwynn, M., Smith, R., & Miller, D. (2002). Tizanidine is effective in the treatment of myofascial pain syndrome. *Pain Physician, 5,* 422–432.

Gill, J. M., & Quisel, A. (2005). Fibromyalgia and diffuse myalgia. *Clinics in Family Practice, 7,* 181–190.

Nelson, L. S., & Hoffman, R. S. (1998). Intrathecal injection: Unusual complication of trigger-point injection therapy. *Annals of Emergency Medicine, 32,* 506–508.

Papadopoulos, E. C., & Khan, S. N. (2004). Piriformis syndrome and low back pain: A new classification and review of the literature. *Orthopedic Clinics of North America, 35,* 65–71.

Rachlin, E., & Rachlin, I. (2002). *Myofascial pain and fibromyalgia: Trigger point management* (2nd ed.). St. Louis, MO: Mosby.

Patellar Dislocation

Presentation

After a direct blow to the medial aspect of the patella or, more commonly, without contact and only after a sudden twisting motion to the opposite side of an outward-pointing planted foot (with a powerful contraction of the quadriceps while the thigh is turning inward), the patient's kneecap dislocates laterally. The patient, who is usually an adolescent, is brought in with the knee guarded and slightly flexed, in severe pain, with the patella situated lateral to the lateral femoral condyle, creating an obvious and dramatic lateral deformity (Fig. 122.1). Most often there will have been a spontaneous reduction, and the patient reports that the knee or kneecap "gave way" or "gave out" with pain and then slipped back into place. A patient with recurrent, acute dislocation is usually able to relate an appropriate history and usually knows exactly what happened.

What to Do

✅ **For a persistent dislocation, provide immediate reduction prior to obtaining x-rays. Pain medications and sedatives may be needed for reduction, but gaining the patient's confidence, while holding and stabilizing the leg and patella, will minimize this need.** Position the patient with the hip flexed to reduce strain on the quadriceps muscle (one way to do this is to have the patient sitting on the edge of the stretcher with legs down). Stand on the lateral side of the patient. **Slowly and gently extend the lower leg at the knee while holding the patella in its original position. While the knee is being extended, control the movement of the patella with your hand so that it slowly slides back into its normal position. If needed, and while firmly holding on to the patella and lifting its most lateral edge, apply continuous gentle anteromedial force to the patella to lift it over the edge of the femoral condyle, never allowing it to snap back into place.**

✅ **Some practitioners have successfully used the following maneuver as well: Gain the patient's confidence and cooperation while gently grasping the patella and stabilizing it by applying mild lateral traction and maintaining its original position to prevent sudden motion. Place the patient in a relaxing semiprone position holding the leg in a position of greatest comfort. Then have the patient allow you to passively and very gradually extend the knee while continuing to hold the patella in its lateral position. When the knee is fully extended, slowly release traction on the patella while maintaining continuous control and gently let it slip back into its normal anatomic position (medial force is generally not required when the knee is fully extended) (See Video 122.1).** With experience, this technique rarely requires any analgesia or sedation, only a calm and reassuring approach.

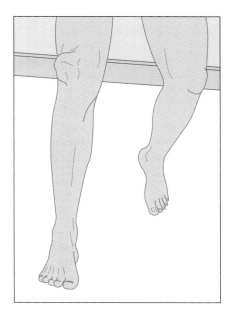

Fig. 122.1 Patellar dislocation.

✓ **If the patella is irreducible**, urgent orthopedic consultation is required.

✓ **After the patella has been reduced and the patient is comfortable, order knee radiographs, including patellar views,** to help rule out an avulsion fracture of the superomedial pole of the patella, an osteochondral fracture of the lateral femoral condyle, or a fracture of the medial posterior patellar articular surface. There are associated fractures in 28% to 50% of patellar dislocations, which can lead to degenerative arthritis. It must be appreciated that plain radiographs do not show a high percentage of osteochondral fractures occurring at the time of patellofemoral dislocation.

✓ **A standard evaluation of the knee ligaments should be performed to rule out concurrent injury** (see Chapter 113).

✓ **Palpate for rents in the vastus medialis obliquus and the medial patellofemoral ligament or for a grossly dislocatable patella** (Fig. 122.2). **Also note the presence of any swelling or effusion.** High-frequency ultrasonography can help in the diagnosis of injuries to medial patellofemoral ligaments and chondral and osteochondral lesions.

✓ **A hemarthrosis can develop from a capsular tear and/or an osteochondral fracture.** Some authors suggest that when a tense and painful hemarthrosis is present, aspiration should be considered to reduce pain and check for fat droplets, indicating an occult osteochondral injury.

✓ **Fit the patient for crutches and a knee immobilizer that will keep the knee straight.**

✓ Provide analgesia as required and instruct the patient on the use of ice and elevation. Teach non–weight-bearing walking with crutches.

✓ **Provide orthopedic follow-up** in 1 to 3 days.

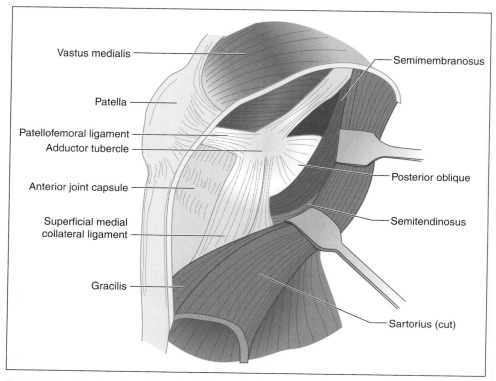

Fig. 122.2 Anatomic structures of the medial patellofemoral ligament and the vastus medialis obliquus and patella.

⊘ Quadriceps isometrics, straight-leg raises, and single-plane motion exercises are begun early and progress as tolerated. Quadriceps strengthening is paramount and kept in balance with adequate extensor mechanism rehabilitation. **Repetition of the injury mechanism or mechanically similar activities must be avoided in the healing period.** Exercises should be done in a pain-free manner. Patellar pain may indicate unrecognized or progressive articular cartilage damage.

⊘ **If pain persists beyond early rehabilitation,** articular cartilage magnetic resonance imaging (MRI) techniques should be used to identify any undiagnosed osteochondral injuries. MRI also has a role in determining the extent and location of injury to the medial patellofemoral ligament.

⊘ As strength and symptoms allow, patients progress out of their brace in physical therapy to single-plane walking, running, cutting, and finally sport-specific activity.

What Not to Do

⊗ Do not try to force the patella to move medially. This may succeed in reduction but is unnecessarily painful and can cause harm.

Discussion

The patella is the largest sesamoid bone in the body, and it resides within the complex of the quadriceps and patellar tendons. It functions as both a lever and a pulley. As a lever, the patella magnifies the force exerted by the quadriceps on knee extension. As a pulley, the patella redirects the quadriceps force as it undergoes normal lateral tracking during flexion.

Most series on patellar dislocation report a greater incidence in women, although some series have reported equal numbers of men and women affected, and others have found a higher incidence in men. Depending on the study, 30% to 72% of dislocations can be expected to be sports related, and 28% to 39% will have associated osteochondral fractures. Concurrent osteochondral injuries are a major contributor to adverse outcomes.

The most common sports involved are football, basketball, and baseball, but it is not unusual in gymnastics, simple falls, cheerleading, and dancing. This injury may occur when patients with normal anatomy are exposed to direct high-energy forces, but most studies find that it occurs more commonly when patients with abnormal anatomy are exposed to indirect forces. Some authors think that anatomic predispositions, such as patella alta, trochlear dysplasia, and ligamentous laxity, play greater roles in recurrent instability.

The average age of these patients is 16 to 20 years old; it is a rare injury for those older than age 30.

The incidence of recurrent dislocation decreases with age: 14-year-olds have a 60% incidence of redislocation; those age 17 to 28 years have an incidence of 30%.

Most patellar dislocations are of the lateral type. Horizontal, superior, and intracondylar patellar dislocations are very uncommon and usually require surgical reduction.

Relative indications for early operative intervention after an acute lateral patella dislocation are controversial, without clear supporting research, but include the following: (1) failure to improve with initial nonoperative care, (2) concurrent osteochondral injury, (3) continued gross patella instability, (4) palpable disruption of the medial patellofemoral ligament–vastus medialis obliquus–adductor mechanism, and (5) high-level athletic demands coupled with mechanical risk factors and an initial injury mechanism not related to contact.

One study suggests that most patients without anatomic abnormality do well whether they are treated conservatively or surgically, and that among patients with anatomic abnormality, half will do well if treated conservatively, whereas up to 80% will do well if treated surgically. Some studies show a trend toward increased osteoarthritis following surgical repair for patella dislocation.

Suggested Readings

Hinton, R. Y., & Sharma, K. M. (2003). Acute and recurrent patellar instability in the young athlete. *Orthopedic Clinics of North America, 34,* 385–396.

Morelli, V., & Rowe, R. H. (2004). Patellar tendonitis and patellar dislocations. *Primary Care, 31,* 909–924, viii-ix.

Zhang, G.-Y., Zheng, L., Shi, H., Quand, S.-H., & Ding, H.-Y. (2013). Sonography on injury of the medial patellofemoral ligament after acute traumatic lateral patellar dislocation: Injury patterns and correlation analysis with injury of articular cartilage of the inferomedial patella. *Injury, 44*(12), 1892–1898.

Plantar Fasciitis

("Heel Spur")

Presentation

Patients seek help because of gradually increasing inferior heel pain that has progressed to the point of inhibiting their normal daily activities. This fasciitis can develop in anyone who is ambulatory but appears to be more common in athletes (especially runners), those older than 30 years of age, those who stand for prolonged periods of time, and the overweight. There is no defining episode of trauma. The most distinctive clue is exquisite pain in the plantar aspect of the heel when taking the first step in the morning. There is gradual improvement with walking, but as the day progresses, the pain may insidiously increase. First-step pain is also present after the patient has been sitting. The heel is tender to palpation over the medial calcaneal tubercle and may be exacerbated by dorsiflexion of the ankle and toes, particularly the great toe, which creates tension on the plantar fascia. Often the midfascia is tender to palpation, too. There is generally no swelling, heat, or discoloration.

What to Do

✓ **Obtain a general medical history in addition to details of the patient's current illness.** Patients with systemic conditions and those with potential infection will have other areas of involvement or bilateral involvement. Other clues might include a history of diabetes, chemotherapy, retroviral infection, a rheumatologic disorder, or another similar chronic condition. A history of focal pain after localized trauma indicates a contusion to the heel (sometimes referred to as "fat pad syndrome").

✓ **Increased levels of activity or exercise may indicate that overuse is the cause of the pain.** Other potential precipitating factors include recent weight gain, a change in footwear, inappropriate or worn-out shoes, or working on cement floors. If the patient describes the sensation as "burning," "tingling," or "numbness," the cause may be peripheral nerve entrapment. Pain that develops in the evening after physical activity is often seen early in stress fracture.

✓ **Perform a careful foot examination** to determine the location of the point of maximal tenderness and to detect any signs of infection, atrophy of the heel pad, bony deformities, bruising, or breaks in the skin. **Diagnosis is made by eliciting pain with palpation in the region of the medial plantar tuberosity of the calcaneus (the origin of the plantar fascia). Pain may be worsened by passive dorsiflexion of the foot.**

✓ **Radiographs can be deferred and are not always required.** However, as clinical findings demand, they may be obtained to look for stress fractures of the metatarsals, tumors, osteomyelitis, calcifications, or spurs, which are located on the leading edge of the calcaneal inferior surface.

✓ **Unless contraindicated, prescribe nonsteroidal anti-inflammatory drugs (NSAIDs) for 2 to 3 weeks.**

✓ **Have the patient wear soft (viscoelastic) heel cushions, such as Bauerfeind Viscoheel (Bauerfeind USA, Kennesaw, GA), and a sports shoe with a firm, impact-resistant heel counter and longitudinal arch support. AirCast (DJO Global, Vista, CA) provides an alternative pneumatic compression dressing for the foot and ankle (AirHeel).**

✓ Use of dorsiflexion night splints may be particularly beneficial in preventing the severe pain that often comes with the first steps in the morning on awakening. However, compliance is low.

✓ **Ice massage can be helpful. The patient can roll the heel over a can of frozen juice concentrate, followed by stretching.**

✓ **Athletes should practice stretching the Achilles tendon before running by placing the sole flat, leaning forward against a counter or table, and slowly squatting while keeping the heel on the ground.** Others may stand, wearing tennis shoes, on the edge of a step, facing up the stairs, slowly lowering the heels until they feel a pulling sensation in the upper calf. Hold for 30 to 60 seconds or until there is pain. Repeat three times daily, increasing the stretch time to a maximum of 3 minutes per session. Although there may be a transient increase in pain after beginning this program, the heel pain usually begins to resolve within several weeks.

Stretching and Strengthening

✓ Stretching and strengthening programs play an important role in the treatment of plantar fasciitis and can correct functional risk factors such as tightness of the gastrocsoleus complex and weakness of the intrinsic foot muscles. Increasing flexibility of the calf muscles is particularly

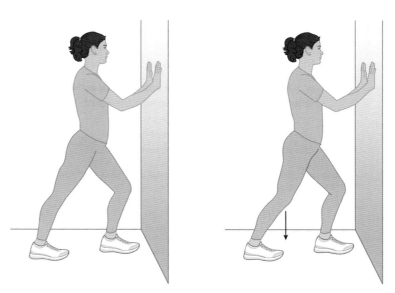

Fig. 123.1 Wall exercises for calf stretching. *(Left)* Soleus stretch. *(Right)* Gastrocnemius stretch.

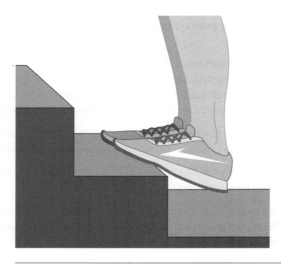

Fig. 123.2 Stair stretch.

important. Frequently used stretching techniques include wall stretches (Fig. 123.1) and curb or stair stretches (Fig. 123.2).

Other effective techniques include use of a slant board (Fig. 123.3) or placing a 2-inch × 4-inch piece of wood (Fig. 123.4) in areas where the patient stands for a prolonged time (e.g., workplaces, kitchen stove) to use in stretching the calf. Dynamic stretches such as rolling the foot arch over a 15-ounce can or a tennis ball are also useful (Fig. 123.5). Cross-friction massage above the plantar fascia (Fig. 123.6) and towel stretching (Fig. 123.7) may be done before getting out of bed and serve to stretch the plantar fascia.

In one study, 83% of patients involved in stretching programs were successfully treated, and 29% of patients in the study cited stretching as the treatment that had helped the most compared with use of orthotics, NSAIDs, ice, steroid injection, heat, heel cups, night splints, walking, plantar strapping, and shoe changes.

In Addition to Stretching and Strengthening

Have the patient reduce ambulatory activities and try to keep weight off the foot whenever possible. Also, have female patients avoid thin-soled flats and high heels. Have runners decrease their mileage by 25% to 75% and avoid sprinting, running on hard surfaces, and running uphill. A program of cross training incorporating swimming and bicycling maintains cardiovascular fitness while decreasing stress on the feet.

Although not often easily applied, recommend weight loss for those patients who are overweight.

Usually, plantar fasciitis can be treated successfully by tailoring treatment to an individual's risk factors and preferences.

When conservative measures have failed and there is an exquisitely tender area on the medial calcaneus, local corticosteroid injection may speed recovery. Use with care because there may be increased risk of plantar fasciitis rupture. Palpate the heel pad to locate the point of maximum tenderness. Place the patient in the lateral recumbent position with

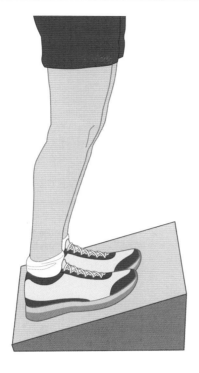

Fig. 123.3 Slant board.

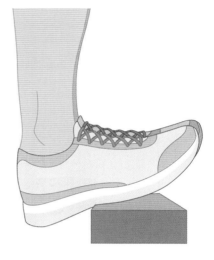

Fig. 123.4 Use of 2-inch × 4-inch piece of wood for stretching.

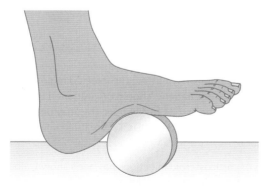

Fig. 123.5 Dynamic stretching with a 15-ounce can.

the lateral aspect of the painful heel resting against the examination surface. Cleanse the skin with povidone-iodine and, using a 25-gauge (1.25–1.5 inch) needle, inject the area with 2 mL of 0.25% or 0.5% of bupivacaine (Marcaine) along with betamethasone (Celestone Soluspan), 1 mL of 6 mg/mL, or methylprednisolone (Depo-Medrol), 1 mL of 40 mg/mL. Enter medially, perpendicular to the skin, and advance the needle directly down past the midline of the width of the foot to the plantar fascia until you can feel its thick and gritty substance. Inject the mixture slowly and evenly through the middle one-third of the width of the foot while the needle is

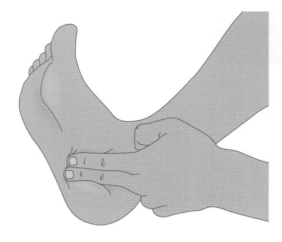

Fig. 123.6 Cross-friction massage above the plantar fascia.

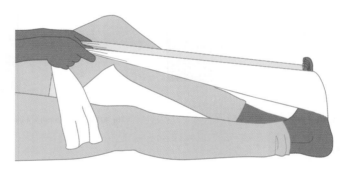

Fig. 123.7 Towel stretching.

being withdrawn (Fig. 123.8). Finish by putting the injected region through passive range of motion to spread the medication. Patients should be cautioned that they may experience worsening symptoms during the first 24 to 48 hours. This may be related to a possible steroid flare, which can be treated with ice and NSAIDs. Two or three injections at intervals of several weeks may be necessary.

✓ The effectiveness of corticosteroid injections has been shown, albeit the effects are short lasting. With respect to other injection modalities, botulinum toxin injections appear better than corticosteroid injections, and corticosteroid injections are better than autologous blood injections. Orthotics devices and corticosteroid injections are reported as the best treatment for plantar fasciitis in many studies. Specific stretching exercises for the treatment of plantar fasciitis are the best statistically significant long-term results.

✓ In all cases, orthopedic follow-up should be arranged.

What Not to Do

✗ Do not inject into the heel pad itself, which may cause fat atrophy.

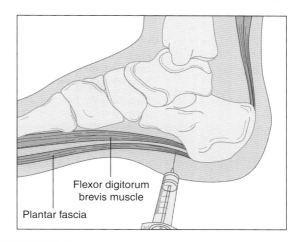

Fig. 123.8 Proper location for injection.

Flexor digitorum
brevis muscle

Plantar fascia

Discussion

Plantar fasciitis is a common problem that 1 in 10 people will experience in a lifetime.

In general, plantar fasciitis is a self-limiting condition. Unfortunately, the time until resolution is often 6 to 18 months, which can lead to frustration for patients and physicians. With proper treatment, 80% of patients with plantar fasciitis improve within 12 months. Early recognition and treatment usually lead to a shorter course of treatment as well as increased probability of success with conservative treatment measures.

The plantar fascia provides an intimate attachment to the overlying skin and functions to provide protection to the underlying muscles, tendons, arteries, and nerves. The fascia assists in the maintenance of the foot arch and keeps the foot in relative supination through the push-off phase of ambulation. During heel strike, the plantar fascia remains supple and allows the foot to adjust to the ground surface and absorb shock. Then, during the toe-off phase of ambulation, the plantar fascia becomes taut and thereby renders the foot a rigid lever, thus facilitating forward movement.

Plantar fasciitis, the most common cause of heel pain in adults, typically results from repetitive use or excessive load on the fascia. Persons who are overweight, female, or older than 40 years or who spend long hours on their feet are especially at risk for developing plantar fasciitis. Athletes, especially joggers and runners, also develop plantar fasciitis.

Tightness of the Achilles tendon contributes to increased tension on the plantar fascia during walking or running and is therefore an important contributor to plantar fasciitis. Stretching of the Achilles tendon can therefore alleviate some of the pain caused by plantar fasciitis. It should be relayed to the patient, however, that this can initially make the discomfort worse.

Mechanical causes of heel pain are generally synonymous with plantar fasciitis, but some cases are enigmatic in etiology and are deemed idiopathic. Although the word *fasciitis* implies inflammation, recent research indicates that it is more likely to be a noninflammatory, degenerative process that might be more appropriately called plantar fasciosis.

Acute onset of severe plantar heel pain after trauma or vigorous athletics may indicate rupture of the plantar fascia. The patient may have heard a "pop" or felt a tearing sensation. Findings suggestive of rupture include a palpable defect at the calcaneal tuberosity accompanied by localized swelling and ecchymosis.

If conservative treatment of plantar fasciitis fails to alleviate symptoms, radiographs, ultrasonography, and magnetic resonance imaging may be advisable to check for other causes of heel pain, such as stress fracture, arthritis, or skeletal abnormality. Radiographs may show a spur on the leading edge of the calcaneal inferior surface, but this radiographic finding is not pathognomonic of the condition,

Discussion continued

nor is it necessary for the diagnosis. It is a common finding in the asymptomatic foot and is generally not the cause of a patient's heel pain.

If a patient with heel pain has persistent bilateral involvement, systemic disease may be the cause. Ankylosing spondylitis, Reiter disease, rheumatoid arthritis, systemic lupus erythematosus, and gouty arthritis all may cause medial calcaneal pain. Calcaneal bursitis and fat pad atrophy are other potential causes of heel pain.

Using injectable steroids for plantar fasciitis is somewhat controversial; therefore, in general, they should be used only when conservative measures have failed. The main concern with the use of steroid injections is delayed rupture of the plantar fascia. Rupture is typically associated with resolution of plantar fasciitis symptoms, but a majority of these patients may go on to

develop long-term sequelae such as longitudinal arch strain, lateral plantar nerve dysfunction, stress fracture, and development of hammertoe deformity.

In most patients with plantar fasciitis, conservative therapy works best. Symptoms will usually resolve, but this may take many weeks or months. For the 10% or fewer with heel pain that persists for at least 1 year despite treatment, surgery should be considered, especially when the symptoms of plantar fasciitis are disabling. Determining the source of repetitive stress to the plantar fascia and addressing it as part of the treatment is crucial to both facilitating recovery and reducing the risk of recurrence. Chronic recurrences may indicate biomechanical imbalances in the foot, which may resolve with custom orthotics from a podiatrist.

Suggested Readings

Aldridge, T. (2004). Diagnosing heel pain in adults. *American Family Physician, 70*, 332–338.

Petraglia, F., Ramazzina, I., & Costantino, C. (2017). Plantar fasciitis in athletes: Diagnostic and treatment strategies. A systematic review. *Muscles, Ligaments, and Tendons Journal, 7*(1), 107–118. https://doi.org/10.11138/mltj/2017.7.1.107

Sheon, R. P., & Buchbinder, R. (2012). *Plantar fasciitis and other causes of heel and sole pain.* UpToDate. http://www.uptodate.com.

Tallia, A. F., & Cardone, D. A. (2003). Diagnostic and therapeutic injection of the ankle and foot. *American Family Physician, 68*, 1356–1362.

Torpy, J. M. (2003). Plantar fasciitis. *JAMA, 290*, 1542.

Williams, S. K., & Brage, M. (2004). Heel pain—plantar fasciitis and Achilles enthesopathy. *Clinics in Sports Medicine, 23*, 123–144.

Young, C. C., Rutherford, D. S., & Niedfeldt, M. W. (2001). Treatment of plantar fasciitis. *American Family Physician, 63*(3), 467–475.

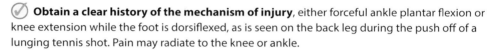

CHAPTER 124

"Plantaris Tendon" Rupture, Gastrocnemius Muscle Tear

(Calf Muscle Tear)

Presentation

The patient will come in limping, having suffered a whiplike sting in the calf while stepping off the foot hard or attempting a lunging shot during a game of tennis or similar activity. The patient may have actually heard or felt a "snap," described as being like the "pop" of a champagne cork, at the time of injury or may think someone actually kicked or shot him in the calf. The deep calf pain persists and may be accompanied by mild to moderate swelling and ecchymosis. Neurovascular function will be intact.

What to Do

⊘ **Obtain a clear history of the mechanism of injury**, either forceful ankle plantar flexion or knee extension while the foot is dorsiflexed, as is seen on the back leg during the push off of a lunging tennis shot. Pain may radiate to the knee or ankle.

⊘ **Perform a physical examination**, which should reveal calf tenderness, especially along the medial musculotendinous junction of the medial gastrocnemius. There may be a defect in the muscle belly itself. Swelling will usually be asymmetric. Over time, any ecchymosis may be found spreading to a more dependent site over the ankle or foot. Dorsiflexion of the foot and resisted plantarflexion are typically painful. Peripheral pulses should be present and symmetric.

⊘ **Rule out an Achilles tendon rupture, as this needs orthopedic evaluation for possible surgery. Palpate the Achilles tendon for a defect or deformity, which represents a torn segment. Perform a Thompson test by squeezing the gastrocnemius muscle just distal to its widest girth, with the patient kneeling on a chair or lying prone on a stretcher with the legs overhanging the end** (Fig. 124.1) (See Video 124.1) **to examine for normal plantar flexion of the foot. Alternatively, the test may be performed with the patient's knees flexed and the feet up while lying supine. Always compare the affected leg with the contralateral limb. <u>The resultant plantar flexion will be totally absent with a complete Achilles tendon tear.</u>** A defect in the contour along the length of the Achilles tendon, pain distal to the body of the gastrocnemius, and lack of pain with palpation of the muscle belly are all typical of Achilles tendon rupture and not plantaris tendon rupture or a gastrocnemius tear.

⊘ **When there is any uncertainty, a definitive diagnosis can be established with ultrasonography or magnetic resonance imaging (MRI). With any Achilles tendon tear, orthopedic consultation is necessary.**

⊘ **If there is excruciating pain** out of proportion to what would be expected with these injuries, the possibility of an acute compartment syndrome must be entertained, and immediate orthopedic consultation should be obtained.

543

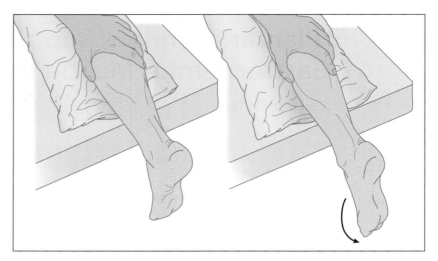

Fig. 124.1 Thompson, Simmonds, or calf squeeze test.

✅ **When serious conditions have been ruled out, and it is assumed that the patient has a plantaris tendon rupture or a tear of the gastrocnemius muscle, provide the patient with elastic support (e.g., Ace bandage, antiembolism stocking, Tubigrip) from the foot to the tibial tuberosity, with or without a posterior splint to provide additional comfort. Gravity equinus (allowing the toe to drop down naturally) is generally the most comfortable position.**

✅ **Patients with severe pain may require crutches for several days.** Some clinicians have begun using rocker-bottom postoperative boots for early ambulation.

✅ **Have the patient keep the leg elevated** above the level of the heart and at rest as much as possible for the next 24 to 48 hours, initially applying cold packs to the calf intermittently.

✅ An opiod analgesic may be helpful initially for 1 to 2 days, as well as nonsteroidal anti-inflammatory drugs (NSAIDs) for a few days, in the absence of contraindication.

✅ **The temporary use of bilateral 1-inch heel wedges may also provide immediate comfort for ambulatory patients. Encourage patients to return to a heel-toe walking sequence as quickly as possible. When this is achieved, they can discontinue using the heel lift.**

✅ Gentle stretching may be initiated as soon as it can be accomplished without pain. Strengthening may begin as soon as 24 hours after the initial injury. Massage is helpful as an adjunct to a strengthening program.

✅ **Patients should be reassured about the generally benign nature of this injury and the excellent chance for a full recovery. They should also be warned about potentially alarming ecchymosis that may develop in the days following the injury and be reassured that this is a benign phenomenon.**

✅ Athletes generally can return to training and competition in 4 to 6 weeks following the injury, although severe tears may take up to 12 weeks to heal. Sports-specific activities can be resumed once the athlete is pain free with full and symmetric range of motion (ROM) and full strength has been regained. Strengthening and stretching should continue for several months to overcome the increased risk for reinjury resulting from the deposition of scar tissue involved in the healing process.

What Not to Do

❌ Do not bother getting radiographs of the area unless there is a suspected associated bony injury. This is a soft tissue injury that is not generally associated with fractures.

❌ Do not attempt to evaluate Achilles tendon function merely by asking the patient to plantarflex the foot. Achilles tendon function is only isolated with the calf squeeze test.

Discussion

The main function of the gastrocnemius muscle is to plantarflex the ankle. The plantaris muscle is a pencil-sized structure tapering down to a fine tendon that runs beneath the gastrocnemius and soleus muscles to attach to the Achilles tendon or to the medial side of the tubercle of the calcaneus. The function of the muscle is of little importance, and, with rupture of either the muscle or the tendon, the transient disability is due only to the pain of the torn fibers or swelling from the hemorrhage. Most instances of tennis leg are now thought to be the result of partial tears of the medial belly of the gastrocnemius muscle or to ruptures of blood vessels within that muscle. Throughout the belly of the muscle, the medial gastrocnemius has several origins of tendinous formation. Most strains or tears occur at this musculotendinous junction. The greater the initial pain and swelling, the longer one can expect the disability to last.

Tendon ruptures typically affect men in their third or fourth decade who are active in sports. The average occurrence of a gastrocnemius muscle tear is in the fourth to sixth decade. A tendon rupture is usually an indicator of intratendinous degenerative changes. Acute ruptures of the musculus plantaris tendon can be associated with a tear of the gastrocnemius or soleus muscle. An injury to the gastrocnemius muscle, soleus muscle, or Achilles tendon can be related to a plantaris tear.

Achilles tendon injury can occur with the identical mechanism of a plantaris tendon or medial gastrocnemius rupture. Because the pain and debility may be similar, clinical differentiation is sometimes difficult.

The diagnosis of Achilles tendon rupture is missed by the initial examiner in up to 25% of patients.

One misleading finding is that the patient is able to plantarflex the foot with no resistance because several other muscles (toe flexors, peroneus) also perform this action. The expected defect in the tendon may also be obscured by edema or hemorrhage. **The squeeze test (Thompson or Simmonds test) is usually an infallible sign of complete rupture, but a false negative might arise if the plantaris tendon is left intact.** Imaging techniques—including real-time high-resolution ultrasonography and MRI—are now used to aid diagnosis. Ultrasonography usually costs less than MRI; however, when limited MRI protocols are available and only a few images of the suspected region of disease are obtained, pricing can be competitive and will give images superior to ultrasonography.

Other entities that can be confused with plantaris tendon and medial gastrocnemius rupture are Baker cyst rupture and deep venous thrombosis. When physical findings are dubious, the history along with Doppler ultrasonography will often help clarify the diagnosis.

Direct injection of steroids and administration of systemic corticosteroids and fluoroquinolone antibiotics are associated with an increase in the risk for Achilles tendon rupture. Other disease processes, such as rheumatoid arthritis, systemic lupus erythematosus, chronic renal failure, hyperuricemia, genetically determined collagen abnormalities, arteriosclerosis, and diabetes mellitus, have been implicated as risk factors for rupture. With age, tendons stiffen from the effects of reduced glycosaminoglycan content and increased collagen concentration. Blood and nutrient supply also are reduced with age.

Suggested Readings

Glazer, J. L., & Hosey, R. G. (2004). Soft-tissue injuries of the lower extremity. *Primary Care, 31,* 1005–1024.

Legome, E., & Pancu, D. (2004). Future applications for emergency ultrasound. *Emergency Medicine Clinics of North America, 22,* 817–827.

Maffulli, N., & Wong, J. (2003). Rupture of the Achilles and patellar tendons. *Clinics in Sports Medicine, 22,* 761–776.

van der Linden, P. D., Sturkenboom, M. C., Herings, R. M., et al. (2003). Increased risk of Achilles tendon rupture with quinolone antibacterial use, especially in elderly patients taking oral corticosteroids. *Archives of Internal Medicine, 163,* 1801–1807.

Zickmantel, B., Krause, F., & Frauchiger, L. (2018). Isolated rupture of the distal plantaris muscle. *Journal of Foot and Ankle Surgery, 57*(5), 995–996.

Radial Head Fracture

Presentation

A patient has fallen on an outstretched hand and has a normal, nonpainful shoulder, wrist, and hand; on careful examination, however, the patient has pain in the elbow joint. Swelling may be noted over the antecubital fossa, and the patient may be able to fully flex the elbow joint, but there is pain and decreased range of motion (ROM) on extension, supination, and pronation of the forearm. The patient will be unable to fully extend the elbow joint. Tenderness is greatest on palpation over the radial head. Radiographs may show a fracture of the head of the radius. Often, however, no fracture is visible, and the only radiographic signs are of an elbow effusion or hemarthrosis pushing the posterior fat pad out of the olecranon fossa and the anterior fat pad out of its normal position on the lateral view (Fig. 125.1). In all radiographic views, a line down the center of the radius should point to the capitellum of the lateral condyle, ruling out a dislocation.

What to Do

⊘ **Obtain a detailed history of the mechanism of injury and do a careful physical examination, looking for the features described, and, when present, obtain radiographs of the elbow, looking for visible fat pads as well as possible fracture lines.** The evaluation should include an assessment of neurovascular status and a comparison with the uninjured elbow for baseline motion, strength, and stability. Examine the shoulder and wrist on the affected side to rule out an associated injury.

⊘ **Radiographs are unnecessary if the patient can fully extend the elbow with the forearm in supination. It can be assumed that there is no elbow fracture,** and no further treatment is necessary other than reassurance and the possible use of acetaminophen or nonsteroidal anti-inflammatory drugs (NSAIDs) when tolerated.

⊘ **For nondisplaced fractures, a sling is all that is necessary.** Refer these patients to an orthopedist within 3 to 5 days for definitive care. The patient should be instructed to not wait longer, because early mobilization is thought to be important for proper healing.

⊘ **If there is a displaced or comminuted radial head fracture, immobilize the elbow in 90% of flexion and the forearm in full supination (preventing pronation and supination of the hand) with a gutter splint extending from the proximal humerus to the hand, and then place in a sling for comfort** (Fig. 125.2). These patients should also receive early orthopedic consultation or follow-up because with displacement of greater than 2 mm or comminution, surgical repair may be recommended.

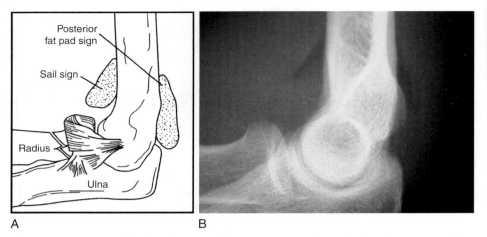

Fig. 125.1 Radiologic evidence of elbow hemarthrosis. (Adapted from Raby, N., Berman, L., & de Lacey, G. [2005]. *Accident and emergency radiology.* Philadelphia, PA: Saunders.)

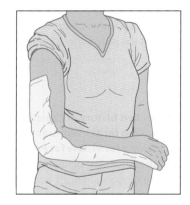
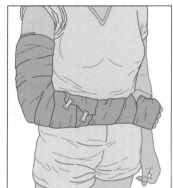

Fig. 125.2 Long-arm gutter splint for complex radial head fractures.

✅ **Provide adequate analgesia,** especially during the first few days. NSAIDs and acetaminophen are first line in the absence of contraindications. Opiate analgesics can be prescribed for the first 2–3 days, if necessary.

✅ **When there is an inability to fully extend the elbow, along with a positive fat pad sign without a visible fracture, explain to the patient the probability of a fracture, despite radiographs that only demonstrate an effusion. Treat it as a nondisplaced fracture (see earlier) and arrange for follow-up.**

✅ **For uncomplicated fractures, ROM exercises should begin as soon as possible and certainly within the first week post-injury** to reduce the risk for developing permanent loss of motion because of elbow joint contractures.

What Not to Do

(X) Do not obtain radiographs on all patients with minimal symptoms after a minor injury. The elbow extension test, as described earlier, can be used as a sensitive screening test for patients with acute injury to the elbow. Patients who can fully extend the affected elbow can be safely treated without radiography.

(X) Do not miss a dislocation of the radial head. Examine all radiographs; a line drawn through the radial head and shaft should always line up with the capitellum (radiocapitellar line).

(X) Do not treat simple radial head fractures (minimal or no displacement without comminuted fragments) with prolonged immobilization. Joint motion is difficult to recover even with extensive physical therapy. Avoiding the problem by providing early mobilization is preferable to attempting to reverse an established joint contracture.

Discussion

The elbow is a hinge (ginglymus) joint between the distal humerus, the proximal ends of the radius and ulna, and the superior radioulnar joint. The lateral capitellum of the distal humerus articulates with the radial head, enabling flexion and extension as well as pronation and supination.

Radial head fractures are relatively common, representing approximately one-third of all elbow fractures. Radial head fractures are the result of trauma, usually from a fall on the outstretched arm. The force of impact is transmitted up the hand through the wrist and forearm to the radial head, which is forced into the capitellum, where it is fractured and possibly deformed.

Outcomes are generally inversely proportional to the amount of force involved in the mechanism of injury, with simple fractures doing better than more comminuted ones. However, the prognosis for these fractures may also be influenced by associated injuries and patient-related factors (age, body index mass, gender, tobacco habit, etc.). One study concludes that patients with associated injuries had a significant loss of extension and total elbow ROM, which were both correlated with worse functional outcome scores. Therefore definitive treatment choice (surgical vs. conservative) should consider all related injuries and specifically address them to favor early mobilization and potentially prevent worse outcomes.

Small nondisplaced fractures of the radial head may show up on radiographs weeks later or never.

Because pronation and supination of the hand are achieved by rotating the radial head on the capitellum of the humerus, very small imperfections in the healing of a radial head fracture that involves the joint may produce enormous impairment of hand function, which may be only partly improved by surgical excision of the radial head. Early orthopedic referral is essential because treatment is controversial.

One other study observes that radial head fractures are associated with a high rate of concomitant ligament tears. The authors recommend viewing radial head fractures not merely as osseous lesions but as osteoligamentous lesions. They conclude that simple fractures displaced less than 2 mm can be treated nonoperatively and that prolonged rehabilitation should raise suspicion of complicating additional injuries. They also note that the treatment of choice for 2 to 5 mm displaced partial articular fractures remains debatable and that several investigators report good results of nonoperative treatment comparable to open reduction and internal fixation (ORIF) but with lower complication rates. However, rate of osteoarthritis seems to be higher with nonoperative treatment.

Always keep in mind that most occult or small radial head fractures are treated symptomatically with early ROM exercises and generally heal without functional loss.

Suggested Readings

Anderson, S. J. (2005). Sports injuries. *Disease-a-Month, 35*, 110–164.

Burkhart, K. J., Wegmann, K., Müller, L. P., & Gohlke, F. E. Fractures of the radial head. *Hand Clinics, 31*(4), 533–546.

Couture, A., Hébert-Davies, J., Chapleau, J., Laflamme, G. Y., Sandman, E., & Rouleau, D. M. (2019). Factors affecting outcome of partial radial head fractures: A retrospective cohort study. *Orthopaedics and Traumatology: Surgery & Research, 105*(8), 1585–1592.

Rosenblatt, Y., Athwal, G. S., & Faber, K. J. (2008). Current recommendations for the treatment of radial head fractures. *Orthopedic Clinics of North America, 39*, 173–185.

Radial Neuropathy

(Saturday Night Palsy)

Presentation

The patient has injured the upper arm, usually by sleeping with the arm over the back of a chair. The patient now presents, usually the next day, holding the affected hand and wrist with the good hand and reports decreased or absent sensation on the radial and dorsal side of the hand and wrist and the inability to extend the wrist (wrist drop), thumb, and finger joints. With the hand supinated (palm up) and the extensors aided by gravity, hand function may appear normal, but when the hand is pronated (palm down), the wrist and hand will drop (Fig. 126.1). Symptoms can also begin several days after the initial insult, leading to a delayed presentation.

What to Do

✓ When there is a history of significant trauma, look for associated injuries. This sort of nerve injury may be associated with cervical spine fracture, injury to the brachial plexus in the axilla, or fracture of the humerus. X-ray imaging can evaluate for fractures, dislocations, and bony tumors that may be the cause of this nerve injury.

✓ **Document all motor and sensory impairment.** When practical, draw a diagram of the area of decreased sensation, and grade muscle strength of various groups (flexors, extensors, etc.) on a scale of 1 to 5. The triceps reflex may be lost and the brachioradialis reflex will be decreased or absent.

✓ Patients with radial palsy often appear to have weakness in addition to radial-innervated muscles. A study of volunteers found decreased strength of handgrip, key pinch, and thumb palmar adduction after radial nerve block. Patients have difficulty spreading the fingers, suggesting weakness of finger abduction, but this is correctable by supporting the fingers or extending the hand when the examiner holds the wrist level with the forearm.

✓ **If there is complete paralysis or complete anesthesia, arrange for early neurologic consultation and treatment. Incomplete lesions may be satisfactorily referred for delayed follow-up evaluation and physical therapy.**

✓ **Construct a splint, extending from proximal forearm to just beyond the metacarpophalangeal joint (leaving the thumb free), which holds the wrist in 90-degree extension** (Fig. 126.2). This and a sling will help protect the hand, also preventing edema and distortion of tendons, ligaments, and joint capsules, which can result in loss of hand function after strength returns.

✓ Explain to the patient the nature of the peripheral nerve injury; if minor, recovery may take place over a few hours; if more significant, there may be a slow rate of regeneration (about 1 mm

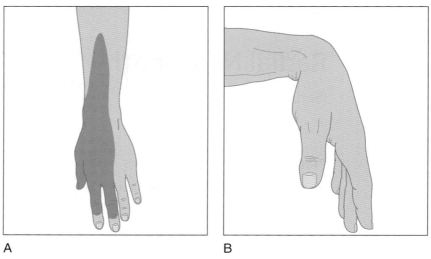

Fig. 126.1 (A) Decreased or absent sensation on the radial and dorsal sides of the hand and wrist. (B) Hand will drop when positioned palm down.

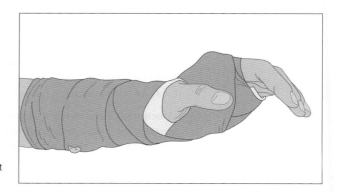

Fig. 126.2 Construct a splint that holds the wrist in 90-degree extension.

per day or approximately 1 inch per month). **Usually, recovery is not rapid, with even mild cases resolving at the earliest in 2 to 4 months and often much longer**.

✅ **Stress the importance of splinting and physical therapy** for preservation of the eventual return of function.

✅ **Arrange for follow-up.**

✅ In follow-up additional diagnostic tools can be helpful in evaluating alternative causes and complications as well as for predicting prognosis. Electromyography and nerve conduction studies are able to localize lesions anatomically, which can help differentiate between cervical radiculopathies, brachial plexopathies, and peripheral neuropathies. Ultrasound can be a low-cost, low-risk modality that can assist with visualizing the nerve and identifying areas of damage or disruption. With more severe trauma, it can also be highly beneficial in early identification of obvious nerve disruption and hastening early surgical intervention for these cases.

What Not to Do

(X) Do not be misled by the patient's ability to extend the interphalangeal joints of the fingers, which may be accomplished by the ulnar-innervated interosseous muscles.

Discussion

Usually there is no difficulty in establishing the diagnosis of radial palsy (also called Saturday night palsy, honeymoon palsy, or Saturday night arm). **This neuropathy is produced by prolonged, direct compression of the radial nerve as it wraps around the humerus at the upper medial arm or axilla,** where its proximity to the bone makes it susceptible to injury. Most commonly, it occurs when a person falls into a deep sleep, either drug-induced or a result of intoxication, and is held up by the arm thrown over the back of a chair or compressed in some other similar fashion. Because depressant drugs and alcohol predispose a person to prolonged sleep in one position (without the movement typical of normal sleep), the weight of the body may exert pressure on the arm for enough time (usually a period of several hours) to produce wallerian degeneration of nerve fibers. Less severe forms may befall the swain who keeps his arm on his date's chairback for an entire double feature, ignoring the growing pain and paresis. **One must be aware that Saturday night palsy can be caused by any unnatural positioning or use of the limbs that can cause compression by a similar mechanism.** This includes but is not limited to compressive clothing or accessories, improper use of crutches, and prolonged blood pressure cuff usage.

If the injury to the radial nerve is in the forearm, sensation typically is spared, despite the wrist drop. The deficient groups will be the wrist ulnar extensors as well as the metacarpophalangeal extensors. A high radial palsy in the axilla (e.g., from leaning on crutches) will involve all of the radial nerve innervations, including the triceps.

In many circumstances, this condition gives rise to a temporary neuropathy or plexopathy, which generally resolves within hours or days. In most cases, the moderate to severe Saturday night palsy resolves spontaneously and completely over the course of a few months. Pain control, a wrist splint, and passive range-of-motion (ROM) exercises are usually sufficient treatment.

Definitive treatment for Saturday night palsy is largely focused on physical rehabilitation.

Physical therapy involves the use of a soft wrist splint that holds the wrist in extension. However, it is important to allow for full passive ROM of the affected extremity during rehabilitation, which can be accomplished by using a dynamic splint. These measures can be supplemented with supportive care, including nonsteroidal antiinflammatory drugs (NSAIDs), systemic corticosteroids, steroid injections, and rest from vigorous use.

It should be kept in mind, though, that if the compression is severe and prolonged, a graver form of this condition known as crush syndrome may occur. Skeletal muscle injury, brought about by protracted immobilization, leads to muscle decay, causing rhabdomyolysis, which may in turn precipitate acute renal failure. This condition is potentially fatal and has an extremely high morbidity.

The prognosis for Saturday night palsy depends on the extent of the injury, which is determined by the force and duration of compression. Mild damage results in neuropraxia, a transient conduction block without nerve degeneration. This type of injury will almost always result in complete recovery. Moderate damage results in axonotmesis, characterized by axonal damage and wallerian degeneration that can have incomplete or late recovery. Severe damage results in neurotmesis, characterized by complete axon degradation and Schwann cell death with a low chance of full recovery.

The management of radial nerve palsy associated with fractures of the shaft of the humerus has been disputed for several decades. The overall prevalence of radial nerve palsy after fracture of the shaft of the humerus in 21 papers was 11.8%. Fractures of the middle and middle-distal parts of the shaft had a significantly higher association with radial nerve palsy than those in other parts. Transverse and spiral fractures were more likely to be associated with radial nerve palsy than oblique and comminuted patterns of fracture. The overall rate of recovery was 88.1%, with spontaneous recovery reaching 70.7% in patients treated conservatively. There was no significant difference in the final results when comparing groups that were initially

Continued

Discussion continued

managed expectantly with those explored early, suggesting that the initial expectant treatment did not affect the extent of nerve recovery adversely and would avoid many unnecessary operations.

Surgical management should be reserved for severe injuries of the radial nerve or for cases in which the compression results from an intrinsic process such as a mass, bone spur, or cyst.

It is interesting to note that the term *Saturday night palsy* may have an origin different than the commonly accepted association of Saturday night with carousing. A group of authors offer an alternate explanation: They think the term *Saturday night palsy* was introduced mistakenly as a simplification of saturnine palsy (much like the way the word *palsy* was shortened from *paralysis*). Saturnine palsy, which is a relatively common complication of lead poisoning, has the same clinical presentation of radial nerve compression, and *Saturday night palsy* even sounds like *saturnine palsy*. Moreover, Saturday, lead, carousing, and alcohol are associated with each other through their connection to *Saturn*, the Roman god of agriculture, which encourages the association of the two syndromes with one another.

Suggested Readings

Ansari, F. H., & Juergens, A. L. (2020). *Saturday night palsy*. StatPearls [Internet].

Devitt, B. M., Baker, J. F., Ahmed, M., et al. (2011). Saturday night palsy or Sunday morning hangover? A case report of alcohol-induced crush syndrome. *Archives of Orthopedic and Trauma Surgery*, *131*, 39–43.

Shao, Y. C., Harwood, M. R., Grotz, W., Limb, D., & Giannoudis, P. V. (2005). Radial nerve palsy associated with fractures of the shaft of the humerus. *The Journal of Bone and Joint Surgery (Britian)*, *87-B*(12).

Spinner, R. J., Poliakoff, M. B., & Tiel, R. L. (2002). The origin of "Saturday night palsy"? *Neurosurgery*, *51*(3), 737–741.

Scaphoid Fracture

Presentation

The patient (usually 14–40 years of age) fell on an outstretched hand (FOOSH) with the wrist held rigid and extended and now complains of decreased range of motion (ROM) and a deep full pain in the wrist, particularly on the dorsal radial side. Physical examination discloses no deformity or ecchymosis but shows pain with motion and palpation and often swelling. Swelling may be seen, especially in the anatomic snuff box, the hollow seen on the radial aspect of the wrist when the thumb is in full extension (between the tendon of the extensor pollicis longus and the tendons of the abductor pollicis longus and extensor pollicis brevis) (Fig. 127.1). The pain, which may be mild, is worsened by gripping or squeezing.

What to Do

✓ For comfort, apply a cold pack and a temporary splint or sling and administer analgesia as needed.

✓ **A thorough history and well-performed physical examination, along with a high index of suspicion,** are necessary to make the diagnosis.

✓ **The classic hallmark of anatomic snuff box tenderness on examination is a highly sensitive (90%) indication of scaphoid fracture, but it is nonspecific (specificity, 40%). A thorough hand and wrist examination should be performed, as well as examination of other parts of the body, as indicated. Tenderness of the scaphoid tubercle (i.e., extend the patient's wrist with one hand and apply pressure to the tuberosity at the proximal wrist crease with the opposite hand) (Fig. 127.2) has a sensitivity of 87% but is more specific than snuff box tenderness (57%). Absence of tenderness with these two maneuvers makes a scaphoid fracture highly unlikely.**

✓ **Pain with the scaphoid compression test (applying a longitudinal axial load to the scaphoid via the proximal phalanx of the thumb through to the first metacarpal) (Fig. 127.3) may also be helpful in identifying an underlying scaphoid fracture. Another maneuver that suggests fracture of the scaphoid is pain in the snuff box with pronation of the wrist, followed by ulnar deviation (52% positive predictive value, 100% negative predictive value) (Fig. 127.4).**

✓ **Be vigilant for associated injuries,** such as fractures of the distal radius, lunate, or radial head at the elbow, scapholunate dissociation, or median nerve injury.

✓ **When any clinical suspicion for a scaphoid fracture is raised, obtain radiographs of the wrist that include a scaphoid (navicular) view (a posteroanterior view in ulnar deviation). Conservative estimates suggest that 10% to 20% of scaphoid fractures are not visible on any view in the acute setting** (Fig. 127.5). An abnormal scaphoid "fat stripe" or "stripe sign" may appear

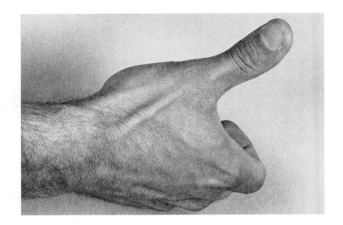

Fig. 127.1 Examine for swelling or tenderness within the anatomic snuff box.

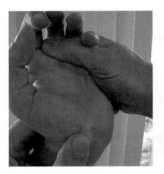

Fig. 127.2 Palpating the scaphoid tubercle while extending the wrist.

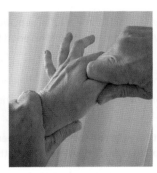

Fig. 127.3 The scaphoid compression test.

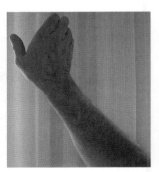

Fig. 127.4 Pronation of the wrist, followed by ulnar deviation.

as an outward bulging radiolucent line in the soft tissue adjacent to the scaphoid, representing bleeding within the joint space, and may indicate the presence of an occult fracture.

✓ **When there is scaphoid tenderness or pain elicited by any of the aforementioned diagnostic maneuvers, but radiographs are negative, the wrist should still be immobilized in a short-arm thumb spica splint with the wrist in mild extension and the thumb interphalangeal joint free** (Fig. 127.6). Follow-up radiographs at 2 weeks may reveal bone resorption adjacent to a fracture site or early callus formation if an occult fracture was present; otherwise, all splinting can be removed. Arrange for follow-up within 5 to 7 days.

✓ **When occult fractures are suspected in athletes, individuals opposed to wearing a splint for 2 weeks, or workers who require a more urgent diagnosis, a bone scan, computed tomography (CT), or magnetic resonance imaging (MRI) may be considered for additional imaging.** A bone scan may be positive 24 hours after the injury; however, it can take 4 days for abnormal uptake to appear at the fracture site. A normal bone scan 4 days after

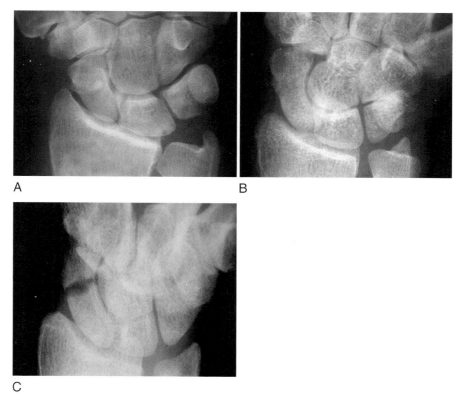

A

B

C

Fig. 127.5 (A–C) Radiograph of the wrist demonstrating a scaphoid fracture—identified (with certainty) on one projection only. (Adapted from Raby, N., Berman, L., & de Lacey, G. [2005]. *Accident and emergency radiology.* Philadelphia, PA: Saunders.)

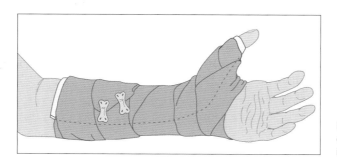

Fig. 127.6 Splint or cast the wrist in mild extension, including the thumb, but leaving the interphalangeal (IP) joint free.

injury is accurate in excluding scaphoid fracture. MRI is very sensitive and will have an abnormal bone marrow signal 48 hours postfracture; however, it may not clarify fracture displacement. **A CT scan gives clearer fracture visualization and is more accurate for determination of displacement. One small study concluded that CT should be used with caution for triage of nondisplaced scaphoid fractures because false-positive results occur, perhaps from misinterpretation of vascular foraminae or other normal lines in the scaphoid. Given the** relative infrequency of true fractures among patients with suspected scaphoid fractures, CT might be better for ruling out a fracture than for ruling one in.

✓ Ultrasound examination with routine equipment is not appropriate in the initial evaluation of suspected scaphoid fractures. **High–spatial-resolution ultrasonography has been shown to be reliable and accurate in identifying occult scaphoid fractures.**

✓ **When initial radiographs demonstrate a scaphoid fracture, the treatment is dictated by the degree of injury.**

✓ **For nondisplaced fractures** (<1 mm of fracture separation without any visible step-off on any radiographic view), **the treatment of choice is a long-arm thumb spica splint, with follow-up with a hand surgeon or orthopedist arranged for 5 to 7 days after treatment.**

✓ **For fractures with significant displacement, angulation, or comminution or for fractures involving the proximal pole of the scaphoid, immediate orthopedic or hand surgeon consultation should be made. (See review of perilunate and lunate dislocations in Discussion box.)**

✓ Patients who are placed in a splint should be given standard cast instructions.

✓ **It is very important to explain to the patient** the common difficulty of visualizing scaphoid fractures on radiographs, the possibility of poor healing in scaphoid fractures because of variable blood supply, and the resultant necessity of keeping this splint or cast in place until reevaluated by a specialist. The importance of this follow-up appointment should be emphasized.

✓ **Provide a sling if needed for comfort and prescribe acetaminophen or nonsteroidal antiinflammatory drugs (NSAIDs), adding a brief course of narcotics when necessary.**

✓ As with any acute injury, have the patient apply ice for 15 to 20 minutes three or four times per day if this provides comfort, and maintain elevation above the level of the heart as much as possible.

What Not to Do

✗ Do not assume a wrist injury is "just a sprain" when radiographs are negative. Any wrist injury with significant tenderness, pain on ROM, and swelling should be splinted and referred for further evaluation.

Discussion

Of all the wrist injuries encountered in the emergency department, fracture of the scaphoid is one of the most commonly missed. Radiographic findings can be subtle or even absent. Accurate early diagnosis of scaphoid fracture is critical, however, because the morbidity associated with a missed or delayed diagnosis is significant and can result in long-term pain, loss of mobility, decreased function, and litigation.

The scaphoid bone is unique for two reasons. First, it spans both the proximal and distal carpal row, making an intact scaphoid imperative for carpal stability. Second, the scaphoid relies on an interosseous blood supply that enters distal to its middle third and provides the sole blood supply to its proximal pole. Therefore fractures through the proximal third disrupt the blood supply and are prone to osteonecrosis and nonunion.

The location of the scaphoid fracture (proximal, middle, or distal third) depends mostly on the position of the forearm at the time of the injury. Fracture of the middle third is most common (80%), followed by fractures of the proximal third (15%), fractures of the distal third (4%), and fractures of the distal tubercle (1%).

In general, the more proximal, oblique, or displaced the fracture, the greater the risk of interrupting the blood supply. Distal fractures heal most rapidly, often within 6 weeks. In contrast, proximal fractures, because of the tenuous blood supply, may take 6 months. Nonunion complicates up to 20% to 30% of proximal-third fractures and 10% to 20% of middle-third fractures. Nonunion of distal-third fractures is relatively rare. In addition to nonunion, patients are also at risk for the development of avascular necrosis of the scaphoid. This outcome occurs in approximately 10% of proximal-pole fractures and 5% of middle-third fractures.

Open reduction and internal fixation have now become standard for all proximal-pole fractures and are required for unstable fractures. Also consider surgical referral for any athlete or manual laborer because many surgeons offer percutaneous screw fixation techniques to these patients to decrease the time of cast immobilization.

Other carpal bone injuries, including carpal dislocations, can also occur typically (but not always) in a high-energy injury. Pay careful attention to the carpal bone anatomy in a swollen, tender wrist particularly in the absence of a fracture. Careful attention should be paid to the distance between the scaphoid and lunate to evaluate for scapholunate disruption. In addition, a triangular appearance of the lunate and in anteroposterior (AP) projection, the so-called "piece of pie sign," is indicative of lunate pathology—either a lunate or perilunate dislocation. A lateral view should be obtained to evaluate for a lunate tilting of the lunate proximally or a so-called "spilled teacup" sign, which would indicate a full lunate dislocation. All of these carpal injuries require urgent hand surgeon evaluation (Figs. 127.7 and 127.8).

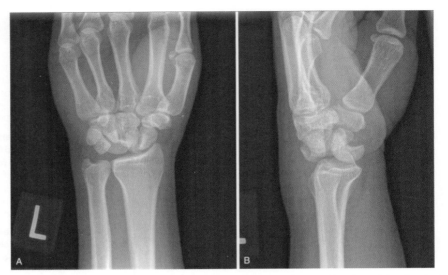

Fig. 127.7 Perilunate dislocation. (A) This posteroanterio r view of the wrist shows an abnormal-appearing lunate bone, obvious disruption of the normal carpal arcs, and commonly associated and, in this case, displaced scaphoid fracture. (B) Lateral view shows a dislocated and dorsally displaced capitate bone in relation to the lunate. Of note, the lunate maintains its articular connection and alignment with the radius, suggesting perilunate dislocation. (With permission from Williams, D. T., & Kim, H. T. [2018]. Wrist and forearm. In: *Rosen's emergency medicine: Concepts and clinical practice* [2nd ed., pp. 508–529]. Philadelphia, PA: Elsevier.)

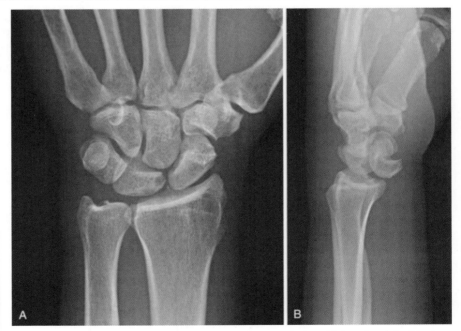

Fig. 127.8 Lunate dislocation. (A) This posteroanterior view shows the characteristic triangular shape of the lunate bone during dislocation. (B) Volar displacement of the lunate resembles a spilled teacup on the lateral view. Note the disrupted articulation between the lunate and distal radius and realignment of the radius, capitate, and metacarpals, suggesting lunate dislocation. (With permission from Williams, D. T., & Kim, H. T. [2018]. Wrist and forearm. In: *Rosen's emergency medicine: Concepts and clinical practice* [2nd ed., pp. 508–529]. Philadelphia, PA: Elsevier.)

Suggested Readings

Breederveld, R. S., & Tuinebreijer, W. E. (2004). Investigation of computed tomographic scan concurrent criterion validity in doubtful scaphoid fracture of the wrist. *Journal of Trauma*, *57*, 851–854.

Brydie, A., & Raby, N. (2003). Early MRI in the management of clinical scaphoid fracture. *British Journal of Radiology*, *76*, 296–300.

Davidson, J. S., Brown, D. J., Barnes, S. N., & Bruce, C. E. (2001). Simple treatments for torus fractures of the distal radius. *Journal of Bone and Joint Surgery (Britain)*, *83*, 1731–1735.

Kaneshiro, S. A., Failla, J. M., & Tashman, S. (1999). Scaphoid fracture displacement with forearm rotation in a short-arm thumb spica cast. *Journal of Hand Surgery*, *24*, 984–991.

Murphy, D. G., Eisenhauer, M. A., Powe, J., et al. (1995). Can a 4-day bone scan accurately determine the presence or absence of scaphoid fracture? *Annals of Emergency Medicine*, *26*, 434–438.

Parmelee-Peters, K., & Eathorne, S. W. (2005). The wrist: Common injuries and management. *Primary Care*, *32*, 35–70.

Perron, A. D., & Brady, W. J. (2003). Evaluation and management of the high-risk orthopedic emergency. *Emergency Medicine Clinics of North America*, *21*, 159–204.

Phillips, T. G., Reibach, A. M., & Slomiany, W. P. (2004). Diagnosis and management of scaphoid fractures. *American Family Physician*, *70*(5), 879–884.

Stanbury, S. J., & Elfar, J. C. (2011). Perilunate dislocation and perilunate fracture-dislocation. *Journal of the American Academy of Orthopedic Surgery*, 19(9), 554–562.

Waeckerle, J. F. (1987). A prospective study identifying the sensitivity of radiographic findings and the efficacy of clinical findings in carpal navicular fractures. *Annals of Emergency Medicine*, *16*, 733–737.

Williams, D. T., & Kim, H. T. (2018). Wrist and forearm. In *Rosen's emergency medicine: Concepts and clinical practice* (2nd ed.) (pp. 508–529). Philadelphia, PA: Elsevier.

Shoulder Dislocation

Presentation

The patient arrives holding one arm with the opposite hand, complaining of severe pain that increases with any movement of the injured shoulder joint. The patient states that the "shoulder is out," and is unable to move it because of the pain. Patients with anterior dislocations typically present with their arm held fixed, slightly internally rotated, and abducted.

Often, the patient had had the arm lifted horizontally to the side ("quarterback position") when it was leveraged posteriorly, causing the dislocation. Another mechanism may have been a fall onto an outstretched arm.

Recurrent dislocations may be the result of relatively minor forces, such as those produced when reaching into the back seat of a car from the driver's seat or rolling over while asleep.

An acute shoulder dislocation is the separation of the humerus from the glenoid fossa of the scapula at the glenohumeral joint.

The deltopectoral groove may show a bulge (caused by the dislocated head of the humerus), and the acromion appears to be prominent laterally, with an emptiness beneath the acromion where the humeral head should be (Fig. 128.1).

Of shoulder dislocations, 90% to 98% are anterior, as just described. Most of the others are posterior and are usually caused by trauma (67% of cases), a seizure (31%), or high-voltage electric shock (2%). Patients arrive complaining only of shoulder pain with their arm held fixed in internal rotation and adduction. Posterior shoulder dislocations can be subtle on anteroposterior (AP) and scapular Y views. A rotation of the humeral head or so-called "light bulb sign" may be the only indication. If AP and scapular Y views are equivocal and there is a high clinical concern, an axillary lateral radiograph should be obtained (Fig. 128.2).

Inferior dislocations (luxatio erecta) are rare and occur with the arm above the head at the time of injury. They are associated with high-energy trauma, specifically grasping a fixed, overhead object while falling. The patient presents with the forearm elevated to the level of the forehead and reports, "I can't put my arm down." Neurovascular injury and fracture often accompany these unusual dislocations, which demand urgent orthopedic consultation.

What to Do

⊘ **Quickly examine the patient to rule out neurologic or vascular deficits.** Although it is rare, arterial damage can be a complication of shoulder dislocation. **Test and record the sensation over the lateral deltoid to establish whether there is an injury to the axillary nerve (approximately 1% incidence).**

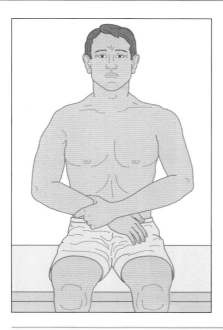

Fig. 128.1 Shoulder dislocation with loss of the normal deltoid bulge. (Adapted from Ruiz, E., & Cicero, J. J. [1995]. *Emergency management of skeletal injuries*. St. Louis, MO: Mosby.)

✓ **Provide analgesia when necessary;** intravenous (IV) narcotics may be needed.

✓ **An alternative is the use of intraarticular lidocaine.** After preparing the skin with povidone-iodine, using a 1.5-inch, 20-gauge needle, inject 20 mL of 1% lidocaine 2 cm inferiorly and directly lateral to the acromion, into the lateral sulcus left by the absent humeral head.

✓ **Often, analgesics are not needed.** This may depend on whether the clinician can gain the patient's trust and apply gentle, stabilizing, pain-relieving traction to the patient's affected arm.

✓ **Reduction should be performed promptly. Obtaining radiographs may be unnecessary** and may serve only to delay this procedure and prolong patient discomfort. There is no need to obtain radiographs when you feel confident about your clinical diagnosis and there was a relatively atraumatic mechanism of injury (especially when there is a history of a previous shoulder dislocation).

✓ **Radiographs should be obtained in patients older than 40 years of age and when significant trauma is involved,** such as from a fall from a height, a sports injury, or a motor vehicle collision.

✓ **Keep in mind that minor fractures are not a contraindication to reduction,** but significant fractures of the glenoid socket or humeral head may preempt attempts at closed reduction and may require a surgical approach.

✓ **If the patient is relatively comfortable and cooperative and there are no contraindications, you can begin reducing the shoulder without first starting an IV for administering analgesics.** Muscle spasm is the main obstacle, and gentle and gradual maneuvers are always more likely to be successful than high-force rapid movement techniques, which are more likely to cause complications.

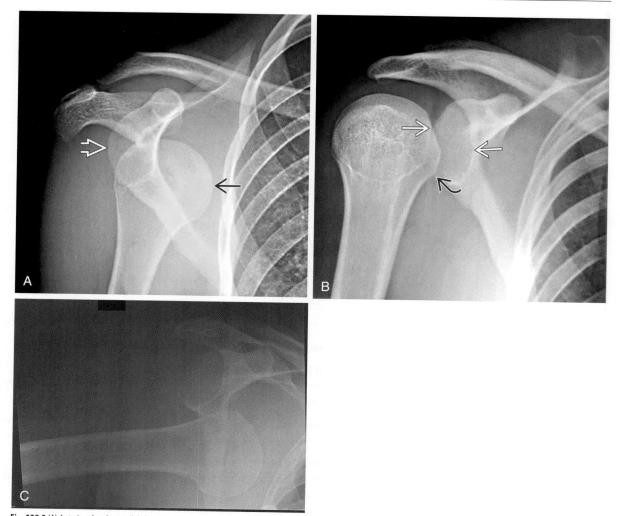

Fig. 128.2 (A) Anterior glenohumeral dislocation. Anteroposterior (AP) radiograph in a patient with shoulder pain after trauma shows inferior and medial displacement of the humeral head *(black arrow)* relative to the glenoid fossa *(white arrow)*. The humeral head in anterior dislocation is usually pulled medially by muscles and is displaced inferiorly under the coracoid process. (B) Posterior glenohumeral dislocation. AP radiograph shows a patient with shoulder pain after a motorcycle accident. Note the wide glenohumeral joint *(white arrows)*, the so-called rim sign, and loss of the normal half-moon overlap. The humerus is also internally rotated, causing the light bulb sign, where the lesser tuberosity *(black arrow)* projects medially. (C) Inferior glenohumeral dislocation (luxatio erecta humeri). AP radiograph of right shoulder showing inferior dislocation of glenohumeral joint. (A–B, With permission from Tuite, M. J. [2016]. Anterior glenohumeral dislocation. In: Blankenbaker, D. G., et al. [Eds.], *Diagnostic imaging: Musculoskeletal trauma* [2nd ed., pp. 68–71]. Philadelphia, PA: Elsevier; C, with permission from Frank, M. A., et al. [2012]. Irreducible luxatio erecta humeri caused by an aberrant position of the axillary nerve. *Journal of Shoulder and Elbow Surgery, 21*[7], e6–e9 [fig. 2].)

⊘ **Patients who cannot relax because of pain should be given either intraarticular lidocaine or procedural sedation and analgesia (PSA)** (see Appendix E).

⊘ **Positioning and patience are more important than strength for reducing a shoulder. Several techniques can be used successfully, and clinicians should be comfortable with several of them.** If one does not work, try another.

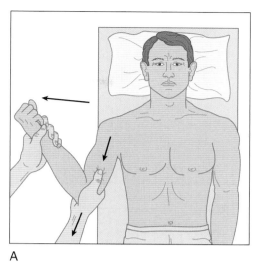
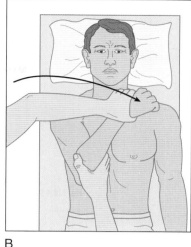

A   B

Fig. 128.3 (A) Slow and gentle external rotation technique. (B) Slow and gentle adduction followed by gradual internal rotation will reduce the majority of dislocations that do not respond to external rotation alone. (Adapted from Ruiz, E., & Cicero, J. J. [1995]. *Emergency management of skeletal injuries*. St. Louis, MO: Mosby.)

✓ **With all techniques, gain patient confidence by holding the arm securely and instructing them to relax. Tell the patient there will not be any sudden movements and that if any pain occurs, you will stop and allow time to get comfortable before starting again. Then, in a very calm and gentle manner, ask the patient to let the muscles go loose so that the shoulder can stretch out "like taffy." This may need to be said repeatedly.**

✓ **Using a modified Hennepin technique** with the elbow flexed at 90 degrees, and the patient resting comfortably on a stretcher with the head elevated 10 to 30 degrees, apply steady traction at the distal humerus. Continue to pull inferiorly and, at the same time, start to externally rotate the forearm very, very slowly. If the patient complains of pain, stop rotating, allow time for the patient to relax, and let the shoulder muscles stretch while traction is maintained along the humerus. Resume external rotation when the patient is comfortable again. Using this method, full external rotation alone will reduce most anterior shoulder dislocations (Fig. 128.3A). (See Video 128.1)

✓ **If the shoulder joint is not felt or seen to reduce**, slowly and gently adduct the humerus while maintaining traction and external rotation until the humerus moves over the chest and is finally resting against the anterior chest wall. You may then, very slowly, internally rotate the forearm until it also meets the anterior chest wall (also demonstrated in above video). Most shoulder dislocations can be reduced comfortably this way, often without the use of any analgesics (see Fig. 128.3B).

✓ **Scapular rotation** is an alternative technique that can be used when the lateral border of the scapula can be palpated. Reduction is accomplished by scapular manipulation. With the patient sitting up, and after providing reassurance as described earlier, have an assistant face the patient and gently lift the patient's outstretched wrist of the affected arm until it is horizontal. The assistant then places the palm of the free hand against the midclavicular area of the injured shoulder as a counterbalance, and then gently but firmly pulls the patient's arm toward oneself while applying slight external rotation to the humerus. The patient should be asked calmly and continuously to

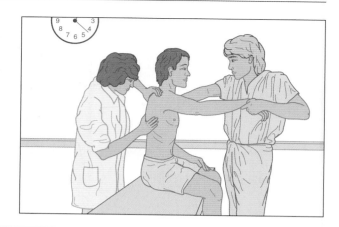

Fig. 128.4 Scapular rotation technique.

relax and let the muscles stretch out. At the same time the assistant is applying traction to the patient's arm, manipulate the scapula by pushing the inferior tip medially and dorsally using both thumbs while stabilizing the superior aspect of the scapula with the upper hand (Fig. 128.4).

This technique can be modified by placing the patient in the prone position with the affected arm hanging dependent over the side of the examination table. Downward traction is applied to the arm with the same slight external rotation of the humerus, and scapular rotation is performed in the same manner as noted earlier.

Scapular rotation without lifting the arm can be an added maneuver performed by an assistant during the Hennepin technique if the patient is positioned sitting upright on the stretcher with the back exposed.

The Spaso technique for reducing anterior shoulder dislocations is simple, requires minimal force, and can be performed by a single clinician. With the patient supine, the clinician grasps the wrist or distal forearm of the affected extremity, very slowly lifts the arm vertically, and, with application of gentle traction, rotates the humerus slightly externally until a "clunk" is felt, indicating a successful reduction.

The Cunningham technique is reported to be painless and fast, using only proper positioning and massage to accomplish reduction. Seat the patient comfortably, as upright as possible, with shoulders relaxed. Supporting the affected arm, slowly and gently move the humerus into full adduction. Gently massage the trapezius and deltoids; this helps to relax the patient and reassures that the doctor is not going to do anything painful.

Then, move on to gently massaging the biceps at the midhumeral level. Ask the patient to shrug the shoulders, continuing the biceps massage. Wait for the patient to relax fully, and the humeral head will slip back into place. Warn the patient that it may feel strange as this happens and not to fight against the movement (Figs 128.5 and 128.6). If the patient cannot relax enough to cooperate, or the arm cannot be adducted, this approach will not work. Videos and detailed instructions can be found at www.shoulderdislocation.net.

For difficult reductions where PSA is being used, the traditional traction against countertraction method can be used. In this method, while the patient lies supine, the clinician grasps the patient's affected arm by the wrist and applies traction at a 45-degree angle of

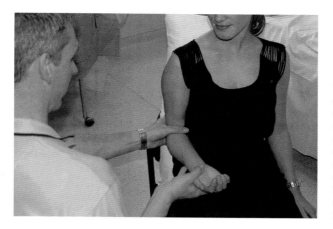

Figure 128.5 Dr. Neil Cunningham demonstrates his technique for reducing shoulder dislocations. Seat the patient comfortably, as upright as possible, with shoulders relaxed. Supporting the affected arm, slowly and gently move the humerus into full adduction. Then gently massage the trapezius and deltoids. (Adapted from Shaw, G. [2011]. Breaking news: Believe it or not: Painless reduction of dislocated shoulders. *Emergency Medicine News*, 33[1], 28.)

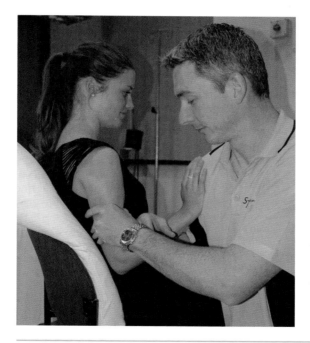

Fig. 128.6 In the second part of the technique, Dr. Cunningham demonstrates how to gently massage the biceps at the midhumeral level. The next step is to ask the patient to shrug her shoulders, continuing the biceps massage. Wait for the patient to fully relax, and the humeral head will slip back into place. (Adapted from Shaw, G. [2011]. Breaking news: Believe it or not: Painless reduction of dislocated shoulders. *Emergency Medicine News*, 33[1], 28.)

abduction while an assistant provides countertraction by wrapping a sheet around the patient's torso and pulls on it in the opposite direction.

✓ **Reexamine the shoulder after it is reduced.** Neurovascular status should again be rechecked.

✓ **Postreduction films are only required if there is uncertainty regarding reduction or if fractures were noted on prereduction radiographs. No studies to date have shown a single iatrogenic postreduction fracture, given the use of more modern, gentler techniques of reduction.**

✅ **When the patient is comfortable and limited range of motion (ROM) has been restored, secure the reduction in a sling and a swathe around the arm and chest. (Although this represents standard postreduction treatment, a recent study suggests that no immobilization at all may actually be the treatment of choice.)**

✅ **After a closed reduction,** discharge the patient (once they are alert) with a prescription for analgesics as needed and an appointment for orthopedic follow-up in 1 week (sooner if there is any problem). Restrictions include no external rotation past neutral and no abduction beyond 90 degrees for 4 to 6 weeks. Most patients experience enough comfort to allow motion after 2 to 3 weeks. Patients may resume all activities, including sports, once there is full ROM without pain and normal strength is regained.

What Not to Do

❌ Do not perform any reduction technique using high-force or rapid movements.

❌ Do not use the forearm as a lever to force reduction and possibly fracture the neck of the humerus.

❌ Do not redislocate the shoulder by repeating the motions of the mechanism of injury.

Discussion

The shoulder is the most mobile joint in the human body. It allows the upper extremity to rotate up to 180 degrees in three different planes, enabling the arm to perform a versatile range of activities. This mobility comes at a cost because it leaves the shoulder prone to dislocation.

In younger patients, most shoulder dislocations are caused by direct trauma and sports injuries. In elderly persons, falls are the predominant cause, and the dislocation often is accompanied by a fracture.

An excessive external rotation or abduction force usually causes anterior dislocations, whereas posterior dislocations usually occur when the humeral head is driven posteriorly with great force and internal rotation, as during a seizure. Posterior dislocations can be subtle and more difficult to diagnose.

The strategy is to relocate the shoulder with minimal damage to the joint capsule and anterior labrum of the glenoid fossa, hoping the patient does not become a chronic dislocator with an unstable shoulder. Chronic dislocators are easier to reduce and come less often to the emergency department because they learn how to relocate their own shoulders. Of patients whose first shoulder dislocation occurs before 20 years of age, 90% will have a recurrent dislocation. Only 14% of first dislocations after 40 years of age recur.

Posterior dislocations can be reduced using traditional in-line traction on the dislocated arm, along with countertraction using a sheet. Posterior pressure on the humeral head may help.

Inferior dislocations can also be reduced using traction/countertraction, but with scapular rotation as an adjunct. Keep in mind though that patients with inferior dislocation are more likely to have associated injuries (e.g., neurovascular injury, humeral and glenoid fractures) and therefore care is typically provided by an orthopedist or trauma surgeon.

Numerous studies have shown that early surgical intervention, rather than conservative treatment (especially in the younger athletic population), provides a reduced incidence of recurrent dislocation. Therefore orthopedic referral is most important for these patients.

Treatment after reduction traditionally includes immobilization of the shoulder for 4 weeks, followed by rehabilitation. One Australian study and a more recent study in *Orthopaedics &*

Discussion continued

Traumatology: Surgery & Research, suggests that putting the arm in internal rotation (the normal sling position) results in more pronounced labral detachment, inhibiting healing of the underlying injury. Additionally, for patients with anterior shoulder dislocation, sling immobilization (internal rotation) provides no benefit, and positioning in external rotation, using an Ultrasling or similar device, might be more effective.

It might be preferable not to immobilize the shoulder at all, and total immobilization may cause worse problems, such as a frozen shoulder, but this remains unproven. After 1 or 2 days, the patient with the uncomplicated shoulder dislocation should be instructed to start gentle ROM exercises to help prevent this complication. It should be stressed to the patient to avoid reproducing the position that originally caused the dislocation.

Suggested Readings

Baykal, B., Sener, S., & Turkan, H. (2005). Scapular manipulation technique for reduction of traumatic anterior shoulder dislocations: Experience of an academic emergency department. *Emergency Medicine Journal, 22,* 336–338.

Blankenbaker, D. G., et al. (Eds.). (2016). Anterior glenohumeral dislocation. In *Diagnostic imaging: Musculoskeletal trauma* (2nd ed.) (pp. 68–71). Philadelphia, PA: Elsevier.

Burton, J. H., Bock, A. J., Strout, T. D., et al. (2002). Etomidate and midazolam for reduction of anterior shoulder dislocation. *Annals of Emergency Medicine, 40,* 496–504.

Garnavos, C. (1992). Technical note: Modifications and improvements of the Milch technique for the reduction of anterior dislocation of the shoulder without premedication. *The Journal of Trauma, 32,* 801–803.

Hendey, G. W. (2000). Necessity of radiography in the emergency department management of shoulder dislocations. *Annals of Emergency Medicine, 36,* 108–113.

Hendey, G. W., & Kinlaw, K. (1996). Clinically significant abnormalities in postreduction radiographs after anterior shoulder dislocation. *Annals of Emergency Medicine, 28,* 399–402.

Kosnick, J., Raphael, E., Malachias, Z., et al. (1999). Anesthetic methods for reduction of acute shoulder dislocations: A prospective randomized study comparing intra-articular lidocaine with intravenous analgesia and sedation. *American Journal of Emergency Medicine, 17,* 566–570.

Matthews, D. E. (1995). Intra-articular lidocaine versus intravenous analgesic for reduction of acute anterior shoulder dislocation: A prospective randomized study. *The American Journal of Sports Medicine, 23,* 54–58.

McNamara, R. M. (1993). Reduction of anterior shoulder dislocation by scapular manipulation. *Annals of Emergency Medicine, 22,* 1140–1144.

Miller, S. L., Cleeman, E., Auerbach, J., & Flatow, E. L. (2002). Comparison of intra-articular lidocaine and intravenous sedation for reduction of shoulder dislocations: A randomized prospective study. *Journal of Bone and Joint Surgery (America), 84,* 2135–2139.

Murrell, G. A. C. (2003). Treatment of shoulder dislocation: Is a sling appropriate? *The Medical Journal of Australia, 179,* 370–371.

Point of care. (2020). *Shoulder dislocation.* Amsterdam, Netherlands: Elsevier BV.

Quillen, D. M., Wuchner, M., & Hatch, R. L. (2004). Acute shoulder injuries. *American Family Physician, 70,* 1947–1954.

Riebel, G. D., & McCabe, J. B. (1991). Anterior shoulder dislocation: A review of reduction techniques. *American Journal of Emergency Medicine, 9,* 180–188.

Shaw, G. (2011). Breaking news: Believe it or not: Painless reduction of dislocated shoulders. *Emergency Medicine News, 33*(1), 28.

Shuster, M., Abu-Laban, R. B., & Boyd, J. (1999). Prereduction radiographs in clinically evident anterior shoulder dislocation. *American Journal of Emergency Medicine, 17*, 653–658.

Shuster, M., Abu-Laban, R. B., Boyd, J., et al. (2002). Prospective evaluation of a guideline for the selective elimination of prereduction radiographs in clinically obvious anterior shoulder dislocation. *Canadian Journal of Emergency Medicine, 4*, 257–262.

Westin, C. D., Gill, E. A., Noyes, M. E., et al. (1995). Anterior shoulder dislocation: A simple and rapid method for reduction. *The American Journal of Sports Medicine, 23*, 369–371.

Yuen, M. C., Yap, P. G., Chan, Y. T., & Tung, W. K. (2001). An easy method to reduce anterior shoulder dislocation: The Spaso technique. *Emergency Medicine Journal, 18*, 370–372.

Zhang, B., Sun, Y., Liang, L., Yu, X., Zhu, L., Chen, S., et al. (2020). Immobilization in external rotation versus internal rotation after shoulder dislocation: A meta-analysis of randomized controlled trials. *Orthopaedics and Traumatology: Surgery & Research, 106*(4), 671–680.

Tendinopathy: Tendinosis, Paratenonitis

(Tendonitis)

Presentation

There is pain along an involved tendon, often poorly localized, that worsens with motion, resisted contraction, or passive stretching. A vibratory crepitus may be felt on palpation over the tendon during tendon movement. Common sites include the posterior heel, the inferior aspect of the patella, the greater tuberosity of the shoulder, the thumb side of the wrist (de Quervain disease, see Chapter 105), and the lateral elbow (tennis elbow, see Chapter 114). There may be a history of repetitive overuse of the tendon or of a single sudden pull. Older patients participating in occasional sports are particularly prone to tendon injuries.

What to Do

✅ **Obtain a history** that includes details of pain onset and potential precipitating factors. Include questions about general health that may reveal sources of a secondary tendinopathy, such as psoriasis, a sexually transmitted disease, a puncture wound, gout, or the use of a fluoroquinolone within the past 3 months.

✅ **Perform a physical examination that includes inspection and careful palpation while gently putting the tendon through its range of motion** (as much as comfort allows). Palpation should reveal focal tenderness that essentially reproduces the patient's pain. At the Achilles tendon, this may be 3 to 5 cm above the calcaneal insertion (classic midportion tendinopathy) or, less commonly, at the insertion (insertional tendinopathy or enthesiopathy) itself. The tenderness of patellar tendinopathy (jumper's knee) is generally found on the inferior patellar pole at the site of the proximal attachment of the patellar tendon and is best palpated when the knee is in about 30 degrees of flexion and the quadriceps muscle is totally relaxed. Calcific tendinitis in or around the rotator cuff tendons of the shoulder usually exhibits specific tenderness over the greater tuberosity of the proximal humerus. This tendinopathy usually has an abrupt onset of pain and can severely limit shoulder movement secondary to the severe pain. The cardinal signs of lateral and medial elbow tendinopathy are tenderness at the origins of the elbow extensors and flexors, respectively. To help rule out cervical disorders, the neck should be examined carefully in all cases of suspected shoulder and elbow tendinopathy.

✅ **If there is swelling, erythema, fever, puncture of the skin, a history of gonorrhea, or marked pain, you must first rule out infection. Send blood for complete blood count (CBC) and erythrocyte sedimentation rate (ESR) and request consultation. If gonococcal infection is suspected, obtain appropriate cultures and tests** (see Chapter 83).

✅ **Radiographs are usually of little diagnostic value. They may reveal calcifications, osteochondritis, or osteophytes that suggest chronic inflammation but do not necessarily**

correlate with symptoms. However, radiographic evidence of calcification within the shoulder, along with the clinical history and physical examination, can help to make the diagnosis of calcific tendinitis. The most common site of calcium deposition is within the supraspinatus tendon.

✔ **In most other cases of tendinopathy, many expert clinicians believe that a confident diagnosis can be made clinically, thus obviating the need for any imaging studies.** Order plain radiographs if there was a traumatic mechanism of injury or if calcific tendonitis is a concern.

✔ **In cases in which the history and examination may not be typical,** both ultrasonography and magnetic resonance imaging provide additional information that may be helpful. The clinician must bear in mind that there are many cases in which abnormal tendon morphology does not parallel pain when interpreting imaging findings.

✔ **Instruct the patient to avoid the precipitating activity and prescribe a nonsteroidal anti-inflammatory drug (NSAID) unless it is contraindicated by allergy, bleeding, gastritis, or renal insufficiency.** The role of oral antiinflammatory therapy, such as NSAIDs or steroids, remains controversial. Although no inflammatory infiltrates have been documented in histologic analyses of tendinopathic samples, **anti-inflammatory medications do help to diminish pain and facilitate rehabilitation in cases of chronic tendinopathy and most certainly have a place in the management of insertional tendinitis and calcific tendinitis of the shoulder. One recent trial suggests that a 7-day treatment course with a once-daily dose of a 100-mg ketoprofen topical patch can provide pain relief without the adverse events associated with systemic delivery of an NSAID.** An alternative is diclofenac sodium "topical" gel. For adults, apply 2 g to the most painful area of the tendon once daily, as needed. (Keep in mind that topical NSAIDs are more expensive than oral NSAIDs.) Steroid injection at the site of the tendinopathy may help pain in the short run but carries a risk of increased pain and delayed healing later in the course of injury.

✔ **Cryotherapy (ice)** has also been shown to be useful to help facilitate therapy in tendinopathy.

✔ **With overuse injuries, occasionally complete rest or cessation of the training that caused the symptoms may be required for a short time to settle severe symptoms. Even splinting with use of a sling or providing crutches may help to prevent or minimize painful motion.**

✔ Because repair and remodeling of collagen fibers are stimulated by loading of the tendon, **only very short courses of complete rest should be prescribed.**

✔ **Heel lifts or the AirCast AirHeel (DJO Global, Vista, CA) pneumatic compression dressing for the foot and ankle can provide pain relief with Achilles tendinopathy.** Night splints are considered for patients who have significant pain on awakening in the morning.

✔ **A patellofemoral brace with a patellar cutout and lateral stabilizer may improve patellar tracking and help in the recovery of jumper's knee.**

✔ More time than expected is required for collagen turnover, repair, and remodeling; therefore **patients and clinicians must understand that these conditions may take months, rather than weeks, to resolve.**

✔ **Appropriate and progressive exercises represent the gold standard for tendon rehabilitation.** The goal of therapy is to increase tolerance to increased load on the tendon through exposure to controlled tendon reloading and graduated strengthening under the guidance of a physical therapist.

✅ Operative treatment is recommended for patients who do not respond adequately to an extended trial of conservative treatment. Surgery for overuse tendinopathies usually involves excision of fibrotic adhesions and degenerated nodules, or decompression of the tendon by longitudinal tenotomies.

What Not to Do

❌ Do not inject corticosteroids directly into the tendon or provide repeat steroid injections, which may potentiate infection, lead to tendon atrophy, weaken the tendon, or cause it to rupture. Repeated subfascial or subcutaneous injections can result in atrophy of the skin and subcutaneous tissue and loss of pigmentation. Because overuse tendinosis is not an inflammatory condition, the rationale for using corticosteroids may need reassessment. Corticosteroids, however, provide short-term pain reduction by mechanisms that are poorly understood and may therefore be indicated to allow for early rehabilitation.

❌ Do not confuse the **Haglund deformity (pump bump),** a superficial bursitis that forms a bony enlargement of the calcaneus where a low-cut shoe rubs over the heel, with Achilles tendinopathy. This is most often seen in adolescent females and is treated with changes in footwear, shoe padding, or, when necessary, orthotics.

❌ Do not miss discovering an avulsion fracture in the setting of recent trauma. Obtain a plain radiograph to exclude a fracture when indicated.

Discussion

Under the light microscope, normal tendon consists of dense, clearly defined, parallel, and slightly wavy collagen bundles. Histopathologic examination of symptomatic Achilles tendons reveals degeneration and disordered arrangement of collagen fibers.

Until recently, if a patient presented with a history of exercise-related pain and tenderness at one of the common sites of tendinopathy (the Achilles, patellar, rotator cuff, or elbow tendons), and if history and examination features suggested that pain was emanating from the tendon, the patient would most likely have been diagnosed as having tendinitis, an inflammatory condition of the tendon. Most of these conditions are truly tendinoses.

As long ago as 1976, Giancarlo Puddu of Rome examined the Achilles tendons of symptomatic runners and showed that inflammatory cells are absent. Others have shown that the major lesion in chronic Achilles **tendinopathy** "is a degenerative process characterized by a curious absence of inflammatory cells and a poor healing response."

New nomenclature is reflective of the underlying histopathologic changes in patients with overuse tendon disorders and favors use of the term **tendinopathy** as a generic descriptor of clinical conditions. These include **tendinosis** (chronic degeneration), **tendinitis** (acute inflammation of the tendon), **paratenonitis** (inflammation of the outer layer of the tendon [paratenon] alone, whether or not the paratenon is lined by synovium), **tenosynovitis** (inflammation of the synovial tendon sheath), and partial and complete **tendon ruptures** (see Chapter 120).

Tendinosis can be associated with paratenonitis. The majority of overuse tendinopathies in athletes are the result of tendinosis, with collagen degeneration and fiber disorientation, increased mucoid ground substance, and an absence of inflammatory cells.

The etiology of **Achilles tendon overuse injuries** is multifactorial. Excessive repetitive overload of the tendon is, however, regarded as the main pathologic stimulus that leads to its tendinopathy. Whereas **paratenonitis** is characterized by **"squeaky"**

Discussion continued

crepitus, exquisite tenderness, and swelling that does not move with tendon action, chronic Achilles **tendinopathy** is notable for **absence of crepitation and swelling**, with focal tender nodules that move as the ankle is dorsiflexed and plantarflexed.

Another cause of posterior heel pain in the setting of overuse injury is **retrocalcaneal bursitis,** in which there is inflammation of the commonly afflicted bursa anterior to the insertion of the Achilles tendon on the calcaneus.

Achilles tendon disorders occur most often in athletes involved in running sports.

Patients suffering from **jumper's knee** are usually tall athletes.

In children and adolescents, tendons are relatively stronger than the bones into which they insert. Osgood-Schlatter lesions are traction **apophysitis** of the tibial tubercle. The condition presents as localized tenderness and radiographic fragmentation in athletic adolescents between the ages of 8 to 13 (in girls) and 10 to 15 (in boys). These lesions are typically self-limiting.

It is thought that **calcific tendinitis of the shoulder** becomes acutely painful only when the calcium is undergoing resorption. This is **one form of tendinopathy for which steroid injection may be beneficial**. Gentle exercises with a physical therapist can help maintain range of motion.

Fluoroquinolone-induced tendinopathy can occur weeks to months following completion of a course of these antibiotics. This tendinitis is similar to the overuse injuries described. The Achilles tendon is most frequently affected, but any tendon complaint warrants inquiry regarding recent or distant fluoroquinolone use. Treatment is the same as it is for overuse tendinopathy, but subsequent fluoroquinolone use should be avoided. When any patient has **tenosynovitis of more than one tendon, consider quinolone tendinopathy as well as gonococcal infection** as possible causes.

For recalcitrant pain, injection of **platelet-rich plasma (PRP)** may prove to be an effective adjunct treatment for these tendinopathies. Ultrasound-guided PRP injection seems to be an effective treatment modality for symptomatic refractory distal biceps tendonitis; it has also been found to be promising for treating patellar tendinopathy as well as lateral epicondylitis. Additional treatment modalities (e.g., extracorporeal shock wave therapy, sclerotherapy [injection of a sclerotic agent], prolotherapy [injection of hypertonic glucose], percutaneous tenotomy [dry needling], and topical nitroglycerine [transdermal patch]) may also be considered, although evidence is lacking for some.

Prognosis for most tendinopathies is good with just conservative treatment.

Suggested Readings

Hurt, G., & Baker, C. L. (2003). Calcific tendinitis of the shoulder. *Orthopedics Clinics of North America, 34,* 567–575.

Khan, K. M., Cook, J. L., Kannus, P., et al. (2002). Time to abandon the "tendinitis" myth. *BMJ, 324,* 626–627.

Khan, K., & Cook, J. (2003). The painful nonruptured tendon: Clinical aspects. *Clinics in Sports Medicine, 22,* 711–725.

Point of Care. (2019). *Tendinopathy.* Amsterdam, Netherlands: Elsevier BV.

Rodriguez-Merchan, E. C. (2013). The treatment of patellar tendinopathy. *Journal of Orthopaedics and Traumatology, 14,* 77–81.

Sanli, I., Morgan, B., van Tilborg, F., Funk, L., & Gosens, T. (2016). Single injection of platelet-rich plasma (PRP) for the treatment of refractory distal biceps tendonitis: Long-term results of a prospective multicenter cohort study. *Knee Surgery, Sports Traumatology, Arthroscopy, 24,* 2308–2312.

Wilder, R. P., & Sethi, S. (2004). Overuse injuries: Tendinopathies, stress fractures, compartment syndrome, and shin splints. *Clinics in Sports Medicine, 23,* 55–81, vi.

Toe Fracture

(Broken Toe)

Presentation

A patient has stubbed, hyperflexed, hyperextended, hyperabducted, or dropped a weight on a toe. The patient presents with pain, swelling, ecchymosis, and decreased range of motion (ROM) or point tenderness. There may or may not be deformity or angulation. Often, after stubbing the toe, there is little discomfort and no deformity, but the toe appears purple, and the patient just wants to be sure that the "toe is not broken."

What to Do

✓ **Examine the toe,** particularly for lacerations that could become infected or could suggest open fractures, subungual hematoma that may require drainage, prolonged capillary filling time in the injured or other toes that could indicate poor circulation, or decreased sensation in the injured or other toes that could indicate peripheral neuropathy and may interfere with healing. When a fracture exists, most patients have point tenderness at the fracture site or pain with gentle axial loading of the digit (i.e., compressing the distal phalanx, in line with the proximal phalanx, inward toward the foot). Most displaced or angulated fractures and dislocations present with a visible deformity.

✓ **Radiographs often are not essential but may be necessary to provide patient satisfaction and to detect open fractures, angulated fractures, and fractures of the great toe.** They may have little effect on the initial treatment of closed nonangulated lesser toe injuries but may help predict the duration of pain and disability (e.g., fractures entering the joint space or Salter-Harris fractures greater than type I or II).

✓ **Adult patients who are simply worried about their "purple" toe** (Fig. 130.1), **when there is little or no pain or swelling and there is no angulation, should be encouraged to forgo the unnecessary irradiation of their foot because the treatment will be essentially the same whether or not a fracture is present. You can still give the autonomy of decision making to the patient by stating, "I'd be glad to order an x-ray if you still want it."**

✓ **With or without a radiograph, a bruise or a stable, nondisplaced fracture of one of the lesser toes should be treated with comfortable footwear,** usually consisting of a semirigid-sole shoe to limit joint movement. They can use whatever footwear provides them with the greatest comfort and protection. Buddy-taping (described next) can be offered to the patient if it provides any improvement in comfort; otherwise, it is an unnecessary inconvenience. If helpful, the patient may also take acetaminophen or over-the-counter nonsteroidal antiinflammatory drugs (NSAIDs), unless contraindicated.

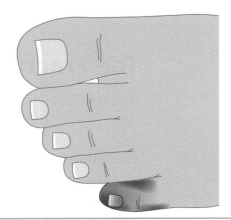

Fig. 130.1 A patient may just be worried about their bruised purple toe.

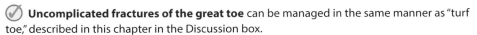 **Uncomplicated fractures of the great toe** can be managed in the same manner as "turf toe," described in this chapter in the Discussion box.

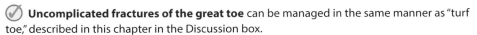 **Displaced or angulated phalangeal fractures must be reduced with strong linear traction after a digital block** (see Appendix B) **or injection of the fracture hematoma.**

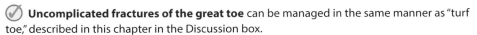 **Angulation can be further corrected by using a finger as a fulcrum to reverse the direction of the distal fragment. The broken toe should fall into its normal position when it is released after reduction.** The nail bed of the fractured toe should lie in the same plane as the nail bed of the corresponding toe on the opposite foot. If it does not, rotational deformity should be suspected and corrected by further manipulation. If any deformity persists, specialty referral is indicated.

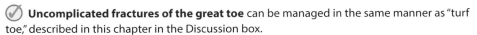 **Postreduction, splint the broken toe by taping it to an adjacent, nonaffected toe (buddy-taping).** Slide one thickness of gauze or Webril cotton pads between the two toes and, using 0.5-inch tape, bind the toes together. Give the patient additional padding and tape to revise the splinting, and (if there is a fracture) advise that the patient will require such immobilization for approximately 1 week, by which time there should be good callus formation around the fracture and less pain with motion. Inform the patient to keep the padding dry between the toes while they are taped together or the skin will become macerated and break down. **If the toe had required reduction**, warn the patient not to forcefully separate the toes when replacing the padding, due to the risk of recreating the original displacement or angulation (See Video 130.1).

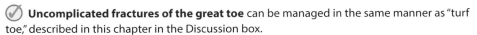 **Also recommend rest, elevation, and mild analgesic medication. A cane, crutches, or hard-soled shoe that minimizes toe flexion may also provide greater comfort.** Let the patient know that, in many cases, a soft slipper or an old sneaker with the toe cut out may be more comfortable.

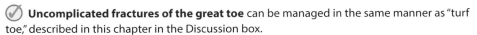 **If the fracture is not of a phalanx but of the metatarsal**, buddy-taping is not effective.

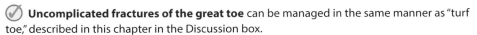 Arrange for follow-up if the toe is not much better within 1 week.

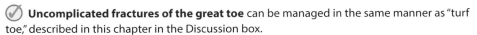 **Orthopedic or podiatric referral is indicated in patients with circulatory compromise, open fractures, significant soft tissue injury, physeal fractures in children, fracture dislocations, displaced intraarticular fractures, or fractures of the first toe that are unstable or involve more than 25% of the joint surface. Otherwise, patients with uncomplicated toe fractures, who need follow-up, can be referred to a primary care physician.**

✅ **Because of the first toe's role in weight bearing, balance, and pedal motion, fractures of this toe require referral much more often than other toe fractures.** Deformity, decreased ROM, and degenerative joint disease in this toe can impair a patient's functional ability.

What Not to Do

❌ Do not tape toes together without padding between them, unless the tape is changed frequently, and the skin is dried thoroughly if it becomes wet. (A hair dryer works well.) Friction and wetness will otherwise macerate the interdigital skin.

❌ Do not let the patient overdo ice, which should not be applied directly to skin and should not be used for more than 10 to 20 minutes per hour. It is questionable whether cryotherapy provides any benefit, and it should be used only if it reduces discomfort.

❌ Do not overlook the possibility of acute gouty arthritis (severe pain in the first metatarsophalangeal [MTP] joint), which sometimes follows minor trauma after a delay of a few hours (see Chapter 112).

Discussion

Toe phalangeal fractures occur most commonly from assaults, motor vehicle accidents, sporting injuries, falls, and direct trauma, with the resulting force causing either direct impact crushing or axial loading stubbing injuries. Toe injuries have also been described as a result of twisting supination injuries, and the most lateral fifth toe is also at risk of horizontal plane abduction injuries (bedroom or nightwalker's fracture). High-energy hyperflexion and hyperextension forces are often associated with joint dislocations or metatarsophalangeal joint capsular injuries (turf and sand toe), which can be characterized by the absence of a fracture despite significant clinical signs of injury (see upcoming discussion).

The first toe has only two phalanges; the second through the fifth toes generally have three, but the fifth toe sometimes can have only two. Sesamoid bones generally are present within flexor tendons in the first toe. In children, a physis (i.e., cartilaginous growth center) is present in the proximal part of each phalanx.

The same mechanisms that produce toe fractures may cause a ligament sprain, contusion, dislocation, tendon injury, or other soft tissue injury. With a clinically significant injury, radiographs are often required to distinguish these injuries from toe fractures. Tendon injuries are uncommon in closed injuries of the toes.

If there is no toe fracture, the treatment is the same, but the pain, swelling, and ability to walk may improve in 3 days rather than 1 to 2 weeks.

Although patients call the emergency department or clinic wanting to know whether their toe may be broken, if there is no deformity, they can usually be managed adequately over the telephone and seen the next day.

Stress fractures can occur in toes. They typically involve the medial base of the proximal phalanx and usually occur in athletes. Stress fractures have a more insidious onset and may not be visible on radiographs for the first 2 to 4 weeks after the injury.

Turf toe is a hyperextension sprain of the first metatarsophalangeal (MTP) joint with resulting subluxation and damage to the joint capsule. Hyperflexion, valgus, and varus stress can also cause MTP injury (Fig. 130.2). Classic signs and symptoms include pain located over the plantar and medial aspect of the first MTP joint with associated swelling and ecchymosis. More severe injuries will exhibit marked swelling, limited ROM, and an antalgic gait. **Radiographs**

(Continued)

577

Discussion continued

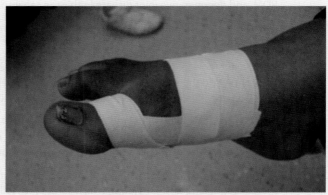

Fig. 130.2 Taping procedure for turf toe injury to allow hallux interphalangeal motion but limit metatarsophangeal dorsiflexion. (With permission from Park, J. S. [2020]. *Turf toe; essential orthopaedics* [pp. 772–775]. Philadelphia, PA: Elsevier.)

should be obtained to rule out associated fractures and possible degenerative arthritis. Treatment should be individualized, depending on the severity of the injury. **Mild sprains respond to supportive care, including elevation, compression, and acetaminophen or NSAIDs. Further hyperextension can be limited with stiff, solid footwear. Moderate sprains require** additional immobilization with cast padding, Ace wrap, and use of a stiff cast boot. **Early ROM and strengthening exercises should be advanced as symptoms permit. Severe injuries warrant complete immobilization, crutches, and NSAIDs (if tolerated), as well as a brief course of narcotic analgesics (if needed) and specialist consultation.**

Suggested Readings

American College of Foot and Ankle Surgeons. (2016). Do broken toes need follow-up in the fracture clinic? *Journal of Foot and Ankle Surgery, 55*(3), 488–491.

Hatch, R. L., & Hacking, S. (2003). Evaluation and management of toe fractures. *American Family Physician, 68,* 2413–2418.

Park, J. S. (2020). *Essential orthopaedics; turf toe*. Philadelphia, PA: Elsevier, 772–775.

Pommering, T. L., Kluchurosky, L., & Hall, S. L. (2005). Ankle and foot injuries in pediatric and adult athletes. *Primary Care, 32,* 133–161.

Shepherd, R. F. J. (2020). *Vascular medicine: A companion to Braunwald's heart disease*. Philadelphia, PA: Elsevier, 609–624.

Torticollis

(Wryneck)

Presentation

The patient, usually a young or middle-aged adult, complains of neck pain and is unable to turn the head, usually holding it twisted to one side, with involuntary spasm of the neck muscles and the chin pointing to the other side. Attempts at movement generally cause the pain to worsen. These symptoms may have developed gradually, after minor turning of the head, after vigorous exercise, or overnight during sleep. Spasm in the occipitalis, sternocleidomastoid, trapezius, splenius cervicis, or levator scapulae may be visible and/or palpable (Fig. 131.1).

What to Do

✓ **Ask the patient about precipitating factors, and perform a thorough physical examination,** looking for muscle spasm, point tenderness, signs of injury, nerve root compression, masses, or infection. Include a careful nasopharyngeal examination as well as a basic neurologic examination.

✓ **When forceful trauma is involved** and fracture, dislocation, or subluxation is possible, obtain lateral, anteroposterior, and odontoid radiographic views of the cervical spine. If there are neurologic deficits, a computed tomography (CT) scan or magnetic resonance imaging (MRI) may be better to visualize nerve involvement (as well as herniated disk, hematoma, or epidural abscess). Consider a CT angiogram if there is concern for a vascular injury.

✓ **With signs and symptoms of infection** (e.g., fever, toxic appearance, lymphadenopathy, tonsillar swelling, trismus, pharyngitis, or dysphagia), especially in the pediatric patient, obtain a lateral neck x-ray or a contrast-enhanced CT scan and consider obtaining a complete blood count and erythrocyte sedimentation rate to help rule out retropharyngeal abscess formation. Arrange for specialty consultation as needed.

✓ **When there is no suspicion of a serious illness or injury, carefully examine the side of the neck in spasm for tender trigger points.** Press the examining finger firmly and deeply into the neck muscles along muscular borders and their origins and insertions, searching for one or two spots approximately the size of the fingertip that cause the patient to wince in pain. **If a localized trigger point is discovered, then consider treating this as for any other source of myofascial pain and thus inject these areas with 5 to 10 mL of bupivacaine (Marcaine) 0.25% to 0.5%, with or without a corticosteroid** (see Chapter 121). Trigger-point injection can often partially or completely relieve the symptoms of the acute and painful form of muscular torticollis.

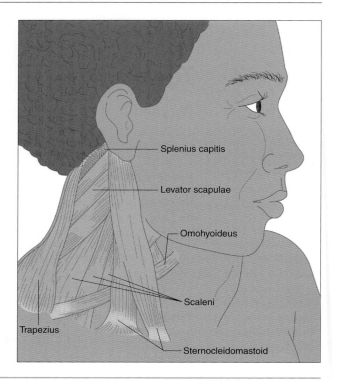

Fig. 131.1 Wryneck.

✅ **After trigger-point injection or when a trigger point cannot be found (or the patient elects not to have the injection),** have the patient apply ice to decrease inflammation and spasm for the first 48 hours; then switch to heat. If not contraindicated, give acetaminophen or anti-inflammatory analgesics (e.g., ibuprofen, naproxen) and a muscle relaxant—consider metaxalone (Skelaxin), cyclobenzaprine (Flexeril), or diazepam (Valium).

✅ Alternating heat with ice massages may also be helpful, as well as gentle range-of-motion exercises and friction massage.

✅ A soft cervical collar can be provided if it affords comfort. This should be worn for as short a period as tolerated. Position the wider segment of the collar on the side that produces the greatest comfort for the patient.

✅ **Inform the patient that with successful trigger-point injection, there may be mild soreness the next day and complete resolution of discomfort over the next week.** Symptoms usually resolve spontaneously within 2 weeks without treatment. If symptoms persist beyond this period, further evaluation is warranted.

What Not to Do

❌ Do not overlook infectious causes presenting as torticollis, especially the pharyngotonsillitis of young children, which can soften the atlantoaxial ligaments and allow subluxation.

(X) Do not fail to consider the unusual disk herniation or bony subluxation that, on occasion, can present as acute wryneck or torticollis.

(X) Do not undertake violent spinal manipulations in the emergency department or clinic, which can make acute torticollis worse and potentially cause other problems.

(X) **Do not confuse torticollis with a dystonic drug reaction**, where (typically) even though the neck may be twisted there is no complaint of pain (see Chapter 1).

Discussion

Torticollis is an involuntary twisting of the neck to one side, secondary to spasm and contraction of the neck muscles. The ear is pulled toward the contracted muscle while the chin is facing in the opposite direction. The term *torticollis* is derived from the Latin words *tortus* ("twisted") and *collum* ("collar" or "neck"). Twisting of the neck may also be accompanied by the elevation of one shoulder up toward the contracted neck muscles.

Although torticollis may signal an underlying disorder, in the acute care setting it is usually a local musculoskeletal problem—only more frightening and noticeable because of the apparent deformity of the neck—and need not always be worked up comprehensively when it first presents to the clinician.

Torticollis can be a symptom as well as a disease, with a host of underlying disorders. Abnormalities of the cervical spine can range from fracture, subluxation, and osteomyelitis to tumor. Infectious causes include retropharyngeal abscess, cervical adenitis, tonsillitis, and mastoiditis. Head tilting can occur to compensate for an essential head tremor, and idiopathic spasmodic torticollis and cervical dystonia should be suspected when symptoms are prolonged.

Suggested Readings

Cersosimo, M. G., & Koller, W. C. (2003). Movement disorders. *Medical Clinics of North America*, *87*, 133–161.

Roberson, D. W. (2004). Pediatric retropharyngeal abscesses. *Clinics in Pediatric Emergency Medicine*, *5*, 1413–1422.

Ulnar Collateral Ligament Tear of the Thumb

(Ski Pole, Skier's, or Gamekeeper's Thumb)

Presentation

The patient fell while holding on to a ski pole, banister, or other fixed object, forcing the thumb radially into abduction and causing pain at the base of the thumb. The metacarpophalangeal (MCP) joint of the thumb is swollen and tender and may be ecchymotic. When tested for stability, it may show varying degrees of joint widening toward the radial (or palmar) aspect more than the MCP joint of the other thumb. The patient's power pinch between the thumb and index finger, if possible at all, is less strong than with the other hand (Fig. 132.1).

What to Do

Obtain a history of the mechanism of injury, and examine the thumb, hand, and wrist thoroughly. Tenderness to palpation should be greatest along the ulnar border of the proximal thumb.

Gentle stress testing of the first MCP joint should be performed. Because the ulnar collateral ligament (UCL) is comprised of two parts, the thumb must also be tested in two positions. First, the patient's thumb is held with the MCP joint in extension, while applying valgus stress to the thumb; then the test is repeated with the MCP joint in 30 degrees of flexion. Laxity of the joint is noted in these two positions. Care must be taken by the investigator to place a thumb on the radial side of the MCP joint to prevent rotational effects.

The patient may not be able to tolerate this part of the examination because of pain, and it can consequently be deferred until specialist follow-up. Likewise, when swelling hinders the physical exam, the patient can be given cast immobilization and the thumb can be tested a few days later when most of the swelling has subsided.

A complete UCL tear may induce the appearance of a palpable mass in the ulnar aspect of the joint, along with instability to valgus stress, reaching an angle of more than 35 degrees during valgus stress with the MCP in extension, more than 20 degrees with the MCP joint in 30 degrees of flexion, and/or more than a 15-degree difference compared to the contralateral side. An alternative measurement could be the presence or absence of a firm end point during testing.

Obtain radiographs, which may be negative or show a small avulsion fracture of the proximal phalanx at the insertion of the UCL. Ultrasound can also be used to demonstrate a UCL tear. For future definitive confirmation, magnetic resonance imaging (MRI) can be seen as the gold standard with a reported sensitivity of 96% to 100% and a specificity of 95% to 100%.

Treat with ice, elevation, rest, acetaminophen, or anti-inflammatory medications, for comfort.

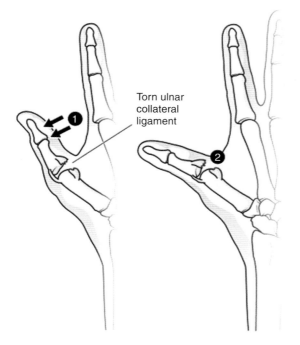

Torn ulnar
collateral
ligament

Fig. 132.1 Rupture of the ulnar collateral ligament (gamekeeper's thumb). *(1)* This injury is caused by forcible abduction. If unrecognized and untreated, progressive metacarpophalangeal (MCP) subluxation may occur *(2)* with interference during grasp, causing significant permanent disability. Suspect this injury when there is a complaint of pain in this region. Look for tenderness on the medial side of the MCP joint. (From Roberts, J. R., & Hedges, J. R. [2009]. *Clinical procedures in emergency medicine* [5th ed.]. St. Louis, MO: Saunders. Adapted from McRae, R. [1981]. *Practical fracture treatment.* Edinburgh, Scotland: Churchill Livingstone. Reproduced by permission.)

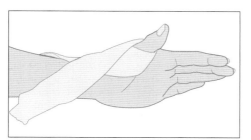

Fig. 132.2 Apply the splint in a cross fashion around the dorsum of the thumb incorporating the metacarpophalangeal (MCP) joint. (Adapted from Hart, R. G., Kleinert, H. E., & Lyons, K. [2005]. A modified thumb spica splint for thumb injuries in the ED. *American Journal of Emergency Medicine, 23,* 777–781.)

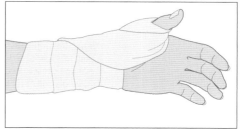

Fig. 132.3 After the thumb and wrist have been positioned comfortably, an elastic bandage can be applied. (Adapted from Hart, R. G., Kleinert, H. E., & Lyons, K. [2005]. A modified thumb spica splint for thumb injuries in the ED. *American Journal of Emergency Medicine, 23,* 777–781.)

⊘ **A thumb spica provides support to the wrist and thumb for the more significant ligament injuries.** The patient's thumb should be positioned in a comfortable neutral position, and a 2-inch padded splint, which can be molded around the thumb, should be applied (Fig. 132.2).

⊘ **A soft dressing with an immobilizing elastic bandage that incorporates the thumb may be adequate for sprains or mild partial tears (Fig. 132.3).**

⊘ **Explain to the patient with a significant partial or a complete ligament tear that this particular injury may not heal with closed immobilization and sometimes requires**

operative repair. Complete tears that require surgical repair should be done 1 to 3 weeks after the injury.

(✓) **Arrange for reexamination** and hand specialist or orthopedic referral after a few days when the swelling has decreased.

What Not to Do

(✗) Do not place excessive abduction or radial deviation force on the first metacarpophalyngeal joint after a mechanism concerning for an ulnar collateral ligament tear, as doing so may cause the ruptured ends of the ligament to displace and become separated by the aponeurosis of the adductor pollicis muscle, leading to a Stener Lesion, the need for surgery, or failure to heal.

(✗) Do not fail to provide orthopedic or hand surgery follow-up for a patient with a suspected ulnar collateral ligament tear, as doing so may result in a missed opportunity to recognize nonhealing or the need for surgery.

Discussion

A skier's thumb is an acute rupture of the UCL of the MCP joint of the thumb. It occurs when a thumb, which is already in abduction, receives an extra valgus stress. The classic trauma mechanism is when a skier falls while holding on to a ski pole. However, this injury can also occur with people playing sports involving a ball or stick, falling from a bicycle when holding on to the handlebars, or simply falling on an outstretched thumb. The estimated incidence of this injury in the United States is approximately 200,000 patients per year.

This same lesion was once produced by the repeated breaking of the necks of rabbits by Scottish hunters or gamekeepers—hence the name.

Injury to the UCL is a frequent lesion that occurs from a radially directed force on the abducted thumb. Rupture of the UCL may be total or partial and usually takes place at its phalangeal point of insertion. The rupture of the thumb UCL can be

an isolated lesion or can occur in combination with other joint structures, such as the volar plate or dorsal capsule. They will present with pain, swelling, and hematoma on the ulnar side of the MCP joint of the thumb. Sometimes a mass can be felt, suggesting a Stener lesion, which is a subtype of complete UCL rupture with the ruptured ligament interpositioned underneath the adductor aponeurosis. However, this mass is not a pathognomonic finding. MRI can detect the torn ligament and reveal displacement, if present.

Nondisplaced UCL tears are usually treated conservatively. Surgical intervention is usually reserved for Stener lesions and complete undisplaced tears with significant instability because conservative treatment leads to chronic instability and arthrosis.

Avulsion fractures involving more than 20% of the articular surface may require pinning.

Suggested Readings

Cerezal, L., Abascal, F., Garciía-Valtuille, R., et al. (2005). Wrist MR arthrography: How, why, when? *Radiology Clinics of North America*, *43*, 709–731, viii.

Hart, R. G., Kleinert, H. E., & Lyons, K. (2005). A modified thumb spica splint for thumb injuries in the ED. *American Journal of Emergency Medicine*, *23*, 777–781.

Mahajan, M., Tolman, C., Würth, B., & Rhemrev, S. J. (2016). Clinical evaluation vs magnetic resonance imaging of the skier's thumb: A prospective cohort of 30 patients. *European Journal of Radiology*, *85*(10), 1750–1756.

PART 10

Soft Tissue Emergencies

■ Philip M. Buttaravoli ■ Kevin J. Brochu

CHAPTER

133

Bicycle Spoke Injury

Presentation

A small child, riding on the back of a friend's bicycle, gets their foot caught between the spinning spokes and the frame. The skin over the lateral and medial aspects of the foot or ankle is crushed and abraded with underlying soft tissue swelling (Fig. 133.1).

What to Do

✅ **Remain cognizant that other injuries could have resulted from a fall off the bicycle** after the incident. Perform a focal examination of the foot and ankle, including distal sensation, motor, and perfusion assessment. Note any laceration(s) and soft tissue crush injuries. Assess for bony tenderness, including the distal tibia and fibula (ankle joint experiences significant torque with this mechanism). Perform a Thompson/Simmond test to assess for Achilles tendon injury, which can occur in up to 20% of patients.

✅ **Cleanse the area with a gentle scrub** of soap and tap water to remove dirt and oil-based lubricant under local anesthesia as needed.

✅ **Provide tetanus prophylaxis, cryotherapy, elevation, and nonopioid analgesics as needed** (see Appendix G).

✅ **Obtain plain film radiographs of crushed and tender areas. Fractures are found in 25% to 31% of patients, most commonly in the distal tibia/fibula.**

✅ **Consider point-of-care ultrasonography of the Achilles tendon.**

✅ **Repair lacerations as indicated. Crushed, nonviable tissue may require debridement. Dress with nonadherent dressing.**

✅ Encourage elevation and cryotherapy, provide weight-based recommendations for nonopioid analgesia.

587

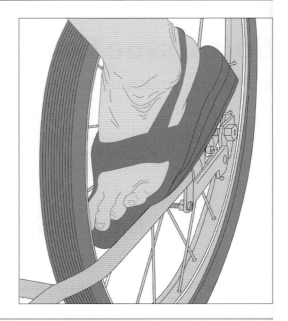

Fig. 133.1 Foot caught in bicycle spokes.

✅ **Arrange for a 48-hour follow-up with podiatric/orthopedic surgery for significant injuries. Crushed tissues should be reevaluated for viability at that time.**

✅ Educate patient/family about proper closed-toe footwear when riding a bicycle, helmet use, and chain/spoke guards to minimize the chance of future injuries.

What Not to Do

❌ Do not underestimate the degree of tissue crush injury, miss fractures due to torque remote from the crush injury, or miss a partial or complete Achilles tendon rupture/laceration.

Discussion

Bicycle and motorcycle spoke injuries can result in significant soft tissue and bony injury. There are no historical or physical exam components that predict fractures. Good follow-up is imperative, as patients may require debridement and skin grafting for significant crush injuries that can result in skin necrosis and ulcerations. Poor prognostic factors include high-energy injury, contamination and infection, and delayed treatment.

Suggested Readings

Chu, G., Vlok, L., Zwaag-Pijls, C., Houser, C. M., & de Groot, B. (2014). Emergency department management and follow-up of children with bicycle spoke injuries. *Journal of Emergency Medicine*, 47(3), 259–267. https://doi.org/10.1016/j.jemermed.2014.04.028

Mak, C. Y., Chang, J. H. T., Lui, T. H., & Ngai, W. K. (2015). Bicycle and motorcycle wheel spoke injury in children. *Journal of Orthopedic Surgery (Hong Kong), 23*(1), 56–58. https://doi.org/10.1177/230949901502300113

Slaar, A., Karsten, I. H. C. M., Beenen, L. F. M., et al. (2015). Plain radiography in children with spoke wheel injury: A retrospective cohort study. *European Journal of Radiology, 84*(11), 2296–2300. https://doi.org/10.1016/j.ejrad.2015.07.013

Contusion

(Bruise)

134

Presentation

The patient has experienced blunt trauma such as a fall or other impact injury. The initial pain has subsided, but point tenderness, swelling, ecchymosis, and pain with use remain after 3 days. On physical examination, there is insignificant loss of function and no bony tenderness, instability, or crepitus.

A contusion is soft tissue damage with diffuse capillary rupture due to focal blunt trauma. Extravasated blood in the subcutaneous tissue produces visible bruising. Blood may form a focal collection that can exert mass effect on surrounding structures.

What to Do

✔️ Consider other injuries depending on the mechanism of injury. Assess sensorimotor function and perfusion distal to the contusion. Screen for antiplatelet/anticoagulant use or known bleeding disorder as part of the obtained history.

✔️ **Ecchymosis and/or swelling out of proportion to the mechanism of injury warrant an investigation of possible bleeding disorders (e.g., hemophilia, idiopathic thrombocytopenia, leukemia) as well as abuse.** Remember: Kids who don't cruise don't bruise.

✔️ Extensive muscle contusion predisposes to rhabdomyolysis. If indicated, point-of-care urinalysis may be used to screen for myoglobinuria, as it cross-reacts with the hemoglobin assay. Patients may report dark urine in the absence of rhabdomyolysis due to increased production of urobilin as a breakdown product of resorbed hemoglobin.

✔️ **Pain out of proportion to the injury combined with tense tissues on exam raises concern for compartment syndrome. Apart from pain, pallor, paresthesias, poikilothermia, and absent pulses are late findings of compartment syndrome.**

✔️ **Obtain radiographs if there is clinical concern for bony injury.**

✔️ Inflammation due to tissue damage will result in increased pain and swelling. This typically peaks 24 hours after the injury. Provide expectation management for patients who present early.

✔️ **Topical cryotherapy with ice packs does not affect hematoma formation but may reduce pain. Animal studies suggest that structures as deep as 4 cm benefit from topical cold application.**

✓ **Provide appropriate nonopioid analgesia.** While nonsteroidal antiinflammatory drugs (NSAIDs) inhibit platelet function, their use does not appear to increase hematoma formation.

✓ **Hematoma evacuation:** Most hematomas will resolve spontaneously. Hematomas that compress adjacent neurovascular structures or produce overlying skin necrosis (due to pressure exceeding capillary pressure) may require drainage. The decision must be carefully weighed, as it allows for introduction of bacteria into an otherwise sterile fluid collection, and the hematoma may reaccumulate. Three techniques are available:

○ **Needle aspiration:** Often inadequate due to viscosity of partially congealed blood

○ **Incision and drainage:** Incision should be made on the lateral aspect of the hematoma along lines of tension

○ **Liposuction:** Requires specialist consultation

✓ **Iliac crest contusion ("hip pointer").** This injury results from blunt trauma to the iliac crest that results in a periosteal hematoma. Treatment consists of periosteal aspiration and injection of dexamethasone (2 cc, 8 mg) and bupivacaine (8 cc, 0.5%) into the periosteal hematoma. Follow-up with orthopedic surgery or sports medicine is encouraged.

✓ **Quadriceps contusion.** This injury results from blunt trauma to the quadriceps muscle group. Patients should receive RICE (rest, ice, compression, elevation) therapy and nonopioid analgesics. Patients with a grade II or III contusion (unable to flex knee past 90 degrees and 45 degrees, respectively) should be referred to sports medicine due to the increased risk of developing myositis ossificans traumatica.

What Not to Do

✗ Do not apply an elastic bandage to the middle of a limb, where it may act as a venous tourniquet. Include the entire distal limb in the wrapping if a compression dressing is necessary.

✗ Do not use systemic corticosteroids to help decrease inflammation, as risks outweigh potential benefits.

Discussion

Contusions are often minor, self-limiting injuries. However, patients with bleeding disorders or who are anticoagulated may be challenging to manage. Antidotal reversal of the anticoagulated status must be carefully considered, balancing the risk of hematoma expansion with the risk of systemic thrombosis. Patients with mechanical heart valves must remain anticoagulated.

Individuals with significant contusions should be reevaluated after 48 hours by their primary care provider. Depending on size and location of the contusion, a subset of patients may benefit from physical therapy to enhance mobility and expedite recovery.

Suggested Readings

Chen, T., & Adamson, P. A. (2009). Comparison of ibuprofen and acetaminophen with codeine following cosmetic facial surgery. *Journal of Otolaryngology and Head and Neck Surgery, 38*(5), 580–586.

Hall, M., & Anderson, J. (2012). Hip pointers. *Clinics in Sports Medicine, 32*(2), 325–330. https://doi.org/10.1016/j.csm.2012.12.010.

Manson, A. L. (1988). Trial of ibuprofen to prevent post-vasectomy complications. *The Journal of Urology, 139*(5), 965–966.

Megson, M. (2011). Traumatic subcutaneous haematoma causing skin necrosis. *BMJ Case Reports, 2011*, bcr0520114273–bcr0520114273. https://doi.org/10.1136/bcr.05.2011.4273.

Pool, S. M. W., van Exsel, D. C. E., Melenhorst, W. B. W. H., Cromheecke, M., & van der Lei, B. (2015). The effect of eyelid cooling on pain, edema, erythema, and hematoma after upper blepharoplasty: A randomized, controlled, observer-blinded evaluation study. *Plastic and Reconstructive Surgery, 135*(2), e277–e281. https://doi.org/10.1097/PRS.0000000000000919.

Walton, M., Roestenburg, M., Hallwright, S., & Sutherland, J. C. (1986). Effects of ice packs on tissue temperatures at various depths before and after quadriceps hematoma: Studies using sheep. *Journal of Orthopedic and Sports Physical Therapy, 8*(6), 294–300.

Fingernail or Toenail Avulsion

Presentation

Blunt trauma to the distal phalanx may result in nail avulsion, nail bed laceration, and distal phalanx fractures. The nail may be completely avulsed, partially held in place by the nail folds, or adhering only to the proximal nail bed (Fig. 135.1). On occasion, an exposed nail bed will have a pearly appearance, with minimal bleeding, making it seem as if the nail is still in place when it actually has been completely avulsed. See the anatomy of the fingernail in Fig. 135.3.

What to Do

✅ Assess vascular and sensory status distal to the injury **prior to performing a digital block.** Ensure preserved function of the extensor digitorum tendon.

✅ **Perform a digital block** (see Appendix B) with bupivacaine for long-lasting relief. Contrary to traditional teaching, epinephrine-containing local anesthetics are safe to use and reduce bleeding.

✅ **Obtain radiographs if there was any crushing or high-velocity shearing force involved.** Radiographs are otherwise unnecessary.

✅ **Cleanse the nail bed with tepid tap water, and remove any loose cuticular debris. Whenever possible, salvage the nail or any remaining fragment for replacement over the nail bed.** This will provide the most comfortable dressing (with the most accurate anatomic and physiologic match) for the patient.

✅ **If the partially avulsed nail is still tenuously attached**, it can be left in place. **If removal is required to facilitate wound cleaning or nail bed repair,** it should be separated from the nail fold with a straight hemostat and/or fine scissors. **Cleanse the nail thoroughly** with normal saline, cut away any contaminated portions of the distal free edge of the nail, and remove only loose cuticular debris from the remainder of the nail. **Do not excise any of the proximal nail root.**

✅ **If bleeding interferes with inspection and wound management,** a finger tourniquet can be applied to provide a bloodless field. If a commercial tourniquet is not available for a finger injury, place a tight surgical glove onto the patient's hand, cut a small opening at the tip of the glove finger, and then roll up the glove finger over the injured digit until it forms a tight band around the base of the finger. **Place a hemostat on this tourniquet** so it is not accidently left on the finger after the procedure is completed.

✅ **Inspect the nail bed for lacerations, and if large or displaced wounds are present, carefully reapproximate with fine (6-0 or 7-0) absorbable sutures. Cyanoacrylate-based tissue adhesives (e.g., Dermabond) are similarly efficacious as sutures.**

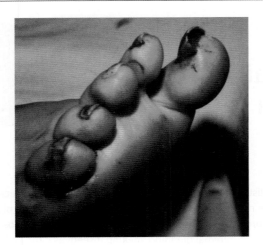

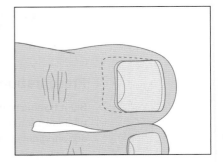

Fig. 135.1 Partially avulsed toenail of the great toe.

Fig. 135.2 Avulsed nail reinserted under the eponychium.

✅ **Reinsert the nail root under the eponychium** (Fig. 135.2) and **apply a fingertip-type dressing** (see Appendix C).

✅ **A loose-fitting nail can also be glued in place using cyanoacrylate topical skin adhesive (Dermabond).** Place several drops of tissue adhesive onto a clean, dry nail bed. Insert the clean, dry nail root first under the eponychium. Lower the rest of the nail onto the nail bed and hold it in place using a swab to apply gentle pressure for 1 minute. Apply a simple protective dressing. Do not apply bacitracin or other antibiotic ointment because this may dissolve the adhesive.

✅ **If the nail is missing, badly damaged, or severely contaminated, replace it with a substitute.** An artificial nail can be cut out of the sterile aluminum foil found in a suture pack or can be cut from a sheet of fine-mesh Vaseline gauze. Cut this substitute nail into the shape and size of the original nail, including the nail root, so that it can completely cover the nail bed, including the germinal matrix. Insert this stent under the eponychium in place of the nail and apply a fingertip dressing after it is in place. The aluminum stent can be secured in place using tissue adhesive as previously described.

✅ **Leave the replaced nail or these stents in place until the underlying nail bed hardens and the original nail or stent separates spontaneously.**

✅ *Unless immunocompromised, patients generally do NOT benefit from prophylactic antibiotics even in the setting of open distal phalanx fractures.*

✅ Provide appropriate tetanus prophylaxis (see Appendix G).

✅ Along with a soft fingertip dressing, a protective fingertip splint can be applied (see Chapter 109).

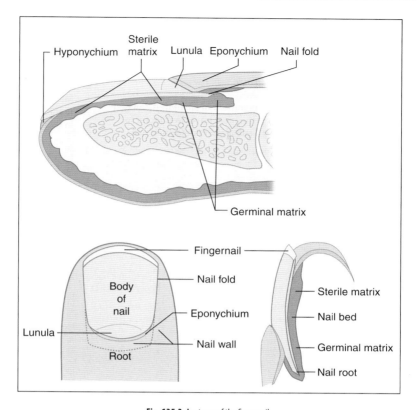

Fig. 135.3 Anatomy of the fingernail.

✓ **The patient should be given standard wound instructions**, and elevation of the injured digit above the level of the heart should be stressed.

✓ Initially, the dressing should be changed every 3 to 5 days, but **the nail (or artificial substitute) should always be left in place.**

What Not to Do

✗ Do not dress an exposed nail bed (where the nail has not been replaced) with an ordinary gauze dressing or any supposedly nonadherent dressing. These dressings will adhere to the nail bed, require lengthy soaks, and usually cause an extremely painful removal.

✗ Do not fail to repair a significant nail bed laceration. Otherwise it may result in a poor cosmetic appearance of the nail and may lead to recurrent ingrown nails.

✗ Do not débride any portion of the nail bed, sterile matrix, or germinal matrix to help prevent future nail deformity. Severely damaged nail bed tissue will usually survive.

✗ Do not use nonabsorbable sutures to repair a nail bed. These would be extremely difficult and painful to remove.

Discussion

Inserting the nail or stent under the eponychium prevents adhesions between the eponychium and the nail bed, which may result in cosmetic and functional deformities or permanent nail loss. **Proper alignment of all injured nail bed structures is the most important factor in preventing a subsequent deformed nail.**

Antibiotic prophylaxis is not needed except in unique circumstances. Before discharge, patients should be counseled on the importance of monitoring carefully for signs of infection, including worsening pain or redness, purulent drainage, red streaking, and fever.

Minimally traumatized avulsed nails can readhere and grow normally if carefully replaced in their proper anatomic positions.

Complete regrowth of an avulsed nail usually requires 4 to 5 months at 1 mm per week.

Suggested Readings

Denkler, K. (2001). A comprehensive review of epinephrine in the finger: To do or not to do. *Plastic and Reconstructive Surgery, 108*(1), 114–124.

Edwards, S., & Parkinson, L. (2019). Is fixing pediatric nail bed injuries with medical adhesives as effective as suturing? A review of the literature. *Pediatric Emergency Care, 35*(1), 75–77. https://doi.org/10.1097/PEC.0000000000000994.

Ilicki, J. (2015). Safety of epinephrine in digital nerve blocks: A literature review. *Journal of Emergency Medicine, 49*(5), 799–809. https://doi.org/10.1016/j.jemermed.2015.05.038.

Metcalfe, D., Aquilina, A. L., & Hedley, H. M. (2016). Prophylactic antibiotics in open distal phalanx fractures: Systematic review and meta-analysis. *Journal of Hand Surgery Europe, 41*(4), 423–430. https://doi.org/10.1097/01.prs.10.1177/17531934156010551

Thomson, C. J., Lalonde, D. H., Denkler, K. A., & Feicht, A. J. (2007). A critical look at the evidence for and against elective epinephrine use in the finger. *Plastic and Reconstructive Surgery, 119*(1), 260–266. https://doi.org/10.1097/01.prs.0000237039.71227.11.

Fingertip Avulsion, Superficial

Presentation

A patient arrives holding a bandage over a missing fingertip. The patient may or may not have brought along the avulsed tissue.

Traumatic finger pad injuries are common. The mechanisms of injury can be diverse: A knife, a meat slicer, a mandolin, a closing door, broken glass, spinning fan blades, and turning gears are a few examples. Depending on the angle of the amputation, varying degrees of tissue loss will occur from the volar pad or the finger tip.

What to Do

✓ Determine the patient's employment as well hand dominance. This information will help guide the need for aggressive intervention. Inquire about tetanus status and provide prophylaxis if indicated (see Appendix G).

✓ Examine whether there is an associated nail or nail bed injury (see Chapter 144), or whether there is bone involvement.

✓ **Obtain a radiograph of any crush injury or injury caused by a high-speed mechanical instrument, such as a hedge trimmer or lawn mower.**

✓ **Wounds that are infected, associated with tendon injuries, associated with fractures (other than tuft fractures), show exposed bone accompanied by digit dislocations, and wounds greater than 1 cm in diameter with absent, destroyed, or heavily contaminated tissue require specialty consultation with a hand surgeon.**

✓ **With wounds that do not require specialty consultation, perform a digital block to obtain complete anesthesia** (see Appendix B).

✓ **Thoroughly irrigate the wound.** High-volume/low-pressure irrigation with tap water is adequate in most instances once the digital block takes effect.

✓ **When active bleeding is present,** provide a bloodless field with a commercial or improvised tourniquet (e.g., a rolled-up surgical glove finger with tip cut off, a Penrose drain—with a tag preventing it from being forgotten at the end of the procedure).

✓ **For wounds with less than 1 cm^2 of full-thickness tissue loss, you may allow the injury to granulate. A small patch of hemostatic gauze (Surgicel, ActCel, GuardaCare) or foam (Gelfoam) can be applied (following thorough irrigation) to reduce further bleeding. A simple nonadherent dressing** (see Appendix C) **with some gentle compression can then be applied.**

✅ **An alternative approach** is to apply a polyurethane film (OpSite) adherent semiocclusive dressing as a wound cover. It is attached to a lacerated partial-thickness wound. It keeps the wound moist and thereby accelerates reepithelization. It can be left in place for 7 to 10 days; it is not painful to remove, which is especially important in treating small children.

✅ **In infants and young children (<2 years of age), fingertip amputations can be sutured back on in their entirety. If the amputated tissue is contaminated or not available, the wound can usually be dressed and allowed to granulate.** Consider using a polyurethane film (OpSite) dressing as noted earlier.

✅ **In older children and adults,** composite grafts will usually fail; therefore it is important to consult a hand surgeon before any significant amputation repair is attempted.

✅ **Consider consultation with a hand surgeon if:**

- ○ **There is massive tissue loss/exposed bone**
- ○ **Any significant injury affects the dominant hand**
- ○ **The patient performs in a high-dexterity profession**
- ○ **The avulsed piece of tissue is available and is not severely crushed or contaminated (the surgeon may be able to convert it to a modified full thickness graft)**

✅ **Schedule a wound check in 2 days.** During that time, the patient should be instructed to keep the finger elevated. Do not encourage application of ice packs if grafted, as this will reduce graft perfusion.

✅ **Apply a protective aluminum splint for comfort** (see Chapter 109).

✅ Unless the bandage gets wet, a dressing change need not be done for 5 to 7 days (7–10 days with a polyurethane dressing), at which time active range of motion can begin.

✅ **Always have the patient return immediately if there is increasing pain, purulent drainage, red streaking extending from the wound, or other signs of infection.**

✅ **Antibiotics are generally not indicated in immunocompetent patients even in the presence of a distal phalanx fracture.**

✅ Recommend nonopioid analgesics. Encourage starting the regimen prior to the digital block losing effect.

What Not to Do

❌ Do not attempt to stop wound bleeding by cautery or ligature, measures that are likely to increase tissue damage and are probably unnecessary.

Discussion

Fingertip injuries are common, but most can be treated without the assistance of a specialist. Treating small and midsize fingertip amputations without grafting is appropriate in most cases. Allowing repair by wound contracture may leave the patient with as good a result and likely better sensation, without the discomfort or minor disfigurement of a split-thickness graft. This open technique is not recommended for wounds greater than 1 cm because healing time will exceed 3 to 4 weeks, and it will significantly delay return to work. In addition, patients may acquire a permanent volume defect in their finger pads in larger avulsions left to heal by secondary intention.

The nature of the wound, the preferences of the follow-up physician, and the special occupational and emotional needs of the patient should determine the technique followed. Explain the options to the patient, who can help decide the course of action.

Suggested Readings

Chao, C., & Runde, D. (2015). Tap water vs. sterile saline for wound irrigation. *American Family Physician, 92*(3), online.

Shabat, S., Sagiv, P., Stern, A., & Nyska, M. (2000). Polyurethane film (OpSite) for superficial fingertip avulsion injuries. *Plastic and Reconstructive Surgery, 106*(2), 512.

Fishhook Removal

Presentation

The patient has been snagged with a fishhook and arrives with it embedded in the skin (Fig. 137.1). This most commonly occurs on the hand, face, scalp, or upper extremity but can involve any body part. Removal of the fishhook is often the sole procedure necessary, except when the injury involves the eye.

Fishhooks have between one and four barbed prongs (Fig. 137.2). By design, they embed into tissue but are not easily removed in retrograde fashion.

What to Do

⊘ All items attached to the hook (i.e., fishing line, bait, and the body of any lure) should be removed.

⊘ Prior to manipulation of the hook for any reason, local anesthesia should be provided by either injecting local anesthetic along the path of the hook, as a field block, or as a digital block.

⊘ **If the fishhook features multiple prongs** (treble fishhook) (Fig. 137.1), all exposed barbs should be covered or clipped to prevent injury to the treating provider (See Video 137.1).

⊘ Radiographs are generally not required. If after removal the fishhook appears incomplete, radiographs are helpful in screening for retained foreign bodies.

⊘ **Any fishhook injury that may involve deeper structures,** such as bone tendons, vessels, nerves, or joints, may benefit from a specialist consultation.

⊘ **Patients with fishhooks that are imbedded in the eye** or in a location in which removal may injure the eye should have the eye covered with a protective metal shield. With an eye injury, an ophthalmologist should be immediately consulted.

⊘ Provide tetanus prophylaxis as needed (see Appendix G).

⊘ **There are four techniques for the removal of fishhooks. The optimal technique depends on the nature, depth, and location of the hook.** Techniques here are listed from superficial to deep hook location (Figs. 137.3, 137.4, 137.5, and 137.6).

⊘ **String-yank technique: A string is attached to the center of the curve of the hook. The provider pushes down on the long arm of the hook to disengage the barb. Once the barb is disengaged, a quick jerk on the string (a loop of fishing line or 1-0 silk) allows retrograde removal** (see Fig. 137.3) (See Videos 137.2 & 137.3). Provider and patient should wear eye protection when using this technique. This technique works best on a stable flat skin surface

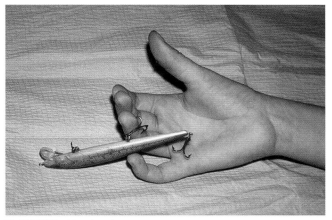

Fig. 137.1 Fishhook impalement.

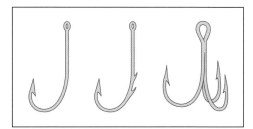

Fig. 137.2 Types of fishhooks. *(Left)* Simple single-barbed fishhook. *(Middle)* Multiple-barbed fishhook. *(Right)* Treble fishhook.

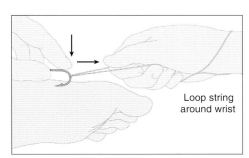

Loop string around wrist

Fig. 137.3 String technique.

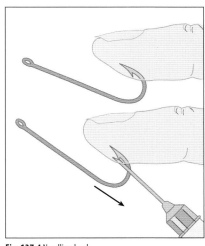

Fig. 137.4 Needling hook.

that will not move when the string is pulled. Therefore the involved skin area should be well stabilized against a flat surface before starting. When done properly, this procedure is painless and can be done in the field without anesthesia. A useful variant of this technique that may require anesthesia is to push down on the hook as described earlier but instead of pulling on a string, use the thumb and middle finger to grasp the shaft of the hook and push the hook out in the same direction as with the string.

Needle cover technique: A hollow-bore needle (≥18 gauge) is inserted parallel to the inner side of the short arm of the hook through the same puncture wound that the hook created. The tip of the needle covers the barb, which allows it to disengage from the tissues. The needle and hook are withdrawn in retrograde fashion simultaneously (see Fig. 137.4) (See Video 137.4). With skin anesthetized, this technique can be made easier

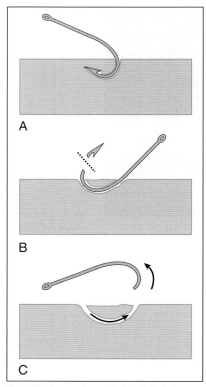

Fig. 137.5 Advance and cut method: single-barbed fishhook.

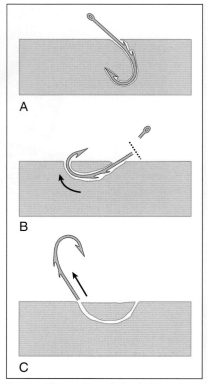

Fig. 137.6 Advance and cut method: multiple-barbed fishhook.

by slightly enlarging the entrance wound with a No. 11 scalpel blade, pushing the point of the blade toward the barb.

✅ **Advance and cut technique: After anesthetizing surrounding tissues, the hook is advanced along its curve until the tip of the hook penetrates the tissue nearby. This is best achieved with a hemostat or needle driver. Once the tip has penetrated, the barb is clipped off with an orthopedic pin cutter or metal snip and the hook is removed in retrograde fashion** (see Fig. 137.5) (See Video 137.5).

✅ **Push-through technique: Best used on a multiple barbed fishhook, this technique is similar to the clip technique (see earlier), but instead of clipping the barb, the end of the shaft is removed and the entire hook is pushed through and taken out of the tissue distant from where it entered** (see Fig. 137.6) (See Video 137.5).

✅ Prophylactic antibiotic therapy is generally not necessary but may be considered for persons who are immunosuppressed or have injuries that involve tendons, cartilage, joints, or bone.

✅ Provide follow-up in 2 days for high-risk patients. Provide immediate follow-up care for any patient who develops signs or symptoms of infection (rare).

What Not to Do

(X) Do not try to remove a treble hook or a fishing lure with multiple hooks without first removing or covering the unembedded hooks.

(X) Do not routinely prescribe prophylactic antibiotics. Even hooks that have been contaminated by fish rarely cause secondary infection.

Discussion

All individuals near bodies of water are at risk for fishhook injuries, either while handling hooks, being injured as a hook is cast by an angler, or by stepping on a discarded hook.

Most embedded fishhooks can be removed with minimal surgical intervention. Often, individuals have tried retrograde removal prior to presentation. For hooks not embedded further than the initial part of the hook's curve, the string-yank technique should be attempted first as it results in the least amount of tissue trauma. The more invasive procedures, such as the advance and cut or push-through techniques, usually are reserved for more difficult cases. Sometimes multiple techniques must be attempted before the fishhook is successfully removed. Let patients know this before you begin.

Suggested Readings

Beasley, K., Ouellette, L., Bush, C., et al. (2018). Experience with various techniques for fishhook removal in the emergency department. *American Journal of Emergency Medicine*, *37*(5), 979–980. https://doi.org/10.1016/j.ajem.2018.09.028.

Gammons, M., & Jackson, E. (2001). Fishhook removal. *American Family Physician*, *63*(11), 2231–2237.

Foreign Body Beneath Nail

Presentation

The patient complains of a paint chip or wooden sliver under the nail. Due to high sensory nerve density, these injuries are often quite painful. Most subungual foreign bodies are completely visible and are lodged under the distal portion of the nail. Occasionally, a wooden sliver will be large and deeply embedded over the proximal germinal matrix.

Often the patient has unsuccessfully attempted to remove the foreign body, which has broken off and could not be grabbed using household tweezers.

What to Do

✓ In general, there are four different techniques to remove a subungual foreign body. Depending on the technique used and the pain/anxiety experienced by the patient**, a digital block may help facilitate the procedure.**

✓ **Nail shaving technique: Starting proximal to the foreign body (this technique works best with a distal paint chip), shave the nail with a No. 15 scalpel blade. Hold the blade at an acute angle (5–10 degrees) to the nail surface and repeatedly shave off thin slices with gentle pressure in a distal direction until the foreign body is fully exposed** (Fig. 138.1). The foreign body can then be lifted away. Irrigate the exposed nailbed with tap water to remove any residual debris. Dress the wound with petroleum gauze to prevent adherence of the bandage material to the exposed nail bed. With distal foreign bodies, this technique is often not painful and can be done without a digital block.

✓ Provide tetanus prophylaxis if necessary (see Appendix G).

✓ **Needle extraction technique: For small nonfriable objects**, it may be possible to take **a needle (23 or 25 gauge) and push it into the exposed end of the foreign body, angling the needle up toward the distal nail plate. Then, when the needle is firmly lodged in the foreign body (while maintaining the same angle), the sliver can be pulled out by using the needle tip for traction** (Fig. 138.2). This technique usually does not work on paint chips, which will simply break off. If significant debris remains, partial removal of the nail will be necessary to facilitate irrigation.

✓ **Hemostat technique: After performing a digital block, insert an open fine tip hemostat underneath the nail with each arm on one side of the foreign body. Grasp the foreign body with the hemostat and apply traction to facilitate removal.** If significant debris remains, partial removal of the nail will be necessary to facilitate irrigation.

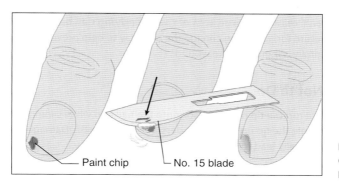

Fig. 138.1 Paint chip removal. This technique creates a U-shaped defect that releases the paint chip foreign body.

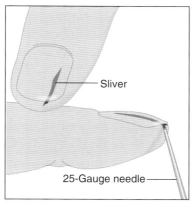

Fig. 138.2 Sliver removal. Push a needle (23 or 25 gauge) into the exposed end of the splinter, angling the needle up toward the distal nail plate. Then, when the needle is firmly lodged in the splinter (while maintaining the same angle), the sliver can then be pulled out by using the needle tip for traction.

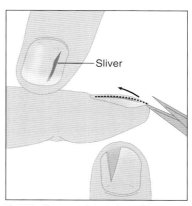

Fig. 138.3 Sliver removal. Angle the tip of the scissor blade up into the nail plate, not down and into the nail bed.

✅ **Partial nail removal technique: When presented with a large or friable foreign body, a more extensive excision of an overlying nail wedge may be required.** Perform a digital block (see Appendix B).

✅ **Slide a small (but strong) straight iris scissor arm between the nail and nail bed on both sides of the sliver and cut out the overlying V-shaped wedge of nail** (Fig. 138.3). The point of the V should be at or near the proximal tip of the splinter. The wedge of nail plate will fall away, and the exposed sliver can then be easily picked away. Irrigate the exposed nailbed with tap water to remove any residual debris. Dress the wound with petroleum gauze to prevent adherence of bandage material to the nail bed.

✅ Provide tetanus prophylaxis (see Appendix G) if needed.

✅ **When a relatively large area of the underlying nail bed has been exposed,** have the patient return for a dressing change the next day to help prevent the non adherent dressing from painfully adhering to the wound.

What Not to Do

❌ Do not run the tip of the scissors into the nail bed while sliding it under the fingernail (instead angle the tip up into the undersurface of the nail). Damage to the germinal matrix could potentially lead to a permanent nail plate deformity.

❌ Do not routinely prescribe antibiotics. When the foreign body has been removed, there is little risk for infection.

Discussion

Very small and minimally painful subungual foreign bodies, particularly the ones composed of nonreactive materials (glass, metal, plastic), may not need to be removed at all and can be managed conservatively. Some clinicians will only provide nonopioid analgesics and allow uninfected slivers to grow out with the nail. The sliver can be removed more easily in 10 to 14 days. These patients should be informed of the possible increased risk for infection, and they require easy access to follow-up care with any increased pain or swelling or subungual purulence.

Suspected but poorly visualized foreign bodies can be revealed by using ultrasound or dermoscopy when available.

A large foreign body made of reactive material (plant matter or animal spines), or one that results in significant discomfort, should always be promptly and completely removed.

Suggested Readings

Chan, C., & Salam, G. A. (2003). Splinter removal. *American Family Physician, 67*(12), 2557–2562.

Schwartz, G. R., & Schwen, S. A. (1997). Subungual splinter removal. *American Journal of Emergency Medicine, 15*(3), 330–331.

Teng, M., & Doniger, S. J. (2012). Subungual wooden splinter visualized with bedside sonography. *Pediatric Emergency Care, 28*(4), 392–394.

You, H.-S., Kim, G.-W., Kim, W.-J., Mun, J.-H., Song, M., Kim, H.-S., et al. (2016). The usefulness of dermoscopy for detection of subungual white foreign bodies. *Annals of Dermatology, 28*(1), 144–145.

Impalement Injuries, Minor

Presentation

A sharp metal object, such as a needle, heavy wire, or nail, is driven into the soft tissue. The patient may arrive with an additional large object attached (e.g., a child who has stepped on a nail going through a board) (Fig. 139.1). Any of these skin-piercing foreign objects, such as impaled Taser darts, can be quite dramatic and can be the cause for emotional distress in both the patient and others involved. These events are not uncommon; there are about 25,000 annual emergency department (ED) visits due to nail gun use alone, half of which involve the hand.

What to Do

✓ **If the patient arrives with an impaled object attached to something that is acting like a lever, either quickly remove or stabilize the object. Any movement of the penetrating portion can cause significant pain. Removal may require cutting off the impaling object where it is exposed outside of the patient's body. An exposed nail or metal spike can usually be cut with an orthopedic pin cutter** (Fig. 139.2).

✓ **Obtain preremoval radiographs only when bone or joint injury that requires surgical removal is suspected. Postremoval radiographs have higher utility** as they allow screening for retained/fragmented foreign bodies as well as fractures at the same time.

✓ **If the impaled object penetrated fabric prior to entering the patient's skin, it may carry debris from the fabric into the patient's wound. After removal, meticulous wound irrigation and exploration in a hemostatic (bloodless) field are paramount.**

✓ **Nail guns fire nails at approximately 300 feet/second (some as high as 1400 feet/second), approximately the muzzle velocity of a 0.22-caliber gun. The kinetic energy creates a tissue shock wave that can injure nearby structures not directly in the path of the nail. Thus carefully examine the extremity for neurovascular and tendon injury.**

✓ **Rapid removal using sudden forceful traction on firmly embedded smooth, straight objects (e.g., fork, nail, or letter spike) is generally the most appropriate method for removing these objects (See Video 139.1). The exceptions are ring-shank nails and Herringbone nails**, which are barbed. Be sure to ask the patient prior to attempting removal whether barbed nails were used.

✓ **For barbed nails, the length of the nail and the anatomic location determine if the push-through method is feasible. If it is not, consultation with a surgeon is advised.**

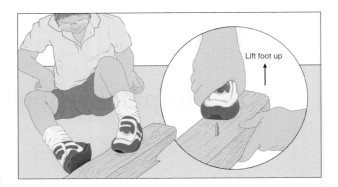

Fig. 139.1 Foot stuck to nail with rapid removal.

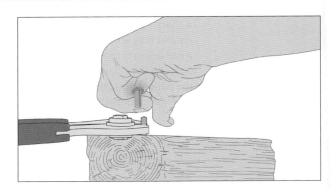

Fig. 139.2 Cut an exposed nail with an orthopedic pin cutter.

✓ **Other barbed foreign bodies (crochet needles, fish spines, Taser darts) that remain only superficially embedded may not require push-through removal. After first anesthetizing the area, apply firm traction until the barb is revealed through the puncture wound. The fibrils of connective tissue caught over the barb can then be cut with a No. 11 scalpel blade or fine scissors.** To provide better exposure, the entrance wound can be enlarged using the No. 11 blade.

✓ **If surgical debridement is anticipated after removal of the object, infiltration of an anesthetic should be provided before removal.** Otherwise, patient preference should determine whether a local anesthetic is used. Local anesthesia will usually not give complete pain relief when a deeply embedded object is removed by quickly pulling it out. Therefore let the patient decide about the painful "numbing shot" before you pull out the foreign body.

✓ Contaminated objects that track superficially under the dermis may be released using the same techniques described in Chapter 153.

✓ **After removal of the impaled object, the wound should be appropriately irrigated as described for puncture wounds** (see Chapter 151).

✓ Tetanus prophylaxis should be provided (see Appendix G).

✓ Except for contaminated wounds, such as a fish spine, contaminated fork, or wood impalement, prophylactic antibiotics should not routinely be prescribed.

✓ Provide early follow-up and/or have the patient seek care with any sign of infection.

What Not to Do

❌ Do not send a patient for a radiograph with a leveraged object impaled, thus creating further pain and possible injury with every movement. When radiographs are necessary, fully immobilize or remove the attached objects.

❌ Do not try to hand saw a board attached to an impaled object. The resultant movement will obviously cause unnecessary pain and possibly harm.

❌ **Do not remove impaled objects within proximity of major vascular structures without having a plan to control hemorrhage if necessary.**

❌ **Do not remove impaled objects near eyes or any other delicate structures without first consulting with an appropriate specialist.**

Discussion

Simple impalement injuries of the distal extremities can usually be treated by direct removal of the object. **Impalement objects in the neck and trunk, groin, or buttock** should not be precipitously removed. **With major impalement injuries (e.g., a metal rod impaled into the abdomen or chest),** careful localization with radiographs is required, and full exposure and vascular control in the operating room are necessary to prevent rapid exsanguination when the impaled object is removed from the heart or a great vessel. Large impalement injuries of the extremities (especially of the groin, thigh, and axilla) also require immediate surgical consultation and thorough consideration of potential neurovascular and musculoskeletal injuries.

Suggested Readings

Lipscomb, H. J., & Schoenfisch, A. L. (2015). Nail gun injuries treated in US emergency departments, 2006-2011: Not just a worker safety issue. *American Journal of Industrial Medicine*, *58*(8), 880–885. https://doi.org/10.1002/ajim.22457.

Rhee, P. C., Fox, T. J., & Kakar, S. (2013). Nail gun injuries to the hand. *Journal of Hand Surgery (America)*, *38*(6), 1242–1246 [quiz, 1246]. https://doi.org/10.1016/j.jhsa.2013.01.037.

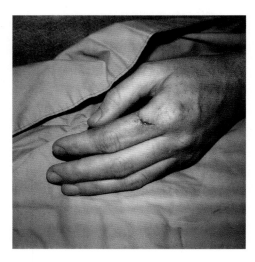

Laceration, Simple

Presentation

Lacerations arise from either a cut with a sharp object or direct blunt trauma that exceeds the tensile strength of the skin. Consequently, lacerations may be linear (Fig. 140.1) or stellate/complex with various amounts of tissue loss. The elderly and patients on chronic steroid therapy may present with "wet tissue paper" skin tears following relatively minor trauma.

What to Do

✓ A history should establish the approximate time of injury as well as the exact mechanism of injury. Traditional teaching associates increased risk with delayed closure, but this is not supported by data. There is no clear cutoff at which wounds are too high risk to repair. However, closure after 19 hours is associated with poorer wound healing. The location of the wound is more predictive of infectious risk, with lower extremity wounds being highest. This may in part be due to reduced circulation as well as bacteria from the anogenital region being washed over the wound during showers.

✓ **Perform a distal neurovascular exam and assess tendon function on all extremity injuries. Put joints through both active and passive range of motion to assess for tendon injuries that may be temporarily outside the field of view. Test tendon function against**

Fig. 140.1 Simple laceration.

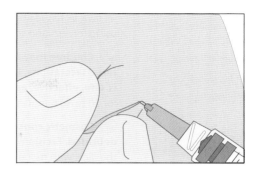

Fig. 140.2 Demonstration of the pinching of the skin with the thumb and forefinger, just behind the area of injection with the anesthetic. Note the perpendicular relationship of the needle to the thumb and forefinger. (Adapted from Fosko, S. W., Gibney, M. D., & Harrison, B. [1998]. Repetitive pinching of the skin during lidocaine infiltration reduces patient discomfort. *Journal of the American Academy of Dermatology, 39*, 74–78.)

resistance. **Significant pain and/or lack of function indicates a partial or complete tendon laceration. Decreased or absent sensation suggests nerve injury.** Tendon and nerve lacerations deserve specialty consultation.

⊘ **The following also require surgical consultation: joint capsule disruptions, vascular injuries, repair of specialized structures (e.g., parotid or lacrimal duct, eyelid margin, tarsal plate), extensive injuries, or those involving significant tissue loss.**

⊘ **Provide either regional or local anesthesia prior to irrigation and wound repair. To help reduce the pain of injection, begin subdermally, inside the wound edge so as to avoid piercing intact skin. Inject slowly while repetitively pinching the skin, just behind the area being injected** (Fig. 140.2).

⊘ **Irrigation is the most important step in preventing infection. It is not necessary to use sterile water; tap water appears to be as efficacious in preventing infection.**

⊘ **Two equally efficacious approaches to irrigation are available: high pressure/low volume (HP/LV) or low pressure/high volume (LP/HV).**

○ **HP/LV: Using a 60-cc syringe or a** *pressurized* **bag of intravenous fluid and an 18-gauge catheter creates an approximate pressure of 8 pounds per square inch (psi). No high-quality data are available regarding the optimal volume of irrigation solution with this technique, but a general guideline is to use 100 cc per centimeter of laceration length.**

○ **LP/HV: Using the pressure generated by the tap of a sink, the patient self-irrigates the wound with tap water. Again, no high-quality data exist regarding optimal volume and duration with this technique, but a general guideline is to irrigate for 1 minute per centimeter of laceration length.**

⊘ **After irrigation and under hemostatic conditions, inspect for embedded foreign bodies and adherent debris.** Keep in mind that with deeper lacerations, upper tissue layers may slide back in place and cover over hidden contaminants. Always use a gloved finger to explore the depth of any wound and expose any hidden debris. Consider bedside ultrasonography or radiographs if concern for foreign bodies persists. If a foreign body is seen, the risk of removal must be weighed against the risk of complications. Glass, metal, and plastic are generally inert, and their removal is not paramount but always recommended. Organic matter (e.g., wood, soil, other plant matter) can have highly immunogenic resin and serve as a nidus of infection. These contaminants must always be removed completely by further high-jet lavage, tissue abrasion with a wet surgical sponge or No. 10 scalpel blade, or sharp excision using forceps and scissors.

✓ **Children may also benefit from a topical anesthetic agent, especially for scalp and facial lacerations. Lidocaine 4% plus epinephrine 1:1000 (0.1%) plus tetracaine 0.5% (LET) is safe, effective, and inexpensive.** Put 3 mL on a cotton ball and press firmly into the wound for 20 to 30 minutes, either with tape or with the parent's gloved hand.

✓ **Cosmetic considerations will influence the degree to which facial lacerations are debrided.** Excision of contaminated nonviable wound edges should be kept to a minimum on the face, with tissue preservation being of primary concern.

✓ **Hair generally does not need to be removed.** When necessary, shorten hair with scissors rather than shaving with a razor.

✓ **Sterile gloves may be used for enhanced dexterity, but they are not necessary and do not reduce the risk of infection.** Of course, routine protective vinyl gloves are required as an alternative.

✓ **Ask about tetanus immunization status and provide prophylaxis where indicated** (see Appendix G).

✓ **In general, prophylactic systemic antibiotics are only indicated in heavily contaminated wounds, lacerations from bites, or in patients who are immunocompromised.**

✓ **After closing the wound with sutures, apply bacitracin antibiotic ointment and a sterile protective nonadherent dressing. While data are scarce, they suggest that topical application of bacitracin or neomycin reduces infection rates. However, neomycin is a highly allergenic compound, thus bacitracin is preferred.**

✓ **Give patients clear, specific discharge instructions** that explain the potential complications of their injuries, and tell patients when and where to go for reevaluation and follow-up care.

✓ **Schedule a wound check in 2 days if the patient is likely to develop any problems with infection, require dressing changes, or need continued wound care.** After 48 hours, most sutured wounds can be redressed with a simple bandage that can be easily removed and replaced by the patient, allowing for a shower each day.

✓ The following discusses various suture and other wound closure techniques. They are meant to refresh memory but are not adequate as instruction for a novice provider.

Wound Closure Options

Steri-Strips

○ **Wound closure tapes (Steri-Strips) and tissue adhesives offer the lowest risk for infection and are most successfully used on simple superficial lacerations with minimal tension. Tape strips are the closure material of choice for "wet tissue paper" skin tears.** Before application, degrease the skin with alcohol wipes, being careful not to get any alcohol into the wound. An adhesive agent such as tincture of benzoin may then be thinly applied to the skin surrounding the laceration (again, avoiding the open wound). Push the wound edges together and apply the tape to maintain approximation (Fig. 140.3).

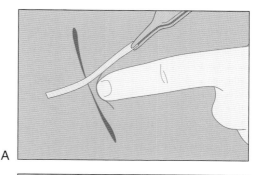

A

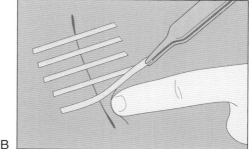

B

Fig. 140.3 (A) The tape is placed on one side of the wound at its midpoint while the clinician grasps it with forceps in the dominant hand. The opposite wound edge is then gently apposed by pushing with a finger of the nondominant hand. (B) The remaining open sections of the wound are bisected by additional tape strips until the strips are within 2 to 5 mm of each other.

Topical Skin Adhesive

○   **Cyanoacrylate topical skin adhesive (Dermabond, Indermil, Epiglu) can be used with small wounds in a location that does not allow the application of a length of wound closure tape.** These adhesives can also be used in combination with the tape strips (Fig. 140.4). **Tissue glues, like tape closures, are rapid and relatively painless to apply; therefore they generally do not require the use of a painful local anesthetic.** There is also no need for suture removal. In addition, cyanoacrylate tissue adhesives have a barrier function against microbial penetration and serve as an optimal wound dressing that creates a moist environment, thus enhancing wound healing.

○   With the wound edges completely dry (degreasing the skin with alcohol wipes) and meticulously approximated, the adhesive is carefully expressed through the tip of the applicator and gently brushed over the wound surface, covering 5 to 10 mm on either side of the wound edges (Fig. 140.5). Initially, only a thin layer should be applied because thicker layers may result in release of unpleasant heat as the glue polymerizes. After allowing the first layer of the adhesive to polymerize for 30 to 45 seconds, two to three additional layers should be applied, waiting 5 to 10 seconds between successive layers. **Usually reserved for low-tension wounds, tape closure strips and tissue adhesives can be used over areas of moderate skin tension if an appropriate immobilizing dressing or splint is applied.** Otherwise, simple wound coverings are optional. Ointments should not be used because they will loosen the adhesive. The patient's wound is allowed to get wet briefly each day during showering or bathing.

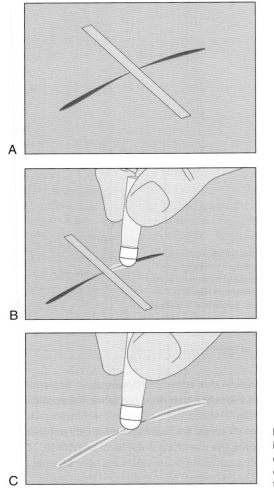

A

B

C

Fig. 140.4 Closing a long or complex wound. (A) The wound is bisected with a strip of surgical tape. (B) The wound limbs on either side of the tape are glued. (C) The strip is removed, and the central portion of the wound is glued. Some practitioners prefer to leave the tape strip and apply the adhesive over it.

Staples

○ **Most scalp lacerations and many trunk and proximal extremity lacerations that are straight, without edges that curl under (invert), can be most easily and rapidly repaired using skin staples.** However, staples do not allow meticulous repairs and should not be used in areas of cosmetic concern. Push wound edges together and staple so that edges evert slightly. Hair does not interfere with this technique and does not cause a problem if caught under a staple.

Hair Approximation Technique

○ With simple linear scalp lacerations, where the hair is at least 3 cm long and there is no active hemorrhage, closure can be obtained without using any anesthesia by using the hair apposition technique with tissue glue (Fig. 140.6). Patients are able to wash their hair 3 days after repair.

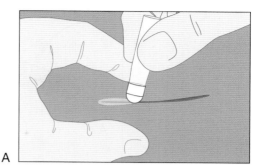

A

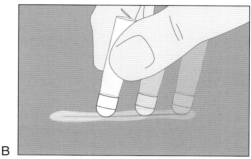

B

Fig. 140.5 (A) To prevent inadvertent runoff of the Dermabond adhesive, position the wound in a horizontal plane. Manually approximate the wound edges with forceps or gloved fingers. Use gentle brushing strokes to apply a thin film of liquid to the approximated wound edges, and maintain proper eversion of skin edges as you apply Dermabond adhesive. The adhesive should extend at least ½ cm on each side of the apposed wound edges. Apply Dermabond adhesive from above the wound. (B) Gradually build up three or four thin layers of adhesive. Ensure that the adhesive is evenly distributed over the wound. Maintain approximation of the wound edges until the adhesive sets and forms a flexible film. This should occur about 1 minute after applying the last layer.

Suture

○ **For deep or irregular lacerations, or lacerations on hands, feet, and skin over joints, use a monofilament nonabsorbable suture, such as nylon (Ethilon) or polypropylene (Prolene) (either 4-0, 5-0, or 6-0), using the smallest diameter with sufficient strength. Deep absorbable sutures (Vicryl, Vicryl Rapide) assist in approximating wound edges by decreasing tension and lessening dead space in which transudate and blood could accumulate** (Fig. 140.7). Because of an increased risk for infection, one relative contraindication to deep suture placement is contamination of the laceration.

○ A good strategy to realign skin and minimize sutures is to begin by approximating the midpoint of the wound and then bisecting the remaining gaps with subsequent sutures. Put known landmarks together first (e.g., vermilion border, flexion creases, wrinkles). Simple interrupted stitches in most body sites should be about 0.5 cm apart, 0.5 cm deep, and 0.5 cm back from the wound edge (Fig. 140.8). Make each dimension 0.25 cm for cosmetic closure on the face. Angle the needle going in and coming out so that it grasps more subcutaneous tissue than skin. The wound edges should evert so that the dermis is aligned level on both sides, thereby minimizing visible scar. Tie each stitch with only enough tension to approximate and mildly evert the edges. The raised edge will flatten out as the healing tissue contracts. A continuous running suture (Fig. 140.9) is a more rapid technique of closing a fairly straight laceration. When there is wound edge inversion (where the wound edge curls under), the length of the wound edge can be completely excised prior to repair. Alternatively, vertical mattress sutures can be placed between simple interrupted stitches, thereby preventing the wound edge from curling under (Fig. 140.10).

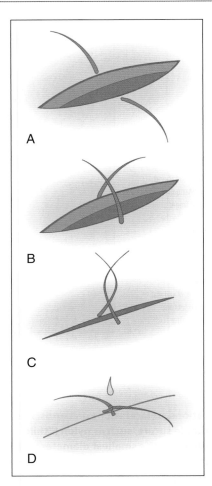

Fig. 140.6 Hair apposition technique. (A) Choose four to five strands of hair in a bundle on either side of the scalp laceration. (B) Using artery forceps, cross the strands. (C) Make a single twist to appose the wound. (D) Secure with a single drop of glue. (Adapted from Ong, M. E., Coyle, D., Lim, S. H., & Stiell, I. [2005]. Cost-effectiveness of hair apposition techniques for suturing. *Annals of Emergency Medicine, 46,* 237–242.)

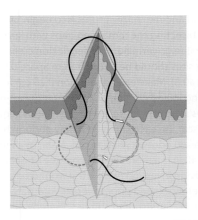 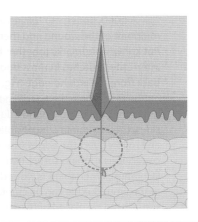

Fig. 140.7 Absorbable intradermal sutures.

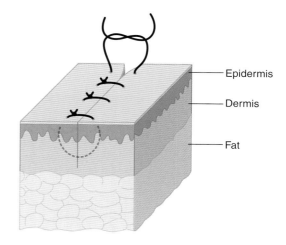

Epidermis

Dermis

Fat

Fig. 140.8 Simple sutures.

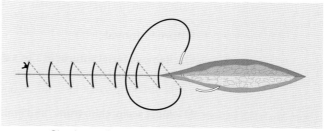

Fig. 140.9 Simple running suture.

Simple running suture (advancing on underside)

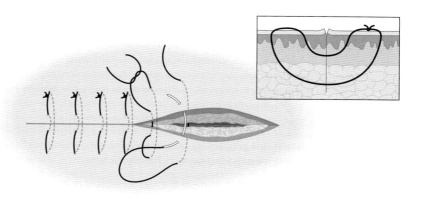

Fig. 140.10 Vertical mattress suture.

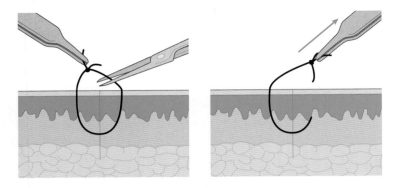

Fig. 140.11 Simple suture removal.

○ **When small children require sutures in a location that will make suture removal very difficult, use polyglactin (Vicryl Rapide) absorbable suture material rather than a monofilament nonabsorbable suture.** Suture removal is thereby unnecessary. Standard polyglactin (Vicryl) is more slowly absorbed and is more likely to cause discomfort or suture abscess than the Rapide material.

Suture Removal

○ **Remove facial sutures in 3 to 5 days to reduce the risk for visible stitch marks.** The epidermis should have resealed by this time, but the dermis will not have developed much tensile strength; so reinforce the wound edges with wound closure strips for a few more days.

○ **Most scalp, chin, trunk, and limb stitches should be removed in 7 days. Sutures may be left in for 10 to 14 days where there is tension across wound edges, as over the extensor surfaces of large joints.** Sutures are easily and painlessly cut with the tip of a No. 11 or 12 scalpel blade or with fine scissors and removed with simple smooth forceps (Fig. 140.11). Cut alternate loops of running sutures when these are ready to be removed.

What Not to Do

Ⓧ Do not prescribe prophylactic antibiotics for simple lacerations. Antibiotics do not reduce infection rates and only select for resistant organisms. Several clinical studies and a meta-analysis have found that there is no benefit to prophylactic antibiotics for routine laceration repair. Most infections can be easily treated when they occur. Limit prophylactic antibiotics to high-risk wounds.

Ⓧ **Do not close a laceration if there is visible or suspected contamination, debris, or nonviable tissue that cannot be adequately removed or if there are any signs of infection. Dress it open for delayed primary closure.**

Ⓧ Do not substitute antibiotics for wound cleansing and debridement.

Ⓧ Do not use undiluted skin cleansing solution, such as 10% povidone-iodine or any skin scrub containing detergents or soap, in an open wound. They are toxic and will delay wound healing.

ⓧ Do not miss a hidden human bite. Any laceration over the knuckles of the hand should be considered a human bite until proven otherwise (see Chapter 142).

ⓧ Do not shave an eyebrow. The hair is a useful marker for reapproximating the skin edges and can take months to years to grow back.

ⓧ Do not remove too much skin or underlying tissue when debriding the face and scalp.

ⓧ Do not place tissue adhesives within a wound or between wound margins.

ⓧ Do not allow tissue glue to drip into the patient's eye. When working near the eye, cover the lid with moistened gauze for protection. When available, high-viscosity Dermabond should be used.

ⓧ Do not use buried absorbable sutures in a wound with a high risk for infection.

ⓧ Do not insert drains in simple lacerations. They are more likely to introduce infection than prevent it.

ⓧ Do not apply ointments or petroleum jelly to wounds closed with tissue adhesives or sterile tape closures. This will cause these products to loosen prematurely and may lead to early wound dehiscence.

Discussion

The most important goal of early wound care is preventing infection while attaining a functional closure with minimal scarring. Patients have these same concerns, along with the desire for the least painful repair.

Nonabsorbable suture material is the standard for percutaneous use, because nylon and polypropylene are low-reactive materials with good tensile strength. This, of course, is also true for **stainless steel staples. Their use should also be delayed if computed tomography (CT) scanning is planned because of the possible scatter artifacts the staples can cause**.

Buried absorbable sutures are more reactive and, in animal studies of contaminated wounds, have been shown to increase the risk for infection. The placement of these sutures, however, has not been shown to increase infection in clean wounds.

Tissue glue is nonreactive and has the added advantage over sutures of being quickly applied and painless (a special benefit when children are involved). The clinician using these tissue adhesives must always use the same care in providing adequate wound cleansing as with sutured wounds. The limitations of the adhesive's tensile strength and tendency toward wound dehiscence must also be taken into consideration. If cyanoacrylates get into undesirable areas, such as the eye, the glue can

be removed with a petroleum-based product (e.g., ophthalmic bacitracin or erythromycin).

Primary closure is the closure of a wound at the time of presentation. Delayed primary closure is the closure of a wound 3 to 4 days after the injury. Delayed primary closure should be used for heavily contaminated wounds or contaminated wounds in a host predisposed to infection. Wounds that are grossly contaminated or infected can be treated with wet to dry dressing or packing changes as often as two to three times per day to provide automatic cleansing and debridement. When the wound appears clean, without signs of infection, it can be closed typically within 3 to 5 days.

Healing by secondary intention is simply allowing a wound to heal without formal closure, other than in some instances applying a protective dressing. The primary advantage to this technique is its ease of use. The disadvantage is the associated delay in wound closure and possible increased scar size.

For some small wounds, this nonclosure technique may be most appropriate. Simple hand lacerations, less than 2 cm in length and without deep structure involvement (distal to the distal volar wrist crease), that have been

(continued)

Discussion continued

left open without repair have been shown to heal without cosmetic or functional difference compared with primary closure.

Suturing therefore may not offer any advantages over simple cleansing and dressing of small hand lacerations. Healing by secondary intention may produce superior aesthetic results on concave surfaces of the face and ears (e.g., the medial canthal area, nasal alar crease, nasolabial area, and concave fossa and concha of the auricle).

Where practical, those wounds may be covered with moistened cotton or gauze and held in place with a dressing to provide better wound edge alignment.

Permanent hyperpigmentation was observed in some wounds, caused by dermabrasion after excessive exposure to sunlight for the 6 months following injury. It is unclear whether this should be extrapolated to simple skin lacerations, but some clinicians recommend that sunscreens be used for several months to prevent hyperpigmentation.

Suggested Readings

Berk, W. A., Osbourne, D. D., & Taylor, D. D. (1988). Evaluation of the "golden period" for wound repair: 204 cases from a third world emergency department. *Annals of Emergency Medicine, 17*(5), 496–500.

Dire, D. J., Coppola, M., Dwyer, D. A., Lorette, J. J., & Karr, J. L. (1995). Prospective evaluation of topical antibiotics for preventing infections in uncomplicated soft-tissue wounds repaired in the ED. *Academic Emergency Medicine, 2*(1), 4–10.

Moscati, R. M., Mayrose, J., Reardon, R. F., Janicke, D. M., & Jehle, D. V. (2007). A multicenter comparison of tap water versus sterile saline for wound irrigation. *Academic Emergency Medicine, 14*(5), 404–409. https://doi.org/10.1197/j.aem.2007.01.007

Perelman, V. S., Francis, G. J., Rutledge, T., Foote, J., Martino, F., & Dranitsaris, G. (2004). Sterile versus nonsterile gloves for repair of uncomplicated lacerations in the emergency department: A randomized controlled trial. *Annals of Emergency Medicine, 43*(3), 362–370.

Pronchik, D., Barber, C., & Rittenhouse, S. (1999). Low- versus high-pressure irrigation techniques in *Staphylococcus aureus*-inoculated wounds. *American Journal of Emergency Medicine, 17*(2), 121–124.

Zehtabchi, S., Tan, A., Yadav, K., Badawy, A., & Lucchesi, M. (2012). The impact of wound age on the infection rate of simple lacerations repaired in the emergency department. *Injury, 43*(11), 1793–1798. https://doi.org/10.1016/j.injury.2012.02.018

Leg Edema

Presentation

A patient presents with swelling of the lower extremity. It may be mildly painful, but there has been no trauma. The patient denies any fever, chest pain, difficulty breathing, or other systemic symptoms.

Peripheral edema can be categorized in two different ways: unilateral versus bilateral and pitting versus non-pitting. The list of differential diagnoses varies; a comprehensive history, physical exam, and target laboratory testing are paramount.

What to Do

✓ **On physical exam, assess symmetry between both lower extremities.** Lifting both heels off the stretcher reduces compression of the calves against the mattress and allows for better visual assessment. Asymmetry may be difficult to appreciate visually but can be objectively measured. A measuring tape can assess circumference of the calf and should be applied to the largest diameter of the gastrocnemius/soleus muscle group.

✓ The extent of the edema should be assessed and documented. This is important to allow subsequent providers to track therapeutic progress. In ambulatory patients, edema is most likely to accumulate in the ankle, pretibial area, and knees. In patients who are bedridden, sacral edema is often the first place of accumulation.

✓ **Determine whether the edema is pitting or non-pitting.** Press gently on the area of edema with the thumb for 5 seconds. If it leaves a palpable depression, it is considered pitting.

✓ Pitting edema is described from "trace" to "4+". Grading the degree of pitting is an inexact science, but in general for each 2 mm of depth of pitting it is assigned the next higher level. Thus trace pitting edema is from minimal to 2 mm depth, 1+ is from 2 mm to 4 mm of depth, and so forth (Figs. 141.1, 141.2, and 141.3).

✓ **For unilateral pitting edema:**

○ **Pitting edema is typically a venous problem rather than a lymphatic problem. Unilateral pitting edema should raise concern for a deep vein thrombosis (DVT).**

○ Obtain a bedside venous duplex ultrasound to assess for DVT, especially if the patient has a history of DVT, has a clotting disorder (e.g., factor V Leiden), is a smoker, is on birth control, had recent surgery, or has experienced prolonged immobility.

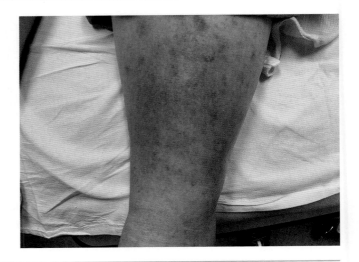

Fig. 141.1 Cellulitis.

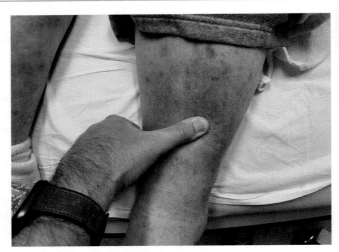

Fig. 141.2 Determine whether the edema is pitting or non-pitting. Press gently onto the area of edema with the thumb for 5 seconds.

○ If an ultrasound is not readily available, a D-Dimer blood test can rule out a DVT (sensitivity of 96% with negative likelihood ratio of 0.09), but due to its low positive likelihood ratio of 1.5, it cannot be used to confirm the diagnosis.

○ **Phlegmasia cerulea dolens results in venous ischemia due to massive iliofemoral occlusion from DVT.**

○ **Cellulitis may result in unilateral pitting edema.** An infrared thermometer can objectively compare surface temperatures between both legs and aid in making the diagnosis.

⊘ **For bilateral pitting edema:**

○ **All the abovementioned etiologies may be present bilaterally or centrally** (e.g., a pelvic DVT) and thus result in bilateral symptoms.

○ **Bilateral pitting edema raises concern for systemic illness.** In general, edema occurs due to increased venous hydrostatic pressure or decreased intravascular oncotic pressure.

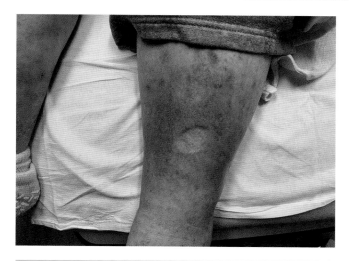

Fig. 141.3 Pitting edema is from minimal 2 mm to 4 mm of depth.

- ○ Increased hydrostatic pressure may be due to heart failure, high-sodium diet (often seen after holidays during which salty food is consumed), or aggressive fluid resuscitation during a recent hospital stay. Recent steroid therapy may have led to increased fluid retention.
- ○ Decreased oncotic pressure is due to reduced albumin synthesis (liver disease, malnutrition) or due to increased protein loss (nephrotic syndrome).
- ○ Heat edema is attributed to microvascular transudate of fluid with prolonged peripheral vasodilatation. This type of edema is not associated with volume overload.

✅ **For unilateral and bilateral non-pitting edema:**

- ○ The pressure on the tissue that results in pitting displaces interstitial fluid into lymphatics. Thus **non-pitting edema is highly concerning for lymphatic obstruction.**
- ○ Inquire if the patient had any surgery or trauma to the lower extremity that may have injured lymphatic ducts.
- ○ In males, perform a testicular exam. Testicular cancer may lead to inguinal lymphadenopathy and thus lymphatic outflow obstruction.
- ○ Inquire about weight loss, night sweats, low-grade fevers that may indicate lymphoma as it may result in decreased lymphatic outflow from a lower extremity.
- ○ Ask about recent travel, as filariasis often presents as non-pitting edema.

✅ **Treatment depends on the underlying pathology.** Fluid overload states are best treated initially with diuretics. A patient who is naïve to diuretics should be started on 20 mg furosemide orally, but further management should be under the guidance of a primary care provider.

✅ **If there is concern for cirrhosis, heart failure, or nephrotic syndrome**, the patient should be referred to the appropriate specialist. Therapy for the respective condition should be discussed with the specialist who will continue caring for the patient.

✅ **If ultrasonography reveals a DVT**, anticoagulant therapy should be initiated unless the patient has contraindications such as recent surgery, metastatic cancer to the brain, or recent gastrointestinal hemorrhage.

✓ **If a patient with a DVT has any recent history of syncope, shortness of breath, hemoptysis, or chest pain**, a computed tomography angiography (CTA) of the chest or ventilation/perfusion (VQ) scan should be obtained to screen for pulmonary embolization.

✓ **Regardless of cause, or with heat edema**, leg elevation and compression with Ace bandages (or compression stockings) will allow for some reduction in the leg swelling and thus lead to symptomatic improvement. When managing heat edema, diuretics have no role.

What Not to Do

✗ Do not confuse chronic venostatic changes with cellulitis. Cellulitis is usually not bilaterally symmetric, but venostatic changes are. In addition, venostasis does not lead to calor (warmth) or systemic fever.

✗ Do not attempt to drain edema by incision. With significant swelling, reapproximation of the skin will be difficult.

✗ Do not discount the possibility of two simultaneous pathologic processes, especially in the elderly and immunocompromised. Patients with peripheral edema are at increased risk of cellulitis.

✗ Do not withhold furosemide (Lasix) from patients with a history of allergy to sulfa-containing antibiotics. There is no significant cross reactivity.

✗ Do not forgo groin examination in a patient with unexplained non-pitting edema. Missing testicular cancer or the matted, immobile lymph nodes of a patient with lymphoma has devastating consequences.

✗ Do not empirically treat DVTs without confirming their presence with imaging (venous Doppler [preferred] or CT with venous phase contrast). Anticoagulants may have life-threatening complications and thus should only be given to patients who can benefit from anticoagulation.

Discussion

Lower extremity edema is common, although due to a heterogenous pathophysiology. If there is concern for heart failure, obtain an electrocardiogram (EKG), brain natriuretic peptide (BNP), and echocardiography. If the patient spills significant protein in the urine, consider nephrotic syndrome. Use imaging and lab studies judiciously to assess for DVT and lymphoma. Advise patients to elevate and compress the lower extremities, and prescribe diuretics if indicated. Most patients will require follow-up with either their primary care provider or a specialist if a specific organ system is suspected as a cause of the peripheral edema.

In elderly patients who are poorly heat acclimated and present with dependent edema during hot weather, consider the more benign etiology of heat edema. Heat edema is lower extremity–dependent edema seen after heat exposure, attributed to microvascular transudate of fluid with prolonged peripheral vasodilatation. It can also present in the hands. This type of edema is not associated with volume overload and is commonly seen in elderly patients with relative hypovolemia caused by inadequate replacement of volume losses in hot environments. Heat edema is commonly found immediately following abrupt transition from a cold to a hotter climate. Elevation and compression stockings are the preferred treatment; diuretics have no role.

Suggested Readings

Atha, W. F. (2013). Heat-related illness. *Emergency Medicine Clinics of North America*, *31*(4), 1097–1108.

Elgendy, I. Y., & Lo, M. C. (2014). Unilateral lower extremity swelling as a rare presentation of non-Hodgkin's lymphoma. *BMJ Case Reports*. https://doi.org/10.1136/bcr-2013-202424.

Phipatanakul, W., & Adkinson, N. F. J. (2000). Cross-reactivity between sulfonamides and loop or thiazide diuretics: Is it a theoretical or actual risk? *Allergy and Clinical Immunology International: Official Organization of the International Association of Allergology and Clinical Immunology*, *12*(1), 26–28.

Stein, P. D., Hull, R. D., Patel, K. C., Olson, R. E., Ghali, W. A., et al. (2004). D-dimer for the exclusion of acute venous thrombosis and pulmonary embolism: A systematic review. *Annals of Internal Medicine*, *140*(8), 589–602.

Mammalian Bites

Presentation

Histories of animal bites are usually volunteered, but the history of a human bite, such as one obtained over the knuckle during a fight, is more likely to be denied or explained only after direct questioning. Dog bites make up about 60% to 80% of all bite injuries, followed by cats (20–30%). Urban medical centers may see human bites more frequently (up to 20%). In the United States the annual incidence of animal bites is 1 to 2 million per year (200/100,000 people per year).

Bites may cause injuries from abrasions, to lacerations, puncture wounds, soft tissue crush injuries, fractures and tendon injuries, and amputations. Patients either will present with a fresh wound soon after the injury or will delay and only seek help after developing painful signs of infection.

What to Do

✓ **All bite wounds require a detailed history to help classify the injury as high risk or low risk.**

✓ **Information regarding the animal:** If known, the species of the animal should be determined, as well its rabies vaccination status. Feline bites are complicated by bacterial wound infections in about 50% to 80% of cases, whereas human bites (20%) and canine bites (≤15%) are at notably lower risk. Rabies is exceedingly uncommon in domesticated animals in the United States, and no prophylaxis is necessary if the animal can be observed for the development of rabies symptoms.

✓ **Information regarding the patient:** Children younger than 2 years, patients with prosthetic heart valves, and those who are immunocompromised (asplenism, chemotherapy, impaired immune system, diabetes mellitus, vasculopathy, etc.) are at high risk of infectious complications.

✓ Assess tetanus vaccination status.

✓ **Information regarding the bite:** Puncture wounds lead to deep inoculation of pathogens. Tissue planes slide relative to each other, and the true depth of the bite is often underappreciated on physical exam. Bites to the hand have the highest risk of infection (18–36%), followed by upper extremity bites (17–20%). Facial bite wounds have a lower rate of infectious complications (4–11%).

✓ **Examination should determine the extent and nature of all skin and soft tissue injuries,** with special attention given to any possible tendon, nerve, joint, or vascular injury. Injuries near joints or involving tendons must be examined through full range of motion (ROM). **A tendon injury sustained with the fingers flexed (as in a fist) will be missed if the hand is** only examined in extension. Bony tenderness, pain on ROM of a joint, swelling, and/or a forceful mechanism (e.g., a large biting animal) indicates a need for radiographs to assess for fractures and retained foreign bodies.

✅ If required by local law or institutional policy, report the bite to appropriate local authorities.

✅ Simple abrasions and contusions that do not break through the dermis require only cleansing with soap and water.

✅ Small puncture wounds can be irrigated by attaching an intravenous (IV) catheter to an infusion bag. Low-pressure irrigation is preferred to prevent inoculation of surrounding tissues with pathogens.

✅ Open lacerations can be cleansed with a standard wound irrigation technique. Devitalized tissue should be sharply debrided.

✅ The wound must be fully explored in a bloodless and well-lit field, looking for foreign bodies or tendon or joint involvement.

✅ Most uninfected facial lacerations should be closed using sutures or tape closures to provide the most effective cosmetic repair. A plastic surgeon, ophthalmologist or otorhinolaryngologist should be consulted for injuries involving the lacrimal or salivary ducts.

✅ Nonhuman animal bite wounds of the scalp, neck, trunk, and proximal extremities that are clean, open, uninfected lacerations may also be closed using tape closures, staples, or nonabsorbable suture material. Buried sutures should be avoided because they serve as a nidus for infection.

✅ Closure of hand bites has traditionally been discouraged. However, for canine bites the rate of infection appears similar between wound closure and healing by secondary intention. The risk of infection must be balanced with optimal functional and cosmetic outcome and should involve shared decision making with the patient.

✅ Patients who have a high risk for infection, such as those with diabetes, immunosuppressed conditions, and renal failure, should have their wounds left open. These wounds can be loosely packed with saline-soaked fine-mesh gauze for delayed primary closure after approximately 72 hours.

✅ Prophylactic antibiotics are indicated for all feline bites; bites of the hand, wrist, or foot; and high-risk patients (see earlier discussion).

✅ Face, scalp, ear, and mouth injuries do not require prophylactic antibiotics.

✅ When a prophylactic antibiotic is indicated, prescribe amoxicillin/clavulanic acid (Augmentin), 875/125 mg twice daily for 5 days, for adults. For children, 45 mg amoxicillin/kg/day, divided into two daily doses.

✅ *If penicillin allergic,* prescribe the following:

Dog Bite

○ Keep in mind that **routine prophylaxis is not recommended** with clean uncomplicated dog bite wounds in patients with a normal risk for infection.

○ **For adults:** metronidazole, 250 to 500 mg three times a day for 5 days, or clindamycin (Cleocin), 300 mg three times a day plus doxycycline, 100 mg twice a day for 5 days

○ **For children:** clindamycin, 10 mg/kg three times a day (oral solution: 75 mg/5 mL) + trimethoprim-sulfamethoxazole (TMP/SMX) (Bactrim, Septra), 8 to 12 mg TMP/kg/day divided into two daily doses (oral solution: 40 mg TMP/5 mL)

Cat Bite

○ Cefuroxime axetil (Ceftin), 500 mg twice a day for 5 days (for children, 15–30 mg/kg/day divided into two daily doses; oral solution 125 or 250 mg/5 mL) or

○ Doxycycline (Vibramycin), 100 mg twice a day for 5 days (adults only)

Raccoon or Skunk Bite

○ Doxycycline (Vibramycin), 100 mg twice a day for 5 days

Human Bite

○ Clindamycin (Cleocin), 300 mg four times a day plus ciprofloxacin (Cipro), 500 mg twice daily (or TMP/SMX [Bactrim, Septra] DS twice daily) for 5 days

✓ **With early signs of infection, the same antibiotic coverage can be used, but it should be continued for a full 10 to 14 days.** In a more worrisome case, you may give an initial parenteral dose of IV Unasyn, 3 g, or ertapenem, 1 g.

✓ **Before antibiotics are started,** reopen the wound and remove all suture material (if previously closed), and obtain aerobic and anaerobic cultures from deep within the wound followed by irrigation.

✓ **Hand infections, joint infections, open fractures, and moderate to severe soft tissue infections require specialty consultation and consideration for hospitalization, IV antibiotics, and possible surgical intervention.**

✓ **Rabies postexposure prophylaxis (PEP) should be based on current Centers for Disease Control and Prevention (CDC) recommendations at** https://www.cdc.gov/rabies/medical_care/index.html. **The decision to give human rabies immune globulin must be weighed carefully considering the significant cost of the treatment. Consider consultation with an infectious disease specialist or the local health department. If not available, help can be obtained through the Division of Viral and Rickettsial Diseases of the CDC. During work hours, call 404-639-1050; after hours and on weekends and holidays, call 770-488-7100. Help is also available at** https://www.who.int/news-room/fact-sheets/detail/rabies.

✓ **Human bites have the potential to transmit bloodborne disease. While the risk of human immunodeficiency virus (HIV) transmission by needle stick is estimated at 0.23%, salivary transmission risk of HIV is between 0.1% and 1%. PEP should be considered if the bite source is known or is high risk to be HIV seropositive. When prophylaxis is indicated,** offer adults and adolescents aged ≥ 13 years, including pregnant women, with normal renal function (creatinine clearance ≥ 60 mL/min) the three-drug cocktail consisting of:

○ tenofovir DF 300 mg **and** fixed dose combination emtricitabine 200 mg (Truvada) once daily **with** raltegravir 400 mg twice daily **or** dolutegravir 50 mg once daily, all PO,

× 4 weeks. Alternative regimens for those with impaired renal function (CrCl <60 mL/min) and children are required. Patients who receive these drugs require baseline and follow-up testing as well as counseling. These medications are not widely available and will be different outside the United States. Under these circumstances, guidance from local Infectious Disease specialists or Health Departments should be sought.

○ Provide hepatitis prophylaxis for patients who have been bitten by known carriers of hepatitis B. Administer hepatitis B immune globulin, 0.06 mL/kg intramuscularly (IM), at the time of injury, and schedule a second dose in 30 days.

✓ **Monkey bites:** These require special consideration. In addition to being highly prone to severe infection, monkey bites may cause an inoculum of the herpes B virus and require antiviral therapy with acyclovir, valacyclovir, or famciclovir.

✓ **Bites near joints may benefit from immobilization to alleviate pain. Provide nonopioid analgesia and encourage icing and elevation.**

✓ **Patients with high-risk bites should return to care within 24 to 48 hours for a wound check. Infection can manifest as early as 12 hours after the bite.**

What Not to Do

Ⓧ Do not overlook a puncture wound.

Ⓧ Do not infiltrate irrigant solution into tissue planes in puncture wounds.

Ⓧ Do not suture debris, nonviable tissue, or a bacterial inoculum into a wound.

Ⓧ Do not use buried absorbable sutures, which act as a foreign body and a nidus for infection.

Ⓧ Do not attempt to treat bite wounds using monotherapy with penicillin, clarithromycin, amoxicillin, or a first-generation cephalosporin. These antibiotics provide inadequate microbial coverage.

Ⓧ Do not obtain cultures and Gram stains from fresh wounds. It is too early to isolate pathogenic bacteria.

Discussion

Children are especially prone to animal bites, especially of the face. Bites occur most commonly among children who disturb the animals while they are sleeping or feeding, separate them during a fight, try to hug or kiss an unfamiliar animal, or accidentally frighten an animal. Women are more often bitten by cats, and young men are commonly bitten by dogs. Dog bites tend to be avulsion injuries with a component of crush. Cat bites more commonly are puncture wounds. Because most cat bites are inflicted by the patient's own animal, cat bite victims tend to delay care until signs of infection develop.

Wound infection is from skin bacteria (*Staphylococcus* and *Streptococcus* spp.) and saliva (*Eikenella corrodens, Moraxella* spp., *Pasteurella* spp., *Fusobacterium* spp., *Bacteroides* spp.). Most infections are polymicrobial. Septicemia is rare and mainly occurs in immunocompromised hosts.

Human bites generally are more severe than animal bites, particularly in clenched-fist injuries. The teeth may cause a deep laceration that implants oral organisms into the joint capsules or dorsal tendons, causing devastating complications that include cellulitis, septic arthritis, tenosynovitis, and osteomyelitis.

A minimal number (~2 cases per year, half from bats) of all animal bites in the United States result in rabies. The incubation period for humans depends on the distance from the bite to the brain, with an

(continued)

Discussion continued

average of 1 to 3 months. Given this relatively long incubation period, **postexposure prophylaxis for rabies is not a medical emergency.** An infectious animal will die of rabies within the human incubation period, and prophylaxis (active and passive) can be delayed if the animal can be observed. Wild animals (e.g., a bat), if caught, can be sacrificed and the brain tested for rabies with immunofluorescence through the local health department.

Suggested Readings

Bula-Rudas, F. J., & Olcott, J. L. (2018). Human and animal bites. *Pediatrics in Review, 39*(10), 490–500. https://doi.org/10.1542/pir.2017-0212.

Kennedy, S. A., Stoll, L. E., & Lauder, A. S. (2015). Human and other mammalian bite injuries of the hand: Evaluation and management. *The Journal of the American Academy of Orthopaedic Surgeons, 23*(1), 47–57. https://doi.org/10.5435/JAAOS-23-01-47.

Pfortmueller, C. A., Efeoglou, A., Furrer, H., & Exadaktylos, A. K. (2013). Dog bite injuries: Primary and secondary emergency department presentations—a retrospective cohort study. *Scientific World Journal,* Article ID 393176.

Rothe, K., Tsokos, M., & Handrick, W. (2015). Animal and human bite wounds. *Deutsches Arzteblatt International, 112*(25), 433–442. [quiz, 443]. https://doi.org/10.3238/arztebl.2015.0433.

Marine Envenomations

Presentation

After coming into contact with marine life, the patient may seek medical attention because of local pain, swelling, or skin discoloration. While more common in coastal areas, envenomation can also occur from handling animals kept in saltwater aquaria. Marine animal envenomations can be divided into two major categories: macropenetration and micropenetration. Macropenetration occurs after contact with spiny fish or mollusks and is due to stingers and spines that leave visible tissue defects (Fig. 143.1). Micropenetration occurs from contact with cnidaria that contain nematocysts (Figs. 143.2–143.4), cellular spring-loaded harpoons designed for venom delivery underneath the epidermis. Management is fundamentally different. Exact identification of the animal is generally not necessary.

Envenomations that cause severe systemic symptoms such as Irukandji syndrome, seizures, and paralysis as well as poisoning due to ingestion of seafood (e.g., ciguatera, paralytic/neurotoxic/amnesic shellfish poisoning) are beyond the scope of this chapter and will not be discussed here.

Macropenetration

This injury typically occurs in individuals who wade through shallow water. Stingrays have a dorsal reflex that results in whiplike propulsion of the tail and typically leads to lower extremity injuries. Anglers are at risk for upper extremity injuries during attempted removal of a stingray from fishing lines. Other animals (scorpionfish, stonefish, catfish, sea urchin, etc.) possess dorsal (and some species pectoral) spines that penetrate the plantar aspect of the patient's foot. In addition to the penetrating injury, injected venom often contains hyaluronidase, arachidonic acid, and serotonin, leading to pain out of proportion to the visible injury (see Fig. 143.1).

Micropenetration

This injury may occur on any part of the body that comes in contact with cnidaria. Common animals in this genus include true jellyfish, anemones, fire coral, and hydrozoa. On the surface of their body or along their tentacles are nematocysts with a spring-loaded, venom-containing harpoon that will fire due to mechanical or chemical stimulation of the cellular organelle. It typically results in intense burning and a linear, frosted-ladder-appearing skin reaction (see Fig. 143.2). Vesication and skin necrosis may follow and can last 24 hours or longer. Occasionally there will be residual hyperpigmentation. Tentacles still may be adherent on patient presentation.

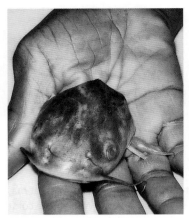

Fig. 143.1 Catfish spine impalement.

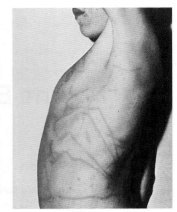

Fig. 143.2 Tentacle prints from the Atlantic Portuguese man-of-war.

What to Do

Macropenetration

✓ **Two approaches are required in the treatment of marine macropenetrative injuries: venom inactivation and wound care.** Virtually all marine venoms are thermolabile and will denature at 45 °C (113 °F).

✓ **Submerse the affected limb in hot (not scalding) water (~45 °C [113 °F]) for 30 to 90 minutes or longer for pain control.** Due to paresthesia induced by some venoms, the patient should also submerse an unaffected (heat-sensitive) body part. This will warn the patient if the water is too hot and thereby prevent thermal tissue damage to the insensitive injured limb.

✓ **Pharmaceutic management of pain should include nonsteroidal antiinflammatory drugs (NSAIDs) and local anesthetics (bupivacaine is preferred due to longer action). Pain can be severe, and patients may require intravenous (IV) opioid analgesia.**

✓ **After pain control has been achieved, remove any remaining stingers. Stingrays have serrated stingers, fragments of which may require surgical removal** (see Chapter 154). **Obtain radiographs or soft tissue ultrasound** after removal to screen for retained foreign bodies such as broken spines.

✓ **Sea urchin spines are fragile and often difficult to remove.** The tissue damage of attempted removal must be weighed against leaving the spines in place (see sliver removal, Chapter 153). Thin retained spines without symptoms generally are absorbed or extruded. If left in place, treatment should include a 7-day to 14-day course of NSAIDs and prednisone if a severe secondary reaction occurs.

✓ **Wounds should be thoroughly irrigated.** Puncture wounds can be irrigated by attaching an 18-gauge catheter to IV fluid bags and gently inserting it into the wound. Use low-pressure irrigation to prevent the spread of venom and pathogens along tissue planes.

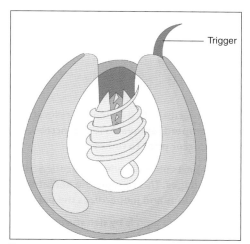

Fig. 143.3 Nematocyst prior to discharging. (Adapted from Stauffer, A. R., & Auerbach, P. S. [2003]. Marine envenomations: Common Florida injuries. *EMpulse, 8,* 12.)

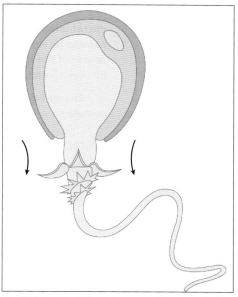

Fig. 143.4 Nematocyst after discharge occurs. (Adapted from Stauffer, A. R., & Auerbach, P. S. [2003]. Marine envenomations: Common Florida injuries. *EMpulse, 8,* 12.)

⊘ **Lightly pack larger wounds open for delayed primary closure** (see Chapter 140).

⊘ While tetanus infection is highly unlikely to occur from marine envenomation injuries (it is a soil bacterium), patients who have lapsed on their tetanus vaccination will likely have a future minor injury for which they may not seek care, and providing tetanus prophylaxis is a good public health practice (see Appendix G).

⊘ **Prophylactic antibiotics are not required for minor abrasions, superficial punctures, and superficial lacerations. Injuries with potential for serious infection include large lacerations, deep puncture wounds (particularly near joints), and wounds with retained foreign material.**

⊘ **These infection-prone wounds, and any wound in an immunocompromised individual of any type, require antibiotic prophylaxis. Ciprofloxacin, 500 mg twice daily, or doxycycline (Vibramycin), 100 mg twice daily for adults, and trimethoprim-sulfamethoxazole (Bactrim/Septra), 8 to 12 mg TMP/kg/day divided into two daily doses for children, all prescribed for 3 to 5 days, are the most appropriate regimens for coverage of pathogenic marine microbes.**

⊘ The genus *Vibrio* is particularly common in the ocean and poses a serious risk for immunosuppressed patients. Rapidly progressive cellulitis or myositis indicates *V. parahaemolyticus* or *V. vulnificus*. Also known to inoculate marine wounds are *Erysipelothrix rhusiopathiae* and *Mycobacterium marinum*. In the more severe wounds, the recommended initial parenteral antibiotics include cefoperazone, ceftazidime, gentamicin, ciprofloxacin, ceftriaxone, and cefuroxime.

✓ **For infected wounds, obtain both aerobic and anaerobic cultures, and alert the clinical microbiology laboratory that standard antimicrobial susceptibility testing media may need to be supplemented with NaCl to permit growth of marine bacteria. Prescribe a course of the above-mentioned antibiotics for 7 to 14 days.** Hospitalization may be required for severe infections and in those individuals who are immunosuppressed.

✓ **Ensure follow-up** on all infected wounds in 1 to 2 days with periodic revisits until healing is complete.

Micropenetration

✓ **Patients often still have tentacles with live nematocysts attached to them. The mechanical stimulation of attempted removal leads to increased venom delivery. Thus nematocyst inactivation must occur prior to removal.**

✓ **Irrigate the affected body parts liberally with 5% acetic acid (vinegar) and cover areas with vinegar-soaked bandages. This renders the nematocysts inactive. Urine is not recommended, as it is not efficacious and jeopardizes the patient/provider relationship.**

✓ **The most effective way to control pain is by denaturing thermolabile venom with hot water (45 °C [113 °F]) immersion.**

✓ **After decontamination and pain control has been achieved,** remove attached tentacles with a credit card (or similar object). This should be done double-gloved in case of any remaining live nematocysts.

✓ If removal causes increased pain, nematocyst inactivation was incomplete. Stop removal and reapply vinegar.

✓ **Residual inflammation can be treated with topical corticosteroids, such as triamcinolone 0.1% or 0.5% cream. Avoid the use on areas of cosmetic importance such as the face, as it can lead to skin discoloration. Systemic antihistamines will also be helpful for pruritus, and on occasion, systemic corticosteroids will be required.**

✓ **Advise the patient about sun avoidance** and the use of sunblocks to prevent possible postinflammatory hyperpigmentation.

What Not to Do

✗ Do not use fresh water or isopropyl (rubbing) alcohol to decontaminate jellyfish stings. The chemical stimulation will cause remaining nematocysts to fire.

✗ Do not use full-strength ammonia as a substitute for vinegar compresses. It is a powerful skin irritant.

Discussion

Many marine animals have developed systems for attack and defense that on accidental exposure to humans result in envenomation. Most envenomations are not life threatening, often presenting only as minor contact dermatitis or a small puncture wound. Venomous marine organisms can be difficult to identify or may not be seen at the time of envenomation.

Marine animals responsible for envenomation can be broken into two large groups—vertebrates and invertebrates. Venomous vertebrate marine animals include stingrays, lionfish, scorpion fish, stonefish, and catfish, whereas venomous invertebrates include jellyfish, anemones, and fire coral.

Treatment can be based on the nature and appearance of the wound when the specific sea creature cannot be identified.

A special case of marine envenomation can occur during saltwater aquarium maintenance. Ornamental zoanthid corals are prone to overgrowing a saltwater tank, but they are easily killed by pouring boiling water over affected rocks. Zoanthids contain palytoxin, one of the few thermostabile marine toxins. The boiling water aerosolizes the toxin, which when inhaled inhibits the Na+/K+ ATPase (similar to digoxin). Patients present with flulike symptoms, eye irritation, and severe bronchospasm. Individuals in other rooms in the same building can be affected. Treatment consists of inhaled bronchodilators and steroids, as well as respiratory support as needed.

Suggested Readings

Hornbeak, K. B., & Auerbach, P. S. (2017). Marine envenomation. *Emergency Medicine Clinics of North America*, *35*(2), 321–337. https://doi.org/10.1016/j.emc.2016.12.004.

Reese, E., & Depenbrock, P. (2014). Water envenomations and stings. *Current Sports Medicine Reports*, *13*(2), 126–131.

Nail Bed Laceration

Presentation

The patient has either cut into the nail with a sharp edge or crushed a finger (commonly in a door). With shearing forces, the nail may be avulsed from the nail bed to varying degrees, and there may be an underlying bony injury. The nail bed is prone to lacerations in these types of injuries.

What to Do

✓ Perform a distal neurovascular exam prior to performing a **digital block.**

✓ Provide appropriate **tetanus prophylaxis** (see Appendix G).

✓ **Obtain radiographs of any crush injury.** Approximately 50% of patients will have a distal phalanx fracture. Severely angulated fractures may require reduction.

✓ **Elevate the nail** by inserting a fine straight hemostat or a delicate spatula between the nail and the hyponychium (Fig. 144.1). For inspection only, try maintaining the nail in the proximal nail fold. If the nail bed cannot be well visualized or requires repair, temporary removal of the nail may be necessary.

✓ **A small nail bed laceration with minimal wound separation can simply be cleansed and sealed with cyanoacrylate tissue adhesive.**

✓ **With a larger or more complicated nail bed laceration, repair is often required** (Fig. 144.2).

✓ A bloodless field may need to be established using a **finger tourniquet.**

✓ **If not already accomplished, use a straight hemostat or periosteal elevator to separate the nail from the nail bed.**

✓ Irrigate the wound thoroughly. Do not debride the germinal or sterile matrix, as tissue loss in these areas will lead to permanent nail deformity (Fig. 144.3).

✓ **Suture with a fine absorbable material** (6-0 or 7-0 Vicryl or Dexon) (see Fig. 144.2).

✓ **When available, replace the nail back into its normal anatomic position (see later).**

✓ **An intact nail should be cleaned and reinserted for protection and proper tissue alignment, or an alternative nail bed dressing can be applied** (see Chapter 135).

✓ **Tissue adhesive can be used to bond the nail to the nail bed and seal open spaces or defects in the nail** (see Chapter 135). Cover with an appropriate fingertip dressing (see Appendix C).

✓ Inform the patient that a new nail will slowly push off the replaced nail or artificial stent.

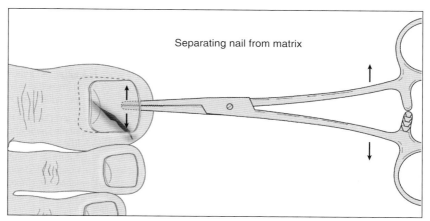

Fig. 144.1 Separate nail from nail bed using a straight hemostat.

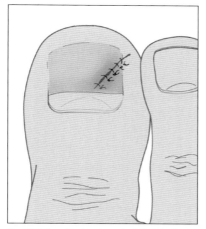

Fig. 144.2 The nail bed can be repaired after it has been fully exposed.

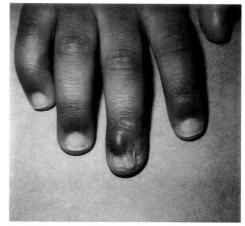

Fig. 144.3 Improper nail bed repair will increase the risk for future fingernail or toenail deformity.

What Not to Do

(X) Do not use nonabsorbable sutures to repair the nail bed. The patient will require a second digital block and nail elevation when the sutures are removed.

(X) Do not place a dressing that requires removal onto an exposed nail bed. Any such dressing will adhere tenaciously to the nail bed and will be extremely painful to remove (even after a short period of time).

Discussion

The objective of a nail bed repair is to provide a flat, smooth surface on which the new nail will grow. It is crucial that the provider is attentive while addressing these injuries because mismanagement can lead to further complications. If a wound is inadequately repaired or if a wound is allowed to heal by secondary intention, additional scar tissue may cause the nail to split or become nonadherent.

It is also necessary to provide separation of the eponychium from the germinal matrix to prevent potential adhesions. Scarring of the eponychium to the germinal matrix can result in deformed or split nail growth. Replacement of the original nail into its normal anatomic position, with the nail root under the eponychium, is the best method of preserving future nail integrity. When the nail has been severely damaged or is missing, an artificial stent can be provided (see Chapter 135).

Significant nail bed injuries can be hidden by hemorrhage and a partially avulsed overlying nail. These injuries must be repaired to help prevent future deformity of the nail (see Fig. 144.3). Surgical consultation should be obtained when nail bed lacerations involve the germinal matrix under the base of the nail.

Suggested Reading

Tos, P., Titolo, P., Chirila, N. L., Catalano, F., & Artiaco, S. (2012). Surgical treatment of acute fingernail injuries. *Journal of Orthopaedics and Traumatology: Official Journal of the Italian Society of Orthopaedics and Traumatology, 13*(2), 57–62. https://doi.org/10.1007/s10195-011-0161-z.

Nail Root Dislocation

Presentation

The patient has caught a finger in a car door or dropped a heavy object on an exposed toe, causing a painful deformity. The base of the nail will be found resting above (on top of) the eponychium instead of in its normal anatomic position beneath. The cuticular line that had joined the eponychium at the nail fold will remain attached to the nail at its original position (Figs. 145.1 and 145.2).

What to Do

✓ Perform a thorough evaluation to ensure that neurovascular status is intact.

✓ **Anesthetize the area using a digital block (see Appendix B).**

✓ **Obtain a radiograph to rule out an underlying fracture (which may require reduction as well as protective splinting). About 50% of these types of injuries are associated with distal phalanx fractures. The nail proper can serve as a splint for the fracture if adequately secured.**

✓ **Lift the proximal end of the nail off the eponychium and thoroughly cleanse and inspect the nail bed.** Attempt to preserve distal adherence of the nail to the sterile matrix. Minimally débride loose cuticular tissue, and test for a possible avulsion of the extensor tendon (see Chapter 106).

✓ **If there are significant nail bed lacerations**, the entire nail will need to be removed and lacerations repaired using tissue adhesive or a fine **absorbable** suture, such as 6-0 or 7-0 Vicryl or chromic gut (see Chapter 144).

✓ **Just replacing the nail root into its normal position will approximate most minor nail bed lacerations.**

✓ **Using a fine hemostat, reinsert the root of the nail under the eponychium. A delicate spatula may be used to raise the eponychium and drape it over the proximal nail root.**

✓ **Reduce any underlying volar angulated fractures** by grabbing the distal phalanx and firmly bending it back into normal alignment. Reduction of volar angulation will help secure the nail under the nail fold. Unstable fractures may require fixation with Kirschner wires or a 21-gauge needle. This should be performed by or in consultation with a specialist.

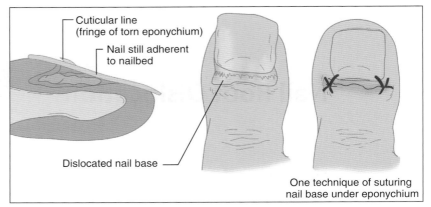

Fig. 145.1 Dislocated nail root.

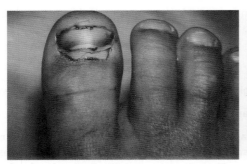

Fig. 145.2 The subtle appearance of a dislocated nail root can be inadvertently overlooked by the clinician.

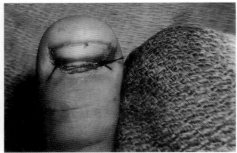

Fig. 145.3 Appearance of the same toenail as shown in Fig. 145.2 after a thorough cleansing, reinsertion of the nail root under the eponychium, and being sutured in place.

✅ **If the nail still tends to drift out from under the eponychium, it can be sutured in place using two 4-0 or 5-0 nylon or Prolene sutures in the proximal corners** (see Figs. 145.1 and 145.3). Avoid central suture, as scarring of the germinal matrix may lead to split nail growth.

✅ Any nonabsorbable sutures should be removed after 1 week.

✅ Cover the area with a fingertip dressing (see Appendix C) and splint any underlying fracture (see Chapter 109).

✅ **Provide tetanus prophylaxis** (see Appendix G).

✅ **Follow-up should be provided in 3 to 5 days.** Patients should be advised to leave the dressing and splint (if applicable) in place until follow-up evaluation. If the dressing becomes wet or soiled, the patient should return immediately for redressing of the wound.

✅ **Instruct patients** to return immediately if there is increasing pain or any other sign of infection (redness, swelling, purulent drainage, or red streaking). The patient should be advised that it is normal to have blood continue to ooze from beneath the nail in the first 1 to 2 days following the injury.

✓ **Prescribe appropriate nonopioid pain management.** Instruct the patient to keep the extremity elevated and if effective, apply a cold pack to further reduce discomfort.

✓ **Prophylactic antibiotics are not routinely required, even with associated fractures of the distal phalanx,** except in immunocompromised patients. Significantly contaminated wounds should receive 3 to 5 days of cephalexin, 500 mg four times daily, after thorough wound cleansing.

What Not to Do

✗ **Do not ignore the nail root dislocation and simply provide a fingertip dressing (Fig. 145.2). Failure to reduce the nail root dislocation may result in scarring of the eponychium to the germinal matrix, thereby leading to permanent nail loss or deformity.**

✗ Do not débride any portion of the nail root, nail bed, sterile matrix, or germinal matrix. Tissue loss in these areas will lead to permanent nail loss or deformity.

✗ **Do not neglect to thoroughly irrigate the injury site to minimize the risks of infection, as well as to meticulously repair significant injuries to the nail bed to prevent complications and to maximize cosmetic appearances.**

Discussion

The germinal matrix lies protected under the eponychium, forming the area from which the nail is produced. Growth takes place in the nail root, or lunula. The lunula is the pale crescent-shaped structure under the proximal portion of the nail.

Because the nail is not as firmly attached at the lunula and root as it is to the distal nail bed, impact injuries can avulse only the base (nail root), leaving the proximal nail lying on top of the eponychium.

It may be surprising that this injury is often missed, but at first glance a dislocated nail root can appear to be in place, and without careful inspection a patient can return from radiology with negative radiographs and be treated as if there is only an abrasion or a contusion. The attachment of the cuticle from the nail fold of the eponychium to the base of the nail forms a constant landmark on the nail. **If any nail is showing proximal to this landmark** (Fig. 145.2), **then the nail is not in its normal position beneath the eponychium.**

Suggested Reading

Tos, P., Titolo, P., Chirila, N. L., Catalano, F., & Artiaco, S. (2012). Surgical treatment of acute fingernail injuries. *Journal of Orthopaedics and Traumatology: Official Journal of the Italian Society of Orthopaedics and Traumatology, 13*(2), 57–62. https://doi.org/10.1007/s10195-011-0161-z.

Needle (Foreign Body) in Foot

Presentation

Although a needle could be embedded under any skin surface, most commonly a patient will have stepped on one while walking without shoes on a carpeted floor. In general, the patient will experience a sharp pain initially and complain of a foreign-body sensation with weight bearing. Patients with peripheral neuropathy may seek care with delay. A very small puncture wound may be found at the point of entry, and frequently a portion of the needle will be palpable. Occasionally the needle goes in eye first, and a thread is hanging out of the puncture.

What to Do

☑ **Tape a radiographic marker or partially opened paper clip as a skin marker to the plantar surface of the foot, with the tip of the opened paper clip over the entrance wound.** The marker must remain in place until the needle is removed (Fig. 146.1A) (See Video 146.1).

☑ **Obtain anteroposterior and lateral radiographs of the foot with the skin marker in place** (see Fig. 146.1B).

☑ **Evaluate the radiographs for both presence and position of the needle.** A superficially located needle can be removed at bedside. Deep or fractured needles may require fluoroscopic guidance.

☑ **Ultrasonography** may be substituted for radiography and a skin marker if you are skilled in the use of soft tissue ultrasonography for locating foreign bodies.

☑ If bedside removal is attempted, limit removal attempts to less than 15 minutes to minimize patient discomfort and damage to the soft tissues of the foot. "Blind digging" is discouraged.

☑ **Establish a bloodless field** by elevation, elastic wraps, and then application of a tourniquet.

☑ **Anesthetize the area. Depending on the location of the foreign body, consider performing a posterior tibial or a sural nerve block. Augment this as needed with locally infiltrated buffered 1% lidocaine.**

☑ The radiographs should reveal an **approximate** location of the needle relative to the radiographic marker.

☑ **With the patient lying prone and the plantar surface of the foot facing upward, using a No. 15 scalpel blade,** make an incision that crosses <u>perpendicular</u> to the needle's apparent position at its midpoint or one-third of the way toward the most superficial end of the needle. Cut down until striking the needle, but do not cut deep to the plantar fascia (see Fig. 146.1C) (See Video 146.1).

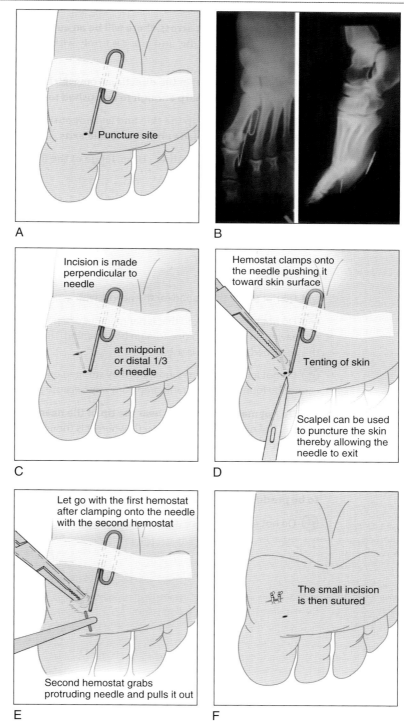

Fig. 146.1 Procedure for removing a needle from the foot.

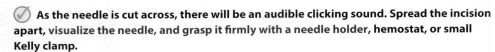

✓ **As the needle is cut across, there will be an audible clicking sound. Spread the incision apart, visualize the needle, and grasp it firmly with a needle holder, hemostat, or small Kelly clamp.**

✓ **Push the needle out in the direction from which it entered.** **Even the eye or back end of a broken needle is sharp enough to be pushed to the skin surface.**

✓ **If the needle tents up the skin and will not push through, nick the overlying skin surface with a scalpel blade until the needle exits** (see Fig. 146.1D).

✓ **Grab this end with another clamp, let go of the first clamp, and remove the needle** (see Fig. 146.1E).

✓ Remove the tourniquet and suture the incision closed. Apply an appropriate dressing (see Fig. 146.1F).

✓ Provide tetanus prophylaxis as indicated (see Appendix G).

What Not to Do

✗ Do not probe the wound for the needle with a gloved finger.

✗ Do not pull on a thread that is hanging out of a puncture wound. It could potentially break off, leaving an infection-prone foreign body behind. The thread will come out with the needle if the described technique is used.

✗ Do not ignore patients who think they stepped on a needle but in whom a puncture wound cannot be found. Obtain a radiograph anyway because the puncture wound is probably hidden.

✗ **Do not make the incision near the tip of the needle or directly over and parallel to the needle.** The needle will not be exactly where it is thought to be, and the incision will very likely miss exposing the needle.

✗ **Do not persist in extensively undermining or extending the incision if the needle is not located within approximately 15 minutes of beginning the procedure. This is unlikely to be productive and may do the patient harm.**

✗ Do not routinely place the patient on prophylactic antibiotics.

Discussion

Plantar embedded needles are difficult to remove, and failure of the procedure is not an unexpected outcome. Ideally, the challenging nature of this procedure should be discussed with the patient prior to attempting bedside removal. While it is tempting to make the incision over the entrance wound and "follow the path" of the needle, this routinely does not yield good results. **The incision must be made in a direction and location best suited for locating the needle, not removing it.**

There are three additional principles to keep in mind. First, the position of the needle on radiographs needs to be correlated with the anatomy of the skin surface rather than the bony anatomy of the foot. Second, the simple geometric principle states that the surest way to intersect a line (the needle) is to bisect it in the plane perpendicular to its midpoint. Third, the only structures of importance in the forefoot or heel that lie plantar to the bones are the flexor tendons, and they lie close to the bones.

If the patient is taken to fluoroscopy, the clinician or radiologist can place a hemostat around the needle under a real-time radiographic image. It can then be pushed out using the same technique described earlier. **Ultrasonography may be an alternative modality for localizing an underlying needle, but it is thought to be technically demanding and requires practice.**

Using the simple technique described, linear foreign bodies, such as needles, can be removed from the sole of the foot without extensive dissection, complex or cumbersome equipment, or repeated radiographic studies.

Suggested Readings

Blankenship, R. B., & Baker, T. (2007). Imaging modalities in wounds and superficial skin infections. *Emergency Medicine Clinics of North America, 25*, 223–234.

Gilsdorf, J. R. (1986). A needle in the sole of the foot. *Surgery Gynecology & Obstetrics, 163*, 573–574.

Hegenbarth, M. A. (2004). Bedside ultrasound in the pediatric emergency department: Basic skill or passing fancy? *Clinics in Pediatric Emergency Medicine, 5*, 201–216.

Lammers, R. L., & Magill, T. (1992). Detection and management of foreign bodies in soft tissue. *Emergency Medicine Clinics of North America, 10*, 767–781.

Leidelmeyer, R. (1976). The embedded broken-off needle. *Journal of the American College of Emergency Physicians, 5*, 362–363.

Needle Stick (Postexposure Prophylaxis)

Presentation

An employee presents for evaluation and treatment after an accidental needle stick injury to the hand obtained in the process of providing patient care. The employee requests postexposure prophylaxis (PEP).

This chapter will discuss the risk of transmission and appropriate PEP of three bloodborne pathogens after accidental occupational needle stick injuries: hepatitis B virus (HBV), hepatitis C virus (HCV), and human immunodeficiency virus (HIV).

What to Do

✅ It is important to obtain the following historical components from the patient: time of injury, tetanus status, source patient (if known), needle type (hollow bore vs. nonhollow bore).

✅ **Determine the medical employee's HBV vaccination status.**

✅ **The type of body fluid that was potentially transmitted** by needle stick (if known) should be determined. Urine, saliva, feces, vomitus, sweat, tears, and respiratory secretions are not known to transmit HBV, HCV, or HIV unless they are visibly bloody.

✅ **If source patient consents for testing**, obtain the following: HIV antibody/antigen (Ab/Ag), HCV ribonucleic acid (RNA) (preferred), or HCV Ab, HBV surface Ag.

✅ **For medicolegal reasons**, consider testing the employee per institutional policy with the same test panel as for the source patient. Please note: This does NOT detect transmission/seroconversion but only documents these infectious diseases were not preexisting in the employee.

HIV Exposures

- **HIV PEP should be initiated** if the source patients' rapid HIV test is positive, if the HIV test is negative but the source patient is believed to have acute retroviral syndrome (i.e., HIV positive but testing negative due to recency of acquiring HIV [the so-called window period]), and if the source patient refuses consent or is not able to give consent. **PEP should be initiated within 1 to 2 hours of exposure.** Animal studies show some benefit within 72 hours.
- **If a rapid HIV test is not available**, PEP should be initiated and discontinued if later testing results are negative.
- **If the source patient is known to have HIV,** past resistance to HIV medications should be considered prior to selecting a PEP regimen.

- **Preferred HIV PEP regimen:** Tenofovir, 300 mg orally daily, plus emtricitabine, 200 mg orally daily (available as combination with brand name Truvada), plus raltegravir, 400 mg orally twice daily. Duration for therapy should be 28 days.
- Tenofovir therapy may lead to nephrotoxicity and hepatotoxicity. **Obtain blood urea nitrogen (BUN), creatinine, and liver function tests (LFTs) at the initial encounter.** Alternative regimens for those with impaired renal function (CrCl <60 mL/min) are required.
- **If PEP is administered**, counsel the patient to expect nausea, vomiting, and diarrhea. Provide prescriptions for antiemetics and antidiarrheal medications.
- **If the employee is pregnant**, the decision to initiate PEP should be based on the same factors as nonpregnant patients. The risk of vertical transmission is high during the acute retroviral syndrome, and the limited available data suggest that PEP is safe even during the first trimester. **Register any pregnant person receiving PEP** at http://www.apregistry.com to further help determine safety of PEP in pregnancy.
- **Breastfeeding is not a contraindication for PEP** and can safely be continued. However, HIV can be transmitted in breastmilk, especially during the acute retroviral syndrome, which features a high HIV serum titer.
- **Unless source patient is documented HIV negative, employee should be retested for HIV at 6 weeks and 3 months.**

HBV Exposures

- **If the source patient is known to be HBV negative or the employee is known to be immune** (full HBV vaccination resinous with postvaccination HBsAb titer > 10 mIU/mL), no treatment is necessary.
- **If the employee is unsure of HBV vaccination status**, obtain HBsAb titers. If greater than 10 mIU/mL, no further treatment is necessary. **Hepatitis B immunoglobin (HBIG) can be delayed by up to 7 days** and still remain effective.
- **If the source patient is known to be HBV positive or cannot be tested AND the employee is not immune,** HBIG 0.06 mL/kg intramuscularly (IM) should be administered now (with a second dose in 1 month).
- **For nonimmune employees**, initiate the HBV vaccination series.

HCV Exposures

- **HCV seroconversion is significantly more likely after needle stick from an HCV-positive source patient (1.8%). It can occur after needle stick with a nonhollow-bore needle (e.g., suture needle).**
- Patients should be advised to **obtain HCV RNA testing 4 to 6 weeks after exposure to screen for seroconversion.**
- Ledipasvir/sofosbuvir (Harvoni) is a treatment available for HCV genotype 1 with 94% to 99% cure rates. However, **at this time no data exist regarding its efficacy in postexposure prophylaxis.** Given the dynamic nature of medical knowledge, **we encourage discussion with an infectious disease specialist if the source patient is known to be HCV positive,** as new data are likely to emerge after publication of this book.

What Not to Do

Ⓧ Do not access the source patient's medical records if the person is not your patient. Doing so is a violation of the Health Insurance Portability and Accountability Act (HIPAA). The source patient should be approached by the treating medical team.

ⓧ Do not order/request testing on the source patient without the explicit consent of the source patient or legal representative.

ⓧ Do not reflexively give PEP to all patients with needle stick injuries. PEP contains drugs with potential toxicities, and the risk of transmission of HIV is low (0.23% if source is known to be positive).

ⓧ There has not been a documented HIV seroconversion from a needle stick outside the health care setting (e.g., child found needle on playground). PEP is not routinely recommended, and patients should be involved in shared decision making by balancing the risk of transmission with the risk of PEP.

ⓧ Do not prescribe antacids or magnesium-aluminum-oxide (MaAlOx), as these reduce the bioavailability of PEP medications. If possible, patients should stop taking these medications if already taking, and discontinue iron and calcium supplementation for the same reason.

Discussion

Needle stick injuries are common among health care providers, with registered nurses making up the majority of exposed individuals. Fortunately, seroconversion to HIV and HCV is relatively rare when the patient is known to be HIV or HCV positive. Most health care workers are immunized against HBV, depending on institutional policy, employee preference, and employee response to the HBV vaccination series.

HIV requires a larger blood volume to be introduced to allow for seroconversion, as is the case with a hollow-bore needle. Accidental injuries from nonhollow-bore needles have not been documented to lead to HIV seroconversion, but may transmit HCV.

"Found needles" inside or outside the hospital that have led to injury are incredibly low risk, with only two HIV seroconversions documented over the past 20 years. This is likely due to the limited life span of HIV outside of the human body. In contrast, recently used needles pose a higher risk.

The decision to initiate PEP should be based on local institutional guidelines/protocols and shared decision making with the employee.

Suggested Readings

Lazarus, R. (2017). Testing for blood-borne viruses after a needle-stick injury in patients who lack the capacity to consent. *Clinical Medicine (London, England)*, *17*(4), 376–377. https://doi.org/10.7861/clinmedicine.17-4-376a.

Tarigan, L. H., Cifuentes, M., Quinn, M., & Kriebel, D. (2015). Prevention of needle-stick injuries in healthcare facilities: A meta-analysis. *Infection Control and Hospital Epidemiology*, *36*(7), 823–829. https://doi.org/10.1017/ice.2015.50.

Paronychia

(Acute)

Presentation

The patient presents with finger or toe pain that has developed rapidly, either over the past several hours or over a few days. This pain is accompanied by a very red, tender swelling of the nail fold (Fig. 148.1A), or this swelling may be less red and tender or has developed granulation tissue and appears chronic in nature (see Fig. 148.1B). Paronychia occur far more frequently in women, likely due to manipulation of the nails and eponychium for cosmetic reasons.

The nail is surrounded by the lateral, medial, and proximal nail folds. Injury (ingrown nail, hang nail, minor trauma) to either of these folds allows bacteria to enter the tissue. This results in local soft tissue infection with or without abscess formation.

Patients may also feature chronic paronychia, often due to chemical exposures seen in a variety of professions. Chronic paronychia is not considered a minor emergency; therefore treatment will not be discussed here. Patients with chronic paronychia should be referred to a hand specialist or podiatrist because more complex surgical procedures may be required. In addition, squamous cell carcinoma may have a similar appearance.

Extension of an acute infection under the nail plate is a subungual abscess (see Fig. 148.1C).

What to Do

Acute Paronychia

✓ **Treatment differs based on the presence of an abscess.** If an abscess is not obvious, obtain a water bath bedside ultrasound by submerging the hand (or foot) in water and hovering with the linear ultrasound probe above the digit. This allows excellent visualization without the difficulty of ultrasonography of highly irregular surface topography of digits.

✓ **If ultrasound is not available, the digital pressure test may be used.** If gentle pressure against the pad of the affected digit causes blanching of the paronychia, an abscess is more likely to be visualized.

✓ **If no abscess is present: Instruct the patient to perform warm water soaks four to five times a day for about 15 minutes** as well as soaks in 1% acetic acid (vinegar). Application of topical antibiotics has been shown to lead to faster resolution (e.g., mupirocin [Bactroban]).

✓ **Patients should return to care in about 3 to 4 days or if pain increases** to monitor for progression and delayed development of an abscess.

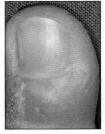
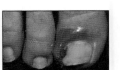

A Acute paronychia B

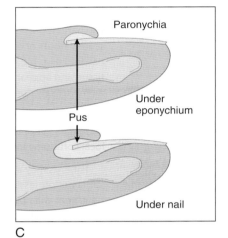

Paronychia

Under
eponychium

Pus

Under nail

C

Fig. 148.1 (A) Acute paronychia of finger with red, hot, tender nail fold showing pus beneath the cuticle. (B) Chronic paronychia with an ingrown toenail. (C) Subungual extension of pus.

Fig. 148.2 (A) Paronychia of right index finger, at presentation. (B) Digital pressure test performed showing blanching of the skin overlying the abscess cavity. (From Turkmen, A., et al. [2004]. Digital pressure test for paronychia. *British Journal of Plastic Surgery, 57*[1], 94.)

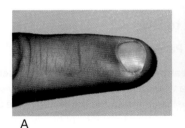
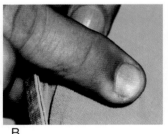

A B

☑ **If an abscess is present, drainage is indicated.** Several techniques exist. The technique described should not be a painful procedure, but if you attempt a more extensive procedure or if you are not skilled in the following painless drainage technique, patients will benefit from a digital block prior to initiation (see Appendix B).

☑ **Slide a large-bore needle (16 or 18 gauge) or a scalpel blade along the hard surface of the nail plate under the affected nail fold. Incise this interior portion of the nail fold where the abscess is located** (Fig. 148.2). When done carefully, gradually separating the nail from the nail fold with the sharp edge sliding back and forth firmly against the nail plate, there should be a painless drainage of pus when the abscess cavity is entered (See Video 148.1).

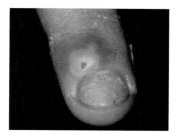

Fig. 148.3 Herpetic whitlow. This acutely painful lesion is due to infection of the finger with herpes simplex virus (HSV). (From Jones, J. [2006]. Infectious diseases. In C. Sproat, et al. [Eds.], *Essential human disease for dentists* [pp. 177–194]. London, England: Churchill Livingstone.)

✓ Once pus is obtained, digitally massage the paronychia proximal-to-distal to aid expression of purulence.

✓ **Instruct the patient to perform frequent warm water soaks**, vinegar soaks, and topical antibiotic application as described earlier.

✓ If a subungual abscess is present (purulence visualized under the proximal nail plate), the patient should undergo trephination. This can be achieved by using a trephination device or simply drilling through the nail plate with a 16-gauge needle (see Chapter 156). In severe cases, partial nail removal is indicated.

What Not to Do

✗ Do not order cultures of expressed purulence. Infections are often polymicrobial and only 4% of paronychial cultures can isolate a specific pathogen. Culture results do not change management.

✗ Do not routinely administer systemic antibiotics, except in patients with significant immunocompromised states.

✗ Do not routinely obtain radiographs.

✗ Do not make an actual (and painful) skin incision while treating acute paronychia. The cuticle needs only to be separated from the nail to release any collection of pus.

✗ Do not remove an entire fingernail or toenail to drain simple paronychia. The patient will be left with a very sensitive exposed nail bed unnecessarily. To relieve more significant purulent subungual fluid collections, an alternative procedure is partial nail plate excision.

✗ Do not attempt to drain a herpetic whitlow (Fig. 148.3). When coalescing vesicles with surrounding erythema are present, assume that the infection is caused by herpes simplex virus. Treatment involves inhibition of viral replication with acyclovir (Zovirax), valacyclovir (Valtrex), or famciclovir (Famvir) (see Chapter 54).

✗ Do not confuse a felon (with a tense tender fingerpad) with a paronychia. Felons will require more extensive surgical treatment.

Discussion

Acute paronychia most commonly results from nail biting, finger sucking, aggressive manicuring, a hang nail, or minor penetrating trauma. **Most infections are minor and can be treated easily with conservative methods.** Patients who have developed an abscess pocket benefit from drainage and are unlikely to improve with conservative management. Drainage can be performed bedside using only landmarks as reference. The ideal approach merely elevates and separates the paronychium from the nail plate to allow purulence to drain, and no skin incision is needed. Full recovery should be expected after approximately 4 days. Patients who fail to improve may have had a missed abscess pocket or have reaccumulated purulence and require repeat drainage.

Suggested Reading

Point of Care. (2019). *Paronychia*. Amsterdam, Netherlands: Elsevier BV.

Pencil Point Puncture

Presentation

The patient presents after being stabbed or stuck with a sharp pencil point. The patient may voice concerns regarding lead poisoning due to retained pencil lead. A small puncture wound lined with graphite tattooing will be present (Fig. 149.1). The pencil tip may or may not be present, visible, or palpable. With palpation of the puncture wound, an underlying pencil point may give the patient a foreign-body sensation.

What to Do

✓ **Reassure the patient that pencil lead does not in fact contain lead.** It is a mixture of graphite (carbon, which functions as pigment) and clay (a complex mixture of phyllosilicates, which functions as a binding agent). Both are nontoxic substances, and poisoning will not occur.

✓ Depending on the location and severity of the injury, test sensory and motor function of the affected area.

✓ Obtain a thorough history relating to the injury, and assess the patient's risk of developing complications, which are rare.

✓ **If retained graphite particles are suspected, given the finding of dark skin discoloration embedded in the wound**, engage the patient in shared decision making regarding their removal. Graphite tattooing may be cosmetically undesirable depending on the location of injury. The patient should weigh this against the mild discomfort of local anesthesia.

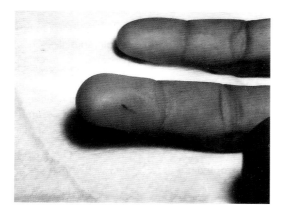

Fig. 149.1 Acute pencil point puncture.

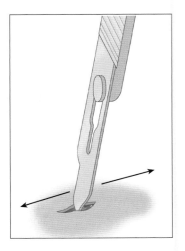

Fig. 149.2 Dermabrade to reduce tattooing.

✓ **If there is uncertainty regarding a retained pencil point foreign body,** radiographs or ultrasonography can assist in confirming its presence or absence. This should not be routinely ordered and only pursued if the patient has a foreign-body sensation when the area is palpated, the examiner feels a foreign body under the skin, or the puncture wound is deep and the pencil point is missing. Graphite and phyllosilicates are relatively inert substances, but granuloma formation has been reported even decades later. This and the possibility of fragments of retained pencil wood should encourage the removal of all detected foreign bodies.

✓ Keep in mind, though, that the vast majority of black wound markings observed are merely graphite particles rather than a broken-off pencil tip.

✓ **If the decision is made to attempt removal of a foreign body or graphitic particles,** administer local anesthesia and then thoroughly scrub the wound.

✓ **To reduce the amount of tattooing, the wound may be scraped back and forth (dermabraded) with the tip of a scalpel blade** (Fig. 149.2). Remove as much of the graphite particles as possible and rinse the wound (See Video 149.1).

✓ **If a pencil tip foreign body is suspected,** a small incision can be made over the puncture wound allowing for blunt dissection and wound exploration (see Chapter 154). Obtain a bloodless field when possible, for this will help in locating the foreign body.

✓ **Warn the patient or family about signs of infection (increasing pain, redness, swelling, red streaking) and inform them that even when there have been attempts to remove the imbedded graphite, there still may be a less apparent but permanent black tattoo.** Let them know that this can be removed later by a specialist if the resulting mark is cosmetically unacceptable (Fig. 149.3).

✓ **Administer tetanus prophylaxis, if necessary** (see Appendix F).

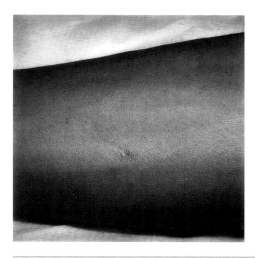

Fig. 149.3 Residual tattoo from old pencil point puncture.

What Not to Do

(X) Do not excise the entire wound on the initial visit.

(X) Do not prescribe prophylactic antibiotics because these are generally not necessary.

Discussion

Traumatic tattoos are caused by unwanted embedding of dirt or debris beneath the skin, which leaves an area of pigmentation after healing. This commonly occurs in "road rash" after bike or motorcycle accidents or puncture injury from a pencil, known as a "graphite or pencil point" tattoo.

It is unwise to excise the entire wound, because the resultant scar might be more unsightly than the tattoo. If a superficial pencil tip foreign body exists, see Chapter 154 (Subcutaneous Foreign Bodies) for an easy removal technique. **Most of these wounds do not contain a foreign body but only the appearance of one. Tattoo prevention should be the clinician's primary concern.**

If tattooing is present and of cosmetic concern, the patient may benefit from a referral to a dermatologist or plastic surgeon for immediate or delayed removal.

Rarely, deep punctures or foreign bodies may require exploratory surgery in the operating room.

Patients who choose to defer removal of a pencil tip foreign body should be counseled on the possible development of a granuloma with graphite staining as well as infection if there are any adherent wood particles.

Clinically, these tattoos can mimic the appearance of a melanoma, but of course it is not malignant.

Suggested Readings

Aswani, V. H., & Kim, S. L. (2015). Fifty-three years after a pencil puncture wound. *Case Reports in Dermatology*, *7*(3), 303–305.

Bittencourt, M. de J. S., Santos, J. E. B. D., Barros, J. N. D. S.J., & Xerfan, E. M. S. (2017). Pencil-core granuloma. *Anais Brasileiros De Dermatologia*, *92*(4), 578–579. https://doi.org/10.1590/abd1806-4841.20176011.

Goldstein, N. (2007). Tattoos defined. *Clinics in Dermatology*, *25*(4), 417–420.

Piercing Complications

Presentation

A patient presents with pain and redness around the piercing site. Upon inspection, there is erythema and some purulence coming from the piercing. The patient is afebrile and denies any other symptoms.

Piercing complications typically fall into two categories: infection or inability to remove. As infections lead to swelling, the edematous surrounding tissue may encase the piercing.

The more usual sites of piercing include ears, eyebrows, glabella, nasal septum, nostrils, lips, tongue, face, mouth (Fig. 150.1), chin, nipples (Fig. 150.2), navel, male and female genitalia, digits, and pocketing or flesh (skin) stapling. There may be a single piercing or multiple piercings. The prevalence of abnormal tooth wear or tooth chipping/cracking is greater for tongue piercing than lip piercing (see Chapter 50).

What to Do

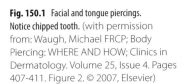 **Obtain a history regarding the piercing**, including how long it was inserted, any recent removal, postpiercing care, and onset of symptoms.

✅ Review with the patient and in the chart any prior methicillin-resistant *Staphylococcus aureus* (MRSA) exposure or infection.

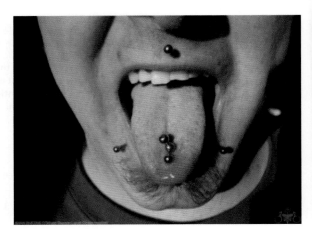

Fig. 150.1 Facial and tongue piercings. **Notice chipped tooth.** (with permission from: Waugh, Michael FRCP; Body Piercing: WHERE AND HOW; Clinics in Dermatology. Volume 25, Issue 4. Pages 407-411. Figure 2. © 2007, Elsevier)

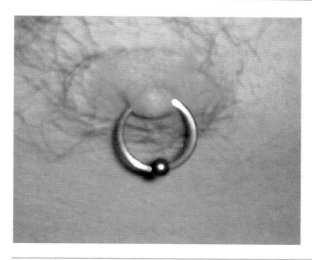

Fig. 150.2 Male nipple ring. (with permission from: Waugh, Michael FRCP; Body Piercing: WHERE AND HOW; Clinics in Dermatology. Volume 25, Issue 4. Pages 407-411. Figure 6. © 2007, Elsevier)

✓ **Screen the patient for immunocompromising conditions** (diabetes, steroids, human immunodeficiency virus (HIV)/acquired immunodeficiency syndrome (AIDS), chemotherapy, etc.).

✓ **For new piercings**, screen if the tetanus vaccination status is up to date, and vaccinate if indicated.

✓ **Piercings that are infected should be removed. For new piercings, this may mean that the pierced canal will close.** However, the foreign body will serve as a nidus for the infection, as it cannot be cleared by the patient's immune system.

✓ **Provide appropriate analgesia.** For piercings in the ear, a great auricular block with bupivacaine 0.5% will provide anesthesia without distorting tissues by avoiding infiltration of local anesthetic near the piercing.

✓ **Removal of the piercing depends on both type and location.** If a hoop cannot be opened for removal, it should be cut in a single location and the free ends bent in opposite directions orthogonal to the two-dimensional plain of the hoop. This allows for easier repair by a jeweler in case the hoop is of large financial or sentimental value.

✓ **If a stud piercing cannot be removed**, the locking mechanism that could not be opened by hand may be opened with hemostats. Hold the front of the stud with one hemostat and use the second hemostat to loosen the back. This may damage the stud.

✓ **Remember that some studs have flat backs, whereas others have screw backs** that require twisting. When available, compare the stud to its twin.

✓ If the back cannot be removed, the shaft of the stud must be cut. This can be done with sturdy wire cutters, ring cutters, and some trauma shears.

✓ **Ear studs may be embedded** when the anterior portion of the stud gets pushed posteriorly into the earlobe. To remove an embedded ear stud, remove the back (or cut the shaft if needed). **After good local anesthesia**, unroof the area over the front of the ear stud. Holding the ear lobe, gently push the stud anteriorly by grasping the shaft with a hemostat. Grab the stud as it exits the anterior side of the ear lobe before letting go of the shaft with your hemostat.

✓ **Transdermals or microdermals** are small implants that consist of a footplate and a post in the shape of the letter L. The post protrudes from the skin's surface and is held in place under the dermis by the small, flat foot plate. Provide local anesthesia with injection of lidocaine. Grasp the outside part of the microdermal with forceps or a hemostat and gently elevate and move the microdermal until the direction of the foot plate can be determined. Using a scalpel, make a small (~2-mm) incision going away from the shaft on the opposite side of the foot plate. Tilt the microdermal toward the foot plate while holding down the surrounding tissue until it releases and comes out.

✓ **Sometimes removal of the piercing and application of warm compresses suffices to allow the infection to subside.** Otherwise, provide oral antibiotic coverage for staphylococcus and streptococcus, and expand to MRSA coverage in patients known to be colonized.

✓ **The most common pathogen in infected cartilage piercings** (nose, ears [does not include earlobe]) is pseudomonas. Ensure appropriate antibiotic coverage.

What Not to Do

✗ Do not cut ear lobe to remove a piercing. It will lead to a poor cosmetic appearance.

✗ Do not leave infected piercing in place. The infection is unlikely to resolve or will immediately return.

✗ Do not cut over the foot plate of a microdermal. It will require a significant incision to remove the microdermal that way and will lead to a poor cosmetic outcome.

✗ Do not treat cartilage piercing infections with antibiotics that do not provide pseudomonal coverage. About 80% of all cartilage piercing infections are infected with pseudomonas.

✗ Do not suture close the cavity of a microdermal after removal. It is a nonsterile cavity that has epithelialized and will predispose the patient to develop an abscess.

Discussion

Piercings are ubiquitous and can be found in a variety of locations ranging from genitals to eyebrows. While typically occurring shortly after the act of getting pierced, infection can occur at any time due to either nonsterile insertion technique or poor patient hygiene. Removal of the piercing remains an integral part of care for most piercing complications. Care must be taken to ensure patient comfort prior to significant manipulation, as infected piercings are painful and often placed in sensitive areas of the body. **Always instruct that jewelry might get damaged during the removal process, and always return the jewelry to the patient rather than discarding it.**

Understanding the basic types of body jewelry may help medical personnel identify and understand how to question patients if they do not volunteer information related to their body piercings. This knowledge may also help to safely remove the jewelry. Each type of jewelry has distinctive features that play a role in keeping the object in place and aid in its removal.

Jewelry Types and Locations

Barbell	Ear, eyebrow, lip, tongue, nostril, navel, genitals
Captive bead	Ear, eyebrow, lip, nostril, navel, genitalia
Dermal	Any flat skin surface
Labret	Lip
Stud or screw	Nose

Barbells

Barbells are straight, curved, or circular rods with a bead or ball closure known as a bell. One or both

(Continued)

Discussion continued

ends of the bar have an outside (i.e., male) thread like that of a metal screw. The bell has an inside (i.e., female) thread like that of a metal nut.

For barbell piercings, removing the bell from the bar is similar to removing a nut from a screw.

Captive Beads

A captive-bead ring is a semicircular piece of metal shaped into an incomplete circle coupled with a dimpled bead that is held captive in the gap in the ring. The tension of the metal ring seizes the ball and keeps it from moving. The mechanism is similar to that of a circular metal ring worn on the finger with a gap cut into it, in which there is a small ball.

Removal of captive beads requires inverted pliers (which may not be available). If such pliers can be obtained, the tip of the inverted pliers should be inserted inside the ring until the ring contacts the pliers' depressed dimples. Slowly squeeze the pliers, spreading the jaws outward, pushing the metal edges of the ring apart until the bead is free. Then, remove the appliance.

Labrets

Labrets are similar to barbells except one end is a flat disc and the other end is a ball.

Labrets have only one spherical ball that sits outside the lip and a flat disc inside the lip opposite the gum line. With gloved hands, grasp the flat surface just behind the lip while holding the ball in front of the lip. Hold the ball in front of the lip and turn it to the left to detach the ball. Then remove the labret.

Nose Studs and Screws

Nose studs are straight lengths of metal with a decorative piece on one end and a small bump on the other end. The small bump at the end of the straight shaft keeps the appliance in position. Nose screws have a distal curvature similar to the end of a corkscrew.

With gloved hands, grasp the top of the nose stud and pull it straight out. Nose screws have a distal curvature similar to the end of a corkscrew and can be removed by grasping the top and twisting it out of the track.

Suggested Readings

Patel, M., & Cobbs, C. G. (2015). Infections from body piercing and tattoos. *Microbiology Spectrum*, *3*(6). https://doi.org/10.1128/microbiolspec.IOL5-0016-2015

Preslar, D., & Borger, J. (2019). *Body piercing infections*. www.europepmc.org.

Smith, F. D. (2007). Caring for surgical patients with piercings. *AORN Journal*, *103*(6), 583–596.

Sosin, M., Weissler, J. M., Pulcrano, M., & Rodriguez, E. D. (2015). Transcartilaginous ear piercing and infectious complications: A systematic review and critical analysis of outcomes. *The Laryngoscope*, *125*(8), 1827–1834. https://doi.org/10.1002/lary.25238

Waugh, M. (2007). Body piercing: Where and how. *Clinics in Dermatology*, *25*(4), 407–411.

Puncture Wounds

Presentation

Puncture wounds are common injuries, especially in children during the summer months when protective footwear may not be worn. The risk of a puncture wound is disproportional to its size, as irrigation is difficult and the tract of the wound is prone to creating an anaerobic environment. As such, patients either present early after the injury or delayed due to the development of infection.

What to Do

✅ **Obtain a detailed history** to ascertain the time interval since injury and the nature of the penetrating object. Inquire whether the injury occurred through the sole of a shoe, as this may change the type of bacteria introduced into the wound. Also, ask about tetanus immunization status and underlying health problems that may potentially diminish host defenses (especially diabetes mellitus).

✅ **Have the patient lie prone, backward on the gurney, so that raising the head of the bed flexes the knee and brings the sole of the foot into clear view.** Place the foot on a pillow. **Clean the surrounding skin, and carefully inspect the wound. Provide good lighting, and take your time.** Examine the foot for signs of deep injury, such as swelling and pain with passive motion of the toes. Although the occurrence is unlikely, test for loss of sensory or motor function.

✅ **If the puncture was created by a slender object, such as a sewing needle or thumb tack that is verified to have been removed intact, no further treatment is necessary.** If there is any question that a piece may have broken off in the tissue, obtain radiographs and/or perform bedside ultrasonography (see Chapter 146).

✅ **Most metal and glass foreign bodies are visualized on plain films, whereas plastic, aluminum, rubber fragments (from rubber-soled shoes that have been penetrated through), thorns, spines, and wood are more radiolucent and may require ultrasonography. Retained foreign bodies increase the potential for infection and should be suspected in patients who present with infection, who are not responding to treatment for infection, who have inordinate pain, or who have a foreign-body sensation when the puncture wound is palpated.** The risks and benefits of the removal of the foreign bodies should be discussed with the patient (see Chapter 154).

✅ **With deep, highly contaminated wounds**, orthopedic or podiatric consultation should be sought. With the most serious of these wounds, consideration should be given to providing a wide debridement in the operating room. This is done to prevent the osteomyelitis or deep space tissue infections. Although controversial, deep wounds such as these may be considered for treatment with a prophylactic antibiotic.

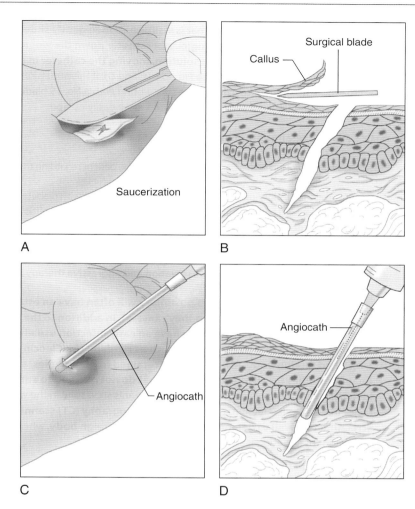

A

Saucerization

B

Callus

Surgical blade

C

Angiocath

D

Angiocath

Fig. 151.1 Simple débridement and irrigation for puncture wounds.

✓ **If there was a deep puncture through a rubber-soled sport shoe, it may be reasonable (although not proven) to provide prophylactic antipseudomonal antibiotic therapy.**

✓ **Most superficial puncture wounds require only simple debridement, possibly with irrigation. In these wounds, prophylactic antibiotics are not indicated.**

✓ **The plantar surface of the foot is exceedingly well innervated**, and even simple debridement is likely to be painful. In appropriate circumstances and depending on the location of the injury/foreign body, **consider performing a posterior tibial or a sural nerve block.**

✓ **Saucerize (shave) across the puncture wound using a No. 10 scalpel blade to remove the surrounding cornified epithelium and expose any debris that may have collected beneath its surface** (Fig. 151.1A and B). Alternatively, the jagged cornified epidermal skin edges overlying the puncture tract may be painlessly trimmed using a scalpel or scissors.

✅ **If debris is found, remove what is visible and then gently slide a large-gauge blunt needle or an over-the-needle (Angiocath) catheter down the wound track and slowly irrigate with a physiologic saline solution, moving the catheter in and out until debris no longer flows from the wound (see** Fig. 151.1C and D). If the puncture wound is small and there is little room for effluent to exit, make a stab wound with a No. 15 blade through the dermis to enlarge the opening and allow the effluent to more easily escape.

✅ **Provide tetanus prophylaxis** (see Appendix G).

✅ Cover the wound with a Band-Aid and instruct the patient regarding the warning signs of infection.

✅ **Arrange for follow-up at 24 hours**, especially in patients with diabetes. Spend some time on documentation and patient education. **Talk about delayed osteomyelitis and the importance of medical attention if there is continued aching or discomfort 1 to 2 weeks postinjury. Explain that even with proper care, foreign material may be embedded deeply in the wound, and infection could occur. Explain that in most cases prophylactic antibiotics do not prevent these infections, and that the best practice is close observation and aggressive therapy if infection occurs.**

✅ **Patients presenting 24 hours postinjury will often have an established wound infection (that is likely the reason they came in). In addition to the debridement procedures described, patients who have an early infection usually respond quickly to an oral antistaphylococcal antibiotic, such as clindamycin (Cleocin), if they do not have a retained foreign body. Always suspect retained foreign bodies, and strongly consider imaging studies for all infected wounds that do not respond to antibiotics.** Retained foreign material (e.g., a piece of sock or a portion of a tennis shoe sole) in the wound is an important factor in persistent infection. **Use computed tomography (CT) scanning when other screening tools fail to demonstrate a suspected foreign body,** when infection is present, or when joint penetration is suspected.

✅ **Provide patients with crutches and/or a surgical shoe if weightbearing is too uncomfortable, and encourage them to soak the infected foot.**

✅ **Consider hospitalization** for patients with severe infection or who have risk factors for serious complications and are unable to have next-day follow-up (e.g., diabetes, peripheral vascular disease, immune suppression).

What Not to Do

❌ Do not be falsely reassured by having the patient soak in Betadine. This does not provide any significant protection from infection and is not a substitute for debridement and irrigation.

❌ Do not attempt a jet lavage within a puncture wound. This will only lead to subcutaneous infiltration of the irrigant and the possible spread of foreign material and bacteria.

❌ Do not perform blind probing of a deep puncture wound. This is not likely to be of any value and may do harm.

❌ Do not obtain radiographs for simple clean nail punctures, except for the unusual case in which large radiopaque particulate debris is suspected to be deeply embedded within the wound or the physical examination suggests bony injury.

Ⓧ **Do not routinely prescribe prophylactic antibiotics. Reserve them for patients with diabetes, peripheral vascular disease, immune suppression, or deep and highly contaminated wounds. In fact, there is insufficient evidence to recommend the use of prophylactic antimicrobials to decrease the incidence of serious infections in any of these puncture wounds.**

Ⓧ **Do not ignore the possibility of a (missed) foreign body in a patient who returns with a recurrent infection.** Obtain an ultrasonogram and/or CT scan and consult an appropriate specialist (orthopedic surgeon vs. podiatrist)

Ⓧ **Do not ignore the patient who is complaining of foot pain long after stepping on a nail.** Osteomyelitis may present weeks or even months after the initial injury. These patients demand special imaging to rule out a retained foreign body, and an erythrocyte sedimentation rate (ESR) and C-reactive protein (CRP) should be obtained. These patients should then be referred to a surgical foot specialist for a bone scan or magnetic resonance imaging (MRI) and, if there is evidence of bone infection, surgical debridement.

Ⓧ Do not begin soaks at home unless there are early signs of developing infection.

Discussion

The most common sites for puncture wounds are the feet. The complication rate from plantar puncture wounds is higher than the rate for puncture wounds elsewhere in the body (with the exception of the hands). Studies suggest that conservative therapy is appropriate in an immunocompetent host (~6% will develop an infection). However, about **one-fourth of patients with diabetes mellitus will develop a complication from the puncture wound**, often with devastating consequences, including sepsis and amputation. Thus prophylactic antibiotic therapy and decoring/debridement are advisable in this group. **Small, clean, superficial puncture wounds uniformly do well. The pathophysiology and management of a puncture wound therefore depend on the material that punctured the foot, the location of the wound, the depth of penetration, the time to presentation, the footwear penetrated, whether there is an indoor versus a more infection-prone outdoor injury, and the underlying health status of the victim. Punctures in the metatarsophalangeal joint area may also be of higher risk for serious wound complications because of the greater likelihood of penetration of joint, tendon, or bone. Early presenters** tend to be children or adults seeking tetanus prophylaxis. These patients tend to have a low incidence of infection. **Patients who present late** usually have increasing pain, swelling, or drainage as evidence of an early or established infection. **Unsuspected retained foreign bodies**, often pieces of a tennis shoe or sock, are a source of serious infection. Other common foreign bodies include rust, gravel, grass, straw, and dirt.

The probability of wound infection is increased with deeper penetrating injuries, delayed presentation (>24 hours), gross contamination, penetration through a rubber-soled shoe, outdoor injuries, injuries that occur from the neck of the metatarsals to the web space of the toes, and decreased resistance to infection. **Specifically, diabetic patients typically present for care later and have higher rates of osteomyelitis (up to 35%). In one study, they were also 5 times more likely to require multiple operations and 46 times more likely to have a lower extremity amputation as a result of a plantar puncture wound.**

Osteomyelitis caused by *Pseudomonas aeruginosa* remains the most devastating of puncture wound complications. The exact incidence of osteomyelitis remains uncertain and is estimated to be between 0.04% and 0.5% in plantar puncture wounds. The metatarsal heads are most at risk for osteomyelitis. **A nail through the sole of a tennis or sport shoe is known to inoculate *Pseudomonas* organisms. Any patient who is considered to have penetration of the bone, joint space, or plantar fascia, particularly over the metatarsal heads, should be warned of the potential for serious infection and then referred to an orthopedic surgeon or podiatrist for early follow-up evaluation.**

Suggested Readings

East, J. M., Yeates, C. B., & Robinson, H. P. (2011). The natural history of pedal puncture wounds in diabetics: A cross-sectional survey. *BMC Surgery, 11*, 27. https://doi.org/10.1186/1471-2482-11-27.

McGee, D. L. (2019). *Podiatric procedures. Roberts and Hedges' clinical procedures in emergency medicine and acute care* (7th ed.) (pp. 1057–1070). Philadelphia, PA: Elsevier. e1, chap. 51.

Volk, A., Zebda, M., & Abdelgawad, A. A. (2017). Plantar and pedal puncture wounds in children: A case series study from a single level I trauma center. *Pediatric Emergency Care, 33*(11), 724–729. https://doi.org/10.1097/PEC.0000000000000615.

Ring Removal

Presentation

Removal of rings from fingers or toes may be required due a variety of conditions that predispose to digital swelling, such as trauma, infection, burns, peripheral edema, or arthropod assault. Sometimes chronic tight-fitting rings begin to obstruct lymphatic drainage, causing swelling and further constriction (Fig. 152.1). Rings often have sentimental and monetary value to the patient. Thus providers should be familiar with a variety of removal techniques.

What to Do

✓ **Removal techniques can be broken down into destructive and nondestructive techniques.** A patient who presents with digital ischemia must have the ring removed emergently. With any disease process or injury to the distal extremities, consider removing rings preemptively prior to the development of local swelling.

✓ **Until removal is initiated**, elevate the limb and apply ice to the affected digit to reduce swelling.

✓ Obtain imaging for suspected fractures in the ring-bearing digit.

Nondestructive Techniques

✓ For analgesia, **consider a local nerve block (e.g., ulnar nerve block)** rather than a digital block. The additional swelling from a digital block increases the risk of digital ischemia and will make removal more challenging.

✓ **Caterpillar technique: Apply lubrication to the affected digit. Apply pressure to the volar aspect of the ring against the digit (creating space between the dorsal aspect of the digit and the ring) and push the dorsal part of the ring distally. Then apply dorsal pressure to the ring and push the volar part distally.** This "walks" the ring down the finger and suffices in most cases. **Applying traction to the skin proximal to the lubricated ring and then twisting the ring while pulling it off also works** (Fig. 152.2) (See Video 152.1).

✓ **Tourniquet/compression technique: Elevate the affected limb. Using umbilical tape or a Penrose drain, tightly wrap the digit from distal-to-proximal and then leave this in place for several minutes** (Fig. 152.3). Then apply an arm tourniquet to prevent blood from returning into the finger. This technique minimizes the edema under the ring, thereby loosening it. Then, after removing the wrap (but not the tourniquet), apply lubricant and use the caterpillar or twisting technique noted earlier. Then, of course, remove the tourniquet (See Video 152.2).

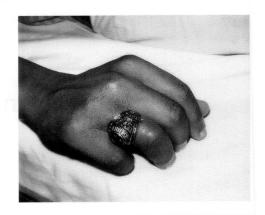

Fig. 152.1 Tight-fitting ring with secondary lymphatic obstruction and swelling.

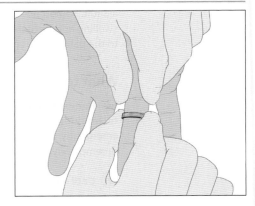

Fig. 152.2 Pull skin taut and twist ring off.

✓ **Winding string technique:** Use a 2-0 or larger suture and pass it proximal-to-distal under the ring. Use the long distal end to circumferentially and tightly wrap the digit proximal-to-distal. Grasp the proximal end and, while applying gentle distal traction, start unwinding the suture thus propelling the ring forward (Fig. 152.4).

✓ **String-loop technique:** Use a 2-0 or larger suture and pass at least two sutures underneath the ring. Our practice is to use five to six sutures spaced at even intervals. Lubricate the digit. Attach hemostats to the distal end of each string pair, and have an assistant apply continuous distal traction on the ring. The strings will help guide the tissue underneath the ring. Combine this with the caterpillar technique noted earlier.

✓ When using only one string loop under a lubricated ring (Fig. 152.5), **apply traction to the string ends while sliding the string around and around under the ring, gradually moving the ring over the skin.** For greater efficiency, traction can be applied to the skin proximal to the ring as seen in (Fig. 152.2).

✓ **Glove technique:** Cut off the finger of an examination glove as well as its tip, creating a tube. Pass it over the affected digit and under the ring. Lubricate the external surface and slide the ring over the gloved part of the digit.

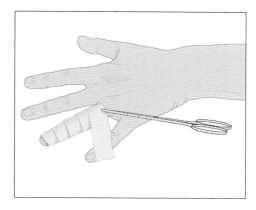

Fig. 152.3 Tourniquet technique.

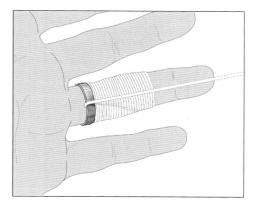

Fig. 152.4 String technique.

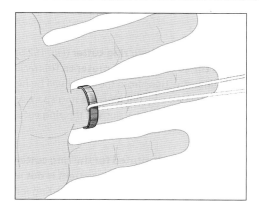

Fig. 152.5 String-loop technique.

Destructive Techniques

✅ **If nondestructive techniques fail or the patient has digital ischemia, the ring should be removed by destructive techniques.** Most rings can be repaired by a jeweler after removal.

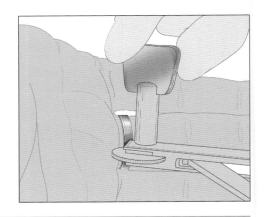

Fig. 152.6 Ring-cutter technique.

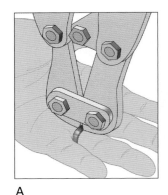 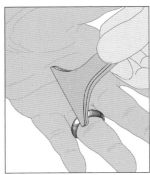

A   B

Fig. 152.7 (A, B) Orthopedic pin-cutter technique.

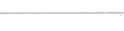 Ring cutter technique: Using a handheld ring cutter (Fig. 152.6), **cut the 3-o'clock and 9-o'clock positions relative to the central gem (if present).** This facilitates easier repair for the jeweler afterward, and any imperfections from the repair will be hidden by the neighboring digits. Avoid making a single cut followed by bending the ring apart, as this is harder to reverse and may distort the setting. There are electric versions of this ring cutter, which can make this process much easier on your fingers (See Video 152.3).

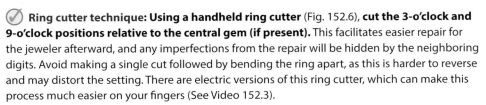 **An orthopedic pin cutter can be substituted for the ring cutter when dealing with thick or hard metal rings. This is especially so if the patient is not worried about any damage to the ring.** A 5-mm wedge can be removed from the ring followed by the insertion of a cast spreader to spread the ring apart (Fig. 152.7). Alternatively, two cuts may be made on opposite sides of the ring, allowing it to be removed in halves (See Videos 152.4 and 152.5).

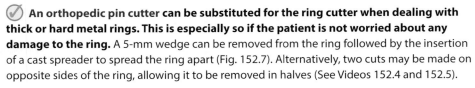 **Tungsten carbide or ceramic rings are quite difficult to cut with ring cutters. However, the hardness of the material predisposes it to shattering under pressure. Attempt removal by cracking them into pieces using a standard vice grip–style locking pliers** (Fig. 152.8). Place the locking pliers over the ring and adjust the jaws to clamp lightly. Release and adjust

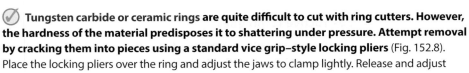

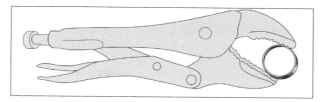

A

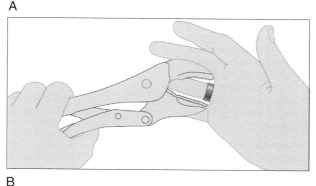

B

Fig. 152.8 (A, B) Vice grip–style locking pliers are used to crack tungsten carbide or ceramic rings. (Adapted from Hajduk, S. V. [2001]. Letter to the editor: Emergency removal of hard metal or ceramic finger rings. *Annals of Emergency Medicine, 37,* 736.)

the tightener one-third turn and then clamp again. Repeat until a crack is heard; then continue clamping in different positions until the hard material breaks away. Return the larger pieces to the patient, to receive a possible replacement ring from the manufacturer, because it is unlikely that a ring removed by this technique is amendable to repair by a jeweler.

⊘ **For a child who sticks a finger into a round hole in a plastic toy, sports helmet, or other plastic product and becomes entrapped, release the finger by first cutting around the hole using a standard orthopedic cast cutter.** This will allow the patient's finger to be released from the large plastic object, leaving a plastic ring around the patient's freed finger. This smaller object can now be removed using any of the earlier techniques or by just protecting the underlying skin and using the cast cutter to cut this plastic ring in half.

What Not to Do

⊗ Do not use nerve blocks unless there is significant tenderness. Most rings can be removed with minimal discomfort. Exercise a judicious approach to using digital blocks. While they provide effective anesthesia for the injured or tender finger, the additional swelling will make ring removal more challenging.

⊗ Do not damage the ring without the patient's consent. Engage in shared decision making with the patient regarding the risks of leaving the ring in place. If the ring cannot be removed and the patient opts to leave the ring in place, provide continued elevation and cooling of the digit. A minor injury may only lead to transient swelling, which will allow the patient to forgo ring removal.

Discussion

The constricting effects of a circumferential foreign body can lead to obstruction of lymphatic and venous drainage, which in turn leads to more swelling and further constriction. Eventually circulation is compromised and ischemia ensues. Thus rings should be removed as early as possible in the clinical course. In patients who present with sepsis and require significant fluid resuscitation, the development of peripheral edema is expected as part of their clinical course. Thus preemptive removal should be considered when feasible. Jewelry is often of significant monetary and sentimental value. Documentation about who receives the removed items (patient, family member, hospital security) avoids disputes in case of loss.

As with all interventions in medicine, the patient should be engaged in shared decision making prior to removal of rings.

Hair-thread tourniquets can become tightly wrapped around an infant's finger, toe, or penis, causing swelling, ischemia, or discoloration distal to the band (Fig. 152.9). Removing this constricting band of one or more fibers can be quite difficult. It usually requires anesthesia, dissection, and severing of the deeply embedded fibers with a large-gauge needle and magnifying loupes. Another technique is to use lysis by a depilatory agent, such as Nair or Neet. By applying hair remover to the hair tourniquet, the constricting bands may be lysed within 10 to 15 minutes. Even when the bands appear to be completely released, provide for a wound check within 24 hours.

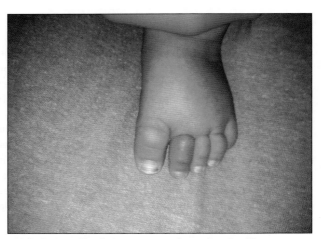

Fig. 152.9 Hair tourniquet with distal venous and lymphatic engorgement on the second toe of a toddler.

Suggested Readings

Boe, C., & Kakar, S. (2018). A modified string technique for atraumatic ring removal. *Journal of Emergency Medicine, 55*(2), 240–243. https://doi.org/10.1016/j.jemermed.2018.05.022.

Gardiner, C. L., Handyside, K., Mazzillo, J., Hill, M. J., Reichman, E. F., Chathampally, Y., et al. (2013). A comparison of two techniques for tungsten carbide ring removal. *American Journal of Emergency Medicine, 31*(10), 1516–1519. https://doi.org/10.1016/j.ajem.2013.07.027.

Kalkan, A., Kose, O., Tas, M., & Meric, G. (2013). Review of techniques for the removal of trapped rings on fingers with a proposed new algorithm. *American Journal of Emergency Medicine, 31*(11), 1605–1611. https://doi.org/10.1016/j.ajem.2013.06.009.

Sliver, Superficial

Presentation

The patient is caught on a sharp splinter (usually wooden) and either cannot grasp it, has broken it trying to remove it, or has found that it is too large and painful to remove. The history may be somewhat obscure. On examination, a puncture wound should be found with a tightly embedded sliver that may or may not be palpable over its entire length (Fig. 153.1A). There may only be a puncture wound without a clearly visible or palpable foreign body.

What to Do

✓ Obtain a history, including patient risk factors (immunosuppression, diabetes), tetanus vaccination status, and suspected nature of the embedded sliver (wood, plastic, metal, etc.).

✓ **If it is unclear whether a foreign body is beneath the skin, obtain a high-resolution ultrasound (US) study using a linear-array transducer that focuses in the near field-of-view. A 7.5- or 10-MHz probe is used to search for small superficial objects, whereas a 5.0-MHz probe is recommended for larger, deeper objects** (Fig. 153.2).

✓ The ultrasound probes first emit ultrasound waves, then switch to record echoes. Soundwaves reflected from very superficial structures may arrive before the switch has completed, thus rendering the most superficial 1 to 2 mm of tissue difficult to evaluate. Spacing the probe away from the skin in a water bath ultrasound or placing a gel-filled gloved finger between the probe and the patient eliminates this problem.

✓ **The clinician who is skilled in ultrasound-guided techniques can use these techniques to assist in sliver removal.**

✓ **If the sliver is visible, very superficial, and easily palpated, it is likely in or just below the epidermis.** The epidermis does not contain nerve endings and can be unroofed over the sliver without the need for local anesthetic.

✓ **For deeper slivers, locally infiltrate with 1% lidocaine (Xylocaine) with epinephrine, and clean the skin with an antiseptic. If the entire length of the sliver is not palpable, when possible, first establish a bloodless field. Then, using a scalpel blade, cut down over the entire length of the sliver (especially if the sliver is friable in nature), completely exposing it. The sliver can now be easily lifted out and completely removed. Cleanse the open track with normal saline** (Fig. 153.3). Debride contaminated tissue and remove any visible debris if necessary. This superficial wound (see Fig. 153.1B) can now be easily closed using wound-closure strips or tissue adhesive. Avoid sutures when possible, especially absorbable buried sutures, because of the increased risk for infection (See Videos 153.1 & 154.1).

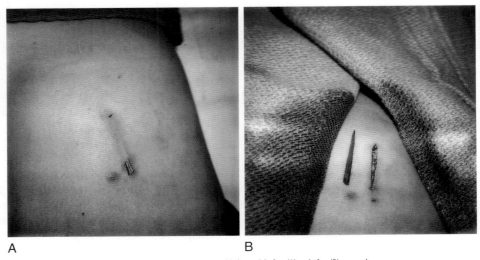

Fig. 153.1 Wooden splinter in child's buttock before (A) and after (B) removal.

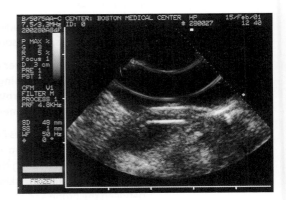

Fig. 153.2 Ultrasonogram of the hand with a wooden toothpick in the superficial soft tissue. (Courtesy A. Dewitz, MD, Boston Medical Center, Boston, MA.)

✅ **A more vertical splinter should be approached in the same manner, but the incision will be straight down along the length of the sliver as deep as possible, thereby releasing the entire foreign body from the surrounding tissue. Be careful not to incise any important anatomic structures such as nerves, vessels, or tendons.**

✅ Patients who have larger organic foreign bodies or foreign bodies located in high-risk areas or patients who are at high risk for infectious complications (e.g., diabetes, peripheral vascular disease, other immunocompromised condition) must have these foreign bodies removed as soon as possible. If unable to remove at bedside, a surgeon should be consulted.

✅ **Give tetanus prophylaxis**, if necessary (see Appendix G).

✅ **Even after the foreign body has been found and removed, some small particles may have remained along the tract.** Warn the patient about the signs of infection and schedule

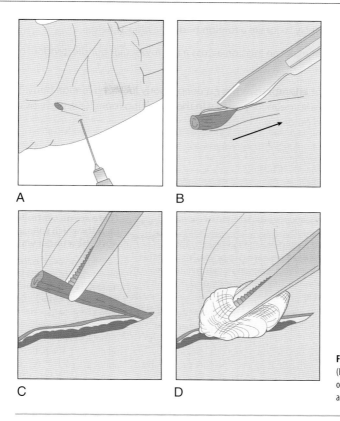

Fig. 153.3 (A) Inject with a local anesthetic. (B) Incise down to the sliver. (C) Lift the sliver out with forceps. (D) Clean the wound track with a wet gauze sponge.

a 48-hour wound check. Prophylactic antibiotics are generally not required when the sliver is thought to be completely removed, but should be considered in high-risk patients, particularly with foot wounds.

✓ **For fine cactus spines, briars, or even multiple small splinters, use fine forceps to remove as many of these slivers as possible. Applying multipurpose glue with overlying gauze to the affected area, allowing it to dry and then pulling off the gauze, can remove many tiny slivers at the same time.** The patient can complete removal at home by using either hair-removal wax or blackhead removal strips.

What Not to Do

🗙 Do not order plain radiographs unless a suspected sliver is made of glass or metal and cannot be found with physical exam, wound exploration, or ultrasound. Wooden foreign bodies are often radiolucent. After approximately 1 day of absorbing water from adjacent tissue, they tend to be isodense on CT scanning as well. In addition, cactus and sea urchin spines, thorns, plastic, and aluminum all tend to be difficult to visualize on plain radiographs.

🗙 Do not try to pull the sliver out by one end unless you feel confident that the material it is composed of will not fragment or be friable. Otherwise, it is likely to break and leave a fragment behind or leave a trail of debris.

(X) Do not try to locate a foreign body in a bloody field.

(X) Do not make an incision across a neurovascular bundle, tendon, or other important structure.

(X) Do not attempt to remove a deep, poorly localized foreign body. Those cases may require referral to a surgeon for removal in the operating room (OR), perhaps with fluoroscopic or ultrasound guidance.

Discussion

Wood, glass, and metallic splinters are among the most common retained foreign bodies. Most superficial splinters may be removed by the patients themselves, leaving to physicians and other clinicians only the deeper and larger splinters or retained splinters that have broken off during an attempt at removal.

The most common error in the management of soft tissue foreign bodies is failure to detect their presence. Signs and symptoms of a hidden foreign body might include sharp pain or a foreign-body sensation with palpation over the puncture wound, dark discoloration beneath the skin, a palpable mass beneath the skin, or a patient's suspicion that a foreign body is present. **An organic foreign body is almost certain to create an inflammatory response and become infected if any part of it is left beneath the skin.** It is for this reason, along with the fact that wooden slivers tend to be friable and may break apart during removal, that complete exposure is generally necessary before the sliver can be taken out.

There are no controlled studies that clearly identify which splinter removal technique works best under which conditions.

If the foreign body is thought to be relatively superficial but cannot be located, explain to the patient that more harm may be caused by exploring and excising further. The splinter will be watched until it forms a "pus pocket," thus making it easier to remove at a later time. If this procedure is followed, it should always be coordinated with a follow-up clinician. The patient should be placed on an antibiotic, such as cephalexin (Keflex), and provided with follow-up care within 48 hours. These retained foreign bodies may also become encapsulated within granulation tissue and can be removed at a much later date. The patient should be so informed.

When a patient returns after being treated for a puncture wound, and there is evidence of nonhealing or recurrent exacerbations of inflammation, infection, or drainage, assume that the wound still contains a foreign body, begin antibiotics, get appropriate imaging studies, and refer the patient for surgical consultation.

Suggested Readings

Chan, C., & Salam, G. A. (2003). Splinter removal. *American Family Physician, 67*(12), 2557–2562.

Ipaktchi, K., Demars, A., Park, J., Ciarallo, C., Livermore, M., & Banegas, R. (2013). Retained palmar foreign body presenting as a late hand infection: Proposed diagnostic algorithm to detect radiolucent objects. *Patient Safety in Surgery, 7*(1), 25. https://doi.org/10.1186/1754-9493-7-25.

Subcutaneous Foreign Bodies
(Metal, Dental Fragments, Glass, Gravel, and Hard Plastic)

Presentation

Small, moderate-velocity metal fragments can be released when a hammer strikes a second piece of metal, such as a chisel. The patient has noticed a stinging sensation and a small puncture wound or bleeding site and is worried that there might be something inside. A BB projectile will produce a more obvious but very similar problem. Another mechanism for producing hard radiopaque foreign bodies is puncturing with glass shards, especially by stepping on glass fragments or receiving them in a motor vehicle collision. Falling onto gravel can also force sharp fragments under the skin through a small puncture wound. Physical findings will show a puncture wound and may show an underlying dark discoloration or a palpable foreign body.

What to Do

✓ **Be suspicious of a retained foreign body in all wounds produced by a high-velocity missile or sharp fragile object. The most common error in the management of soft tissue foreign bodies is failure to detect their presence.**

✓ Obtain a thorough mechanism of injury history and determine if the patient suspects that there is a foreign body in the wound or has a foreign-body sensation. A high index of suspicion for occult foreign bodies is advised in cases of seizure, syncope, abuse, and assault, as well as in self-inflicted wounds.

✓ **Engage in shared decision making with the patient regarding the attempt to locate and remove a suspected foreign body.** Some inert foreign bodies, which may be difficult to locate and remove, can be safely left in place with a low risk for infection or later complications. The decision should be guided by the nature of the foreign body, the location, and the invasiveness of the removal procedure.

✓ **Wound irrigation and exploration will locate and lead to the removal of the majority of foreign bodies.**

✓ **Radiographs may help locate radiodense foreign bodies only.** Organic matter (e.g., wood) is often isodense to surrounding tissues, especially if the presentation is delayed. Radiographs are often not necessary for superficial wounds (yield ~1.4%).

✓ **Ultrasonography allows for localization of most foreign bodies** as hyperechoic structures with posterior acoustic shadowing (Fig. 154.1). Metal objects tend to produce reverberation or comet-tail artifact. Unlike radiographs, organic matter is well visualized by ultrasonography.

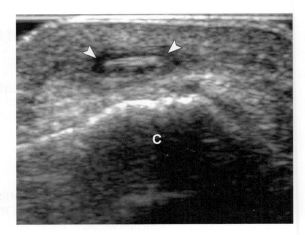

Fig. 154.1 A 47-year-old woman with rose-thorn foreign body. Ultrasound image shows linear hyperechoic foreign body *(arrowheads)* with surrounding hypoechoic halo of inflammation. *C,* Calcaneus.

✅ **If it is unclear whether a foreign body is beneath the skin, obtain a high-resolution ultrasound (US) study using a linear-array transducer that focuses in the near field-of-view. A 7.5- or 10-MHz probe is used to search for small superficial objects, whereas a 5.0-MHz probe is recommended for larger, deeper objects.**

✅ The ultrasound probes first emit ultrasound waves, then switch to record echoes. Soundwaves reflected from very superficial structures may arrive before the switch has completed, thus rendering the most superficial 1 to 2 mm of tissue difficult to evaluate. Spacing the probe away from the skin in a water bath ultrasound or placing a gel-filled gloved finger between the probe and the patient eliminates this problem.

✅ **The clinician who is skilled in ultrasound-guided techniques can use these techniques to assist in subcutaneous foreign body removal.**

✅ **After the presence of a foreign body has been established, the nature and location of the foreign body should guide the risk/benefit discussion of its removal.** Most metals, plastics, and glass are biologically inert. If not removed, the body may form a granuloma around the foreign body and may eventually expel it. On the other hand, the resin in most wood is highly immunogenic, and organic matter in general serves as a nidus for infection. Thus metal, plastic, and glass can potentially be left behind whereas organic matter should always be removed.

✅ **The risk and tissue destruction needed to reach a deep inert foreign body** often negate any potential benefits of its removal. **Do not attempt removal for more than 15 minutes.** If unable to locate and remove the foreign body in this time, surgical consultation and exploration may be necessary.

✅ **Clearly visible and palpable embedded objects, such as windshield glass in the forehead or gravel in a knee, can usually be grasped with fine, smooth forceps and simply picked out of the puncture wound.**

✅ **If the foreign body is in an extremity, it is preferable and sometimes essential to establish a bloodless field. For all cases, provide optimal lighting** conditions and arrange comfortable positioning of both the patient and the clinician (See Video 154.1).

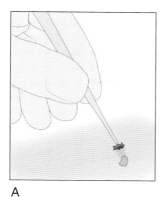 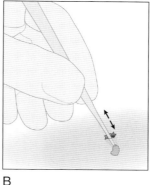

A   B

Fig. 154.2 (A) Puncture wound. (B) Fan probe until foreign body is struck.

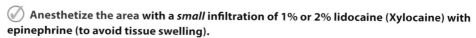

✓ **Anesthetize the area with a *small* infiltration of 1% or 2% lidocaine (Xylocaine) with epinephrine (to avoid tissue swelling).**

✓ **Take a blunt stiff metal probe (not a needle) and gently slide it down the apparent track of the puncture wound. Move the probe back and forth (in and out), fanning it in all directions, until a clicking contact between the probe and the foreign body can be felt and heard.** This should be repeated several times, until it is certain that contact is being made with the foreign body (Fig. 154.2) (See Video 154.2).

✓ **After contact is made, fix the probe in place by resting the hand that is holding the probe against a firm surface. Then, with the other hand, cut down along the probe with a No. 15 scalpel blade until the foreign body is reached. Do not remove the probe** (Fig. 154.3).

✓ **While continuing to hold the probe in place, reach into the incision with a pair of forceps, using the opposite hand, and remove the foreign body (located at the end of the probe)** (Fig. 154.4). This technique works best with small hard objects and will not work as well with softer foreign bodies, such as organic matter.

✓ **After the foreign body is removed and the wound is irrigated,** close the wound loosely with strip closures or tissue adhesive.

✓ **If the foreign body is very superficial and easily palpable** beneath the skin, it may be advantageous to eliminate the probe and just cut down directly over the foreign body while stabilizing it between the fingers of your nondominant hand.

✓ **If the entrance wound is large, the probe may also not be required. Instead, a hemostat may be inserted using a spreading technique to search for, locate, and then remove the foreign body.**

✓ **A small puncture may be enlarged** by using a No. 15 blade to make a stab wound into the opening of the puncture.

✓ **Provide tetanus prophylaxis** (see Appendix G).

✓ **Warn the patient about the signs of a developing infection.** Antibiotics are not routinely prescribed but may be justified when foreign-body removal must be postponed; when there is

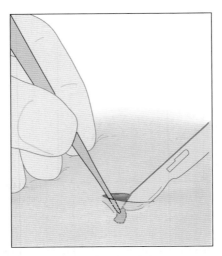

Fig. 154.3 Cut down probe to foreign body.

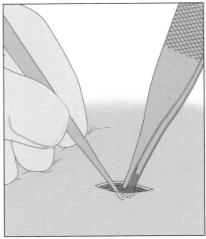

Fig. 154.4 Foreign body removed with forceps while probe remains in contact with it. (Reprinted from Jacobson JA: Musculoskeletal ultrasound: focused impact on MRI, *AJR Am J Roentgenol* 193:619–627, © 2009.)

suspected penetration of bones, joints, or tendons; or in patients who are highly susceptible to infection. Always inform the patient, and document when a retained foreign body is suspected or identified.

✅ **If the wound is in a complex area**, such as the palm of the hand or periorbital region, consultation for removal in the operating room, on an immediate or delayed basis, may be appropriate.

✅ **Always provide the patient with the name of a clinician who can perform the necessary follow-up care.** High-risk patients should have a wound check in 48 hours.

What Not to Do

❌ Do not disregard a patient's suspicion that a foreign body may be present, especially when organic matter may be involved.

❌ Do not cut down on the metal probe if there is any possibility of cutting across a neurovascular bundle, tendon, or other important structure.

❌ Do not attempt to cut down to the foreign body unless it is very superficial or there is a probe in place and in contact with the object. Often a blind incision will be unproductive and may only extend the injury.

❌ Do not blindly grab for something in a wound with a hemostat. An important anatomic structure may be damaged.

Discussion

Every effort should be made to identify the presence of a foreign body during the initial visit. When a foreign body is discovered in a wound, the clinician must weigh the risk of leaving it in place against the potential harm of attempting to remove it. The patient should be engaged in shared decision making. Small, inert, deeply embedded objects that cause no symptoms can usually be left in place. Organic matter causes intense inflammation and should always be removed as soon as possible. **Even inert foreign bodies that are heavily contaminated should be removed as soon as possible.** Glass, metal, and plastic are relatively inert, and removal of relatively clean objects can be postponed if necessary.

Any patient who complains of a foreign-body sensation should be assumed to have one, even if nothing can be seen radiographically.

Almost all glass is visible on plain radiographs, but small fragments, between 0.5 and 2.0 mm, may not be visible, even when left and right oblique projections are added to the standard anteroposterior and lateral views. Sensitivity of radiographs for a 2-mm glass fragment is approximately 87%.

Needle localization under fluoroscopy or ultrasound guidance may be required for those objects that must be removed, if the simple probe technique described (or alternative technique [see Chapter 146]) fails to deliver the foreign body.

The benefit of prophylactic antibiotics for retained foreign bodies has not been studied. Clinical experience suggests that wound infections associated with a retained foreign body are resistant to antibiotics. These wound infections often resolve spontaneously once the foreign bodies are removed.

Suggested Readings

Matsuno, H., Watanabe, T., Tada, S., Sekine, A., Nohisa, Y., Shinoda, K., et al. (2016). Sonographic detection of subcutaneous foreign bodies in 3 cases. *Acta Dermatovenerologica Croatica*, *24*(4), 299–302.

Orlinsky, M., & Bright, A. A. (2006). The utility of routine x-rays in all glass-caused wounds. *American Journal of Emergency Medicine*, *24*(2), 233–236. https://doi.org/10.1016/j.ajem.2005.06.008.

Subungual Ecchymosis

(Tennis Toe)

Presentation

The patient had a mild to moderate crushing injury to a fingernail, such as being caught in a closing drawer or being struck by a heavy object. The pain was initially intense but rapidly subsided over the first few minutes to 0.5 hour. Usually, by the time the patient is examined, there is only mild pain and tenderness. There is a light brown or blue-brown discoloration beneath the nail (Fig. 155.1). The patient may be concerned about the need to have the blood drained.

A similar but painless condition can occur with repeated minor trauma to a toe nail. This can occur inside a sport shoe when rapid thrusting of the athlete's toes into the toe box occurs as a result of abrupt stops, such as on a tennis or basketball court ("tennis toe"). Jogging may also be the cause of such a toe injury. The patient may state that the toe hurt for a brief period of time, but the pain has since resolved. On examination, there is a light brown or light blue-brown discoloration beneath the nail (Fig. 155.2).

What to Do

✓ Radiographs have very limited utility in either of these injuries. Unless there is a history of a significant crushing injury, x-rays can usually be deferred. The unlikely presence of a tuft fracture might warrant a protective fingertip splint on discharge.

✓ **Distinguish between a subungual hematoma and a subungual ecchymosis (see Chapter 156). The major difference is that a dark blue-black hematoma is space occupying and subsequently exerts a persistent, painful mass effect on the sterile matrix. A light blue-brown ecchymosis, on the other hand, occupies minimal space, thus the pain improves significantly after about 30 minutes postinjury.** Repetitive minimal trauma (e.g., runner's toes hitting the toe box of the running shoe) often experience no pain at all.

✓ **Trephination is not indicated for subungual ecchymosis (as opposed to subungual hematoma). Patients with prior subungual hematoma (or know someone who has had one) may expect trephination. Such patients should be counseled that this procedure would most likely be very painful and not benefit them. It might even expose them to the risk of developing a subungual infection.**

✓ Inform the patient that with a larger or repetitive injury, the nail may spontaneously fall off as it loses its attachment to the sterile matrix. Typically, this is not painful. The germinal matrix remains intact during the injury, therefore the nail will regrow.

✓ **With subungual ecchymosis due to a minor crush injury, the patient only needs reassurance** and rarely a protective fingertip splint for comfort.

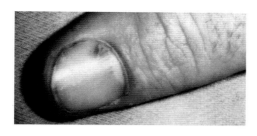

Fig. 155.1 Subungual ecchymosis.

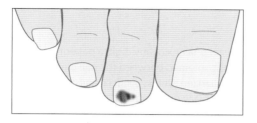

Fig. 155.2 Transverse black-brown discoloration of the second toenail. (Adapted from Adams, B. B. [2003]. Jogger's toenail. *Journal of the American Academy of Dermatology, 48*[Suppl 5], S58–S59.)

✅ **With tennis or "jogger's" toe, the patient's condition will resolve without intervention.** Recurrence can be prevented by wearing correct footwear and keeping nails trimmed short.

What Not to Do

❌ Do not perform trephination of the nail for subungual ecchymosis. This procedure is reserved for drainage of a hematoma that causes a mass effect on the sterile matrix.

❌ Do not prescribe prophylactic antibiotics. If the nail plate remains intact, the ecchymotic area is sterile. Only inappropriate trephination would put the patient at risk for infection.

❌ Do not obtain routine radiographs unless there is a reasonable risk for fracture (which is highly unlikely with tennis toe).

❌ Do not attribute all nail discolorations to a subungual ecchymosis. There should be some trauma to the patient's nail, and the condition should resolve, and the discolored part of the nail should grow out. **See Discussion box.**

Discussion

Unlike the painful space-occupying subungual hematoma, the subungual ecchymosis represents only a thin extravasation of blood beneath the nail or a mild separation of the nail plate from the nail bed. Trephination will not relieve any pressure or pain and may indeed cause excruciating pain, as well as opening this space to possible infection.

Bear in mind that **not all dark patches under the nail are subungual ecchymoses or hematomas. Diagnoses such as malignant melanoma, Kaposi sarcoma, and splinter hemorrhages (often associated with infective endocarditis) should be considered when the history of trauma and the physical examination are not consistent with a simple subungual ecchymosis.**

Suggested Readings

Adams, B. B. (2003). Jogger's toenail. *Journal of the American Academy of Dermatology, 48*(Suppl. 5), S58–S59.

Wang, Q. C., & Johnson, B. A. (2001). Fingertip injuries. *American Family Physician, 63*, 1961–1966.

Subungual Hematoma

Presentation

After blunt trauma to the distal phalanx of any digit, a patient can develop a subungual hematoma. The hematoma is contained between the nail plate and the sterile matrix of the nail bed, which is highly vascularized. Unless artificial nails are present, the collecting blood is easily visualized as a dark blue-black discoloration under the nail (Fig. 156.1). The bleeding into the potential space underneath the nail plate compresses the sterile matrix, which can cause significant discomfort.

What to Do

✅ **Only entertain the diagnosis of a subungual hematoma if the patient had recent trauma.** While subungual hematomas can rarely occur spontaneously, other diagnoses should be considered (subungual melanoma, Kaposi sarcoma).

✅ Blunt trauma to the distal phalanx can produce an avulsion injury of the extensor tendon. Have the patient fully extend the distal phalanx. If it cannot be completely extended, a mallet finger injury should be ruled out. If present, the distal interphalangeal (DIP) joint requires splinting (see Chapter 106).

✅ **If little discomfort is present, when the patient initially seeks care, protective splinting and an analgesic may be all that is required.** The only benefit of nail trephination is pain relief. If there is minimal or no pain, the risk of opening the nail bed to possible infection can be avoided.

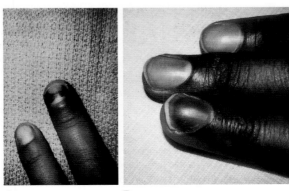

A   B

Fig. 156.1 (A, B) Subungual hematomas.

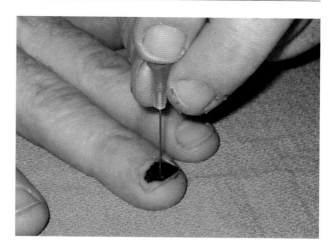

Fig. 156.2 Trephination with a sterile, disposable, 23-gauge, double-bevel, 1-inch needle. (From Bonisteel, P. S. [2008]. Practice tips. Trephining subungual hematomas. *Canadian Family Physician, 54,* 693.)

✅ **Radiographs of the injured digit may reveal a distal phalanx fracture.** Often, obtaining the radiograph does not lead to a change in management. Thus, unless the finger is severely injured, radiographs are not routinely recommended. The patient should understand and be included in this decision making.

✅ **If significant pain is present, disinfect the nail with an antiseptic solution and perform trephination with an electric cauterizing lance or carbon laser. A single-bevel 18-gauge needle or 23-gauge double bevel may also be used with a boring technique** (Fig. 156.2).

✅ **When trephination is performed quickly with a hot cauterizing lance or paperclip, patients do not feel the heat before the relief of pressure. Tap rapidly a few times with the cautery or drill in the same spot at the base of the hematoma until the hole is through the nail.** When resistance from the nail gives way, blood under pressure will spurt out with immediate pain relief. Reflexively, stop further downward pressure to avoid damaging the underlying nail bed (Fig. 156.3).

✅ **Persistent bleeding from this opening can be controlled by simply having the patient hold a folded 4 × 4 gauze pad firmly over the trephination site while holding the hands over the head.**

✅ **To prevent infection, instruct the patient to NOT SOAK the finger. Water may introduce bacteria into the sterile space. The open trephination should be protected with a simple Band-Aid.**

✅ The patient should be instructed to monitor for signs of infection (worsening pain, redness, swelling, red streaking, fevers) and to return immediately if these occur.

✅ **A protective aluminum fingertip splint may also be comforting, especially if the bone is fractured** (see Chapter 109).

✅ **Instruct the patient that trephination will not fully resolve the discoloration of the nail. Also inform the patient that the old nail will eventually separate and come off while a new nail will grow out with time.**

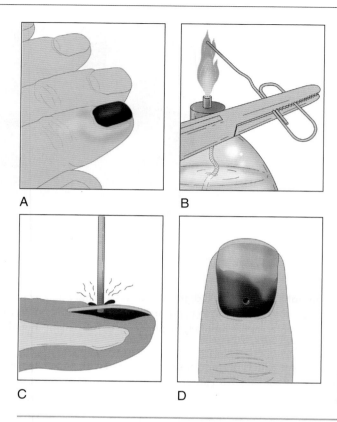

Fig. 156.3 Trephination with a red-hot paper clip. (A) Subungual hematoma. (B) Heating metal. (C) Nail trephination. (D) Result.

What Not to Do

(X) Do not confuse a subungual ecchymosis with a subungual hematoma. This subungual bruising never requires a nail trephination (see Chapter 155).

(X) Do not remove an intact fingernail. The patient likely has a small nail bed laceration, but the intact nail plate already serves as a splint to approximate the wound edges. Traditionally it was taught that a nail should be removed for subungual hematomas that take up more than 50% of the nail to repair the nail bed. However, cosmetic outcomes are the same as trephination alone, but nail removal increases discomfort and cost.

(X) Do not routinely perform a digital block. The digital block procedure is more painful than the trephination, which is often the only required intervention to reduce the patient's pain.

(X) Do not perform trephination on a patient who is no longer experiencing any significant pain at rest. A mild analgesic and protective splint will usually suffice.

(X) Do not make such a small opening that free drainage does not occur. A slender electrocautery tip may have to be bent to the side or spread apart for it to produce a wide enough hole in the nail.

(X) Do not hold a cautery wire on the surface of the nail without applying enough pressure to melt through the nail. Just holding the hot tip adjacent to the nail can heat up the hematoma and increase the pain without making a hole to relieve the pressure.

(X) Do not use tissue adhesive to "seal" the trephination in an attempt to prevent infection. The hematoma may reaccumulate. Just protect with a Band-Aid.

(X) Do not send a patient home to soak the finger after trephination. This may introduce bacteria into this previously sterile space.

(X) Do not routinely prescribe antibiotics. Even when opening a subungual hematoma with an underlying fracture of the distal phalanx, antibiotics have not been shown to be of any value in preventing infection.

Discussion

The subungual hematoma is a space-occupying mass that produces pain secondary to increased pressure against the very sensitive nail bed. Given time, the tissues surrounding this collection of blood will stretch and deform until the pressure within this mass equilibrates. Within 24 to 48 hours, the pain therefore subsides. Although the patient may continue to complain of pain with activity, performing trephination at this time may not improve the discomfort to any significant extent and will potentially expose the patient to a small risk for infection. If trephination is not performed, explain this to the patient, who may be requesting trephination too late. The patient is often the best judge whether the pain is sufficient to warrant taking on this very small risk for infection.

Though many clinicians use a heated paper clip as a cautery device, it may be contraindicated in many settings because it involves the use of an open flame to heat the material. Many paper clips are also made of metals that do not heat sufficiently to penetrate the nail. However, if it is the only device available, it is usually sufficiently effective (see Fig. 156.3). An alcohol wipe that is partially pulled from its foil package, when lit with a match, can serve as a readily available flame for heating up a paper clip.

When there are associated lacerations, open hemorrhage, broken nails, or disruption of the nail plate borders, perform a digital block and remove the nail to inspect the nail bed and repair any lacerations as necessary (see Chapter 144).

Suggested Readings

Patel, L. (2014). Management of simple nail bed lacerations and subungual hematomas in the emergency department. *Pediatric Emergency Care*, *30*(10), 742–745 [quiz 746–748].

Pingel, C., & McDowell, C. (2019). Subungual hematoma drainage.

Superficial Thrombophlebitis/Bleeding Varicosity

Presentation

A patient may present with focal tenderness, a palpable cord, and mild erythema over the course of a superficial vein. The risk factors for the development of a superficial venous thrombosis (superficial thrombophlebitis [ST]) are similar to those of deep venous thrombosis (DVT) and include smoking, estrogen, prolonged immobility, malignancy, clotting disorders, pregnancy, and recent surgery/trauma. Varicose veins are likely the most significant risk factor, with 88% of cases of ST being associated with varicosities.

Superficial venous thrombosis may broadly be divided into four categories: sterile, traumatic (including from venous cannulation or infusion of irritant drugs), infective, or migratory (recurrent, often due to carcinoma of the pancreas).

The risk of venous thromboembolic events (VTE) from ST is very low overall. About 1.3% of patients experience symptomatic VTE from ST. In about 3.4% of patients there is significant proximal extension of the ST, and about 1.6% of patients will have recurrence of this condition after treatment.

Varicose veins not only predispose to ST but may also bleed spontaneously or after minimal trauma. Patients, who are often upset, present with uncontrollable bleeding streaming from a punctate opening over a varicosity in the lower leg. Several techniques are available to control this bleeding.

What to Do

Superficial Venous Thrombosis

✅ **Establish the diagnosis** through physical exam, ultrasonography (Fig. 157.1), and lab testing (D-dimer). Focal pain and a palpable cord are often clues to this diagnosis.

✅ **Identify the etiology if possible**, as certain causes (e.g., infection) warrant additional treatment in addition to treatment provided for ST.

✅ **Evaluate the extent of the ST with ultrasonography.** Physical exam significantly underestimates the proximal extent in 77% of cases. Commonly, lower extremity ST occurs in the greater saphenous vein. If the thrombosis extends to within 10 cm of the saphenofemoral or saphenopopliteal junction (or any other junction with the deep venous system), treat this as a DVT (Fig. 157.2).

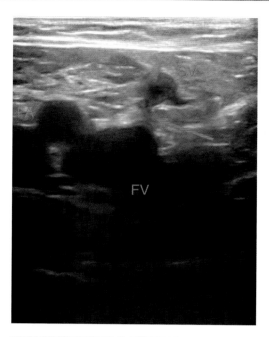

Fig. 157.1 Thrombosis with central recannulation of the saphenous vein. *FA,* Femoral artery; *FV,* femoral vein; *SV,* saphenous vein. Arrow indicates central recannulation of the saphenous vein.

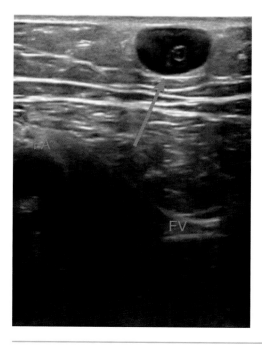

Fig. 157.2 Extension of the thrombosis of the saphenous vein to the saphenofemoral junction. *FA,* Femoral artery; *FV,* femoral vein; *SV,* saphenous vein. Arrow indicates clot in the saphenous vein.

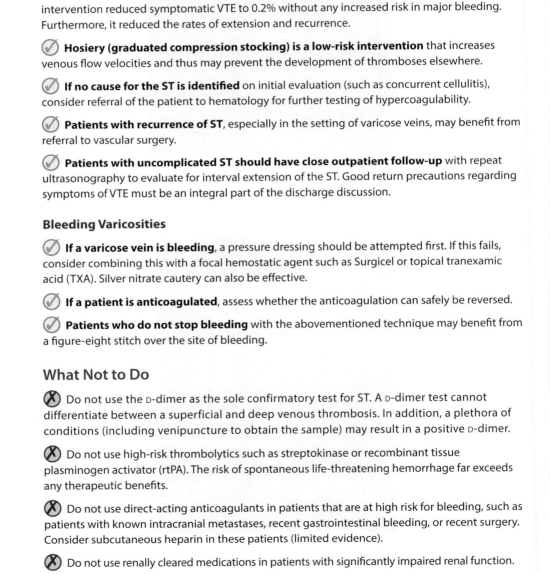

✅ **Evaluate the deep venous system with ultrasonography.** Between 5% and 53% of patients with ST have concurrent DVT, likely due to the shared risk factors between these conditions.

✅ **Discuss treatment options with the patient.** When the diagnosis of ST has been established, aspirin and warm compresses are commonly prescribed. It should be noted, though, that there is only limited supporting evidence for this treatment. While this therapy reduces both extension and recurrence, no data exist to suggest that it prevents VTE.

✅ **A Cochrane review (2018) only found significant supporting evidence for the use of fondaparinux at prophylactic dosing for 45 days (>50 kg: 2.5 mg SC once daily).** This intervention reduced symptomatic VTE to 0.2% without any increased risk in major bleeding. Furthermore, it reduced the rates of extension and recurrence.

✅ **Hosiery (graduated compression stocking) is a low-risk intervention** that increases venous flow velocities and thus may prevent the development of thromboses elsewhere.

✅ **If no cause for the ST is identified** on initial evaluation (such as concurrent cellulitis), consider referral of the patient to hematology for further testing of hypercoagulability.

✅ **Patients with recurrence of ST**, especially in the setting of varicose veins, may benefit from referral to vascular surgery.

✅ **Patients with uncomplicated ST should have close outpatient follow-up** with repeat ultrasonography to evaluate for interval extension of the ST. Good return precautions regarding symptoms of VTE must be an integral part of the discharge discussion.

Bleeding Varicosities

✅ **If a varicose vein is bleeding**, a pressure dressing should be attempted first. If this fails, consider combining this with a focal hemostatic agent such as Surgicel or topical tranexamic acid (TXA). Silver nitrate cautery can also be effective.

✅ **If a patient is anticoagulated**, assess whether the anticoagulation can safely be reversed.

✅ **Patients who do not stop bleeding** with the abovementioned technique may benefit from a figure-eight stitch over the site of bleeding.

What Not to Do

❌ Do not use the D-dimer as the sole confirmatory test for ST. A D-dimer test cannot differentiate between a superficial and deep venous thrombosis. In addition, a plethora of conditions (including venipuncture to obtain the sample) may result in a positive D-dimer.

❌ Do not use high-risk thrombolytics such as streptokinase or recombinant tissue plasminogen activator (rtPA). The risk of spontaneous life-threatening hemorrhage far exceeds any therapeutic benefits.

❌ Do not use direct-acting anticoagulants in patients that are at high risk for bleeding, such as patients with known intracranial metastases, recent gastrointestinal bleeding, or recent surgery. Consider subcutaneous heparin in these patients (limited evidence).

❌ Do not use renally cleared medications in patients with significantly impaired renal function.

Discussion

Superficial venous thrombosis may occur spontaneously, as a result of focal trauma, infection, or due to a provoked or inherited hypercoagulable state. Treatment is controversial, and evidence is limited regarding the available therapeutic options. **Overall, the strongest evidence exists for fondaparinux, but this pharmacologic intervention is rather expensive. Informed, shared decision making with the patient should take into consideration financial abilities and insurance coverage, especially in the United States.**

Patients with ST seldom require admission to the hospital unless an underlying condition that caused the ST warrants this. However, good return precautions regarding symptoms of VTE must be an integral part of the discharge discussion.

Suggested Readings

Di Nisio, M., Wichers, I. M., & Middeldorp, S. (2018). Treatment for superficial thrombophlebitis of the leg. *The Cochrane Database of Systematic Reviews*, *2*, CD004982. https://doi.org/10.1002/14651858.CD004982.pub6.

Nasr, H., & Scriven, J. M. (2015). Superficial thrombophlebitis (superficial venous thrombosis). *BMJ (Clinical Research Ed.)*, *350*, h2039. https://doi.org/10.1136/bmj.h2039.

Taser Injuries

Presentation

A patient is brought in by police officers after being subdued with a Taser. A Taser is a type of conducted electrical weapon (CEW) that fires two barbed darts using a compressed nitrogen charge. The darts penetrate light clothing and embed in the skin. Electricity is conducted through fine insulated copper wires, resulting in neuromuscular incapacitation.

What to Do

✓ **Three different diagnostic approaches must be taken simultaneously:** injury from the CEW darts, injury from the fall after incapacitation, and underlying psychiatric or toxicologic conditions that resulted in the patient requiring incapacitation.

✓ **Dart injury:** CEW dart injuries are similar to fishhook injuries, but removal differs slightly. As the darts are often uniform externally, it is difficult to determine which direction the barb is facing (Figs. 158.1 and 158.2). Thus techniques used for fishhooks (e.g., string technique, needle technique) often do not work as well. **The authors' experience with Taser removal found that attaching a needle driver/hemostat orthogonal (at right angle) to the axis of the dart and exerting traction along the path of entry usually suffices.**

✓ **A second hemostat may then be used to hold down the soft tissue. Rarely, patients may benefit from focal lidocaine infiltration and widening of the puncture wound with a scalpel.**

✓ Providers must take care not to accidentally injury themselves when the dart releases from the patient.

✓ **No convincing cases exist in the literature that the electrical current for a CEW causes significant injuries.** Cardiac dysrhythmia would be expected immediately, but an electrocardiogram (ECG) may provide reassurance to both the patient and the provider. Deaths in police custody are more likely due to excited delirium syndrome than delayed effects of CEW exposure.

✓ **Ensure that the patient's tetanus vaccination status is updated.**

✓ **Several case reports exist of significant injuries from CEW darts, including ocular, lacrimal duct, or testicular injuries. If darts are embedded in an area with important structures located within 13 mm (length of the dart from point to hilt) of the skin surface, specialist consultation may be required prior to dart removal.** A case report of cranial penetration exists.

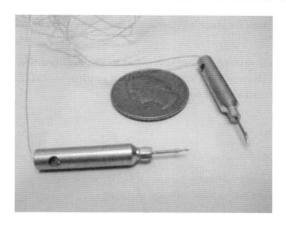

Fig. 158.1 Metallic barbed TASER darts. (From Theisen K, et al. Taser-Related Testicular Trauma. Urology 2016, 88:e5.)

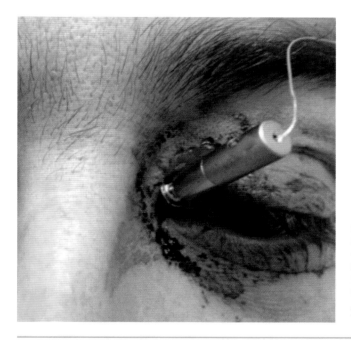

Fig. 158.2 Embedded TASER dart in a location requiring removal by a specialist. (With permission from: de Runz, A.; Minetti, C.; Brix, M.; Simon, E.; New TASER injuries: lacrimal canaliculus laceration and ethmoid bone fracture. *International Journal of Oral & Maxillofacial Surgery*. Vol 43, Issue 6. Pages 722-724. © 2014 Elsevier Inc.)

⊘ **Fall injury: At the time of CEW exposure, patients often suffer a fall. Due to incapacitation, the fall is typically unbraced.** Thus a thorough physical with appropriate skin exposure is necessary to screen for fall injuries.

⊘ **Reason for CEW exposure**: A complex psychiatric or toxicologic evaluation is beyond the scope of this book, but certain aspects are worth highlighting.

⊘ **Screen the patient for suicidal/homicidal ideations and consult psychiatric services as appropriate.**

⊘ **A patient who is restrained and continues to display agitation and keeps fighting against the restraints may have excited delirium syndrome (ExDS). This condition, if unrecognized and untreated, can be rapidly fatal.**

What Not to Do

⊗ Do not twist the darts during removal. Rotation of the barb will worsen the tissue damage.

⊗ Do not remove darts without a hemostat. Significant traction may be required, which may be difficult to generate with a solid "grip" on the dart.

⊗ Do not remove darts embedded in the patient through clothes without first cutting the clothes circumferentially around the dart.

⊗ Do not disregard the potential for head injury after an unbraced fall from standing, especially in patients who are older or anticoagulated.

Discussion

Patients who were subdued by CEW devices may present to care for removal of darts still embedded. Unless the darts are near sensitive structures (eyes, testicles, facial structures), it is unlikely that the patient suffered significant injuries from the penetrating injury. Most injuries associated with CEW exposure are from the fall or previous/subsequent restraint attempts by law enforcement. **Patients who present to care under arrest should be considered a vulnerable population as their ability to seek follow-up care or a second opinion may be restricted due to incarceration.** Therefore a thorough examination is paramount prior to reaching the decision of discharging a patient to police custody.

The primary concern for both patients and providers is often cardiac dysrhythmias secondary to the "electrocution" component of CEW injuries. Depending on spacing and location of the dart in the patient, this risk is overall extremely unlikely. Cardiac "capture" has been documented in a few cases, where the electric pulses of the CEW served as an external pacemaker, resulting in tachycardia between 200 and 250 beats per minute for the duration of the CEW being activated by its user. In a patient who is likely under significant adrenergic drive and potentially stimulating drugs, the concern is that the capture will degenerate to ventricular fibrillation.

Newer models of CEW devices modulate the delivery of electricity to minimize cardiac exposure. If a dysrhythmia were to occur it is most likely to be temporally related (<1 minute) to the CEW exposure and does not occur in a delayed fashion.

Suggested Readings

Hoskin, A. K., & Mackey, D. A. (2014). Eye injuries and tasers. *The Medical Journal of Australia, 201*(2), 89–90. http://doi.org/10.5694/mja14.00256

Kaloostian, P., & Tran, H. (2012). Intracranial taser dart penetration: Literature review and surgical management. *Journal of Surgical Case Reports, 2012*(6), 10. http://doi.org/10.1093/jscr/2012.6.10

Kroll, M. W., Lakkireddy, D. R., Stone, J. R., & Luceri, R. M. (2014). TASER electronic control devices and cardiac arrests: Coincidental or causal? *Circulation, 129*(1), 93–100. http://doi.org/10.1161/CIRCULATIONAHA.113.004401

Torn/Split Earlobe

Presentation

A patient comes to the emergency department or clinic with an earlobe torn by a sudden pull on an earring. Contributing factors might include previous lengthening of the earlobe hole because of long-term use of relatively heavy or dangling ear jewelry, or the original earring hole may have been placed in an excessively low position. Patients with this type of injury require lobuloplasty to maximize cosmetic outcomes.

What to Do

✓ **Engage in shared decision making with the patient. Preservation of the original piercing tract potentially results in several complications,** including increased risk of elongation after repair as well as dermal inclusion cysts if epithelium is enclosed in the repair.

✓ **If cosmetic appearance is of great concern, it may be advisable to consult with a plastic surgeon before attempting the primary repair.**

✓ **Perform a greater auricular nerve block** to anesthetize the ear lobe without distorting the anatomy as would be the case with local anesthetic infiltration.

✓ **Pierce each flap of the torn earlobe with a 6-0 prolene suture.** An assistant can hold gentle traction to stabilize the flaps during the procedure without hindering the repair.

✓ **Use a No. 11 or No. 15 blade to score the wound edges. Use iris scissors to excise the wound edges along the scored tract.**

✓ Place a deep, absorbable suture in the plane of the earlobe to decrease the risk of deep hematoma formation and to provide initial approximation.

✓ Using 6-0 prolene sutures, perform a side-to-side closure with exaggerated wound edge eversion.

✓ Dress the area with a petroleum gauze dressing and arrange for suture removal in approximately 7 days.

✓ **Patients should be instructed that repiercing, if desired, should not be done through the scar but should be placed adjacent to the repair site. This will create a stronger piercing that is less prone to cleft formation. Preferably, replacement of the earring site should be delayed by 3 months.**

✓ Provide tetanus prophylaxis if needed.

What Not to Do

✖ Do not close an earlobe tear when remnants of the old earring track are known to be inside. This old epithelial track will eventually form an inclusion cyst, which will often require excision later.

✖ Do not attempt to suture the epithelialized borders of an old, elongated earlobe piercing together. These old borders (which are now covered with skin) cannot heal together unless they are first completely excised.

✖ Do not use ointment containing neomycin. The neomycin provides no advantage and can often produce severe contact dermatitis.

Discussion

Torn earlobes also are referred to as split or cleft earlobes in the literature; these can be repaired with a variety of techniques. The side-to-side closure is likely the easiest for the provider not trained in plastic surgery. Other approaches such as Casson technique (Z-plasty) (Fig. 159.1) or Effendi technique (rotational flap) are best performed by individuals trained in these procedures.

Repiercing can be done safely after healing has completed (~3 months). The new piercing site should be placed in a nonscarred area of the lobe, preferably in a central location. Patients who have had multiple infections at the piercing site should not have the earlobe repierced.

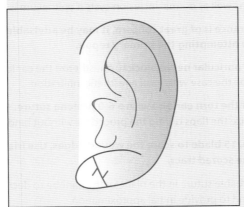
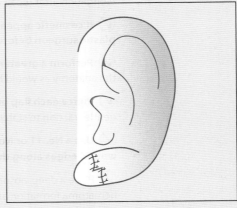

A   B

Fig. 159.1 Straight-line closure with inferior rim modification by Casson. (A) Incisions for a Z-plasty on inferior margin. (B) Z-plasty flap transposition and closure. (Adapted from Watson, D. [2002]. Torn earlobe repair. *Otolaryngology Clinics of North America, 35,* 187–205, vii–viii.)

Suggested Readings

Beschloss, J. K., Toren, K. L., & Bingham, J. L. (2011). Earlobe stabilization with 6-0 suture for repair of a complete split. Official Publication for American Society for Dermatologic Surgery [Et Al.] *Dermatologic Surgery, 37*(6), 848–849. https://doi.org/10.1111/j.1524-4725.2011.02011.x

Raveendran, S. S., & Amarasinghe, L. (2004). The mystery of the split earlobe. *Plastic and Reconstructive Surgery, 114*(7), 1903–1909.

Sharma, R., Krishnan, S., Kumar, S., & Verma, M. (2014). Rotation flap lobuloplasty: Technique and experience with 24 partially torn earlobes. *International Journal of Oral and Maxillofacial Surgery, 43*(10), 1206–1210. https://doi.org/10.1016/j.ijom.2014.04.009

Traumatic Tattoos and Abrasions

Presentation

The patient has fallen onto a coarse surface, such as a blacktop or macadam road. Most frequently, the skin of the face, forehead, chin, hands, and knees is abraded. When pigmented foreign particles are impregnated within the dermis, tattooing will occur. An explosive form of tattooing can also be seen with the use of firecrackers, firearms, and homemade bombs.

What to Do

✓ **Cleanse the wound** with tap water, normal saline, or other products that are not destructive to epidermal and dermal skin cells.

✓ **Provide tetanus prophylaxis as needed** (see Appendix G).

✓ With explosive tattooing, **particles are generally deeply embedded and will require plastic surgery consultation.** Any particles embedded in the dermis may become permanent tattoos. Abrasions that are large (more than several square centimeters), deep into the dermis, or into the subcutaneous tissues may also require consultation and/or skin grafts.

✓ With superficial abrasions and abrasive tattooing, **the area can usually be adequately anesthetized by applying 2% viscous lidocaine, 4% lidocaine solution, or gauze soaked with LET (lidocaine 4%, epinephrine 1:2000, tetracaine 0.5%) directly onto the wound for approximately 5 minutes.**

✓ **If this is not successful,** locally infiltrate with 1% or 2% lidocaine using a spinal needle (25–27 gauge, 1.5–3 inches) for large areas. **Before infiltrating local anesthetics over large and/or painful areas, consider parenteral opioid analgesia, or even procedural sedation.**

✓ **For wounds containing tar or grease,** application of bacitracin ointment before debridement will help dissolve and loosen these contaminants.

✓ **The wound should then be cleansed** with a gauze sponge with saline or 1% (dilute) povidone-iodine (Betadine) solution. For heavily contaminated wounds, **use a surgical scrub brush,** even one impregnated with chlorhexidine (as long as the chlorhexidine is rinsed thoroughly from the injured areas because, over time, it is associated with mild tissue toxicity in wounds).

✓ **When entrapped material remains, use a sterile stiff toothbrush to clean the wound or use the side of a No. 10 or No. 15 scalpel blade to scrape away any debris (dermabrasion)** (Fig. 160.1). While working, continuously cleanse the wound surface with gauze soaked in normal saline to reveal any additional foreign particles. Large granules may be removed with the tip of the scalpel blade (See Video 160.1).

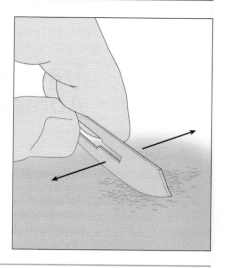

Fig. 160.1 Dermabrasion with a No. 10 scalpel blade.

✅ **Small wounds should be left open and lubricating ointment or petroleum jelly applied. The patient should be instructed to gently wash (not scrub) the area two or three times per day and continue applying the ointment until the wound becomes dry and comfortable under a new coat of epithelium, which may require a few weeks.** Use of ointments over excessively long periods can lead to maceration of tissue, rather than normal healing.

✅ **When a larger wound has been adequately cleansed, one alternative is to use a nonadherent dressing such as Adaptic (oil emulsion) gauze plus ointment with a protective dry gauze covering. Schedule a dressing change within 2 to 3 days.**

What Not to Do

❌ Do not ignore embedded particles. If they cannot be completely removed, inform the patient about the probability of permanent tattooing and arrange for a plastic surgery consultation.

Discussion

The technique of tattooing involves painting pigment on the skin and then injecting it through the epidermis into the dermis with a needle. As the epidermis heals, the pigment particles are ingested by macrophages and permanently bound into the dermis. The best approach in managing patients with traumatic tattoos is the immediate removal of particles during the initial care. Immediate care is important because once the particles are embedded and healing is complete, it becomes much more difficult to remove them. It is advisable for a patient to protect a dermabraded area from sunlight for approximately 1 year to minimize excessive melanin pigmentation of the site.

Traditionally, destructive methods of delayed tattoo removal, including surgical excision, dermabrasion, cryosurgery, and chemical peels, have all produced disappointing cosmetic results with unacceptably high rates of scarring. With the development of Q-switched laser technology, however, tattoo removal has become much safer and more reliable, and the tattoos typically clear within a few laser treatments. The wavelengths emitted by these lasers are absorbed by pigmented particles, breaking them into smaller pieces that are less visible. The smaller particles are then taken up by inflammatory cells and eliminated by the lymphatic system or transepidermally. Tattoo removal with Q-switched lasers is moderately painful; a local anesthetic may be necessary. Transient or permanent hypopigmentation can occur, especially in dark-skinned patients.

Suggested Readings

El Sayed, F. (2005). Treatment of fireworks tattoos with the Q-switched ruby laser. *Dermatologic Surgery, 31,* 706–708.

Graudenz, K. (2003). Diffused traumatic dirt and decorative tattooing: Removal by Q-switched lasers. *Der Hautarzt, 54,* 756–759.

Tanzi, E. L., Lupton, J. R., & Alster, T. S. (2003). Lasers in dermatology: Four decades of progress. *Journal of the American Academy of Dermatology, 49,* 1–31.

Zipper Entrapment

(Penis or Chin)

Presentation

Usually a child (or parent) has dressed (the child) too quickly and, possibly not wearing underpants, has accidentally pulled penile skin into his zipper (Fig. 161.1). The skin becomes entrapped and crushed between the teeth and the actuator (slide) of the zipper, thereby painfully attaching the article of clothing to the body part involved (most often the penis, or less often the area beneath the chin). There is generally little or no bleeding, but it is very uncomfortable for the patient.

What to Do

✅ **First, lubricate the entrapped skin and zipper with mineral oil.** In a significant percentage of cases, the entrapped skin may be released with lubrication and gentle lateral traction. This may obviate the need for painful local anesthesia, systemic analgesia, and more complicated interventions.

✅ If this is unsuccessful, **consider systemic analgesics before local infiltration, which will be distressing and painful, especially in children**. Intranasal fentanyl may be a good option. In some cases, procedural sedation may be necessary (see Appendix E).

✅ **Paint the area with a small amount of povidone-iodine (Betadine) and infiltrate the entrapped skin with 1% buffered lidocaine (without epinephrine)** (Fig. 161.2)**.** As an alternative, perform a dorsal penile block. This will also allow for comfortable manipulation of

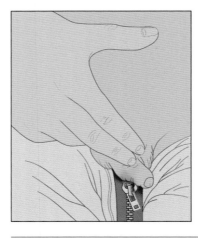

Fig. 161.1 Penis caught in zipper.

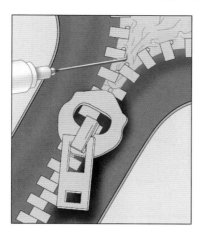

Fig. 161.2 Injection of lidocaine.

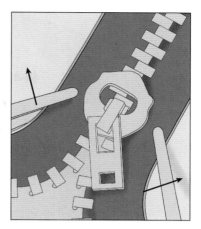

Fig. 161.3 Opening zipper from rear.

the zipper and the article of clothing. A more time-consuming alternative that sometimes may be more acceptable to the patient (and parents) is to first use a eutectic mixture of lidocaine and prilocaine (EMLA) to provide dermal anesthesia through the intact skin. This may take 45 to 60 minutes to become effective and therefore should be applied as soon as the patient arrives.

✅ **Cut the zipper away from the article of clothing.** This will improve access/visualization and will reduce the pain associated with the weight of the clothing on the entrapped skin.

✅ **The method of removal selected will depend on where in the zipper the skin is entrapped.**

○ **Between the teeth of the zipper: this technique may work without elaborate pain control strategies.** Simply cut across the zipper teeth above and below the area of entrapment. **It may even be possible just to cut the closed zipper teeth below the actuator, permitting the unzipping of the zipper from the rear.** Pull the teeth gently apart to release the skin (Fig. 161.3) (See Video 161.1).

○ **Within the slide (actuator): cut the median bar (which holds the anterior and posterior halves, or faceplates, of the actuator together) with a pair of metal snips, a bone cutter, or an orthopedic pin cutter** (Fig. 161.4A). The patient is less likely to be frightened if this procedure is kept hidden from view (See Video 161.2).

○ **If unable to break the two halves of the slide apart using a metal cutter, take two heavy-duty surgical towel clamps** and place their tongs into the side grooves at both ends of the slide. Grip one clamp firmly in each hand and twist your wrists in opposite directions. This often will pop the two halves of the actuator apart, releasing the entrapped skin (see Fig. 161.4B).

○ **Alternatively, insert the head of a small slotted (flathead) screwdriver between the anterior and posterior faceplates of the slide**, and rotate the head 90 degrees. This may increase the gap between the faceplates enough to facilitate release of the skin.

✅ **After the zipper slide has been removed, pull the exposed zipper teeth apart, cleanse the crushed skin, and apply an ointment such as bacitracin** (Fig. 161.5).

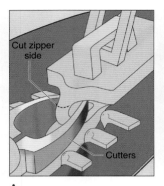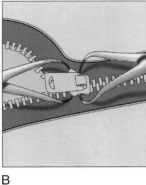

A   B

Fig. 161.4 Cut zipper actuator bar with a metal snip bone cutter or an orthopedic pin cutter (A), or use two heavy-duty surgical towel clamps to break the actuator apart (B).

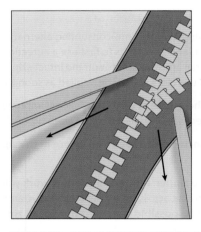

Fig. 161.5 Pull exposed zipper teeth apart.

✓ Tetanus prophylaxis should be administered as needed (see Appendix G).

✓ **In the rare case when none of the described maneuvers is effective, consult a urologist**. The urologist may elect to perform an elliptic incision or emergency circumcision in the operating room.

What Not to Do

❌ Do not cut and damage clothing if mineral oil releases the zipper.

❌ Do not fail to provide appropriate pain control.

❌ Do not destroy the entire article of clothing by cutting into it. Only the zipper needs to be cut away, allowing repair of the clothing.

ⓧ Do not excise an area of skin or perform a circumcision unless absolutely necessary and in consultation with a urologist. Such skin excision will create potentially unnecessary morbidity for the patient.

Discussion

Penile injuries (trauma) are relatively uncommon, but when they occur, zipper entrapment is involved in 3% to 14% of the cases. This injury usually occurs in children who are between 3 and 6 years of age, and many of the victims are not wearing underpants.

Newer plastic zippers have made this problem less common than in the past, but it still occurs, and it is a very grateful patient who is released from this entrapment.

Suggested Readings

Bothner, J. (2019). *Management of zipper injuries. UptoDate.* http://www.uptodate.com.

Burns, E. (2019). *Penile zipper entrapment! Life in the fast lane.* [blog] http://www.Lifeinthefastlane.com.

Dubin, J., & Davis, J. E. (2011). Penile emergencies. *Emergency Medicine Clinics of North America, 29,* 485–499.

Inoue, N., Crook, S. C., & Yamamoto, L. G. (2005). Comparing 2 methods of emergent zipper release. *American Journal of Emergency Medicine, 23,* 480–482.

Kanegaye, J. T., & Schonfeld, N. (1993). Penile zipper entrapment: A simple and less threatening approach using mineral oil. *Pediatric Emergency Care, 9,* 90–91.

Nolan, J. F., Stillwell, T. J., & Sands, J. P. (1990). Acute management of the zipper-entrapped penis. *Journal of Emergency Medicine, 8,* 305–307.

Raveenthiran, V. (2007). Releasing of zipper-entrapped foreskin: A novel nonsurgical technique. *Pediatric Emergency Care, 23,* 463–464.

Stone, D. B., & Levine, M. R. (2010). Foreign body removal. In J. R. Roberts, & J. R. Hedges (Eds.), *Roberts and Hedges' clinical procedures in emergency medicine* (5th ed.) (pp. 651–653). Philadelphia, PA: WB Saunders.

Strait, R. T. (1999). A novel method for removal of penile zipper entrapment. *Pediatric Emergency Care, 15,* 412–413 (1999).

PART 11

Dermatologic Emergencies

■ Mark Bisanzo ■ Kurt Eifling

Allergic Contact Dermatitis 162

Presentation

Patients present with a very pruritic, eczematous-like rash at sites of skin exposure to allergens. Lesions may consist of small papules, vesicles, or bullae that may be confluent. Inflammation may exist with erythema, edema, oozing, or crusting. Dermatitis may remain localized at contact sites or, in severe cases, can spread to involve distant body areas. Sites with thin skin (e.g., eyelids [Fig. 162.1], lateral neck, dorsum of hands, genitals) show greater susceptibility, whereas areas with a thick stratum corneum (palms and soles) have more resistance. Because this is a delayed hypersensitivity reaction, the pruritus and rash may not become evident for 24 to 48 hours or longer after exposure to the allergenic substance. Although a substance new to the patient in the past few weeks is more likely to be the precipitating agent, patients have been known to react to products that they have been using for years.

The one uniformly present feature of allergic contact dermatitis (ACD) is pruritus, without which the diagnosis of ACD is virtually excluded.

What to Do

⊘ **Attempt to determine the offending agent.** Skin lesion distribution often provides a clue to the offending allergen. Question patients about potential exposure to topical medications

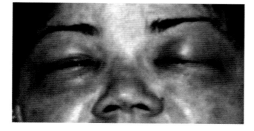

Fig. 162.1 Marked eyelid swelling may mimic the angioedema of anaphylaxis, but with ACD there is only localized pruritus and no associated systemic signs or symptoms. This case was caused by contact with the allergen in hair dye. (Adapted from Mark, B. J., & Slavin, R. G. [2006]. Allergic contact dermatitis. *Medicine Clinics of North America, 90*, 169–185.)

(such as neomycin or benzocaine) or other potential allergens (such as sunscreens, moisturizing lotions, perfumes and other fragrances, nail polish, artificial nails, cosmetics, soaps, shampoos, hair dyes, household cleaners, laundry products, paints, rubbers, latex, adhesives, footwear, clothing, and plants such as poison ivy [*Rhus toxicodendron*]) (see Chapter 184). Metals in jewelry (e.g., nickel, chromium, cobalt) (Fig. 162.2) and chemicals in clothing and footwear (e.g., resins, crease-resistant finishes, leather dyes, rubber accelerators) (Fig. 162.3) can be sources of cutaneous allergens. Vulvitis and balanitis may occur in patients who have an allergy to latex in condoms or ingredients in douches, contraceptive jellies, feminine hygiene products, or toilet paper.

✅ **Evaluate for possible occupational exposure.** Industries in which workers are at the highest risk for occupational skin diseases include food production, construction, printing, metal plating, machine tool operation, engine service, leatherwork, health care, cosmetology, and forestry. Specific chemical agents encountered on the job may reveal the underlying cause.

✅ **Examine the involved skin. The appearance of the lesions in ACD often corresponds to the stage at which the patient presents.** During the acute stage, there is marked erythema, edema, and vesicle formation. Edema predominates in areas of loose connective tissue, such as the eyelids or genitalia. Vesicles are usually multiple, may coalesce, and eventually will rupture during the subacute stage, leading to oozing and eroded skin with a characteristic eczematous appearance. Vesicles may be replaced by papules, crusting and scaling become more prominent

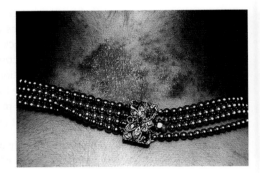

Fig. 162.2 The classic erythematous papulovesicular eruption of ACD on the back of this patient's neck is caused by contact from nickel-plated jewelry. (Adapted from Mark, B. J., & Slavin, R. G. [2006]. Allergic contact dermatitis. *Medicine Clinics of North America, 90,* 169–185.)

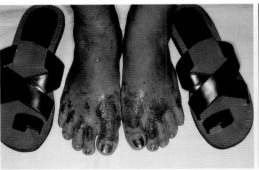
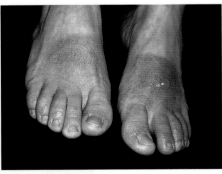

A   B

Fig. 162.3 (A, B) Allergic contact dermatitis to leather shoes. Note the correspondence to sites of exposure. (Adapted from Bolognia, J., Jorizzo, J., & Rapini. R. [2003]. *Dermatology.* St. Louis, MO: Mosby.)

than the erythema and edema, and (over time) lichenification and further scaling predominate during the chronic stage. These stages often overlap, and there is no sharp delineation between them.

✓ **Have the patient remove the offending allergen from the environment to avoid reexposure, and thoroughly wash the skin with a hypoallergenic soap.**

✓ **For acute reactions with significant edema and erythema, especially those with inflamed, oozing, or crusted lesions, supportive care with cold compresses soaked with aluminum acetate solution (Domeboro) has cooling, soothing, and antiseptic effects.** Cool baths with starch or oatmeal (Aveeno) may also be soothing.

✓ **For severe reactions,** if there are no contraindications or relative contraindications (tuberculosis, peptic ulcer, diabetes, herpes, or severe hypertension), **prescribe systemic corticosteroids, such as oral prednisone, 60 mg (or 1 mg/kg) for approximately 5 days, and then taper prednisone over at least 2 weeks.**

✓ **Systemic oral antihistamine therapy,** such as hydroxyzine (Vistaril) or diphenhydramine (Benadryl), 25 to 50 mg up to four times per day, helps control pruritus. The benefits may be nominal in the delayed-type reactions of ACD, but any reduction in pruritus will be appreciated by the patient. The side effect of drowsiness may also be appreciated (especially at bedtime), but other potential deleterious side effects should also be considered when prescribing these medications.

✓ **For mild and localized reactions, topical corticosteroids have anti-inflammatory and antipruritic effects. They are usually effective within a few days and should be continued for 2 weeks. A low-potency preparation such as hydrocortisone 1% is adequate for many presentations. More severe local reactions can be treated with a midpotency steroid such as triamcinolone 0.05%, while the very potent topical steroids such as fluocinonide (Fluonex; Lidex) cream/ointment/gel 0.05% should be reserved for extremely severe presentations. Topical steroids may be potentiated with occlusive dressings.** Avoid long-term use (>10–14 days) of fluorinated corticosteroids such as fluocinonide on the face and genitalia, where they can cause atrophy. In general, higher-potency steroids should be reserved for the extremities and torso.

✓ **With respect to the delivery form of topical steroids,** consider using gels only if the affected area is weeping and will benefit from the drying effect of a gel. Steroid creams may have greater cosmetic appeal than steroid ointments, but creams typically contain more potentially allergenic preservatives and fragrances. Ointments, on the other hand, penetrate more deeply into the skin, increasing their potency.

✓ **When impetigo is present resulting from superimposed bacterial infection** (see Chapter 174), **treat with systemic antibiotics.** First-line agents are cephalexin or dicloxacillin; erythromycin can be used in those with beta-lactam allergies. Consider antibiotics effective against community-acquired methicillin-resistant *Staphylococcus aureus* (MRSA) according to the patient's risk factors. **Avoid topical medications as these are frequent allergic sensitizers.**

✓ When a precipitating agent cannot be determined, the patient should be referred for epicutaneous patch testing, which is considered the gold standard for diagnosing ACD. If patch testing fails to incriminate a likely allergen and the diagnosis of ACD is still strongly considered, a detailed diary of the patient's daily activities may help discover patterns of allergen exposure.

✅ When the allergen cannot be avoided, wearing protective barriers is the next best preventive option. Gloves may be the most effective means of allergen protection. Vinyl gloves are ideal for most applications—they are waterproof and can be worn atop cotton gloves for greater comfort.

✅ The offending objects may sometimes be modified to become less allergenic themselves, such as nickel-plated fasteners and jewelry that is painted with a clear polyurethane varnish.

What Not to Do

❌ Do not allow patients to apply fluorinated corticosteroids for more than 10 to 14 days to the face or genital area, as they can produce premature aging of the skin with thinning and striae.

❌ Do not prescribe a prepackaged steroid dose pack that is tapered over 6 days. It is usually inadequate for treatment of ACD (which will often last for ~2 weeks) and frequently results in an apparent rebound dermatitis and patient dissatisfaction.

❌ Do not prescribe systemic steroids when secondary infections, such as cellulitis or erysipelas, are present. Also do not start steroids if there is a history of infectious disease or other systemic illness (e.g., diabetes) that makes systemic steroids a relative contraindication.

❌ Do not recommend desensitization protocols (allergy shots). They have no role in treating delayed-type hypersensitivities to contact allergens.

Discussion

Allergic contact dermatitis is a delayed cutaneous hypersensitivity or cell-mediated immune reaction to small-molecular-weight chemicals, which act as haptens. To date, more than 3000 chemicals have been described to cause allergic dermatitis in human beings. Approximately 50 chemicals cause 80% of the reactions seen in clinical practice. ACD begins with a sensitization phase, in which these small molecules pass through the stratum corneum and are processed by Langerhans cells in the epidermis. Antigen-coupled Langerhans cells then leave the epidermis and migrate to the regional lymph nodes via the afferent lymphatics and present this antigen to naïve CD4+ T cells. These T cells proliferate into memory and effector T cells, which are capable of inducing ACD after repeat exposure to the allergen. Upon repeat exposure, the elicitation phase has a latency period that corresponds to the travel time for Langerhans cells to present the allergen to T cells plus the time for these T cells to proliferate, secrete cytokines, and home with other inflammatory cells to the site of contact. A contact allergic reaction normally appears 12 to 72 hours after exposure in a previously sensitized individual.

In addition to the history and appearance of the rash, its anatomic distribution may help distinguish ACD from other types of dermatitis. Because the more exposed areas of skin are more open to allergen encounter, the hands and face are the most common body parts presenting with ACD.

Head and Neck

The skin of the scalp tends to be thicker and have greater resistance to ACD than the face, ears, and neck. Hair dyes and shampoos often spare the scalp but involve the thin skin of the eyelids, ears, cheeks, and neck. Facial cosmetics may cause similar symptoms, and products applied to the hands, particularly nail polish, may be inadvertently transmitted to the face. Metals from jewelry piercings anywhere on the face and ears and topical antibiotics for the eyes and ears are common triggers of ACD.

Extremities

More than half of all cases of contact dermatitis involve the hands. The list of household and occupational materials that are frequently

Discussion continued

handled is extensive but should include supposed innocuous items such as foods, moisturizers, musical instruments, and protective gloves. ACD frequently occurs on the dorsal side of the hands, where the skin is thinner and the density of Langerhans cells is greater. Bracelets, watches, and rings may lead to ACD from metal exposure or exotic wood. Metals from keys and coins, and even the striking surfaces of matchboxes in pants pockets, may be the culprits in ACD of the upper legs.

Torso and Groin

Deodorants may cause ACD involving the entire axillary vault, whereas formaldehyde, detergents, and dyes from clothes may preferentially involve the torso and axillary folds, with sparing of the vault. Rubber chemicals in the elastic of undergarments may affect the bra line and waistline. ACD of the periumbilic region is often caused by the metallic fasteners of belts and pants. Medicines, douches, and spermicides may cause contact dermatitis in the genital area, principally the vulva and adjacent thighs rather than the vaginal mucosa.

Knowledge of the common contact allergens will also be helpful in identifying a source of an ACD rash.

Poison Ivy

See Chapter 184.

Metals

Nickel is the most common metal allergen in the United States. Other frequent causes of metal allergy include chromium, cobalt, gold (gold sodium thiosulfate), and organic forms of mercury.

Medications

Topical antibiotics, such as neomycin and (to a much lesser extent) bacitracin, induce more ACD than any other class of medicines. Mupirocin may be a safe alternative. Topical anesthetics of the ester class (benzocaine and tetracaine) are frequently implicated in ACD. The amide class of anesthetics (lidocaine, dibucaine, and mepivacaine) is a rare sensitizer. Surprisingly, topical corticosteroids may be altered to induce allergenicity through both metabolism in the skin and degradative reactions within the pharmaceutic preparation. A preservative with the highest prevalence of positive skin patch tests is thimerosal, found principally in vaccines and numerous topical medicines for the eyes, ears, and nose.

Formaldehyde and Fragrances

Formaldehyde and formaldehyde releasers, such as quaternium-15, are the most common preservatives responsible for ACD other than thimerosal. These two preservatives are found in numerous cosmetics, moisturizers, and fabrics. Fragrances are widely used in cosmetics, fabrics, and topical medicines; in flavorings of foods, drinks, spices, and oral hygiene products; and in perfumes and colognes. Balsam of Peru is the fragrance most often implicated in ACD. In addition to the previously mentioned products, balsam of Peru is also found in sunscreens and shampoos.

Latex and Rubber Chemicals

Chemical accelerators and antioxidants are added to natural rubber latex during its vulcanization process. These chemicals are the primary sensitizers of ACD in rubber products. Of all the rubber products manufactured, latex gloves are the leading cause of ACD reactions.

Until patch testing can identify the specific offending agent, the patient should be instructed about avoidance of the most likely source of allergen that is inferred by the history and the distribution of the rash. A patient with facial dermatitis should be advised to avoid all cosmetics, hair products, facial creams, and lotions until the exact allergen has been identified.

Contact with blister fluid does not spread the allergen, but transfer of allergen remaining under the fingernails or reexposure to allergen persisting on fomites, such as clothing, can continue to spread the dermatitis.

Because corticosteroids halt lymphocyte proliferation and decrease cytokine production, they have become the mainstay of ACD therapy.

Local corticosteroid therapy is not necessary when systemic therapy is used. **When using a topical steroid on the face,** however, a less potent agent, such as hydrocortisone ointment 2.5% or desonide ointment 0.05%, is recommended.

It has been reported that 80% of cases of occupational contact dermatitis are attributable to irritant contact dermatitis (ICD) and 20% to ACD. ICD results from skin barrier disruption and subsequent release of inflammatory mediators without the requirement of previous sensitization. Mild irritants, such as water, soaps,

(continued)

Discussion continued

and detergents, typically cause chronic subclinical irritation, which is cumulative and eventually leads to clinically perceptible dermatitis. Work that requires frequent immersion in water causes maceration, and with frequent wetting and drying, proteins leach from the stratum corneum, which in turn causes breaks with chapping, scaling, and fissuring. Wetting and drying alone is a common cause of ICD, and soaps and detergents accentuate these reactions. Other industrial materials that may cause ICD include petroleum distillates, alkalis, acids, organic solvents, alcohols, chlorinated hydrocarbons, and glycols.

It is often impossible to use appearance to differentiate between allergic and irritant contact reactions. Acute ICD may present within minutes to hours after exposure, with sharply delineated areas of erythema, vesicles, and/or bullae. Chronic cumulative ICD presents with more scaling, fissuring, and lichenification (thickening of the epidermis with marked accentuation of the skin creases).

The mainstay of treating ICD is frequent moisturization and avoidance of irritants. The best agents for this purpose include plain petrolatum or other hypoallergenic skin creams. Data regarding the efficacy of topical steroids on ICD have been mixed in the past, but the results of a recent study support the traditional use of topical steroids to treat the inflammation associated with ICD.

Photocontact dermatitis is caused by the interaction between an exogenous chemical in the skin and the ultraviolet (UV) component of sunlight. The photosensitive agent may be a recently ingested drug, such as a sulfonamide, fluoroquinolone, tetracycline, oral contraceptive, or nonsteroidal anti-inflammatory drug, or may be a topically applied substance, such as cold tar extract. Clinically, only sun-exposed areas, such as the face, arms, and upper chest, are affected, whereas the skin under the chin, behind the ears, and on the upper eyelids is noticeably spared. A **phototoxic reaction** manifests as macular and tender erythema, which can resemble severe sunburn. With a **photoallergic reaction**, a delayed hypersensitivity reaction is induced by UV light, which chemically alters the sensitizing allergen in the skin. This reaction may produce a pruritic, papulovesicular, eczematous dermatitis similar to ACD.

Phytophotodermatitis

Furocoumarins in many plants may cause a phototoxic reaction when they come in contact

with skin that is exposed to UVA light. This is called phytophotodermatitis. Several hours after exposure, a burning erythema occurs, followed by edema and the development of vesicles or bullae. An intense residual hyperpigmentation results that may persist for weeks or months.

Exposure through limes used to flavor gin and tonics and Mexican beer may result in phototoxic reactions in outdoor bartenders and their customers. The intensity of the initial phototoxic reaction may be mild and may not be recalled by the patient despite significant hyperpigmentation.

Tourists in the tropics may rinse their hair with lime juice outdoors, and streaky hyperpigmentation of the arms and back will result where the lime juice runs down (Fig. 162.4).

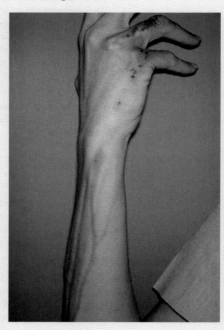

Fig. 162.4 Phytophotodermatitis; the patient had rinsed her hair with lime juice on the beach in Mexico. (With permission from James, W. D., Elston, D. M., Treat, J. R., et al. (2020). *Andrews' diseases of the skin* (pp. 18–45, fig. 3.20). Philadelphia, PA: Elsevier.)

Blistering phytophotodermatitis must be differentiated from rhus dermatitis. The vesicles and bullae of rhus are not necessarily limited to the sun-exposed areas, and itching is the most prominent symptom. Lesions continue to occur in rhus dermatitis for a week or

Discussion continued

more. In phytophotodermatitis, the reaction is limited to sun-exposed sites, a burning pain appears within 48 hours, and marked hyperpigmentation results. The asymmetry, atypical shapes, and streaking of the lesions are helpful in establishing the diagnosis. These features may lead to a misdiagnosis of child abuse.

Treatment of a severe, acute reaction is similar to the management of a sunburn, with cool compresses, mild analgesics if required, and topical emollients. Use of topical steroids and strict sun avoidance immediately after the injury may protect against the hyperpigmentation. The hyperpigmentation is best managed by "tincture of time."

Two types of contact urticaria have recently been recognized as subsets of contact dermatitis. In its nonallergic form, the urticaria remains localized to the site of contact and may be caused by direct mast-cell mediator release from fragrances, food preservatives, insect stings, caterpillar hairs, or topical medicines. Allergic contact urticaria requires previous exposure to sensitizing allergens, such as foods, metals, animal saliva, latex, industrial products, or topical medicines. Both forms of contact urticaria resemble noncontact urticaria, and their classic wheal and flare response usually appears within 30 minutes of exposure and may be relieved or reduced by simple washing. Although allergic contact urticaria may become generalized and even progress to angioedema or anaphylaxis, most cases of generalized urticaria, angioedema, and anaphylaxis result from ingested or internal causes rather than from contact or physical triggers (see Chapter 185).

Suggested Readings

Bains, S., Nash, P., & Fonacier, L. (2019). Irritant contact dermatitis. *Clinical Reviews in Allergy and Immunology, 56*, 99–109.

Cohen, D. E. (2004). Contact dermatitis: A quarter century perspective. *Journal of the American Academy of Dermatology, 51*, S60–S63.

Gober, M. D., Decapite, T. J., & Gasppari, A. A. (DATE). Contact dermatitis. In N. F. Adkinson (Ed.), *Middleton's allergy: Principles and practice* (7th ed., pp. 1105–1116). Philadelphia, PA: Mosby Elsevier.

James, W. D., Elston, D. M., Treat, J. R., et al. (2020). *Andrews' diseases of the skin.* (pp. 18–45, fig. 3.20). Philadelphia, PA: Elsevier.

Kostner, L., Anzengruber, F., Guillod, C., et al. (2017). Allergic contact dermatitis. *Immunology and Allergy Clinics of North America, 37*, 141–152.

Leung, D. Y. M., Diaz, L. A., DeLeo, V., et al. (1997). Allergic and immunologic skin disorders. *Journal of the American Medical Association, 278*, 1914–1923.

Lurati, A. (2015). Occupational risk assessment and irritant contact dermatitis. *Workplace Health and Safety*, 81–87.

Arachnid Envenomation

(Spider Bite)

Presentation

Occasionally patients will come in with a dead or captured spider after having rolled over it in bed or finding it in their clothing while dressing. They may have felt a minor pinprick sensation or no discomfort at all. Early presentations may show only mild erythema at the suspected bite site. Burning pain, pruritus, and swelling may develop within a few hours of the bite.

More commonly, patients come in with a raised erythematous painful lesion with central vesiculation, possibly hemorrhagic, or a darkened or bluish area of early skin necrosis. The patient or companion may suspect that this is a "spider bite," even though a biting spider was never observed.

Brown recluse spider bites vary from mild local reactions to severe ulcerative necrosis with eschar formation (necrotic arachnidism) (Fig. 163.1). The bite often appears as a central blister with mottling and a blanched halo, with surrounding erythema that sometimes makes it look "red, white, and blue." Bites usually are found under clothing and on the thigh, lateral torso, or

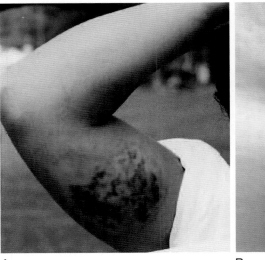
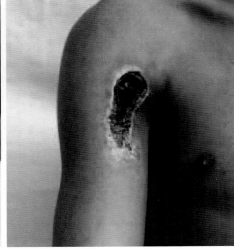

A   B

Fig. 163.1 Appearance of presumptive loxoscelism. (A) Local damage 48 hours after being bitten. (B) Another patient seeking medical care for necrotic scab 26 days after a suspected spider bite. (Adapted from Hogan, C. J., Barbaro, K. C., & Winkel, K. [2004]. Loxoscelism: Old obstacles, new directions. *Annals of Emergency Medicine, 44,* 608–624.)

upper arm. They are uncommon on the neck and are rare on the hands, feet, or face. Transient and mild constitutional signs and symptoms, such as myalgias, malaise, fever, chills, nausea, vomiting, generalized rashes, and headaches, may accompany these bites. A small subset of patients can have a more severe systemic response.

Lesions from other arthropod species and a variety of medical conditions may mimic bites of the brown recluse spider.

What to Do

✓ Ask about the conditions that existed that would raise suspicion for an arachnid bite.

✓ **Determine whether there have been personal contacts with individuals having similar lesions or if the lesions are purulent and consistent with community-acquired methicillin-resistant** *Staphylococcus aureus* **(CA-MRSA) infection. Today, most patients presenting with the complaint of a "spider bite" and who do not have direct evidence of such a bite are actually presenting with a MRSA infection** (see Chapter 165). Culture suspicious lesions and provide appropriate antibiotic coverage and/or incision and drainage when appropriate.

✓ **Consider other possible diagnoses** (especially outside areas endemic to the brown recluse spider), such as burns, cutaneous anthrax, erythema nodosum, focal vasculitis, foreign body, hemorrhagic gonococcal lesion, herpes simplex, Lyme disease (erythema migrans), malignancy, and necrotizing fasciitis.

✓ Cleanse the bite site, and thoroughly irrigate any open wound.

✓ **When there is suspicion that a spider bite has actually occurred, provide and recommend cold compresses, immobilization, and elevation.**

✓ **Confirmed bites are defined as bites associated with a captured or recovered spider found in close proximity to the bite and correctly identified by a qualified person. Most confirmed bites require no treatment and resolve without incident.**

✓ **Provide appropriate analgesics to control pain.**

✓ Provide antibiotics for any secondary infection. Brown recluse spider bites only infrequently become infected; therefore prophylactic antibiotics have not been found to be useful.

✓ Provide tetanus prophylaxis if indicated.

✓ **Evaluation of patients with systemic symptoms should include a complete blood count, electrolytes, blood urea nitrogen, creatinine, prothrombin time, partial thromboplastin time, platelet count, and urinalysis.** There is no cost-effective or time-effective diagnostic test to confirm envenomation.

✓ **Systemic symptoms in the very young and very old most often require admission; and severe symptoms or extensive necrosis in any patient requires admission.**

✓ Patients with mild to moderate local findings can be managed as outpatients with close follow-up in 24 to 48 hours.

✓ **Warn patients of the potential for skin necrosis, with resultant scars requiring possible surgery.** The absence of a lesion 2 to 3 days after the bite usually indicates that necrosis will not

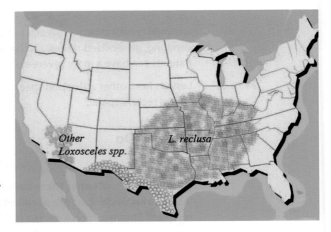

Fig. 163.2 Reported distribution of *Loxosceles* species in the United States. (Adapted from Furbee, R. B., Kao, L. W., & Ibrahim, D. [2006]. Brown recluse spider envenomation. *Clinics in Laboratory Medicine*, *26*, 211–226.)

develop. **Necrotic wounds can take weeks to heal, the average time being 15 days (range, 0–78 days). Appropriate referral to a general or plastic surgeon should be considered with large and nonhealing lesions.**

What Not to Do

❌ Do not apply heat or recommend hot compresses to suspected spider bites. Application of heat to these wounds results in more severe damage.

❌ Do not inject the wound with antihistamines, corticosteroids, and/or vasodilators. This has not been shown to be of any benefit.

❌ Do not perform early skin excision or debridement. Any debridement and/or skin grafting should be delayed until the wound has stabilized (6–8 weeks).

Discussion

Throughout the United States, dermonecrotic wounds of uncertain cause are often attributed to the brown recluse spider, *Loxosceles reclusa*. Many such diagnoses occur in parts of the country where the spider is not native and its populations are not known. The brown recluse has a fairly limited range (Fig. 163.2). Even inside endemic areas, these bites are very uncommon. The incidence of fearing a brown recluse bite is much higher than that of the bites themselves.

Necrotic wounds can be caused by many different factors. Today, patients frequently present with CA-MRSA skin infections that they have self-

diagnosed as a spider bite. Misdiagnosing a necrotic wound as a brown recluse spider bite can lead to delays in appropriate care, with adverse outcomes. In general, spider bites have been overdiagnosed as the cause of necrotic lesions. In addition to MRSA, other important misdiagnosed conditions include neoplasms, vasculitis, Lyme disease (see Chapter 182), cutaneous anthrax, gonococcemia, and perhaps the worst-case scenario—necrotizing fasciitis.

Corroborative evidence should be sought before attributing the cause to a spider or other arthropod bite. Although general wound care may be sufficient

(continued)

Discussion continued

for most similar wounds, it will be ineffective for conditions such as MRSA, neoplasms, Lyme disease, cutaneous anthrax, gonococcemia, and necrotizing fasciitis, in which case a delay in treatment can have grave consequences.

Although all spiders are harmful to their prey, few are dangerous to human beings, and even fewer are capable of causing significant morbidity or mortality. *Loxosceles* spiders are the only globally distributed arachnid species capable of causing necrotizing skin lesions. Rarely, a more severe systemic reaction can occur, causing hemolysis, with subsequent renal failure and significant morbidity. There is no definitive treatment. Diagnosis remains difficult at best, with no specific test available to ensure that a lesion is attributable to the bite of a brown recluse.

The brown recluse is an appropriately named nonaggressive spider that typically seeks shelter in undisturbed places such as attics, closets, and storage areas for bedding and clothing. Humans may be bitten after donning clothing that has recently been taken out of storage.

***L. reclusa* has several distinguishing characteristics** that may not be visible without magnification. The dark-colored, violin-shaped markings on the dorsal aspect of the cephalothorax (hence the name "fiddleback") (Fig. 163.3) may not always be visible because of the variable color of the spider. A helpful identifying feature is the presence of six eyes arranged in three pairs (dyads) as opposed to the more common arrangement of eight eyes found in most spiders.

The current mainstay of therapy is supportive care. Even in the rare case of a confirmed bite, treatment should be supportive. Despite multiple trials, early surgical excision, electric shock, steroids, hyperbaric oxygen therapy, colchicine, antihistamines, vasodilator drugs, anticoagulants, prophylactic antibiotics, and dapsone remain unproven therapies for brown recluse envenomation. All have variable degrees of risk. Antivenin and specific Fab fragments have been shown to be of some benefit but are not available commercially.

In areas of high *Loxosceles* density, the public should be educated about avoidance of bites (inspecting clothing and bed linen) and should be reminded to bring the suspected organism for identification, even if crushed. Should a person find a spider on oneself, it should be brushed off, not crushed.

Like the brown recluse, the maligned black widow spider (most commonly *Latrodectus mactans*) is a shy creature that bites only when provoked. Most of the 26 species of widow spiders are jet black and often can be identified from their characteristic red "hourglass" marking on the undersides of their abdomens. Because webs can be found around outdoor toilet seats, bites may occur on or near the genitalia. These bites may be painful but are usually associated with only mild dermatologic manifestations. Black widow venom causes depletion of acetylcholine at motor nerve endings and release of catecholamine at adrenergic nerve endings. Consequently, black widow bites may produce agonizing abdominal pain and muscle spasm, which may mimic acute abdomen. Other signs and symptoms include headache, paresthesias, nausea, vomiting, hypertension, and sometimes paralysis; fortunately, death is not common. Black widow bites may be misdiagnosed as drug withdrawal, appendicitis, meningitis, or tetanus. Treatment is supportive, and wound care is not typically necessary. Calcium gluconate was formerly recommended, but it has now been shown to be ineffective.

Equine-derived black widow spider antivenin has been considered highly effective, even when given late. However, it has also been reported to cause hypersensitivity reactions. In one case series of 163 bite patients, 1 of the 58 treated patients died of bronchospasm. Therefore some experts will never use antivenin, whereas others may give it only for severe cases, when the patient is very old or very young.

Although antivenin is still available for the treatment of redback spider bites, in Australia it is no longer recommended based on the RAVE-II study. The RAVE-II study showed that antivenin did not provide additional benefit to simple analgesia, for both pain and systemic effects. There continues to be controversy over the effectiveness of redback spider antivenin. A recent meta-analysis found a small overall benefit of intravenous antivenin over intramuscular antivenin or placebo, for pain in widow spider bites. Consult your regional poison control center for further guidance.

With the increasing trend toward having exotic pets, a practitioner may find a patient presenting with a **tarantula bite**. While dramatic in size and appearance, these patient spiders are not likely to bite, and their envenomation is generally no worse than that of a hymenoptera sting. Several species do have irritant hairs on their abdomen, which they may fling outward, causing cutaneous or ophthalmic irritation.

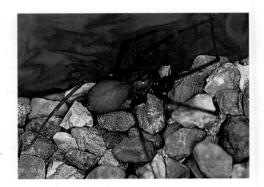

Fig. 163.3 *Loxosceles reclusa* displays classic violin markings on the cephalothorax. (Adapted from Furbee, R. B., Kao, L. W., & Ibrahim, D. [2006]. Brown recluse spider envenomation. *Clinics in Laboratory Medicine, 26,* 211–226.)

Suggested Readings

Boyer, L. V., Binford, G. J., & Degan, J. A. (2016). Spider bites. In T. Cushing, & N. S. Harris (Eds.), *Auerbach's wilderness medicine* (7th ed.) (pp. 993–1016). St. Louis, MO: Mosby-Year Book.

Furbee, R. B., Kao, L. W., & Ibrahim, D. (2006). Brown recluse spider envenomation. *Clinics in Laboratory Medicine, 26,* 211–226.

Isbister, G. (2019). Spider bite. chap. 26.3. In *Textbook of adult emergency medicine* (5th ed.) (pp. 827–830). Philadelphia, PA: Elsevier.

Isbister, G. K., Page, C. B., Buckley, N. A., et al. (2014). Randomized controlled trial of intravenous antivenom versus placebo for latrodectism: The second Redback Antivenom Evaluation (RAVE-II) study. *Annals of Emergency Medicine, 64,* 620–628.

Osterhoudt, K. C., Zaoutis, T., & Zorc, J. J. (2002). Lyme disease masquerading as brown recluse spider bite. *Annals of Emergency Medicine, 39,* 558–561.

Steen, C. J., Carbonaro, P. A., & Schwartz, R. A. (2004). Arthropods in dermatology. *Journal of the American Academy of Dermatology, 50,* 819–842.

Stoecker, W., Vetter, R., & Dyer, J. (2017). Not recluse—a mnemonic device to avoid false diagnoses of brown recluse spider bites. *JAMA Dermatology, 153,* 377–378.

Swanson, D. L., & Vetter, R. S. (2005). Bites of brown recluse spiders and suspected necrotic arachnidism. *New England Journal of Medicine, 352,* 700–707.

Vetter, R. S., & Isbister, G. K. (2004). Do hobo spider bites cause dermonecrotic injuries? *Annals of Emergency Medicine, 44,* 605–607.

Arthropod Bites

(Bug Bites, Insect Bites)

Presentation

Patients with bug or insect bites seek medical help because of itching, secondary infection, or anxiety about secondary effects such as communicable diseases or infestation.

Skin lesions generally consist of single or multiple pruritic wheals or papules, which may include excoriations from scratching (Fig. 164.1).

Mosquito bites most often occur on skin-exposed areas in the summer in mosquito-infested environments (Fig. 164.2). Other biting flies include **midges, horse flies, deer flies, and black flies**.

In tropical and temperate climates, across all socioeconomic strata, **bedbugs** come out of hiding when their victim has retired to bed (Fig. 164.3). Bites are painless and, unlike lice, the bedbug does not remain on the body after feeding. Bites are usually multiple and may be arranged in an irregular linear fashion. The wheals and papules that form have a small hemorrhagic punctum at the center (Fig. 164.4). Blood that oozes from the wounds may be seen as flecks on the bed sheets. Bullous reactions may follow. There is an apparent resurgence of bedbugs in the United States recently. They are hard to avoid because they may survive without feeding for months even in apparently hygienic circumstances. Avoiding residences with frequent turnover (shelters, hostels, etc.) may mitigate the risk of exposure. Permethrin-sprayed bedclothes or sheets may be effective in prevention.

Kissing bugs are found in the southwestern United States, especially from Texas to California. These large (up to 3 cm in length) winged insects are brown to black, with small stripes of red or orange in some species. The bites of these nocturnal insects occur almost exclusively in rural areas. The painless bite occurs only while the host is sleeping, because the blood meal takes 10 or more minutes to complete. Bites have been associated with papular, urticarial, and bullous reactions, and hemorrhagic wounds that resemble bites of the brown recluse spider have also been reported.

Fleas are small (3 mm long), wingless bloodsuckers capable of jumping to a height of 7 inches. Flea saliva is highly antigenic and is capable of producing a pruritic papular rash. Cat and dog fleas also readily bite people, and thus pets infested with fleas are generally the source of the human rash (Fig. 164.5).

Chigger bites are caused by the harvest mite or red bug, which commonly is found in grasslands of the southeastern United States. The larval form of the mite attaches to the patient's skin (usually during summer and fall) and sucks up lymph and tissue dissolved by the mite's

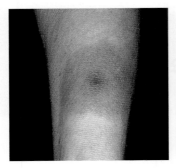

Fig. 164.1 General arthropod bite. (From White, G., & Cox, N. [2006]. *Diseases of the skin* [2nd ed.]. St. Louis, MO: Mosby.)

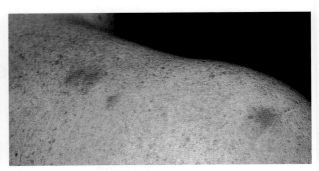

Fig. 164.2 Mosquito bite. (From White, G., & Cox, N. [2006]. *Diseases of the skin* [2nd ed.]. St. Louis, MO: Mosby.)

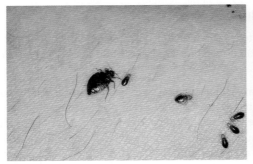

Fig. 164.3 Bedbugs. (From Bolognia, J., Jorizzo, J., & Rapini, R. [2003]. *Dermatology*. St. Louis, MO: Mosby.)

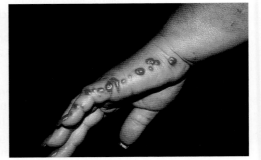

Fig. 164.4 Bedbug bite. (From White, G., & Cox, N. [2006]. *Diseases of the skin* [2nd ed.]. St. Louis, MO: Mosby.)

proteolytic saliva. Frequently, the only signs of exposure are intensely pruritic papules, 1 to 2 mm in size, on the ankles, legs, or belt line, because the bright red mites typically fall off after feeding. The erythematous papules may persist for up to 3 weeks.

A common hypersensitivity response to arthropod bites (most often caused by fleas or bedbugs) is papular urticaria. The condition consists of small (3–10 mm) pruritic urticarial papules that are present on exposed areas and affect predominantly children between the ages of 2 and 7 years. The papules form in clusters and are characteristically distributed on the extensor surfaces of the arms and legs. The lesions generally persist for 2 to 10 days and may result in temporary hyperpigmentation once they resolve.

Caterpillars have hairs (setae) with irritant and allergenic properties that can cause stinging pruritic erythematous papules, often arranged in linear streaks. Symptoms last a few days to 2 weeks. Whereas pruritus is characteristic of caterpillar dermatitis, the hallmark of the sting of the asp or puss caterpillar is intense pain out of proportion to the size of the lesion produced. A characteristic train-track pattern of purpura often appears at the site of the sting (Fig. 164.6). The range of the puss caterpillar is from Maryland down the eastern seaboard to Florida and across the states bordering the Gulf of Mexico.

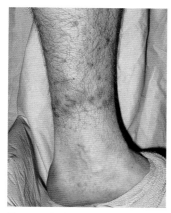

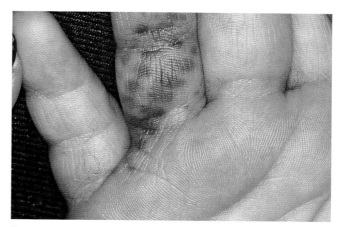

Fig. 164.5 Flea bite. (From White, G., & Cox, N. [2006]. *Diseases of the skin* [2nd ed.]. St. Louis, MO: Mosby.)

Fig. 164.6 Caterpillar sting. (From Bolognia, J., Jorizzo, J., & Rapini, R. [2003]. *Dermatology*. St. Louis, MO: Mosby.)

What to Do

✅ Take a careful history that includes any underlying medical conditions or medications that might produce a papular rash. Also perform a physical examination that provides a detailed description of the rash and its distribution. Attempt to uncover specific circumstances of biting arthropods, from the patient's history as described previously.

✅ **Pruritic lesions can be treated with local application of mild to moderate topical steroids (hydrocortisone cream 1–2.5%).**

✅ **An antipruritic, such as hydroxyzine (Atarax, Vistaril) 25–50 mg may be comforting.**

✅ Treat any infectious complications with appropriate topical or systemic therapy (see Chapters 165, 168, and 174).

✅ **Promote prevention through good clothing choices and the use of insect repellents, and help the patient choose the best product for a situation. Mosquito bites and other fly bites can be prevented outdoors by covering exposed skin with clothing and by the use of insect repellents on skin and clothing.** Clothing is most protective if it has a tight weave and is loose and baggy. Diethyltoluamide (DEET) remains a highly effective repellent. The American Academy of Pediatrics recommends concentrations of 30% or less in products intended for use in children. DEET 25% (in aerosol) or 33% (in cream) is a polymer formulation that provides complete protection against mosquitoes for 6 to 12 hours. DEET can be sprayed on clothing, but the insecticide permethrin, in a formula that can be sprayed on clothing, remains effective for several weeks through at least five or six launderings and can be used in combination with DEET for increased protection. **A 20% solution of picaridin (or icaridin), long used in Europe, has been available in the United States since 2005. It is reported to be tolerated better than DEET and may replace DEET in the future (see Discussion box, later in this chapter).**

✅ Use of permethrin-impregnated mosquito nets while sleeping can be helpful when rooms are not screened or air conditioned. **"No-see-ums" and sand flies are biting flies that are**

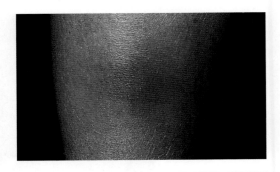

Fig. 164.7 Erythema nodosum. (From White, G., & Cox, N. [2006]. *Diseases of the skin* [2nd ed.]. St. Louis, MO: Mosby.)

small enough to pass through the mesh of standard window screens and mosquito nets, but they may be blocked with fine-mesh screens or with ones that have been treated with permethrin.

✅ **Eradication of bedbugs** often requires protracted and costly treatments for the infested premises.

✅ **Fleas** must be eradicated from the environment to effectively end the problem of **flea bites.** Eliminating cat and dog fleas depends on treating the definitive animal hosts and premises, not just the transient human host.

✅ **To prevent chigger bites, your patient should avoid sitting or lying in grass or weeds in endemic areas during the warm months of the year. Using DEET or spraying clothes with permethrin will also help.**

✅ **Caterpillar dermatitis may require moderate-potency to high-potency topical steroids to help alleviate itching in some cases.** Systemic steroids should be reserved for severe reactions. **Caterpillar hairs (setae) can be removed from the skin by "stripping" with adhesive tape or instruct the patient to apply nontoxic household glue with a cotton swab and top it with a single layer of gauze. Instruct the patient to let the glue dry, then remove the gauze and glue. The setae will usually come out with the glue and gauze. Alternatively, the patient can use blackhead-removal strips following the same directions as to remove blackheads.**

✅ **Intractable pain** caused by the sting of the puss caterpillar may require oral or parenteral narcotic analgesics.

What Not to Do

❌ Do not mistake the multiple painful nodules of erythema nodosum for bug bites (Fig. 164.7). These erythematous nodules are not pruritic and usually develop over the anterior legs, occasionally over the torso, and infrequently over the extensor surfaces of the arms. This condition requires a thorough medical investigation.

❌ Do not recommend antihistamine creams. They are of little value and can irritate the skin.

❌ Do not perpetuate myths about repellents. DEET and picaridin have good safety records. For patients insisting on herbal or natural remedies, make sure they know geraniol shows by far stronger performance than citronella or eucalyptus in clinical trials. None of these offer a plume of protection when applied topically, so every surface must have the substance applied.

 Do not apply DEET near the eyes or mouth, on broken skin, or under clothing.

Discussion

In general, the diagnosis of arthropod bites is dependent on maintenance of a high index of suspicion and familiarity with the arthropod fauna, not only in one's region of practice but also in the travel regions of one's patients. Taking a thorough history and determining the distribution of the rash will aid in the diagnosis.

Mosquitoes are responsible for the recent outbreaks of West Nile virus in the United States. **West Nile** fever develops in approximately 20% of infected humans and is accompanied by a flulike illness. A rash occurs in 20% of patients. Fortunately, severe neurologic manifestations of West Nile fever, including meningitis and encephalitis, are rare. Patients should be so informed and reassured.

Bedbugs are spread chiefly through the clothing and baggage of travelers and visitors, secondhand beds, and laundry.

DEET has been found to be safe and effective, but some patients dislike its odor and find it irritating or uncomfortably oily or sticky on the skin. At high concentrations, DEET can damage clothes made from synthetic fibers, such as nylon or rayon, and can also damage leather and plastics on eyeglass frames and watch crystals. Picaridin 20% is recommended as an alternative to DEET. Unlike DEET, it is odorless, does not feel greasy or sticky, is less likely to irritate the skin, and does not damage plastics or fabrics.

Suggested Readings

Afify, A., Betz, J. F., Riabinina, O., Lahondère, C., & Potter, C. J. (2019). Commonly used insect repellents hide human odors from *Anopheles* mosquitoes. *Current Biology, 29*(21), 3669–3680, e5.

Elston, D. M. (2004). Prevention of arthropod-related disease. *Journal of the American Academy of Dermatology, 51,* 947–954.

Goddard, J., & deShazo, R. (2009). Bed bugs *(Cimex lectularius)* and clinical consequences of their bites. *Journal of the American Medical Association, 301* 1368–1366.

Pollack, R. J., & Marcus, L. C. (2005). A travel medicine guide to arthropods of medical importance. *Infectious Disease Clinics of North America, 19,* 169–183.

Porter, A., Lang, P., & Huff, R. (2004). Persistent pruritic papules. *American Family Physician, 69,* 2640–2642.

Steen, C. J., Carbonaro, P. A., & Schwartz, R. A. (2004). Arthropods in dermatology. *Journal of the American Academy of Dermatology, 50,* 819–842.

Cutaneous Abscess or Pustule

Presentation

A patient with an **abscess** presents with localized pain, swelling, and redness of the skin. The patient may or may not have a history of minor trauma (such as an embedded foreign body or a small skin puncture). The area is tender, warm, firm, and usually fluctuant to palpation. Sometimes there is surrounding cellulitis or lymphangitis and, in the more serious case, fever. If the abscess is close to the skin surface, pointing may occur where the skin is thinned, and pus may eventually break through to drain spontaneously. With the advent of community-acquired methicillin-resistant *Staphylococcus aureus* (MRSA), there may be a central or underlying darkened necrotic area, with the patient often incorrectly reporting a "spider bite." These abscesses generally are extremely tender and inflamed.

A **pustule** will appear only as a cloudy tender vesicle surrounded by some redness and induration, and it will occasionally be the source of ascending lymphangitis.

What to Do

✅ A history and physical examination should include inquiries about immune status, artificial joints or heart valves, valvular heart disease, previous occurrence of similar abscesses, and close contact with people having similar lesions, as well as evidence of systemic symptoms such as fever and tachycardia.

✅ **A pustule should not require any anesthesia for drainage. Very small pustules can be opened or unroofed using an 18-gauge needle.** For larger pustules, simply snip open the cutaneous roof with fine scissors or an inverted No. 11 scalpel blade, grasp an edge with pickups, and excise the entire overlying surface (Fig. 165.1). Cleanse the open surface with normal saline and cover it with ointment and a dressing. The patient should be instructed to use warm compresses or soapy soaks at home.

✅ **When a simple abscess is suspected but the location of the abscess cavity is uncertain, the clinician can attempt to locate it using bedside ultrasonography or by aspirating pus from the cavity with an 18-gauge needle after preparing the area with povidone-iodine.** When using ultrasonography, placing the suspected abscess site in a water bath (such as a bedpan filled with water) will eliminate the need for ultrasound gel or contact between the ultrasound transducer and the patient's skin, thus eliminating discomfort. **If an abscess cavity cannot be located, release the patient on antibiotics and intermittent warm, moist compresses. Instruct the patient to be reevaluated in 24 hours to again check for abscess cavity formation.**

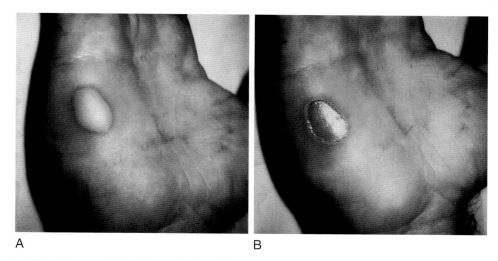

Fig. 165.1 (A) Large pustule before débridement. Local anesthesia is not required. (B) Pustule after débridement and cleansing.

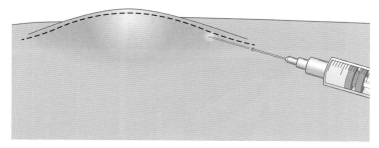

Fig. 165.2 Anesthetizing the incision site of a small abscess. The anesthetic is injected in the subcutaneous plane under the area of the planned incision.

✅ **In patients who are immunocompromised, have valvular heart disease, or have artificial heart valves or joints,** administer empirical antibiotic prophylaxis before performing an incision and drainage (I&D).

✅ **When the abscess is small (2–4 cm) with a thin roof or is beginning to point, prepare the overlying skin for incision and drainage with povidone-iodine solution. Inject lidocaine** superficially into the roof of the abscess along the line of the projected incision (Fig. 165.2). The larger abscesses may require a circumferential infiltration of lidocaine (see later).

✅ **Incise with a No. 11 or 15 scalpel blade at the most dependent and thin-roofed area of fluctuance.** The incision should be large but directed along the relaxed skin-tension lines to reduce future scarring. Alternately, the loop drainage technique can be used. **The loop drainage technique, in which a loop of rubber material is placed through the abscess cavity after I&D, seems to be the new state-of-the-art technique for promoting ongoing drainage** (Fig. 165.3). **Most of the data are retrospective, but a recent prospective trial comparing loop drainage with incision and drainage without packing found better resolution with loop drainage. In addition, it is likely less painful than packing, may reduce**

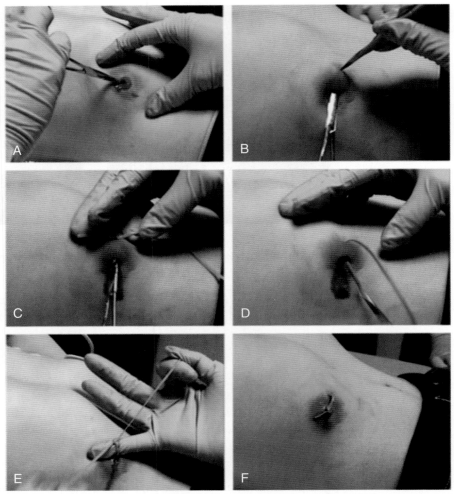

Fig. 165.3 Loop drainage technique. (A) Step 1: Prepare the area and administer local anesthesia. Make a central incision and use a hemostat to break up loculations within the abscess. The abscess may be irrigated now or after the vessel loop is placed. (B) Step 2: Use the hemostat to tent the skin near the farthest edge of the abscess cavity, and make a second incision over the tip of the hemostat. (C) Step 3: Once the second incision is made, push the hemostat through the new incision, and use it to grab the vessel loop and pull it through the abscess cavity. (D) Step 4: Pull vessel loop through the abscess cavity. (E) Step 5: Tie the vessel loop, using a finger or hemostat to keep it loose over the surface of the skin. (F) Step 6: Appearance of final vessel loop placement. (From Ladde J. G., Baker, S., Rodgers, C. N., et al. [2015]. The LOOP technique: A novel incision and drainage technique in the treatment of skin abscesses in a pediatric ED. *American Journal of Emergency Medicine, 33*[2], 271–276.)

scarring because two smaller incisions can be made, and requires fewer if any return visits because patients can cut the loop and remove it painlessly themselves once drainage stops. Most important in the view of these authors is that the sturdy rubber drains allow the patient to immediately begin soaking and washing the incised abscess.

⊘ In larger, more complex abscesses, provide systemic analgesia or procedural sedation (see Appendix E). In addition to infiltration across the dome of the abscess, perform a field block by injecting a ring of subcutaneous 1% lidocaine around the abscess, approximately

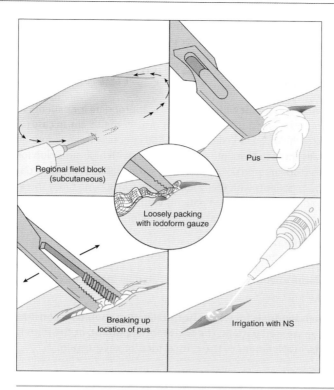

Fig. 165.4 Abscess drainage procedure. *NS,* Normal saline.

1 cm peripheral to the erythematous border. As explained previously, an incision is made across the entire length of the fluctuant area. A hemostat may then be inserted into the cavity to break up any loculated collections of pus. The cavity may be gently irrigated with normal saline and, when deep or expansive, loosely packed with iodoform or plain gauze (Fig. 165.4). Leave a small wick of this gauze protruding through the incision to allow continued drainage and easy removal after 48 hours. Mounting evidence suggests that packing a wound is superfluous, but this should be decided on a case-by-case basis. **Remember that the primary purpose of packing is to keep the wound open and that a small amount of gauze suffices. Overpacking an abscess is both painful and counterproductive;** it fails to allow the wound to drain. In addition, iodoform gauze may cause the patient excessive pain.

⊘ **To prevent recurrence, patients who have infected epidermoid (or sebaceous) cysts containing foul-smelling cheesy material should be referred for complete excision of the cyst after the infection and inflammation have resolved.**

⊘ **Instruct the patient to use intermittent warm water soaks or compresses for a few days when there is no packing used or after the packing is removed. This will encourage further drainage when needed.**

⊘ **The prevalence of MRSA is quite high. However, in the majority of patients with an abscess who have no systemic toxicity, aerobic cultures and sensitivities are not necessary.**

⊘ **There is some debate over the need for antibiotics after I&D. A large, well-done study did show a marginally higher cure rate and a decrease in recurrent lesions. However, this needs to be weighed against potential side effects. In general, trimethoprim-sulfamethoxazole**

(TMP-SMX) is the current agent of choice for community-acquired cases. Clindamycin and doxycycline are alternatives for patients with sulfa allergies. Most abscesses in immunocompetent individuals, if not associated with lymphangitis or extensive cellulitis, probably do not need antibiotics at all; I&D is normally curative. This is as true of MRSA as it is with non-MRSA lesions.

✓ **Empirical treatment** with antibiotics is appropriate for patients with induration surrounding the abscess of total diameter greater than 5 cm. In cases with low suspicion or prevalence of MRSA, include dicloxacillin 500 mg orally three to four times a day; cephalexin 500 mg orally three to four times a day; in cases with high suspicion for MRSA, treat with trimethoprim-sulfamethoxazole 160/800 mg, one tab orally twice a day or two tabs orally twice a day in obese patients with BMI > 40; clindamycin 300 mg orally three times a day or 450 mg orally three times a day in obese patients with BMI > 40. Resistance to these drugs may develop in the future, so refer to the local antibiogram for further guidance.

✓ **Severe infections** should be treated with vancomycin, 1 g twice daily, or 15 to 20 mg/kg twice daily intravenously (IV) in the inpatient setting.

✓ **Very large abscesses** or deep abscesses may require hospitalization and surgical drainage in the operating room.

✓ **Other individuals for whom hospitalization should be considered include the immunosuppressed patient, the toxic febrile patient, or the patient who has a large area of cellulitis, involvement of the central face, or severe pain.**

✓ Provide a dressing to collect continued drainage.

✓ Have outpatients reexamined within 48 hours.

✓ **When multiple family members are involved or the abscesses are recurrent with MRSA, stress the importance of good personal hygiene, recommend use of hexachlorophene soap for bathing, and prescribe mupirocin nasal ointment 2%, 1/2 tube in each nostril twice a day for 5 days to eradicate colonization and the carrier state for the patient and any contacts with positive nasal cultures.** (Push nostrils closed and release multiple times over 1 minute to disburse ointment.) Athletes should be encouraged not to share personal equipment or towels and to regularly clean their sports gear.

What Not to Do

✗ Do not inject anesthetic into a closed abscess cavity, as the pain from pressurizing that space is excruciating.

✗ Do not incise an abscess that is pulsatile or lies in close proximity to a major vessel, such as in the axilla, groin, or antecubital space, without first confirming its location and nature by needle aspiration or, preferably, ultrasonography.

✗ Do not treat deep infections of the hands as simple cutaneous abscesses. When significant pain and swelling exist or there is pain on range of motion of a finger, seek surgical consultation.

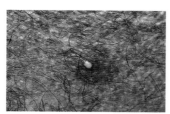

Fig. 165.5 Folliculitis. (From White, G., & Cox, N. [2006]. *Diseases of the skin* [2nd ed.]. St. Louis, MO: Mosby.)

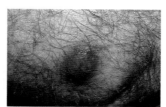

Fig. 165.6 Furuncle. (From White, G., & Cox, N. [2006]. *Diseases of the skin* [2nd ed.]. St. Louis, MO: Mosby.)

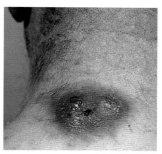

Fig. 165.7 Carbuncle. (From White, G., & Cox, N. [2006]. *Diseases of the skin* [2nd ed.]. St. Louis, MO: Mosby.)

Ⓧ Do not fully pack an abscess cavity with ribbon gauze. This may actually trap pus within the cavity, inhibit drainage, and enlarge the eventual scar. The goal is to insert the gauze across all the surfaces of the cavity and provide some degree of debridement when the gauze is removed.

Ⓧ Do not give one dose of IV vancomycin if you intend to discharge a patient home—a single dose is not effective due to its slow bactericidal effect.

Discussion

Either trauma or obstruction of glands in the skin can lead to cutaneous abscesses. In the past, incision and drainage were considered the definitive therapy for most of these lesions, and therefore routine cultures and antibiotics were generally not indicated. In the past few years, however, there has been an increasing incidence worldwide of MRSA skin infections. Strains of MRSA usually carry a gene encoding the Panton-Valentine leukocidin toxin, which causes necrosis. These strains of *S. aureus* are able to colonize the skin or nares and can produce spontaneous lesions.

There have been **community outbreaks of MRSA** among prisoners and athletic teams. Direct transmission of the skin infection may occur through poor hygiene practices, close living quarters, and shared contaminated objects, such as athletic equipment, towels, and benches. Other risk factors include skin trauma from turf burns and shaving.

Currently there are few research data to provide a scientifically proven regimen for managing these infections. I&D is still a basic tenet for managing an abscess, although there are some randomized controlled trials that indicate the addition of antibiotics to I&D should be considered.

Folliculitis is a superficial infection of the hair follicle that results in mild pain or itching with a small red papule or pustule surrounding a hair shaft (Fig. 165.5). Common sites for folliculitis usually include areas where short, coarse hair predominates, such as the beard, upper back, chest, buttocks, and forearms. Minor uncomplicated cases can be treated with warm compresses, gentle cleansing with antibacterial soap, and, if this alone is ineffective, 2% mupirocin ointment. **Refractory folliculitis** will require MRSA-specific antimicrobials. Advising the patient to avoiding shaving these areas may be warranted.

Hot tub folliculitis may be caused by *Pseudomonas aeruginosa*. A patient usually presents within 72 hours after being in a hot tub with itchy red papules that will be most prominent on parts of the body covered by a bathing suit. Local treatment will usually suffice, but for severe cases, 7 to 10 days of ciprofloxacin, 500 mg q12h, will usually clear up this rash.

A furuncle or boil is an extension of a folliculitis infection into the subcutaneous tissue. This forms a deep red, painful nodule that surrounds the hair shaft (Fig. 165.6). Furunculosis is the most frequently reported presentation of MRSA infections. The syndrome is characterized by the spontaneous development of primary necrotic lesions of the skin and soft tissues. These are the lesions that are often mistaken for spider bites by the patient. Crusted lesions and plaques progress to abscesses or cellulitis but may also present as impetigo, nodules, or pustules. Abscesses may become fluctuant and may drain spontaneously or require I&D and warm compresses. MRSA-specific antimicrobials are now generally initiated.

(continued)

Discussion continued

A carbuncle results when individual furuncles coalesce, resulting in a large painful nodule with deep interconnected sinus tracts and multiseptate abscesses that often are draining pus from a cluster of pores (Fig. 165.7). These are usually found on the back of the neck and generally require I&D with blunt dissection using a hemostat to break up the interconnected loculations of pus. Warm compresses and antibiotics are required.

Hidradenitis suppurativa is a chronic inflammatory condition of the apocrine glands in the axilla and groin. Treatment for early lesions includes intralesional steroid injections, oral antibiotics, and isotretinoin. Secondary infection typically results in formation of abscess and fistula, often requiring I&D and antibiotics. Local care with cleansers and compresses of Burow solution is recommended, and patients should be encouraged to

stop the use of antiperspirants. Recurrent I&Ds cause significant scarring, and extensive surgical procedures are eventually indicated. These patients require referral to a surgeon for long-term management.

A pilonidal cyst abscess is a relatively common finding in the sacrococcygeal region. Drainage should include a search for and removal of hair and follicular tissue at the base of the abscess cavity. To prevent recurrence after the initial infection has cleared, excision of the entire cyst cavity with marsupialization will eventually be required. Surgical referral is therefore necessary.

True brown recluse spider bites are actually very rare (see Chapter 163).

Suggested Readings

Blaivas, M., Lyon, M., Brannam, L., et al. (2004). Water bath evaluation technique for emergency ultrasound of painful superficial structures. *American Journal of Emergency Medicine, 22*, 589–593.

Breyre, A., & Frazee, B. W. (2018). Skin and soft tissue infections in the emergency department. *Emergency Medicine Clinics of North America, 36*(4), 723–750.

Daum, R. S., Miller, L. G., Immergluck, L., et al. (2017). A placebo-controlled trial of antibiotics for smaller skin abscesses. *New England Journal of Medicine, 376*(26), 2545–2555.

Frazee, B. W., Lynn, J., Charlebols, E. D., et al. (2005). High prevalence of methicillin-resistant *Staphylococcus aureus* in emergency department skin and soft tissue infections. *Annals of Emergency Medicine, 45*, 311–320.

Gottlieb, M., DeMott, J. M., Hallock, M., & Peska, G. D. (2019). Systemic antibiotics for the treatment of skin and soft tissue abscesses: A systematic review and meta-analysis. *Annals of Emergency Medicine, 73*, 8–16.

Gottlieb, M., & Peksa, G. D. (2018). Comparison of the loop technique with incision and drainage for soft tissue abscesses: A systematic review and meta-analysis. *American Journal of Emergency Medicine, 36*(1), 128–133.

Huang, S. S., Singh, R., McKinnell, J. A., et al. (2019). Decolonization to reduce postdischarge infection risk among MRSA carriers. *New England Journal of Medicine, 380*, 638–650.

Ladde, J. G., Baker, S., Rodgers, C. N., & Papa, L. (2015). The LOOP technique: A novel incision and drainage technique in the treatment of skin abscesses in a pediatric ED. *American Journal of Emergency Medicine, 33*(2), 271–276..

Llera, J. L., & Levy, R. C. (1985). Treatment of cutaneous abscess: A double-blind clinical study. *Annals of Emergency Medicine, 14*, 15–19.

Naimi, T. S., LeDeell, K. H., Como-Sabetti, K., et al. (2003). Comparison of community- and health care–associated methicillin-resistant *Staphylococcus aureus* infection. *Journal of the American Medical Association, 290*, 2976–2984.

Talan, D. A., Mower, W. R., Krishnadasan, A., et al. (2016). Trimethoprim-sulfamethoxazole versus placebo for uncomplicated skin abscess. *New England Journal of Medicine, 374*, 823–832.

Cutaneous Larva Migrans

(Creeping Eruption)

Presentation

Patients present with intensely pruritic, thin, erythematous, serpiginous, raised eruptions on the sole of the foot, hand, or buttock (Fig. 166.1). The patient may remember recently walking barefoot or sitting in the sand or soil in an area frequented by dogs or cats. Most commonly, this is seen in travelers returning from tropical or subtropical locations in the Caribbean, Central America, and South America, as well as in the southeastern United States.

The etiology of these symptoms is from dog or cat hookworm infections. Beaches and sandboxes provide reservoirs for these parasites. Humans become a dead-end host for the microorganisms by walking through contaminated areas with bare feet or with open footwear or by sitting in the tainted sand or soil.

What to Do

✓ **Thiabendazole is considered a first-line agent in the treatment of cutaneous larva migrans. Because of the toxicity that may be associated with oral administration, topical application is currently the formulation of choice for the treatment of localized cutaneous larva migrans. Topical dosage in adults and children is as follows:**

○ **10% to 15% suspension applied topically to lesions four to six times per day for 2 to 5 consecutive days. Topical preparations will be pharmacist compounded. (This may be the safest treatment, but it may not be the most effective.** See the upcoming discussion).

✓ **For management with oral medication prescribe ivermectin 200 µg/kg, one single dose (typically supplied as a 3-mg tablet).**

✓ **Alternatively, prescribe albendazole 400 mg once per day (supplied as a 200-mg tablet or in a 200-mg/mL suspension) for 3 days.**

✓ For patients with associated folliculitis, give a 2-day course of ivermectin and arrange follow-up as this form of infestation often requires repeat courses of oral medication.

✓ Although it is only mildly effective, it may still be helpful to prescribe diphenhydramine (Benadryl) or hydroxyzine (Atarax, Vistaril), 25 to 50 mg, up to four times per day as needed to reduce itching.

What Not to Do

✗ Do not refer patients for cryotherapy. This was a historical treatment but has been shown to be ineffective and sometimes locally harmful.

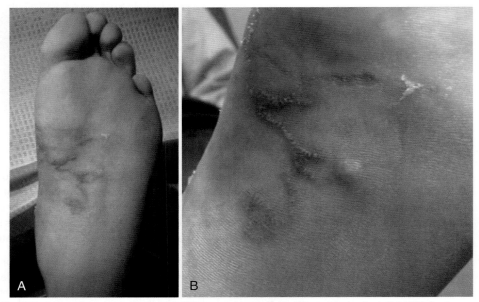

Fig. 166.1 Cutaneous larva migrans. (A) Sole of foot. (B) Close-up photograph of lesion. (With permission from Swartz, M. H. [2021]. *The skin: Textbook of physical diagnosis: History and examination* [pp. 108–155]. Philadelphia, PA: Elsevier Saunders.)

Discussion

This disease is now usually referred to as "creeping eruption" or cutaneous larva migrans. The term *hookworm-related cutaneous larva migrans* has been proposed to describe the cutaneous migration of larvae of animal hookworms in humans.

These lesions result from infestation by the skin-penetrating filiform larvae of hookworms (*Ancylostoma braziliense, A. caninum, Uncinaria stenocephala,* and others) that hatch from eggs that are passed in dog and cat feces. If a human accidentally comes into contact with soil or sand contaminated by these animal droppings, these larvae may then penetrate into the skin. The incidence of this rash is greatest in warm, moist, sandy areas such as tropical beaches.

Migration of the larvae at several millimeters per day results in the characteristic meandering, snakelike burrows in the epidermis. During larval migration, a local inflammatory response is provoked, which causes moderate to intense pruritus. Humans are not the normal host for these parasites, and the

microorganisms lack the necessary collagenase to disrupt the basement membrane beneath the epithelial cells. Therefore the larvae are confined to the skin and usually die within 2 to 8 weeks, even without treatment, but may persist for up to 1 year. Lesions are mostly localized on the feet, but they also appear on the buttocks and thighs, trunk, and knees. The diagnosis of this parasitosis is clinical and relies entirely on history and physical findings.

The use of topical compounds (e.g., 10% thiabendazole) is all too frequently accompanied by irritation, recurrence, and poor patient compliance. Ivermectin and albendazole are effective and fast: A period of 24 to 48 hours is enough to stop the larvae from migrating, with consequent regression of pruritus. The skin heals in 2 to 3 weeks, and adverse reactions are rare. Although hookworm-related cutaneous larva migrans is self-limited, medical treatment shortens the duration and may prevent complications such as impetigo that results from excoriation.

Suggested Readings

Albanese, G., & Venturi, C. (2003). Albendazole: A new drug for human parasitoses. *Dermatology Clinics, 21*, 283–290.

Caumes, E. (2000). Treatment of cutaneous larva migrans. *Clinical Infectious Diseases, 30*(5), 811–814.

Caumes, E., & Danis, M. (2004). From creeping eruption to hookworm-related cutaneous larva migrans. *Lancet, 4*, 659–660.

Chen, S. I., & Singh, A. (2019). Man with a pruritic rash. *Annals of Emergency Medicine, 73*(1), 17–21.

Chen, T. M., & Paniker, P. (2005). An unpleasant memento. *American Journal of Medicine, 118*, 604–605.

del Mar Sáez-De-Ocariz, M., McKinster, C. D., Orozco-Covarrubias, L., et al. (2002). Treatment of 18 children with scabies or cutaneous larva migrans using ivermectin. *Clinical and Experimental Dermatology, 27*, 264–267.

Moon, T. D., & Oberhelman, R. A. (2005). Antiparasitic therapy in children. *Pediatric Clinics of North America, 52*, 917–948.

Diaper Dermatitis

(Diaper Rash)

Presentation

Irritant Diaper Dermatitis

Infants may develop irritation and erythema that is most evident on the prominent parts of the buttocks, medial thigh, and vulva or scrotum. Occurrence is greater in the setting of inconsistent diaper changes or diarrheal illness. Margins are not always well demarcated. There may be papules or small superficial erosions, and skin folds are spared or involved last (Fig. 167.1).

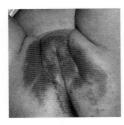

Fig. 167.1 Irritant diaper dermatitis. (Adapted from White, G., & Cox, N. [2006]. *Diseases of the skin* [2nd ed.]. St. Louis, MO: Mosby.)

Candidal Diaper Dermatitis

Frequently following a course of antibiotics, a mild diaper rash may suddenly worsen, with clusters of erythematous papules and pustules coalescing into a beefy red, confluent painful rash with sharp borders that are surrounded by small satellite lesions. The skin folds are commonly involved (Fig. 167.2).

What to Do

✓ **For a mild irritant rash, recommend frequent diaper changes (the most important intervention) and have the parents avoid excessive rubbing, especially with baby wipes that contain alcohol or fragrance, which may actually add to the irritation.** Have the parents rinse the baby's bottom with clear water at each diaper change. They can use a sink, tub, or water bottle for this purpose. Gentle cleansing with soft moist washcloths and cotton balls also can be helpful. Have them pat the baby dry rather than rubbing the infant down with a towel.

✓ **Tell the parents to loosen the baby's diapers** or use oversized diapers to allow airflow and prevent chafing at the waist and thighs. Have them switch to superabsorbent diapers.

✓ **They may also apply a barrier over-the-counter agent—many products are available.** Zinc oxide is the active ingredient in many diaper rash creams, or use petroleum-based ointments. These products are usually applied in a thin layer to the irritated region several times throughout the day. A magnesium/aluminum antacid solution has also been used.

✓ **For a more severe or persistent rash, also instruct the parents to allow the child to go bare (wear no diapers) as much as possible until the rash has healed.** Although at times inconvenient, this allows the skin to dry, avoids physical trauma, and restores natural defenses.

✓ **More severe cases will also benefit from the application of a 1% hydrocortisone cream or ointment twice per day.**

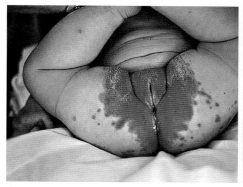
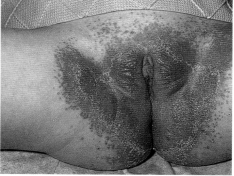

A   B

Fig. 167.2 Two examples of *Candida* diaper rash. (Adapted from White, G., & Cox, N. [2006]. *Diseases of the skin* [2nd ed.]. St. Louis, MO: Mosby.)

✓ **For a mild candidal infection, or for a diaper rash lasting more than 3 days, have the parents apply a topical antifungal cream or ointment such as OTC 2% miconazole (Micatin, Monistat), 1% clotrimazole (Lotrimin, Mycelex), 2% ketoconazole (Nizoral - requires prescription), or 1% naftifine (Naftin - requires prescription) after each diaper change until the rash resolves.**

✓ **With increased inflammation, a combination antifungal-steroid agent, such as triamcinolone/nystatin (Mycolog II - requires prescription), can be applied twice per day.**

✓ **For a severe *Candida* diaper rash, or if there is oral thrush, perianal candidiasis, or repeated bouts of candidal infection, prescribe oral treatment with nystatin to clear the gastrointestinal tract. Use nystatin oral suspension (Mycostatin - requires prescription) to eradicate the infection (see Chapter 53).**

✓ **Recommend the same local measures as noted previously for irritant diaper rash.**

✓ **For secondary bacterial infection (e.g., crusting, vesicles, bullae), prescribe mupirocin 2% ointment three times a day for 10 days.** For severe infections, a broad-spectrum systemic antibiotic, such as amoxicillin/clavulanate, will be required.

✓ **Encourage parents to practice hand washing after changing diapers to prevent the spread of bacteria or yeast to other parts of the baby or to other children.**

✓ Make sure that the family can access outpatient follow-up.

What Not to Do

✗ Do not recommend talcum powder or talcum-free powders for use when diapers are changed. They add little in terms of medication or absorbency and are occasionally aspirated by infants as the diaper is changed.

✗ Do not recommend using cornstarch to protect the baby's skin. Cornstarch helps promote the growth of yeast and bacteria.

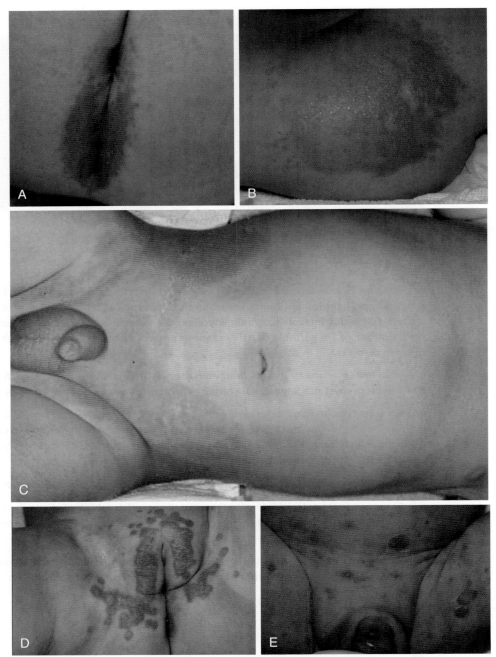

Fig. 167.3 (A) Group A streptococcal infection involving perianal area. Moist erythema of the folds is characteristic. (B) Allergic contact diaper dermatitis from disposable diaper components; called "Lucky Luke dermatitis" by the authors after a cartoon character who carries his holster in the same area. (C) Seborrheic dermatitis, a cause of diaper rash in young infants. This type of dermatitis is difficult to distinguish clinically from infantile psoriasis but tends to be less erythematous, to have thinner scaling, and to respond more quickly to topical anti-inflammatory medications. (D) Typical diaper involvement of psoriasis. (E) Staphylococcal infection with both pustules and bullae in an 11-day-old infant. (A, With permission from Krol, A. L., et al. [2015]. Diaper area eruptions. In: L. F. Eichenfield et al. [Eds.], *Neonatal and infant dermatology* [3rd ed., pp. 245–264 (fig. 17.14B)]. Philadelphia, PA: Elsevier; B, with permission from Krol, A. L., et al. [2015]. Diaper area eruptions. In: L. F. Eichenfield et al. [Eds.], *Neonatal and infant dermatology* [3rd ed., pp. 245–264 (fig. 17.11)]. Philadelphia, PA: Elsevier; C, with permission from Paller, A. S., et al. [2016]. Eczematous eruptions in children. In: A. S. Paller et al. [Eds.], *Hurwitz clinical pediatric dermatology* [5th ed., pp. 38–72 (fig. 3.38)]. Philadelphia, PA: Elsevier; D, with permission from Krol, A. L., et al. [2015]. Diaper area eruptions. In: L. F. Eichenfield et al. [Eds.], *Neonatal and infant dermatology* [3rd ed., pp. 245–264 (fig. 17.9A)]. Philadelphia, PA: Elsevier; E, with permission from Krol, A. L., et al. [2015]. Diaper area eruptions. In: L. F. Eichenfield et al. [Eds.], *Neonatal and infant dermatology* [3rd ed., pp. 245–264 (fig. 17.13A)]. Philadelphia, PA: Elsevier.)

Discussion

Irritant contact diaper dermatitis is a very common disorder during infancy that predisposes the baby to developing a secondary infection with *Candida* organisms. Excessive moisture accompanied by chafing, elevated ammonia and pH levels within the diaper, and proteolytic enzymes present in the stool all irritate and damage the baby's skin. **Superinfection with *Candida* organisms are common enough to treat presumptively in every case of a diaper rash present for longer than 72 hours and severe enough to bring the baby for medical treatment.**

Patients with atopic dermatitis are more susceptible to *Staphylococcus aureus* infection. A culture may help guide therapy in complicated cases. Cases not responding to the usual treatments warrant investigation for psoriasis, seborrheic dermatitis, nutritional deficiencies, and allergic or irritant contact dermatitis.

Some patients may develop perianal group A streptococcus infection. This is characterized by erythema in the perineal or perianal area, painful defecation, stools with blood streaks, and a history of streptococcus infection in the patient or close contacts. The rash is usually pruritic, and perirectal fistulas may be present (Fig. 167.3).

Suggested Readings

Blume-Peytavi, U., & Kanti, V. (2018). Prevention and treatment of diaper dermatitis. *Pediatric Dermatology, 35,* S19–S23.

Cohen, B. Differential diagnosis of diaper dermatitis. *Clinical Pediatrics (Philadelphia), 56,* S16–S22.

Elsevier Point of Care. (2020). *Diaper dermatitis*. Amsterdam, Netherlands: Elsevier BV.

Erysipelas, Cellulitis, Lymphangitis

Presentation

Erysipelas is a superficial cutaneous infection commonly found on the legs or face and generally does not have an inciting wound or skin lesion. Erysipelas appears as a painful, fiery-red induration with raised and sharply demarcated borders, at times giving the skin a pitted appearance like an orange peel (peau d'orange) (Fig. 168.1). In contrast, **cellulitis** involves the subcutaneous connective tissue and has an indistinct advancing border. This deeper infection is characterized by pain and tenderness and by warmth and edema, giving the skin a light red or pink appearance (Fig. 168.2). Cellulitis can occur on any part of the body but is most common on the legs, face, feet, and hands. **Lymphangitis** has minimal induration and an unmistakable erythematous linear pattern ascending along lymphatic channels (Fig. 168.3).

These relatively superficial skin infections (Fig. 168.4) are often preceded by minor trauma, such as an abrasion or the presence of a foreign body. All three conditions are more common in patients with predisposing factors (e.g., diabetes, substance abuse, alcoholism, immunosuppression, vascular insufficiency, and lymphatic drainage obstruction). These conditions may be associated with an abscess or other dermatologic abnormality, such as tinea pedis, impetigo, or folliculitis. The etiology is often unclear. With any of these skin infections, the patient may have tender lymphadenopathy proximal to the site of infection and may or may not have signs of systemic toxicity (fever, chills, rigors, and listlessness).

What to Do

✓ **Perform a careful history and physical examination** to determine if there are any underlying factors that would predispose the patient to such an infection. History of a previous injury, suspicion of a retained foreign body, or knowledge of previous infections may help clarify a possible cause. Underlying illness, such as diabetes, renal failure, chronic dependent edema, immunosuppression, or postoperative lymphedema, will give clues to an underlying predisposition to developing these infections and the need for inpatient management.

✓ **Elucidate a possible source of infection and eliminate it if possible. Debride and cleanse any wound, remove any foreign body, and drain any abscess.**

✓ **Toxic patients** with rapid progression of the erythema, persistent tachycardia, severe pain, or other signs of toxicity require admission. Other indications for hospitalization include coexisting morbidity or cellulitis overlying a medical device such as prosthetic joint or dialysis catheter. In these cases, obtain blood cultures and other relevant labs, and consider obtaining radiographs to look for gas-forming organisms. **Air in the soft tissues on plain radiographs, while not sensitive, is specific for necrotizing fasciitis, and rapid surgical debridement is**

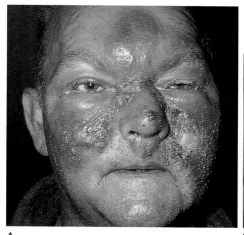
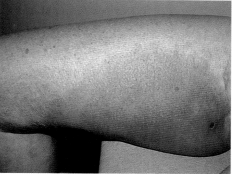

A   B

Fig. 168.1 Erysipelas on the face (A); erysipelas of the leg (B). (Adapted from White, G., & Cox, N. [2006]. *Diseases of the skin* [2nd ed.]. St. Louis, MO: Mosby.)

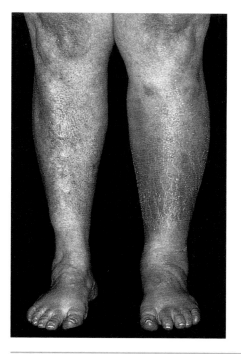

Fig. 168.2 Cellulitis with tender erythema, swelling, and warmth of the patient's left leg. (Adapted from Knoop, K. [2002]. *Atlas of emergency medicine* [2nd ed.]. New York, NY: McGraw-Hill.)

indicated. Ultrasound can also be used to assess for gas in the soft tissues or presence of fluid collections. Obtain cultures from any associated wounds. Cultures, however, are often unsuccessful in establishing a bacteriologic diagnosis. Hospitalization should also be strongly considered for central facial erysipelas/cellulitis, deep infection of the hand, or failure to respond after 72 hours of oral antibiotic therapy.

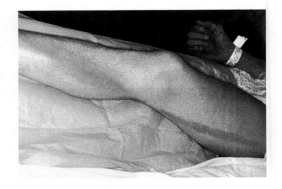

Fig. 168.3 Lymphangitis. (Adapted from Knoop, K. [2002]. *Atlas of emergency medicine* [2nd ed.]. New York, NY: McGraw-Hill.)

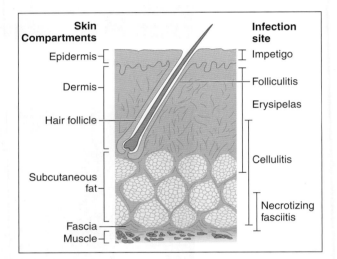

Fig. 168.4 Cutaneous anatomy and sites of infection. (Adapted from Gorbach, S. L. [2003]. *Infectious diseases* [3rd ed.]. Philadelphia, PA: Lippincott Williams & Wilkins.)

☑ If there is little or no fever and the patient is nontoxic and has no significant comorbidity, the patient may be treated as an outpatient. In general, antibiotics prescribed for cellulitis have very good oral bioavailability. Therefore it is not necessary to give a dose of intravenous (IV) antibiotics prior to prescribing oral antibiotics. Options include dicloxacillin, 500 mg four times a day for 5 to 7 days; cephalexin, 500 mg four times a day for 5 to 7 days; or, in penicillin-allergic individuals, doxycycline, 100 mg twice a day for 7 days.

☑ Community-acquired methicillin-resistant *Staphylococcus aureus* (MRSA) has become a common source of infection. Although typically forming abscesses, cellulitis can occur as well. A clue to MRSA infection is an area of central necrosis often reported as a "spider bite" without objective evidence of exposure to spiders. Opening all pockets of purulence is essential to successful treatment. In general, there is little utility to obtaining a wound culture unless the patient has unusual risk factors or exposures to unusual infectious agents, such as an animal bite. In patients who have signs of systemic toxicity, admission to the hospital and coverage with vancomycin, 15 to 20 mg/kg IV, or clindamycin, 900 mg IV, is indicated. Because of a high odds ratio for development of

Clostridium difficile infection, clindamycin should only be used for the treatment of cellulitis when other alternative agents are contraindicated. **Addition of gram-negative and anaerobic coverage is indicated if the lesion is in the perineal area or in cases when there is concern for bloodstream or necrotizing infection. This coverage should also be provided for human or animal bites, surgical wound infections, traumatic aquatic injuries, chronic diabetic foot wounds, involvement of IV illicit drug use, and the presence of neutropenia or severe cell-mediated immunodeficiency.** A local antibiogram should be consulted when deciding on the most appropriate antibiotic.

⊘ **Oral antibiotics alone may be used in less worrisome infections (e.g., trimethoprim-sulfamethoxazole, 160 mg TMP twice a day for 5 days). In cases of isolated abscess, provider discretion may be used with regard to antibiotic coverage (see Chapter 165).**

⊘ Provide tetanus prophylaxis as indicated; prescribe analgesics for pain as needed.

⊘ **Outline the leading edges of the infection with a pen or marker so that the patient and follow-up clinician may monitor the effectiveness of the treatment with the understanding that mild progression within 24 to 48 hours does not necessarily reflect treatment failure.** The intensity of the erythema is often a more important variable, with improving cases resulting in less intensely red inflammation.

⊘ Instruct the patient to keep the infected part at rest and elevated and to use intermittent warm compresses.

⊘ Follow up within 24 to 48 hours to ensure that the therapy has been adequate. Moderate infections worsening after 24 to 48 hours of outpatient treatment will require either culture-guided change in antibiotic therapy or hospital admission for better immobilization, elevation, and IV antibiotics.

What Not to Do

✗ Do not obtain blood cultures or try to aspirate the border of a lesion for bacterial culture in uncomplicated cases. The yield is very low, and it produces unnecessary pain and expense.

✗ Do not overlook a case of necrotizing fasciitis, myonecrosis, or pyomyositis. These patients generally have comorbid conditions, systemic toxicity, and, in the case of pyomyositis, a prolonged course (see Discussion box, later).

✗ Do not mistake deep venous thrombosis (DVT), venous stasis dermatitis, venous insufficiency, lymphedema, contact dermatitis, gout, herpes zoster, noninfectious phlebitis, or insect bite hypersensitivity for cellulitis. These conditions generally do not require antibiotics. **A simple physical examination skill that can help differentiate true cellulitis from other etiologies of erythema of the lower extremity is the passive leg raise. During this examination, the patient lies horizontally on the examination table/bed and the leg is manually elevated to a 45-degree angle or higher. The leg is held aloft for 1 to 2 minutes while observing whether the erythema abates. Cellulitis erythema will persist upon elevation, whereas erythema due to other etiologies, such as stasis dermatitis and lymphedema without superimposed cellulitis, usually disappears with elevation.**

Discussion

Erysipelas (known in the Middle Ages as St. Anthony's Fire) is a rapidly progressing, erythematous, indurated, painful, and sharply demarcated area of superficial skin infection that is usually caused by *Streptococcus pyogenes*. Other causes include *Staphylococcus aureus* (including MRSA) and *Streptococcus pneumoniae*. The initial site of entry is often trivial or not apparent. Systemic symptoms, such as chills and fever, are common. Predisposing factors include venous stasis, diabetes mellitus, alcoholism, and chronic lymphatic obstruction. Erysipelas may progress to cellulitis.

Cellulitis is a deeper skin infection extending through the subcutaneous tissue. It appears as a painful, tender, erythematous, warm area that spreads along indistinct borders. Fever, chills, rigors, and sweats are frequent. There is often an extension via the lymphatic system, producing lymphangitis (formerly referred to as blood poisoning). Causative organisms include group A β-hemolytic streptococci, *S. aureus* (including MRSA), and *S. pyogenes*. Predisposing factors are similar to erysipelas, but look for tinea pedis with fissures, which can serve as a common portal of entry.

All of these infections are typically diagnosed by clinical presentation and treated empirically. **The recent increase in MRSA infections must influence the clinician to maintain a cautious skepticism regarding the use of a traditional antibiotic regimen for treatment of erysipelas, cellulitis, and lymphangitis. Penicillinase-resistant penicillins and cephalosporins would not be expected to be effective against these microorganisms. In general, for patients who appear to have uncomplicated cellulitis, first-generation cephalosporins are still the preferred empiric therapy.**

Alternative conditions exist that can mimic uncomplicated cutaneous infections and may not be apparent until follow-up. These may include abscess, herpes zoster, septic bursitis, gout, and septic arthritis.

Three conditions that should never be confused with uncomplicated cellulitis are necrotizing fasciitis, myonecrosis, and pyomyositis.

Necrotizing fasciitis is a polymicrobial infection that results in the progressive destruction of fascia and fat. This condition is most commonly found in patients with impaired circulation, immune compromise, or in IV drug users. These patients rapidly become very ill with signs and symptoms of systemic toxicity. The affected area (most often the extremities, particularly the legs) is initially erythematous, swollen, hot, shiny, exquisitely tender, and painful. Skin changes progress from red-purple to patches of blue-gray, then to bullae (with clear fluid) associated with marked swelling and edema. These patients develop anesthesia over the affected area, the result of destruction of superficial nerves caused by thrombosis of small blood vessels. It is essential to distinguish necrotizing fasciitis from the less dangerous cellulitis or erysipelas. Urgent surgical debridement and antibiotic therapy are required for patient survival. **The presence of marked systemic toxicity, severe pain, numb skin surface, color changes (red to blue-gray), tendon or nerve impairment, crepitation, and bullae formation point to necrotizing fasciitis.**

Myonecrosis or gas gangrene is a *Clostridium perfringens* infection characterized by gas in a gangrenous muscle group. Currently this is an unusual infection but remains devastating and also requires rapid surgical intervention, IV antibiotics, and hyperbaric oxygen, if available. Pain is the earliest and most common symptom and is accompanied by fever and tachycardia. The patient appears pale, sweaty, and sick. Edema and tenderness may be the only local symptoms. The wound discharge, if present, is typically serosanguineous and dirty and has a foul odor. *Escherichia coli* and *Klebsiella* spp. can also produce gas under anaerobic conditions.

Pyomyositis is often referred to as "tropical pyomyositis" because it is endemic in the tropics. These patients may have a predisposing condition or comorbidity, such as diabetes mellitus, alcoholic liver disease, concurrent corticosteroid therapy, or immunosuppression. This is an infection of skeletal muscle, usually caused by *S. aureus*. One or more muscles may be affected, most frequently the thigh and buttocks. The muscles initially feel achy or crampy, and examination reveals a woody, deep induration of the muscle belly. This is usually a slowly progressive disease; if untreated, within 2 weeks fluctuation, erythema, and then boggy swelling will develop. Tenderness is minimal initially, but fever and marked muscle tenderness develop as the infection progresses. Magnetic resonance imaging (MRI) shows enlargement of the involved muscles along with any fluid collection. Surgical drainage is essential for treatment, along with empiric antibiotic therapy.

Suggested Readings

McCreary, E. K., Heim, M. E., Schulz, L. T., Hoffman, R., Pothof, J., & Fox, B. (2017). Top 10 myths regarding the diagnosis and treatment of cellulitis RSS. *Journal of Emergency Medicine, 53*(4), 485–492.

Mills, A. M., & Chen, E. H. (2005). Are blood cultures necessary in adults with cellulitis? *Annals of Emergency Medicine, 45*, 548–549.

Moran, G. J., Krishnadasan, A., et al. (2006). Methicillin-resistant *S. aureus* infections among patients in the emergency department. *New England Journal of Medicine, 355*, 666–674.

Perl, B., Gottehrer, N. P., Raveh, D., et al. (1999). Cost-effectiveness of blood cultures for adult patients with cellulitis. *Clinics in Infectious Diseases, 29*, 1483–1488.

Powers, R. D. (1991). Soft tissue infections in the emergency department: The case for the use of "simple" antibiotics. *Southern Medical Journal, 84*, 1313–1315.

Stulberg, D. L., Penrod, M. A., & Blatny, R. A. (2002). Common bacterial skin infections. *American Family Physician, 66*, 119–124.

Wong, C. H., Khin, L. W., Heng, K. S., Tan, K. C., & Low, C. O. (2004). The LRINEC (laboratory risk indicator for necrotizing fasciitis) score: A tool for distinguishing necrotizing fasciitis from other soft tissue infections. *Critical Care Medicine, 32*, 1535–1541.

Fire Ant Stings

Presentation

Usually the patient has experienced multiple burning stings (the so-called fire in the fire ant) and is seeking help because of local swelling, itching, and/or pain. Twenty-four hours after the initial wheal and flare at the sting site, there is formation of a small (2 mm), sterile, round pustule on an erythematous base, which is virtually pathognomonic for a fire ant sting (Figs. 169.1 & 169.2). These lesions often occur in clusters. Sometimes there are large local reactions, and it is not unusual for an entire extremity to be affected. Systemic reactions in previously sensitized individuals are analogous to those caused by hymenopteran stings (see Chapter 173).

The appearance of the sting site changes over time. Within 1 week, the pustule often ruptures, forming a small crust or superficial ulcer, which then may become secondarily infected. After 1 month, small visible scars will be persistent.

What to Do

✅ **Examine the patient for any signs of an immediate systemic allergic reaction (anaphylaxis),** such as decreased blood pressure, generalized urticaria or erythema, or wheezing. Treat with 0.3 to 0.5 mL of intramuscular epinephrine 1:1000 (may repeat every 10 to 15 minutes, as needed, to reverse the symptoms) along with boluses of intravenous (IV) normal saline (see Chapter 173).

✅ **Reassure patients who present for treatment after 12 to 24 hours** that anaphylaxis is no longer a cause for concern.

✅ **Relieve itching and burning with cold compresses.**

✅ **Treat minor reactions with topical steroids, such as triamcinolone (Aristocort A), 0.1% or 0.5% cream, or desoximetasone (Topicort) emollient cream, 0.25% or gel 0.05%. Dispense 15 g to apply three or four times daily. These topical medications may help with local pruritus but have no effect on the pustule formation.**

✅ **For severe pruritus**, prescribe an antihistamine such as hydroxyzine (Atarax, Vistaril), 25 to 50 mg orally four times a day.

✅ **When swelling is severe or there are other signs and symptoms of a local allergic component to the stings, and there are no signs of infection or other contraindications to systemic corticosteroids, prescribe a brief course of prednisone, 40 to 60 mg daily for 4 to 5 days, or give one dose of triamcinolone (Aristocort Forte, Kenalog-40), 40 mg intramuscularly.**

✅ Have the patient return or seek follow-up immediately with any sign of infection.

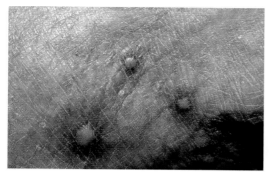

Fig. 169.1 Fire ant sting. (Adapted from White, G., & Cox, N. [2006]. *Diseases of the skin* (2nd ed.). St. Louis, MO: Mosby.)

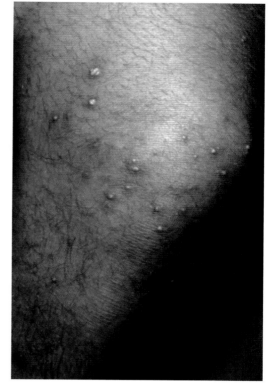

Fig. 169.2 Fire ant stings. Multiple pustules in a cluster. (with permission from Dinulos, James G.H., Habif's Clinical Dermatology; Fig 15.70; Pages 571–630. e1. © 2021, Elsevier.)

✓ **If there are signs of infection** with surrounding swelling, tenderness, heat, and erythema, treat with cephalexin (Keflex), 500 mg four times a day; cefadroxil (Duricef), 500 mg twice a day for 5 days; or doxycycline (Vibramycin), 100 mg twice a day for 7 days. Always consider the possibility of community-acquired methicillin-resistant *Staphylococcus aureus* (CA-MRSA) infection (see Chapter 168).

✓ **Advise all of these patients about avoiding future fire ant stings by wearing shoes (not sandals) when walking outside and to add socks, long pants, and work gloves when working outside. If there are infestations of fire ants around homes or businesses, have professional exterminators help with their removal.**

What Not to Do

✗ Do not open pustules. They are initially sterile, and opening them only sacrifices the remaining barrier function of the skin, increasing the chance of infection.

❌ Do not prescribe prophylactic antibiotics. Antibiotics are of no value unless there are later signs of infection.

❌ Do not send a patient out less than 1 hour after the initial sting. Observe for possible anaphylaxis.

❌ Do not apply heat, even if an infection is suspected. The swelling and discomfort will worsen.

Discussion

The term *imported fire ant* refers to several members of the genus *Solenopsis* (order Hymenoptera), which includes *Solenopsis invicta* (Figs. 169.3 and 169.4), the most widespread of the species. They were first introduced to Mobile, Alabama, from Brazil in the late 1930s. They rapidly migrated and now occupy approximately 310 million acres in at least 12 states. Their current territory covers much of the South Atlantic seaboard from North Carolina to Florida, extends throughout the southern United States and across Texas, and stretches into portions of New Mexico, Arizona, and California. Compared with most native ants, imported fire ants are aggressive and will actively sting intruders.

When their anthill is disturbed, they will swarm and sting any passerby with the venomous apparatus at the tail end of their abdomens. Stings occur most frequently on the ankles and feet. The ants can inflict several painful burning stings within seconds, and each ant can inflict multiple stings. They use their mandibles to grasp the skin, then sting and pivot around their mandibles, inflicting stings that eventually produce the distinctive circular pustules. Unlike stings from bees and wasps, fire ant venom contains hemolytic factors that induce the release of vasoactive amines from mast cells and thereby create these sterile lesions. In heavily infested areas, approximately 30% of the population is stung by fire ants each year, with consequences ranging from local reactions to rare life-threatening anaphylaxis. Secondary infection, which can be severe, especially in diabetics and other infection-prone individuals, is an additional threat, even when the immediate reaction is relatively minor.

Increasingly, fire ants have been implicated in indoor attacks on persons in extended care facilities, where patients typically have sustained hundreds or thousands of stings. Immobility is also a risk factor for infants and persons who are inebriated and who fall asleep on or near an ant mound. Patients who are not allergic have sustained thousands of stings without complication.

Studies have shown, on the basis of allergic-specific IgE, that imported fire ants may be the arthropod posing the greatest risk for anaphylaxis to adults who live in endemic areas. Systemic reactions typically occur in patients previously sensitized to fire ant stings, but because their venom contains allergenic proteins that are antigenically similar to other hymenopteran venom, initial sensitization may occur with a bee or wasp sting. Densensitization may be helpful to protect patients who have experienced generalized allergic reactions. Conventional and rush immunotherapy performed with imported fire ant whole-body extract has proved effective and safe for the treatment of this form of hypersensitivity.

The fire ant gets its name from the fierce burning discomfort caused by its sting, not from its color, which ranges from dark red to brown or black (see Figs. 169.3 and 169.4). Most stings occur during the late spring and early summer, when the ants are most active and their venom is most potent. Public health efforts to diminish the impact of imported fire ants in the United States are focused on introducing predators and pathogens to reduce the overall population of the ants.

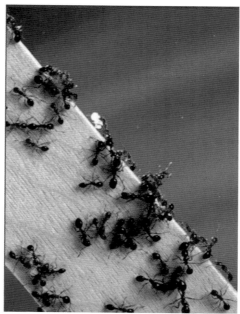

Fig. 169.3   Fire ants *(Solenopsis invicta)*. (Photo by Scott Bauer, USDA Agricultural Research Service, Image Number K5388-1.)

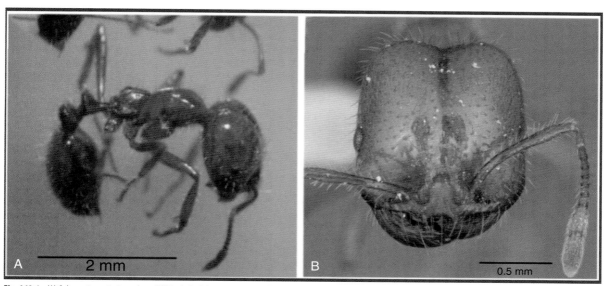

Fig. 169.4   (A) *Solenopsis geminata* workers. (B) Head of a *Solenopsis geminata*. (A, Photograph by Dr. R.K. Sriyani Dias BSc, MSc, PhD. B, Photograph by April Nobile. Used with permission from AntWeb. Version 8.41. California Academy of Science, online at https://www.antweb.org. Accessed 6 October 2020.)

Suggested Readings

Bernaba, M., Power, E., Campion, J., et al. (2019). Unconscious woman in shock and covered with ants pulled from an abandoned automobile. *The American Journal of Medicine, 132*(10), 1239–1241.

Caplan, E. L., Ford, J. L., Young, P. F., et al. (2003). Fire ants represent an important risk for anaphylaxis among residents of an endemic region. *The Journal of Allergy and Clinical Immunology, 111*, 1274–1277.

Erickson, T. B., & Cheema, N. (2017). Arthropod envenomation in North America. *Emergency Medicine Clinics of North America, 35*(2), 355–375.

Goddard, J., Jarratt, J., & de Castro, F. R. (2000). Evolution of the fire ant lesion. *Journal of the American Medical Association, 284*, 2162–2163.

Moffitt, J. E., Golden, D. B., Reisman, R. E., et al. (2004). Stinging insect hypersensitivity: A practice parameter update. *The Journal of Allergy and Clinical Immunology, 114*, 869–886.

Nugent, J. S., More, D. R., Hagan, L. L., et al. (2004). Cross-reactivity between allergens in the venom of the common striped scorpion and the imported fire ant. *The Journal of Allergy and Clinical Immunology, 114*, 383–386.

Porter, S. D., Oi, D. H., Valles, S. M., et al. (2013). Mitigating the allergic effects of fire ant envenomation with biologically based population reduction. *Current Opinion in Allergy and Clinical Immunology, 13*, 372–378.

Steen, C. J., Carbonaro, P. A., & Schwartz, R. A. (2004). Arthropods in dermatology. *Journal of the American Academy of Dermatology, 50*, 819–842.

Friction Blister

Presentation

After wearing a pair of new or ill-fitting shoes or having gone on an unusually long hike or run, the patient complains of an uncomfortable open or intact blister on the posterior heel or ball of the foot. Occasionally these blisters will be hemorrhagic. Secondary infection may be the cause of the visit, after painful pustules, cellulitis, or lymphangitis develops.

What to Do

✅ **For torn or open blisters or blisters that have become infected, remove the overlying cornified epithelium with fine scissors and forceps. Clean the area thoroughly with a nontoxic skin cleanser (e.g., 1% [dilute] povidone-iodine solution). Cover the wound with antibiotic ointment that does not contain neomycin and with a simple strip bandage (Band-Aid). Have the patient wash the area and repeat the dressings until complete healing has taken place.** It usually takes about 5 days for a new stratum corneum to form.

✅ When cellulitis or lymphangitis is present, provide appropriate antibiotics (see Chapter 168).

✅ **For small (<1 cm) untorn or closed blisters that are not infected, the skin may be left intact and covered with a protective dressing.**

✅ **For large intact friction blisters with a fluid bolus inside that is forcibly dissecting the planes of nearby healthy skin, or simply causing discomfort due to bulk, they can be safely drained. Cleanse the area with chlorohexidine. Use a 25-g needle to aspirate or make a small stab incision through the portion that will allow the most natural ongoing drainage of fluid.** Provide a protective covering as noted below.

✅ **Ongoing care of a blister after drainage to avoid contamination and infection depends on the demands you expect to be placed on the skin in the next few days.**

✅ **If further high-friction use such as hiking or working is inevitable, then the dressing should be designed to minimize bulk and transfer friction out of the skin.** In this approach, padding or moleskin will generate a high-friction environment due to the bulk. Paper tape (3M Micropore) followed by spray adhesive (Mueller Pre-tape) then elastic fabric tape (Johnson & Johnson Elastikon) creates a clean, durable, low-friction barrier that can last for days, even with demanding use by ultramarathon runners in tropical climates.

✅ **If high-friction use can be avoided, then a simple wound dressing with antibacterial ointment (bacitracin) and strip bandage protection should be adequate. Alternatively, cover the punctured blister with a polyurethane film (such as OpSite) or a hydrogel dressing (such as Spenco 2nd Skin or Vigilon), or seal the drainage site with cyanoacrylate**

(Dermabond). Other acceptable protective coverings include the hydrocolloid, Duoderm; the occlusive dressing; or the over-the-counter (OTC) liquid bandage, New-Skin.

✓ **Instruct the patient about friction blister prevention.** A properly fitting shoe is essential, and even comfortable shoes need to be broken in gradually. Walking and running activities should be slowly increased day by day. Good socks with moisture wicking and padded insoles can also help prevent friction blisters. Wearing two pairs of socks that are made of different materials may reduce skin friction and prevent blisters. Paper tape (3M Micropore) placed preventively over "hot spots" decreased blister formation by 40% in one study of ultramarathon runners. US military academy cadets who applied an antiperspirant solution containing 20% aluminum chloride to their feet for at least 3 consecutive days reduced their risk for developing foot blisters during a 21-km hike by approximately 50%. The use of such antiperspirants unfortunately causes a high incidence of skin irritation.

What Not to Do

✗ Do not use neomycin-containing ointments because of the potential for allergic reactions.

✗ Do not unroof intact sterile blisters. This will lead to unnecessary discomfort from the denuded area as well as increase the risk for infection.

✗ Do not add bulky dressings to blistered skin that will be subjected to additional high-friction use. Build a slim, low-friction dressing instead.

Discussion

Blisters result from frictional forces—compounded by perspiration—that mechanically separate epidermal cells at the level of the stratum spinosum. This usually occurs when there is inadequate time to develop the protective epidermal hyperplasia that normally occurs with gradual increases in friction stress. Hydrostatic pressure causes the resultant separation to fill with a fluid that is similar in composition to plasma but has a lower protein level.

Active people often develop friction blisters on their feet. Although such blisters rarely cause significant medical problems, they can be quite painful and hinder athletic performance. Treatment goals include maintaining comfort, promoting healing, and preventing infection.

Blister prevention is largely focused on behavior modification and early intervention. Taping with paper tape before activity is effective, cheap, and easy. Once activity starts, paying attention to one's skin allows early intervention for hot spots that have a characteristic overheated feeling or irritation. Hot spots commonly precede blister formation on hands, nipples, feet, or underneath hip belts or shoulder straps. Teach patients to "never tolerate a hot spot" and know how to adjust their gear's fit, change socks, apply paper tape, or make other changes proactively to avoid blisters.

Suggested Readings

Freiman, A., Barankin, B., & Elpern, D. J. (2004). Sports dermatology part 1: Common dermatoses. *Canadian Medical Association Journal, 171,* 851–853.

Heymann, W. R. (2005). Dermatologic problems of the endurance athlete. *Journal of the American Academy of Dermatology, 52,* 345–346.

Lipman, G. S., & Krabak, B. J. (2017). Foot problems and care. In T. A. Cushing & N. S. Harris (Eds.), *Auerbach's Wilderness Medicine* (7th ed.). Philadelphia, PA: Elsevier.

Lipman, G. S., Sharp, L. J., Christensen, M., et al. (2016). Paper tape prevents foot blisters: A randomized prevention trial assessing paper tape in endurance distances II (Pre-TAPED II). *Clinical Journal of Sport Medicine, 26*, 362–368.

Pratte, M. K., Mustafa, M. A., & Stulberg, D. (2003). Common skin conditions in athletes. *Clinical Family Practice, 5*, 653–666.

Frostnip, Frostbite, and Mild Hypothermia

Presentation

Frostnip occurs when skin surfaces, such as the tip of the nose and ears, are exposed to an environment cold enough to freeze the epidermis. These prominent exposed surfaces become blanched and develop paresthesia and numbness but remain pliable. As they are rewarmed, they become hyperemic and are usually very painful. Pernio (chilblains) is an inflammatory skin injury caused by exposure to cold (often repeatedly) above the freezing point and may be idiopathic or secondary to connective tissue disease or cryoglobulinemia.

Superficial frostbite can be either a partial-thickness or a full-thickness freezing of the dermis. The frozen surfaces appear white or mottled, feel doughy or hard, and are insensitive. With rewarming, these areas become erythematous and edematous, with severe pain (Fig. 171.1). Blistering occurs within 24 to 48 hours with deeper partial-thickness frostbite.

Patients who have core body temperatures between 32 and 35 °C are considered to suffer from mild hypothermia and may demonstrate tachypnea, tachycardia, dysarthria, and shivering.

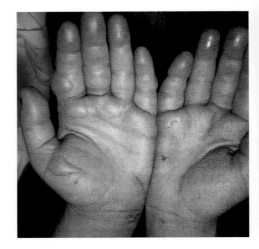

Fig. 171.1 Early frostbite. (Adapted from Marx, J. A., Hockberger, R. S., & Walls, R. M. [2006]. *Rosen's emergency medicine* (6th ed.). Philadelphia, PA: Mosby.)

What to Do

✓ **Obtain an accurate history** of the severity and length of exposure as well as a history of any underlying preexisting medical disorders. Examine the sensitivity of any affected parts of the body. The ability to sense light touch and noxious stimuli helps determine the prognosis. **Favorable prognostic indicators suggesting superficial injury are normal skin color, development of clear fluid in blisters, and the ability of the skin to deform under pressure. Dark color, hemorrhagic blisters, cyanosis, and hard nondeforming skin suggest deep injury.**

✓ **Prior to rewarming, give ibuprofen (Motrin), 400 mg orally, or aspirin, 325 mg orally. This may improve tissue salvage.**

✓ **When there is no longer any danger of reexposure and refreezing, rapidly warm the affected part with heated blankets (or someone else's warm skin in the case of frostnip) or, preferably, in a warm whirlpool bath (at 40–42 °C [104–108 °F]) for 15 to 30 minutes or until capillary refill returns and the tissue is supple.**

✓ A strong parenteral analgesic, such as morphine, may be required to control pain.

✓ **Mild hypothermia can be treated with passive external rewarming, which consists of placing the patient in a warm dry environment after removal of wet clothing. The patient is then covered with blankets.** This alone can be expected to raise the core temperature approximately 0.5 to 2 °C per hour. Adding heating blankets or a forced heated air system (active external rewarming) will increase the rate of recovery.

✓ **When blistering occurs, bullae should not be ruptured, although this is somewhat controversial. If the blisters are open, however, they should be debrided and gently cleansed with normal saline. Silvadene cream or bacitracin ointment may be applied, followed by a sterile absorbent dressing.** Although topical aloe vera is now often recommended, it has not been proven to improve tissue viability. Injured tissue should be handled gently, and dressings must be loose, noncompressive, and nonadherent.

✓ **For anything more than first degree, consider consultation with a burn center to help determine whether treatment with tissue plasminogen activator (tPA or alteplase) is appropriate.** Also consider hospitalization for wound care and analgesia. Hands and feet should be splinted and elevated to reduce edema, and the digits must be separated by nonadherent gauze.

✓ **Intravenous hydration** with crystalloid will theoretically reduce blood viscosity and capillary sludging.

✓ **Tetanus prophylaxis** should be instituted when indicated.

✓ **Outpatients should be provided with follow-up care and warned that healing of the deeper injuries may be slow and produce skin that remains hypersensitive for weeks.** Late sequelae of superficial frostbite include cold hypersensitivity (53%), numbness (40%), decreased sensation (33%), and impaired ability to work (13%).

What Not to Do

✗ Do not warm the injured skin surface while in the field if there is a chance that refreezing will occur. Reexposing even mildly frostbitten tissue to the cold without complete rewarming can result in additional severe damage.

(X) Do not rub the injured skin surface in an attempt to warm it by friction. This further damages the injured tissue.

(X) Do not allow the patient to smoke. Smoking causes vasoconstriction and may further decrease blood flow to the frostbitten extremity.

(X) Do not confuse frostnip and superficial frostbite with deep frostbite. Severe frostbite, when the deep tissue or extremity is frozen with a woody feeling and lifeless appearance, requires inpatient management and could be associated with life-threatening hypothermia.

Discussion

Current scientific knowledge suggests that localized cold injury represents a continuous spectrum ranging from minimal to severe tissue destruction and loss. Frostbite has been categorized into four degrees of severity. First-degree frostbite is characterized by an anesthetic central white plaque with peripheral erythema. Second-degree injury reveals blisters filled with clear or milky fluid surrounded by erythema and edema, which appear in the first 24 hours. Third-degree injury is associated with hemorrhagic blisters that result in a hard black eschar, seen over the course of 2 weeks. Fourth-degree injury produces complete necrosis and tissue loss.

In general, treatment for the four categories of frostbite is the same until demarcation occurs within 3 to 4 weeks after injury.

Hypothermia is classified as being either mild (as previously described) or moderate—with temperatures between 28 and 32 °C, loss of shivering, and diminished level of consciousness— or severe, with core temperatures below 28 °C and loss of reflexes, coma, and, eventually, ventricular fibrillation and death. Moderate to severe hypothermia is a medical emergency necessitating maintenance of airway, breathing, and circulation. High-risk populations include the mentally ill, alcoholics, the urban poor, wilderness enthusiasts, and winter sports participants.

Frostbite is more common in persons exposed to cold at high altitudes. The areas of the body most likely to suffer are those farthest from the trunk or large muscles: ear lobes, nose, cheeks, fingers, hands, toes, and feet. Touching cold metal with bare hands can cause immediate frostbite, as can the spilling of gasoline or other volatile liquids on the skin when the temperature is very low. For those who participate in winter outdoor recreational and sports activities, direct exposure of skin and wearing constricting clothing, such as tight-fitting footwear, will predispose them to frostbite.

Frostnip is a superficial freezing of the skin, a precursor to frostbite, and produces reversible skin changes, including blanching and numbness that resolve with warming. It is important to treat frostnip early to avoid progression to frostbite. With gentle rewarming, the frostnip-affected area becomes hyperemic, and the sensation of pain returns rapidly.

Frostbite occurs when tissue freezes and crystals form in the extracellular space between cells. This occurs at ambient temperatures below 32 °F (0 °C). With dehydration, vasoconstriction, and low epidermal temperature, circulation is limited as blood viscosity increases, and water, hydrostatically pulled out of cells, begins to freeze. Close to 60% of frostbite injuries involve the lower extremities, in particular the great toe and feet. Predisposing diseases can include Raynaud disease, peripheral vascular disease, and diabetes mellitus. Tobacco smoking is another factor that can increase the likelihood of developing frostbite.

Planning for the threat of hypothermia can prevent cold injury. Individuals in cold and isolated areas should never be alone, or they should carry communication devices, such as cell phones or walkie-talkies, close to the body to prevent cold-induced battery dysfunction. They should limit heat loss by insulating and dressing appropriately. Many layers are better than one thick layer. Waterproofed outer clothing is essential. Clothing materials should be wool, wool blends, or polypropylene. Cotton should be avoided. All extremities and the head should be covered. The face should be covered, especially with high wind chill. Dual-layer socks should only be used if the boots are appropriately sized to accommodate their bulk—tight boots will compress fluffy socks, diminishing their insulation factor.

Suggested Readings

Biem, J., Koehncke, N., & Dosman, J. (2003). Out of the cold: Management of hypothermia and frostbite. *Canadian Medical Association Journal, 168,* 305–311.

Dow, J., Giesbrecht, G. G., Danzi, D. F., et al. (2019). Wilderness Medical Society clinical practice guidelines for the out-of-hospital evaluation and treatment of accidental hypothermia: 2019 update. *Wilderness and Environmental Medicine, 30,* S47–S69.

McIntosh, S. E., Freer, L., Grissom, C. K., et al. (2019). Wilderness Medical Society clinical practice guidelines for the prevention and treatment of frostbite: 2019 update. *Wilderness and Environmental Medicine, 30,* S19–S32.

Petrone, P., Kuncir, E., & Asensio, J. A. (2003). Surgical management and strategies in the treatment of hypothermia and cold injury. *Emergency Medicine Clinics of North America, 21,* 1165–1178.

Seto, G. K., Way, D., & O'Connor, N. (2005). Environmental illness in athletes. *Clinics in Sports Medicine, 24,* 695–718.

Ulrich, A. S., & Rathlev, N. K. (2004). Hypothermia and localized cold injuries. *Emergency Medicine Clinics of North America, 22,* 281–298.

Herpes Zoster

(Shingles)

CHAPTER

172

Presentation

The most common presentation is a dermatomal rash and pain. Prodromal symptoms, which occur infrequently, may include malaise, nausea and vomiting, headache, and photophobia. Less commonly there may be fever. During the prodromal stage, which can last several days, patients commonly experience preherpetic neuralgia.

Patients complain of symptoms that range from an itch or tingling to severe lancinating pain, tenderness, dysesthesias, paresthesia, or hypersensitivity that covers a specific dermatome. This discomfort may be precipitated by minor skin stimulation from the patient's clothes and is characteristic of this type of neurologic pain. After 1 to 5 days, the patient may develop a characteristic unilateral rash. The discomfort may be difficult for the patient to describe, often alternating between an itch, a burning, and even a deep aching pain. Prior to the onset of the rash, zoster can be confused with pleuritic or cardiac pain, cholecystitis, or ureteral colic. The pain may precede the eruption by as much as a few weeks, and occasionally pain alone is the only manifestation (zoster sine herpete). Although almost exclusively a unilateral disease, in one study approximately 1% of patients had bilateral involvement.

The early rash consists of an eruption of erythematous macules and papules that usually appear posteriorly first and then spread anteriorly along the course of an involved nerve segment. In most instances, clusters of clear vesicles on an erythematous base will appear within the next 24 hours (Figs. 172.1, 172.2, and 172.3). These continue to form for 3 to 5 days and then evolve through states of pustulation, ulceration, and crusting.

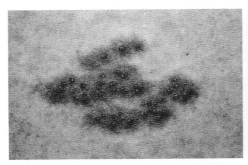

Fig. 172.1 Herpes zoster. Classic appearance of grouped vesicles. (From White, G., & Cox, N. [2006]. *Diseases of the skin* [2nd ed.]. St. Louis, MO: Mosby.)

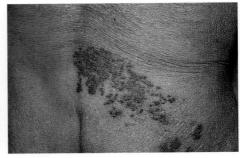

Fig. 172.2 The vesicles of herpes zoster may at times be hemorrhagic. (From White, G., & Cox, N. [2006]. *Diseases of the skin* [2nd ed.]. St. Louis, MO: Mosby.)

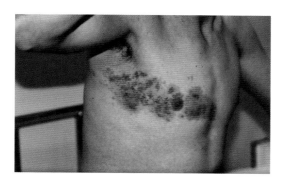

Fig. 172.3 Herpes zoster infection, typically involving a single unilateral dermatome. (From White, G., & Cox, N. [2006]. *Diseases of the skin* [2nd ed.]. St. Louis, MO: Mosby.)

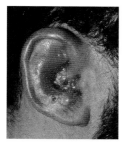

Fig. 172.4 Ramsay Hunt syndrome. (From White, G., & Cox, N. [2006]. *Diseases of the skin* [2nd ed.]. St. Louis, MO: Mosby.)

The skin eruption usually is limited to a single dermatome; the most commonly involved dermatomes are the thoracolumbar region and the face. Lesions may involve more than one dermatome and occasionally may cross the midline. **With seventh cranial nerve involvement** (causing weakness of all facial muscles on one side), the rash will be found in the ipsilateral external ear (called zoster oticus) (Fig. 172.4), or vesicles may be seen on the hard palate. **Bell palsy (see Chapter 5) following zoster dermatitis of the external ear canal is well known and can be part of the Ramsay Hunt syndrome.** The virus invades the facial nerve, especially the geniculate ganglion, and occasionally the auditory nerve, and can produce the peripheral seventh-nerve palsy, along with hearing loss, vertigo, and taste dysfunction.

What to Do

⊘ **If it has been 3 days or less since the onset of the rash, prescribe valacyclovir (Valtrex), 1000 mg three times a day for 7 days; famciclovir (Famvir), 500 mg three times a day for 7 days; or the much less expensive but more inconvenient acyclovir (Zovirax), 800 mg five times per day for 7 days. If a patient presents later than 72 hours after onset, antivirals may still be considered if new lesions are being formed.**

⊘ **Prescribe analgesics appropriate for the level of pain the patient is experiencing.** Nonsteroidal anti-inflammatory drugs (NSAIDs) may help, but opioids are often required (e.g., morphine IR every 6–12 hours). When prescribing opioids for the elderly, remember to warn them that they are likely to suffer constipation as a side effect and treat concurrently with senna (sennosides 8.6-mg tablets, two tabs at bedtime; see Chapter 68). Other side effects of opioids include nausea, decreased appetite, and sedation. If the pain is severe, consider referring the patient for an epidural nerve block, which has been successful in relieving the acute pain and may decrease the incidence of postherpetic neuralgia (PHN).

⊘ **There is not strong evidence that treating older patients (≥60 years) with amitriptyline (Elavil), 25 mg once daily for 90 days, will reduce the risk for PHN. Although one study indicated there was a 50% decrease in pain prevalence at 6 months compared with placebo, this study was small and had other limitations. Coordinate such** treatment with a follow-up physician and be aware of the sedative side effects of the medication itself.

✓ **Cool compresses** with Burrows solution can be comforting (e.g., Domeboro powder, two packets in 1 pint of water).

✓ Dressing the lesions with gauze and splinting them with an elastic wrap may also help bring relief. **Superficial infection may be prevented by the use of a topical antibiotic ointment,** such as mupirocin (Bactroban) 2% ointment applied twice a day.

✓ **Secondary infection should be treated with systemic antibiotics,** such as cephalexin, 500 mg four times a day for 7 to 10 days, or doxycycline, 100 mg twice a day for 7 to 10 days. Always keep in mind the possibility of an infection with community-acquired methicillin-resistant *Staphylococcus aureus* (CA-MRSA) (see Chapter 174).

✓ **Ocular lesions should be evaluated by an ophthalmologist and treated with oral antivirals in combination with topical ophthalmic corticosteroids.** Although topical steroids are contraindicated in herpes simplex keratitis because they allow deeper corneal injury, this does not appear to be a problem with herpes zoster ophthalmicus (Fig. 172.5). **If the rash extends to the tip of the nose (the Hutchinson sign), the eye will probably be involved because it is served by the same nasociliary branch of the trigeminal nerve.** Look for punctate keratopathy on slit-lamp examination with fluorescein staining, although patients may have only pain, lacrimation, conjunctivitis, or scleritis. Herpes zoster ophthalmicus can result in corneal scarring, uveitis, glaucoma, corneal perforation, or blindness. Patients with acquired immunodeficiency syndrome (AIDS) are at risk for developing acute retinal necrosis.

✓ **Systemic corticosteroids are suggested as adjunct treatment in patients with Ramsay Hunt syndrome or severe pain and cranial nerve palsies.**

✓ **Until all lesions are crusted,** instruct patients to stay away from immunocompromised individuals and pregnant women who have not had chickenpox (or the vaccine). Explain that they can transmit varicella (chickenpox) to a susceptible individual.

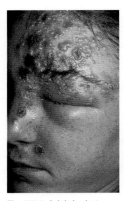

Fig. 172.5 Ophthalmologic zoster vesicles and crusting of the top and side of the nose in herpes zoster implies involvement of the nasociliary branch of the trigeminal nerve and eye involvement. (From White, G., & Cox, N. [2006]. *Diseases of the skin* [2nd ed.]. St. Louis, MO: Mosby.)

What Not to Do

✗ Do not prescribe systemic steroids to prevent PHN, especially for patients who are at high risk (i.e., with latent tuberculosis, immunocompromise, peptic ulcer, diabetes mellitus, hypertension, or congestive heart failure), although they are sometimes recommended to reduce acute symptoms. **There is some evidence that steroids in conjunction with antiviral agents hasten resolution of pain, normal sleep, and resumption of normal activity.** Oral corticosteroids given during the acute phase of the illness have not been shown to reduce the incidence or severity of PHN.

✗ Do not initiate a comprehensive diagnostic workup to look for an occult malignancy simply on the basis of zoster. The incidence of cancer among patients with zoster is no greater than that of the general population. Patients with cancers, particularly lymphomas, are, however, at increased risk for zoster. Usually the cancer diagnosis is already known when zoster occurs.

 Do not use topical antiviral agents. They are not effective and are not recommended.

Discussion

Herpes zoster can usually be readily diagnosed from its clinical appearance of typical lesions in a dermatomal distribution. One well-known diagnostic caveat is that the pain and rash do not cross the midline; however, it is not impossible for the disease to be bilateral and involve more than one dermatome, and multidermatomal zoster may be the presenting finding for human immunodeficiency virus (HIV).

Antiviral therapy has been shown to shorten the duration of viral shedding, halt the formation of new lesions more quickly, accelerate the rate of healing, and reduce the severity of acute pain.

Herpes zoster ophthalmicus is a particularly important variant, and these patients should definitely receive antiviral therapy early with the goal of preventing ocular complications.

Antiviral treatment is generally recommended for all patients of any age with severely symptomatic herpes zoster and for patients older than age 50 years with zoster of any severity. The benefit of antiviral therapy for immunocompetent patients who are younger than 50 years of age who have mild acute symptoms is less well established.

When the diagnosis is in doubt, the Tzanck test can help. Select an intact early vesicular lesion, unroof it, and, using the belly of a No. 15 scalpel blade, scrape the floor of the vesicle to obtain as much exudate as possible. Gently transfer this material to a clean glass slide and allow it to air dry. A Wright or Giemsa stain will reveal multinucleated giant cells.

If available, polymerase chain reaction (PCR) techniques are the most sensitive and specific diagnostic tests for detecting the varicella deoxyribose nucleic acid (DNA) in fluid taken from the vesicles. The direct immunofluorescence antigen-staining test provides an alternative diagnostic modality when PCR is not available, but it carries a lower sensitivity (77–82% vs 94–95% with PCR) and a lower specificity (70–76% vs 100% with PCR).

Herpes zoster affects 10% to 20% of the US population. It results from reactivation of latent herpes varicella-zoster (chickenpox) virus residing in dorsal root or cranial nerve ganglion cells. The virus migrates peripherally along axons into the skin. Two-thirds of the patients are older than 40 years of age. **Herpes zoster is contagious to those who have not had varicella or have not received the varicella vaccine.** Although shingles is not as contagious as chickenpox, it can be transmitted by contact with secretions from the vesicles. A patient with zoster can give chickenpox to a susceptible individual. A patient with chickenpox cannot give any other patient herpes zoster.

In addition to increasing age, other risk factors for reactivation of varicella zoster virus include conditions in which there is altered cell-mediated immunity, including diabetes, cancer, administration of immunosuppressive drugs (including corticosteroids), HIV, and organ transplantation. In immunocompetent patients, zoster is usually a self-limiting localized disease and heals within 3 to 4 weeks. Most patients can be reassured that their disease will abate without permanent problems. The incidence in immunocompromised patients is up to 10 times higher than in immunocompetent hosts, and usually their treatment must be more aggressive.

In immunocompromised patients, herpes zoster can become disseminated, with lesions appearing outside the primary dermatomes. Other significant complications can occur, including bacterial superinfection, aseptic meningitis, and visceral involvement, which is the most common cause of

Discussion continued

fatal outcomes. These patients generally require hospital admission for IV antiviral therapy.

The most common complication of herpes zoster is PHN (i.e., pain along cutaneous nerves, persisting >30 days after the lesions have healed). This is more likely to occur in older patients (≥60 years), those in whom the degree of skin surface involved is larger, and those with severe pain at time of presentation. Both the incidence and the duration of PHN are directly correlated with the patient's age; nearly half of patients 60 years of age or older will develop enduring neuropathic pain. Pain can persist for months and in some patients for many years and can be debilitating, with considerable physical and psychosocial morbidity.

The tricyclic antidepressant amitriptyline (Elavil) can be used to treat such pain. It can be started at 12.5 to 25 mg daily and increased by 12.5 to 25 mg every 3 to 5 days, to a maximum of 150 mg daily. The most common side effects are dry mouth, constipation, and sedation, which are generally not a major problem at the relatively low doses needed for effect (average dosage being 70 mg daily).

At present, there is not good evidence to support the preventative use of any agent to reduce the incidence of PHN. If this condition develops, treatment with amitriptyline or gabapentin (Neurontin; starting dose 100 mg three times a day) or pregabalin (Lyrica; 75 mg twice a day) can be initiated. Sometimes, PHN is severe enough to require opioid analgesics (morphine IR, starting at 7.5 mg every 4–6 hours as needed pain).

Topical treatment of PHN includes the relatively inexpensive capsaicin cream (Zostrix) 0.075%, which needs to be applied four times a day and can cause burning and stinging that usually subsides after the first week. An alternative is the more expensive 5% lidocaine patch (Lidoderm), which is applied to intact skin covering the most painful area. These topical treatments may be used to complement systemic analgesia.

Intrathecal methylprednisolone is an option for PHN patients with persistent pain.

It is interesting that most immunosuppressed individuals who develop zoster, even those with disseminated disease, do not develop PHN.

The new live attenuated varicella-zoster vaccine (Zostavax), which is a more powerful version of the vaccine currently given to children for chickenpox, is approved for adults age 60 years and older. It is expected to reduce the incidence of herpes zoster by about 50% and greatly reduce the severity and duration of the disease in those cases that do occur after vaccination. Its efficacy overall in preventing PHN was 67%. The Centers for Disease Control and Prevention considers Zostavax treatment to be protective for 5 years from administration.

Suggested Readings

Dworkin, R. H., Johnson, R. W., Breuer, J., et al. (2007). Recommendations for the management of herpes zoster. *Clinics in Infectious Disease, 44*(Suppl. 1), S1–S26.

Goh, C. L., & Khoo, L. (1998). A retrospective study on the clinical outcome of herpes zoster in patients with acyclovir or valaciclovir vs. patients not treated with antiviral. *International Journal of Dermatology, 37*, 544–546.

Herpes zoster vaccine (Zostavax). (2006). *The Medical Letter on Drugs and Therapeutics, 48*, 73–74.

Mounsey, A. L., Matthew, L. G., & Slawson, D. C. (2005). Herpes zoster and postherpetic neuralgia: Prevention and management. *American Family Physician, 72*, 1075–1080.

Pascuzzi, R. M. (2003). Peripheral neuropathies in clinical practice. *Medical Clinics of North America, 87*, 697–724.

Point of Care. (2019). *Herpes zoster infection (shingles)*. Amsterdam, Netherlands: Elsevier BV.

Rowbotham, M., Harden, N., Stacey, B., et al. (1998). Gabapentin for the treatment of postherpetic neuralgia: A randomized controlled trial. *Journal of the American Medical Association, 280*, 1837–1842.

Schmader, K. (2018). Herpes zoster. *Annals of Internal Medicine, 169*, ITC19–ITC31.

Shafran, S. D., Tyring, S. K., Ashton, R., et al. (2004). Once, twice, or three times daily famiciclovir compared with acyclovir for the oral treatment of herpes zoster in immunocompetent adults. *Journal of Clinical Virology, 29*, 248–253.

Tenser, R. B., & Dworkin, R. H. (2005). Herpes zoster and the prevention of postherpetic neuralgia: Beyond antiviral therapy. *Neurology, 65*, 340–350.

Thomas, S. L., & Hall, A. J. (2004). What does epidemiology tell us about risk factors for herpes zoster? *The Lancet Infectious Diseases, 4*, 26–33.

Hymenoptera (Bee, Wasp, Hornet) Envenomation

173

Presentation

Sometimes a patient comes to a hospital emergency department (ED) or urgent care center immediately after a painful sting because of alarm at the intensity of the pain or worry about developing a serious, life-threatening reaction. Sometimes the patient seeks help the next day because of swelling, redness, and itching. Parents may not be aware that their child was stung by a bee and may be concerned only about the local swelling.

The usual local reaction to a hymenopteran sting is immediate burning pain, followed by an intense local erythematous wheal, which usually subsides within several hours. Often there is a central punctate discoloration at the site of the sting or, uncommonly, a stinger may be protruding (only honeybees leave a stinger).

A more extensive delayed hypersensitivity reaction can occur, producing varying degrees of edema and induration, which can be quite dramatic when present on the face and may involve all of an arm or leg (Fig. 173.1). These local hypersensitivity reactions can last as long as 7 days. Tenderness and (occasionally) ascending lymphangitis can occur.

Symptoms of a severe anaphylactic reaction may include generalized urticaria, angioedema, generalized pruritus, shortness of breath, chest constriction, wheezing, stomach pain, nausea, vomiting, dizziness, hoarseness, thickened speech, inspiratory stridor, weakness, confusion, and feelings of impending doom or even loss of consciousness.

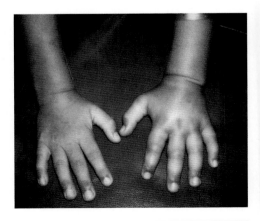

Fig. 173.1. Edema due to local reaction to bee sting.

What to Do

✓ **If an imbedded honeybee stinger is present** at the time the patient is stung, it is most important to remove the stinger quickly, even if it is grasped and pulled off, rather than delaying finding a hard edge to scrape it off with. The entire honeybee venom load is injected in less than 20 seconds. Because of regulation valves on the sting apparatus, the venom does not flow freely when the sting bulb is compressed.

✓ **Examine the patient for any signs of an immediate systemic allergic reaction (anaphylaxis)** such as decreased blood pressure, generalized urticaria or erythema, wheezing, tongue swelling, pharyngeal edema, or laryngeal spasm.

✓ **Treat any anaphylaxis findings aggressively—epinephrine is the keynote of these interventions.** Manage anaphylaxis with epinephrine, 0.3 to 0.5 mg intramuscularly (IM) (with severe reactions, every 10–20 minutes), airway support, and supplemental O_2. Intravenous (IV) fluids (20 mL/kg normal saline bolus infused rapidly) should also be used for hypotension, but epinephrine is the critical intervention. Adjunctive treatments with corticosteroids (e.g., methylprednisolone [Solu-Medrol], 0.2 mg/kg or 125 mg IV); antihistamines (e.g., diphenhydramine [Benadryl], 1–2 mg/kg, or 25–50 mg/dose IV); and an H_2 blocker (e.g., famotidine [Pepcid], 0.25 mg/kg or 20 mg IV) should be considered secondary and should not distract attention from repeated doses of epinephrine, which are often required for anaphylaxis secondary to these envenomations. Additionally, glucagon in patients with beta blockade (0.05 mg/kg, maximum 1 mg IV every 5–10 minutes) can be added if patients on beta blockers are not responding to epinephrine. Glucagon's catecholamine-like action occurs by directly increasing cellular cyclic adenosine monophosphate (cAMP).

✓ **Patients with milder generalized reactions** that rapidly clear after treatment with epinephrine, steroids, antihistamines, and H_2 blockers may be observed for 3 to 6 hours and released if their symptoms have completely cleared. Patients with more serious reactions or with recurrent signs and symptoms of anaphylaxis should be admitted to the hospital for continued treatment and further observation.

✓ **On discharge from acute care after an anaphylactic reaction, prescribe an epinephrine autoinjector to carry at all times (e.g., EpiPen, 0.3 mg; Epi Pen Jr, 0.15 mg) and refer the patient to an allergist for possible venom immunotherapy. There is no clear evidence to support use of a short course of steroids. For mild itching, patients can use antihistamines as needed** (see Chapter 185). Instruct patients on the use of epinephrine autoinjector and instruct them to return to the ED after its use. While subsequent reactions may reach the same intensity, it is rare for a subsequent reaction to be more severe than the original reaction.

✓ **Apply a cold pack to an acute sting to give pain relief and reduce swelling. Try ibuprofen or acetaminophen for analgesia.**

✓ **For a minor sting, give an oral antihistamine, such as diphenhydramine, 25 to 50 mg, or hydroxyzine (Atarax, Vistaril), 25 to 50 mg, to reduce subsequent itching.**

✓ **Prescribe additional antihistamine four times a day for further itching. A minor local reaction will also benefit from a topical steroid cream, such as hydrocortisone, 1% to 2.5%, or triamcinolone (Kenalog, Aristocort), 0.1% to 0.5%.**

✅ **For a severe local reaction with no contraindications, you may prescribe a systemic corticosteroid such as prednisone, 50 mg once daily for 3 to 4 days.** This is a common practice and a reasonable treatment, although steroids have no proven benefit. Be aware of common side effects from steroids: insomnia, agitation, some immune suppression, and a slightly higher incidence of tendon rupture.

✅ **Observe the patient with an acute sting for approximately 1 hour** to watch for the rare onset of delayed anaphylaxis. Delayed anaphylaxis can occur 2 to 6 hours after the stinging; therefore patients should be instructed to return with any generalized symptoms.

✅ **Reassure the patient who has come in after 12 to 24 hours** that anaphylaxis is no longer a potential problem.

✅ **Large, local reactions often have the appearance of cellulitis with swelling, erythema, and (on occasion) warmth and ascending lymphangitis. These reactions most often represent chemical cellulitis and are pruritic and nontender.** Reactions such as these do not require antibiotics but only supportive care with elevation, cooling compresses, and oral antihistamine therapy.

✅ **When there is delayed erythema, tenderness, and pain to suggest rare bacterial cellulitis** at a sting site, it is reasonable to treat the patient with an appropriate antibiotic such as cefadroxil (Duricef), 1 g once daily; cephalexin (Keflex), 500 mg three times a day; or doxycycline 100 mg twice a day 7 to 10 days.

✅ **Provide tetanus prophylaxis** as for a clean minor wound.

✅ **In all situations, if an extremity is involved, have the patient keep it elevated and instruct that the swelling may worsen if the hand or foot is held in a dependent position. Warn patients who have been recently stung that swelling and redness may increase over the next 24 to 48 hours** and may involve a large area and continue for several days. Preparing them for this potentially alarming development may prevent unnecessary worry and an unneeded revisit. Reassure them that even the worst swelling will resolve with time and elevation.

✅ **Promptly remove any rings distal to the sting** (see Chapter 152).

✅ **To help prevent future stings,** instruct patients to wear shoes and avoid wearing brightly colored clothing and using fragrances when outside, and to avoid recreational activities when yellowjackets or hornets are nearby. Hives and nests around a home should be exterminated, and good sanitation should be practiced, because garbage and outdoor food, especially canned drinks, attract yellowjackets. Unfortunately, insect repellents have little or no effect.

What Not to Do

❌ Do not send the patient with an acute sting home less than 1 hour after the sting.

❌ Do not apply heat, even if an infection is suspected—the swelling and discomfort will worsen.

❌ Do not prescribe the Epi-Pen or another anaphylaxis treatment for patients who have only had a localized reaction.

Discussion

Forty to 50 people in the United States die from identified hymenopteran sting anaphylaxis each year where 4% of the population is susceptible to systemic allergic sting reactions. Beekeepers or their relatives have the highest risk of being sensitized.

Only stinging insects of the Hymenoptera order cause anaphylaxis with any frequency. A sting is an injection of venom by the female of each species through a modified ovipositor. Honeybees and bumblebees are relatively nonaggressive and generally sting only when caught underfoot. The barbs along the shaft of the honeybee stinger cause it to remain embedded at the sting site. Africanized honeybees have expanded northward and are present in most of Florida, Texas, and Arizona and southern areas of Nevada, California, and New Mexico. Referred to as "killer bees," they do not have increased venom potency or allergenicity but rather a tendency to attack en masse. Fortunately, even massive stinging incidents of 50 to 100 stings are not usually fatal. Most deleterious effects are estimated to occur in the range of 500 to 1200 stings. Older victims are more susceptible to the toxic effects of the venom.

The family Vespidae includes hornets and wasps, which make papier-mâché–like nests of wood fiber, as do the yellowjackets. Yellowjackets, which cause most of the allergic sting reactions in the United States, usually nest in the ground or in decaying logs. Hornets build teardrop-shaped nests that hang in trees or bushes. Both yellowjackets and hornets are extremely aggressive, especially in the late summer when crowded conditions develop in the nests. Not quite as aggressive as the other vespids, the thin-bodied paper wasps build nests in the eaves of buildings.

Hymenopteran venoms contain a number of interesting constituents. Most of the venoms contain histamine, dopamine, acetylcholine, and kinins, which cause the characteristics of burning and pain. The allergens in the venoms are mostly proteins with enzyme activity.

Systemic allergic reactions (anaphylaxis) may be mild with only cutaneous symptoms (pruritus, urticaria, and angioedema of the eyes, lips, hands) or severe with potentially life-threatening symptoms of laryngeal edema, bronchospasm, and hypotension. Systemic allergic reactions are, in general, less severe in children than adults, although children are more likely to develop isolated cutaneous reactions.

Large local reactions are usually late-phase IgE-mediated allergic reactions with severe swelling developing over 24 to 48 hours and resolving in 2 to 7 days.

Bee stings by themselves are very painful and frightening. **There are many misconceptions about the danger of bee stings**, and many patients with previous localized reactions have been instructed unnecessarily to report to an ED or clinic immediately after being stung. **Patients who have suffered only localized hypersensitivity reactions in the past are not at a significantly greater risk than the general public for developing anaphylaxis, which is defined as an immediate generalized reaction.** Other than some relief of pain and itching for the acute sting, there is little more than reassurance to offer these patients.

Anaphylactic reactions generally occur within a few minutes to 1 hour after the sting. Most victims have no history of bee sting allergy.

Patients with a history of systemic sting reactions have been found on average to have a 50% risk for experiencing another systemic reaction to a challenge sting. Some patients who do not react to a first sting challenge react to a subsequent sting. Systemic reactions usually do not become progressively more severe with each sting. Often, the stinging insect allergy is self-limited. The risk for reaction declines from more than 50% initially to 35% by 3 to 5 years after the sting reaction, to approximately 25% by 10 years or more after the sting reaction. In some instances, unfortunately, the risk for anaphylaxis persists for decades, even with no intervening stings.

Patients with a history of systemic reactions should carry a kit containing injectable epinephrine and chewable antihistamines to be used at the first sign of a generalized reaction.

Venom-specific immunotherapy for hymenopteran allergy can markedly reduce the risk for repeat systemic reaction approximately 30% to 60%. Patients who have had extensive local reactions, but not general ones, tend to react the same way to subsequent stings despite venom immunotherapy.

Although at times it may seem most prudent to treat ascending lymphangitis with an antibiotic, it should be realized that after a bee sting, the resultant local cellulitis and lymphangitis are usually chemically mediated inflammatory reactions and are not affected by antibiotic therapy.

Suggested Readings

Anchor, J., & Settipane, R. A. (2004). Appropriate use of epinephrine in anaphylaxis. *American Journal of Emergency Medicine*, *22*, 488–490.

Chiu, A. M., & Kelly, K. J. (2005). Anaphylaxis: Drug allergy, insect stings, and latex. *Immunology and Allergy Clinics of North America*, *25*, 389–405.

Graft, D. F. (2006). Insect sting allergy. *Medical Clinics of North America*, *90*, 211–232.

Simons, F. E. (2010). Anaphylaxis. *The Journal of Allergy and Clinical Immunology*, *125*, S161–S181.

Visscher, P. K., Vetter, R. S., & Camazine, S. (1996). Removing bee stings. *Lancet*, *348*, 301–302.

Warrell, D. A. (2019). Venomous bites, stings, and poisoning. *Infectious Disease Clinics of North America*, *33*(1), 17–38.

Impetigo

Presentation

Parents will usually bring their children (most commonly aged 2–5 years, although it can occur in any age group) to be checked because they are developing unsightly skin lesions. **The lesions are usually painless but may be pruritic and are found most often on the face** (Fig. 174.1) or other exposed areas. Parents may be worried that their young child has "infant-tigo," the common lay eggcorn for this condition. **Nonbullous lesions** consist of irregular or somewhat circular red oozing erosions (sores), often **covered with a yellow-brown honeylike crust** (Fig. 174.2). These may be surrounded by smaller erythematous macular or vesiculopustular areas. **Bullous lesions** (Fig. 174.3) present as large thin-walled bullae, which quickly rupture and are replaced by a thin, shiny, varnishlike coating over the denuded area on an erythematous base. More than one area may be involved, and a mix of bullous and nonbullous findings can exist. Generally, there is an absence of surrounding erythema.

What to Do

✅ **For a few lesions involving a relatively small area, prescribe mupirocin 2% (Bactroban) cream or ointment to be applied to the rash two to three times a day for 5 to 10 days.** This may be covered with a sterile gauze dressing. Have parents soften and cleanse crusts with warm soapy compresses before applying the antibiotic cream or ointment. There is little scientific evidence regarding the value of any disinfecting measures, such as the use of povidone-iodine

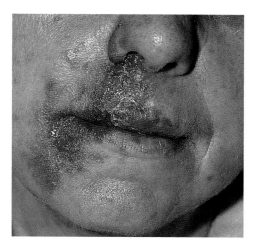

Fig. 174.1 Impetigo of the face. (From White, G., & Cox, N. [2006]. *Diseases of the skin* [2nd ed.]. St. Louis, MO: Mosby.)

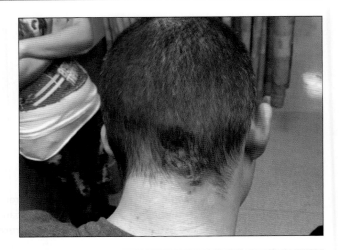

Fig. 174.2 Kerion with surrounding impetigo.

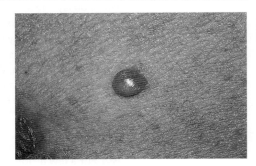

Fig. 174.3 Bullous impetigo. (From White, G., & Cox, N. [2006]. *Diseases of the skin* [2nd ed.]. St. Louis, MO: Mosby.)

and chlorhexidine. A newer antibiotic, retapamulin (Altabax) (ointment 1%, apply twice a day for 5 days), was approved by the US Food and Drug Administration (FDA) in 2007 and, although expensive, appears to be effective even against methicillin-resistant *Staphylococcus aureus* (MRSA) strains.

✅ **For large areas of involvement or resistant cases, add an oral antibiotic with activity against *S. aureus* and group A beta-hemolytic streptococcal infections:** cephalexin (Keflex), 250 to 500 mg three to four times a day (25–50 mg/kg/day); dicloxacillin, 250 to 500 mg four times a day (25–50 mg/kg/day divided every 6 hours) for 7 days. For those with allergies to penicillin or cephalosporins, consider erythromycin (base), 250 mg four times a day (40 mg/kg/day divided every 8 hours). **In communities where community-acquired MRSA (CA-MRSA) is** prevalent, prescribe trimethoprim/sulfamethoxazole (Bactrim, Septra), 160 mg TMP twice daily (8–10 mg/kg/day divided every 12 hours) for 7 days, or clindamycin (Cleocin), 150 to 300 mg four times a day (10–30 mg/kg/day divided every 8 hours) for 7 days. Alternative options should be based on local susceptibility results.

✅ **Consider obtaining cultures if CA-MRSA is prevalent in your area.**

✅ **Impetigo is a highly contagious infectious disease.**

(✓) **To prevent the spread of this infection**, have the patient and family wash their hands frequently, change towels and bed linens every day, and keep infected schoolchildren home until the acute phase has cleared (for 1–2 days after antimicrobial therapy starts; 3 days when contact activities are involved).

(✓) Nasal carriage of *S. aureus* has been implicated as a source of **recurrent disease** and can be reduced by the topical application of mupirocin within the nares twice daily for 5 days (nasal ointment 2%).

(✓) **In patients with a history of atopic dermatitis**, assess for evidence of disseminated bullous impetigo, which needs systemic antibiotics.

What Not to Do

(✗) Do not use bacitracin, neomycin, or similar antibacterial ointments on these lesions. They are less effective than mupirocin and may cause unnecessary contact dermatitis.

Discussion

Impetigo is a common superficial skin infection that is mostly seen during the summer in temperate climates and throughout the year in warm, humid tropical regions worldwide.

Nonbullous impetigo was historically thought to be a group A streptococcal process, and bullous impetigo was primarily thought to be caused by *S. aureus*. Studies now indicate that both forms of impetigo are primarily caused by *S. aureus*, with *Streptococcus* usually being involved in the nonbullous form. Bullous impetigo is always caused by *Staphylococcus aureus*.

If the infection is a toxin-producing phage group II type 71 *Staphylococcus* (the same toxin seen in scalded skin syndrome), large bullae will form as the toxin produces intradermal cleavage. Otherwise, smaller bullae develop, and the honey-crusted lesions predominate.

Diagnosis is determined by history and physical examination; cultures are advisable if identification of causative agent is essential (e.g., persistent or recurrent infection).

Impetigo is thought to be self-limiting, but studies on its natural history do not exist. It may resolve over 2 to 3 weeks if untreated.

It is thought that antibiotic treatment does not alter the subsequent low incidence of **secondary glomerulonephritis**, especially in children aged 2 to 6 years. Presenting signs and symptoms of glomerulonephritis include edema and hypertension; about one-third of patients have smoky or tea-colored urine.

Impetigo is very contagious among infants and young children and may be associated with poor hygiene, a break in the skin, or predisposing skin eruptions, such as herpes simplex, angular cheilitis, insect bites, scabies, and atopic and contact dermatitis. When lesions occur singly, they may be mistaken for herpes simplex. *S. aureus* can directly invade the skin and cause a de novo infection.

Suggested Readings

Bass, J. W., Chan, D. S., Creamer, K. M., et al. (1997). Comparison of oral cephalexin, topical mupirocin, and topical bacitracin for treatment of impetigo. *The Pediatric Infectious Disease Journal, 16*, 708–710.

Hartman-Adams, H., Banvard, C., & Juckett, G. (2014). Impetigo: Diagnosis and treatment. *American Family Physician, 15*, 229–235.

Iyer, S., & Jones, D. H. (2004). Community-acquired methicillin-resistant *Staphylococcus aureus* skin infection. *Journal of the American Academy of Dermatology, 50,* 854–858.

McVicar, J. (1999). Oral or topical antibiotics for impetigo. *Journal of Accident & Emergency Medicine, 16,* 364.

Point of Care. (2019). *Impetigo.* Amsterdam, Netherlands: Elsevier BV.

Sanfilippo, A. M., Barrio, V., & Kulp-Shorten, C. (2003). Common pediatric and adolescent skin conditions. *Journal of Pediatric and Adolescent Gynecology, 16,* 269–283.

Partial-Thickness (Second-Degree) Burns and Tar Burns

Presentation

Partial-thickness burns can occur in a variety of ways. Spilled or splattered hot water and grease are among the most common causes, along with hot objects, explosive fumes, and burning (volatile) liquids. The patient will complain of excruciating pain, and the burn will appear erythematous with vesicle formation. Some of these vesicles or bullae may have ruptured before the patient's arrival, whereas others may not develop for 24 hours. Tar burns are special in that the tar adheres aggressively to the burned skin and therefore makes the burns difficult to evaluate and very unsightly.

What to Do

⊘ **To stop the pain, immediately cover the burned area with sterile towels that have been soaked in iced normal saline, or just use cold tap water.** Continue irrigating the burn with the iced or cold solution for the next 20 to 30 minutes or until the patient can remain comfortable without the cold compresses.

⊘ **Complete a primary survey for trauma with attention to airway, breathing, and circulation before performing a nuanced and distracting evaluation of the burns.**

⊘ **Determine the mechanism of injury and the extent and severity of the burn.** The patient's palm represents approximately 1% of total body surface area and can be used to estimate the total area burned. **Consider transfer to a burn center** and start fluid resuscitation if there are third-degree (full-thickness) burns over 5% of the total body surface, second-degree (partial-thickness) burns alone or in combination with third-degree burns of over 15% of the total body surface (or 5–10% in children <10 years of age), or extensive burns involving the face, hands, feet, joints, or genitalia.

⊘ **Consider and report any burn injuries suggestive of child abuse.** A supposed mechanism of injury that does not fit the injury or is not consistent with the child's level of development warrants investigation. Specific injuries that should trigger consideration for reporting include burns to the face, dorsum of the feet, or genitalia; cigarette burns; imprint burns such as those from a hot iron or grill; stockinglike burns with a sharp line of demarcation from immersion in hot water; or any burns to the extremities that are circumferential or symmetric.

⊘ **Provide the patient with any necessary tetanus prophylaxis.**

⊘ **Administer potent pain medication (e.g., morphine, fentanyl) as required.**

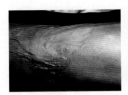

Fig. 175.1 Open second-degree burn bullae may be left in place as a physiologic burn dressing.

✅ **When the pain has subsided, with burns having intact vesicles,** gently cleanse the area with dilute (1%) betadine solution, or **if bullae or vesicles are open**, gently cleanse with plain normal saline.

✅ The providers participating in débridement and wound dressing should wear sterile gowns, gloves, and masks, generally following universal precautions for wound care.

✅ **If the bullae or vesicles are not perforated,** there is some controversy over whether they should be left intact. **With small burns** patients can be sent home to continue cold compresses for comfort. Otherwise, these vesicles should be protected from rupture and contamination with a bulky sterile dressing.

✅ **Once ruptured** (Fig. 175.1), **open bullae or vesicles that are fresh and clean should be cleansed with normal saline and, when possible, the detached epithelium can be easily pulled back into its original position to cover the burn surface and then left in place as a physiologic burn dressing.** This area should then be covered with a standard sterile burn dressing to hold this thin layer of epithelium in place and absorb any leaking plasma. This dressing will also protect the burn from contamination as well as provide comfort.

✅ **Bullae or vesicles that are open and contaminated, old, or whose walls are so friable and damaged that they cannot be used as a biologic burn dressing should be completely débrided. Then the burn surface should be flushed with saline.** Using fine scissors and forceps, strip away any of this loose epithelium from the burn. A dressing should then be applied (see later).

✅ **For small clean burns that have been débrided, covering them with a transparent film of polyurethane with an adhesive coating (OpSite, Bioclusive, Tegaderm) provides a moist environment that enhances reepithelization and is comfortable.** There needs to be intact skin surrounding the area being dressed so that the dressing will adhere. Exudate collects under these film dressings and frequently leaks out. An outer absorbent dressing with dressing changes is required when this occurs. The synthetic film is left in place.

✅ **For larger débrided areas, a simple dressing with oil emulsion gauze (Adaptic) covered with sterile fluffed gauze is an effective acceptable burn dressing. A soft silicone dressing (Mepitel, Mölnlycke Healthcare) can also be applied directly to the burn, with an overlying absorbent sterile dressing that will provide adequate padding to exclude voids beneath this polyamide net.** Mepitel may be left in place for up to 7 to 10 days, but the outer absorbent layer should be changed more frequently as required.

✅ Although unnecessary for most superficial partial-thickness burns in outpatients, silver sulfadiazine (Silvadene) cream was traditionally commonly used to cover open burn wounds. When this cream is used, it is only necessary to provide an absorbent protective gauze dressing over the burn area (without Adaptic); alternatively, the area can be left open and gently washed twice daily, followed by reapplication of the cream.

✅ **For greater patient convenience, but greater expense, an alternative to silver sulfadiazine cream is to use a silver-impregnated dressing (Acticoat), which is occlusive, promotes a moist healing environment, and eliminates the need for frequent dressing changes.** The Acticoat dressing is placed on the wound and is kept moist by applying sterile water, which activates the release of the silver ions into the wound. An outer layer of plain gauze bandage can be used to protect the wound and keep the Acticoat in place. The Acticoat dressing does not require changing more frequently than every 3 days.

✓ **Biobrane collagen Silastic is an alternative synthetic dressing that is designed to be placed tightly against the wound with a compressive gauze dressing wrapped over it.** Within 2 days, as long as the wound is clean and has no seroma formation, the collagen side of the dressing adheres to the surface of the burn and effectively seals it. The dressing acts as a skin substitute and allows the underlying skin to heal and reepithelialize more comfortably. Biobrane may be left in place for 1 month.

✓ **Dressings in general** are used to absorb secretions, protect the burn from bacterial contamination, and prevent the wound from rubbing against clothing or other objects. When simple sterile dressings are used with Adaptic gauze or Mepitel, the frequency of dressing changes will vary depending on the amount of secretions. When Silvadene cream is used, washing and reapplication require that the dressing be changed once daily. **The first dressing change should be done at a return visit to provide teaching instructions and additional dressing material.** If available, continued burn management can be provided at a local burn clinic.

✓ **Facial and neck burns cannot be easily dressed and generally require only the soothing topical application of bacitracin ointment.** These burns will do well without any topical agents and require only gentle washing with a mild soap twice a day.

✓ **Tar burns do not require removal of solidified residual tar. The tar is not toxic to the skin and often forms a sterile wound dressing. By covering the burn and tar with bacitracin ointment and performing daily washing and repeated dressing changes with more ointment, the tar will gradually dissolve away.** Neomycin sulfate/polymyxin ointment (Neosporin) has been recommended as a preferred tar emulsifier, but it carries the potential of causing allergic contact dermatitis. When tar burns on the face are unsightly, the hardened tar can usually be mechanically débrided or cleaned off with repeated applications of creams or ointments. Petrolatum jelly (Vaseline), butter, or mineral oil can also be used to slowly wipe away the tar. The facial burns are then treated like any other facial burn.

✓ **Car radiator and brief flash burns of the face,** such as when patients attempt to light a gas stove, are not associated with inhalation injuries (even with singed facial hair) and are also treated in the standard manner.

✓ Patients should be instructed to keep extremity burns elevated to reduce swelling.

✓ When necessary, prescribe adequate opioid analgesics to provide adequate pain relief over the next 24 hours.

✓ Patients can be reassured that superficial partial-thickness burns will generally heal in 7 to 21 days with full function, and, unless there are complications (such as infection), patients do not have to worry about scarring. Most superficial burns heal within 3 weeks, and long-term follow-up is unnecessary.

What Not to Do

✗ Do not use large ice-containing packs or compresses that might increase tissue damage. Iced compresses should also be avoided on large burns (>15% of total body surface) because they may lead to problems with hypothermia. When pain cannot be controlled with compresses, use strong parenteral analgesics such as morphine sulfate.

(X) Do not provide prophylactic systemic antibiotics. They have not been shown to reduce the incidence of wound infection and are generally not indicated.

(X) Do not use neomycin-containing creams or ointments when avoidable. They have the potential to cause a very unpleasant allergic contact dermatitis.

(X) Do not confuse partial-thickness burns with full-thickness burns. With full-thickness burns, there is no sensory function or skin appendages, such as hair follicles, remaining. They do not form vesicles and may have evidence of thrombosed vessels. If areas of full-thickness burn are present or suspected, seek surgical consultation because these areas will later require skin grafting.

(X) Do not discharge patients with suspected respiratory burns or extensive burns of the hands, feet, or genitalia. These patients require special inpatient observation and management.

(X) Do not use caustic solvents in an attempt to remove tar from burns. It is unnecessary and painful and will cause further tissue destruction.

(X) Do not use synthetic dressings on old or contaminated burns, which have a high risk for infection.

Discussion

The ideal burn dressing is one that promotes wound healing at a rapid pace, minimizes pain during dressing change, absorbs excessive exudate, controls bacterial burden, and prevents any local or systemic adverse reactions.

There are numerous types of dressings for partial-thickness burns. Silver sulfadiazine (SSD) cream has been widely used since the 1960s to prevent wound infection. However, recent studies have shown that SSD has a damaging effect on regenerating keratinocytes and delays wound healing. In addition, traditional dressings with SSD require daily dressing changes that adhere to the wound causing a disruption in the granulation process. There is limited evidence to support the superiority of SSD compared to placebo or nonantibiotic controls (such as wet gauze) in improving wound healing or reepithelialization rates.

Most foam dressings are impregnated with silver (Ag), as this element has been shown to decrease the tissue bacterial bioburden and potentially accelerate wound healing. Despite the growing number of silver-containing dressings for a variety of wounds (burns, chronic ulcers, etc.), the evidence

supporting their clinical use in burn patients is not based on solid evidence.

In another study the authors concluded that nano silver–containing foam dressings were more efficacious for reepithelialization, healing, ease of application, and tolerance when compared to silver-nanoparticle gel and collagen dressings in the treatment of partial-thickness burns. All the dressings were found to be safe and comparable in cost and scar quality.

First-degree or superficial burns involve only the epidermis. These burns are usually painful and erythematous and do not blister. The pain usually resolves in 1 to 2 days and generally does not require anything more than cool compresses. These burns usually occur with brief contact with hot liquids.

Second-degree or partial-thickness burns involve the epidermis and portions of the dermis. Damaged dermal vessels leak serum into the stratum spinosum layer of the epidermis, forming the identifiable blisters or bullae. These burns are particularly painful. They heal spontaneously by reepithelization within 10 to 14 days, providing that no infection occurs.

Discussion continued

Third-degree or full-thickness burns involve all layers of the epidermis and dermis. These burns take on a "waxy white" appearance, and, with prolonged heat exposure, the skin takes on a yellow-brown "leathery" appearance. These burns are painless because of the damaged nerve endings, but the penumbra of partial-thickness burns may still cause the patient to have significant pain.

Simple partial-thickness burns will do well with nothing more than cleansing, débridement, and a sterile dressing. All other therapy, therefore, should be directed at making the patient more comfortable. Silvadene cream is not always necessary or recommended, but it is soothing. Bacitracin ointment may also be used on small burns and burns in areas with good perfusion (i.e. face).

When it is possible to leave vesicles intact, the patient will have a shorter period of disability and will require fewer dressing changes and follow-up visits. Studies suggest that leaving the burn blisters intact results in more rapid reepithelization than when the blisters are debrided.

If the wound must be débrided, the closed-dressing technique may be more convenient and less of a mess than the open technique of washings and cream applications.

Some physicians believe that it is important to remove all traces of tar from a burn. Removal can be accomplished relatively easily by using a petroleum-based antibiotic ointment such as bacitracin, which will dissolve the tar. This can be mixed with an equal amount of Unibase (ingredients: water, cetyl alcohol, stearyl alcohol, white petrolatum, glycerin, sodium citrate, sodium laurel sulfate, propylparaben). Others have found the citrus-and–petroleum distillate industrial cleanser Medi-Sol (Orange-Sol, Chandler, AZ) effective, as well as nontoxic and nonirritating. Other effective solvents include polysorbate and Tween 80. **It should be emphasized that aggressive measures to remove the tar are unnecessary.**

It is interesting to note that raw honey has been used as a successful burn dressing for centuries. One study demonstrated that honey was actually better than Silvadene for superficial burns.

Suggested Readings

American College of Surgeons. (2006). Guidelines for the operation of burn centers. In *Resources for optimal care of the injured patient* (pp. 79–86). Chicago, IL: ACS.

Chaganti, P., Gordon, I., Chao, J., et al. (2019). A systematic review of foam dressings for partial thickness burns. *American Journal of Emergency Medicine, 37*(6), 1184–1190.

Erring, M., Gaba, S., Mohsina, S., et al. (2019). Comparison of efficacy of silver-nanoparticle gel, nano-silver-foam and collagen dressings in treatment of partial thickness burn wounds. *Burns, 45*(8), 1888–1894.

Gotschall, C. S., Morrison, M. I., & Eichelberger, M. R. (1998). Prospective, randomized study of the efficacy of Mepitel on children with partial-thickness scalds. *Journal of Burn Care & Rehabilitation, 19*, 279–283.

Griffin, B. R., Frear, C. C., Babl, F., Oakley, E., & Kimble, R. M. (2020). Cool running water first aid decreases skin grafting requirements in pediatric burns: A cohort study of two thousand four hundred ninety-five children. *Annals of Emergency Medicine, 75*(1), 75–85.

Levy, D. B., Barone, J. A., York, J. M., et al. (1986). Unibase and triple antibiotic ointment for hardened tar removal. *Annals of Emergency Medicine, 15*, 765–766.

Lionelli, G. T., & Lawrence, W. T. (2003). Wound dressings. *Surgical Clinics of North America, 83*, 617–638.

Stratta, R. J., Saffle, J. R., Kravitz, M., et al. (1983). Management of tar and asphalt injuries. *The American Journal of Surgery, 146*, 766–769.

Subrahmanyam, M. (1998). A prospective randomized clinical and histological study of superficial burn wound healing with honey and silver sulfadiazine. *Burns, 24*, 157–161.

Pediculosis

(Lice, Crabs)

Presentation

Patients arrive with emotions ranging from annoyance to sheer disgust at the discovery of an infestation with lice or crabs and request acute medical care. There may be extreme pruritus, and the patient may bring in a sample of the creature to show you. Head lice generally affect children aged 3 to 12 years.

The adult forms of head lice (*Pediculus humanus capitis*) can be very difficult to find, but their oval, light gray eggs (nits) can be readily found firmly attached to the hairs above the ears and toward the occiput. Secondary impetigo and furunculosis can occur.

The adult forms of pubic lice (*Pthirus pubis* or crab lice) are more easily found, but their light yellow-gray color still makes them difficult to see. Small black dots present in infested areas represent either ingested blood in adult lice or their excreta. Maculae ceruleae (bluish-brown macules), which represent intradermal hemorrhage at sites where lice have fed, can sometimes be found. Pubic lice are not limited to the pubic region and may be found on other short hairs of the body, such as body hair, eyebrows, and eyelashes (pediculosis ciliaris).

Identification of lice or viable nits with a magnifying glass makes the diagnosis (Fig. 176.1).

What to Do

✔ **For head lice, instruct the patient and other close contacts regarding the use of nonprescription louse treatments. The most effective is 1% permethrin (Nix), which should be applied undiluted to clean, towel-dried hair until the affected area is entirely wet. After 10 minutes, shampoo and rinse with warm water.** It is not necessary to remove nits. To kill newly hatched nymphs, a second treatment should be given 7 to 10 days later.

✔ **Itching or mild burning of the scalp** caused by inflammation of the skin in response to topical therapeutic agents can persist for many days after lice are killed, and the condition is not a reason for retreatment. Topical corticosteroids and oral antihistamines may be beneficial for relieving these signs and symptoms.

✔ A second over-the-counter (OTC) choice is a preparation combining piperonyl butoxide and pyrethrin extracts (RID), which is applied in the same fashion. This product does not kill all of the unhatched eggs and has no residual activity, is less effective, and is more allergenic than permethrin.

✔ **For severe or resistant infestations, combining 1% permethrin treatment with oral trimethoprim/sulfamethoxazole (TMP/SMX), 5 mg/kg twice a day for 10 days, will have a higher cure rate than permethrin alone at 4 weeks (93% vs. 72%).** TMP/SMX is not toxic to the louse; instead, it acts by killing essential bacterial flora in the insect's gastrointestinal tract.

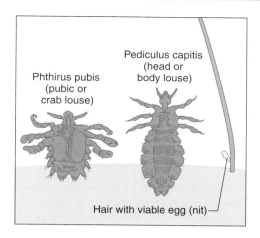

Phthirus pubis
(pubic or
crab louse)

Pediculus capitis
(head or
body louse)

Hair with viable egg (nit)

Fig. 176.1 Lice and nits.

As lice have become resistant to OTC treatments, some clinicians have had to escalate to prescription-strength 5% permethrin cream (Elimite) applied to clean, dry hair and left on overnight (8–14 hours) under a shower cap. Resistance still occurs even at these higher concentrations of permethrin.

Benzyl alcohol lotion 5% (Ulesfia, Sciele Pharma, Atlanta, GA) is a prescription medicine that was approved by the US Food and Drug Administration (FDA) in April 2009 for treatment of head lice in children older than 6 months. The product is not neurotoxic and kills head lice by asphyxiation. Patients receive two 10-minute treatments 1 week apart, but consideration should be given to retreating in 9 days or using three treatment cycles (days 0, 7, and 13–15).

Resistant infestations with treatment failures are most commonly treated with the prescription formula of malathion (Ovide) 0.5% lotion. Apply it to dry hair and then shampoo. It may be reapplied 7 to 9 days later if necessary. Although a lengthy application time is specified on the product's label (8–12 hours), a recent study found that malathion 0.5% was 98% effective with just one or two 20-minute applications. Because of potential flammability, patients should be instructed to avoid using a hair dryer or curling iron during treatment with malathion. Malathion can only be used in people who are 24 months of age or older, when resistance to permethrin or pyrethrins is documented, or when treatment with these products fails despite their correct use.

Spinosad is a topical suspension derived from bacterial fermentation products that causes nervous system excitation, paralysis, and death of lice and eggs. It is appropriate for use on resistant infestations but is expensive.

Removal of all topical pediculicides should be accomplished by rinsing the hair over a sink rather than in the shower or bath. This limits skin exposure. Using warm rather than hot water will minimize absorption attributable to vasodilation.

For head lice that are resistant to all other treatments, give a single oral dose of ivermectin (Stromectol), 200 to 400 µg/kg, repeated once after 7 to 10 days. Most recently, a single oral dose of 400 µg/kg repeated in 7 days has been shown to be more effective than 0.5% malathion lotion. Ivermectin should not be used for children who weigh less than 15 kg.

Instruct families to disinfect sheets and clothing by machine washing in hot water, machine drying on the hot cycle for 20 minutes, ironing, dry cleaning, or just storing in plastic bags for 2 weeks. Combs and brushes should be soaked in 2% Lysol or heated in water to about 65 °C for 10 minutes.

✅ **Nit removal is recommended for aesthetic reasons and can help identify if there is a later recurrence.** Removal of the eggs is not necessary to prevent spreading the infestation. Application of a 1:1 solution of white vinegar and water may help to loosen nits before removal with a fine-toothed comb.

✅ **Pubic lice are most commonly sexually transmitted, so sexual contacts must also be treated. In addition, this finding should prompt an evaluation for other sexually transmitted diseases.**

✅ **Treatment is the same as that for pediculosis capitis, with the exception that pediculosis of the eyelashes should be treated with an occlusive ophthalmic ointment applied to the eyelid margins** for 10 days.

✅ **Patients often want to use "natural," less toxic products or techniques for their children or themselves.** Some occlusive products, such as petroleum jelly (Vaseline), mayonnaise, and olive oil, have been used in place of traditional pediculicides, but their effectiveness has not been established in controlled trials. One OTC product, HairClean 1-2-3, consisting of anise oil, ylang ylang oil, coconut oil, and isopropyl alcohol, was more effective than 1% permethrin in an uncontrolled study.

✅ A "nonneurotoxic" suffocation-based pediculicide ("Nuvo lotion," which is actually Cetaphil Gentle Skin Cleanser) produced a high cure rate in children with head lice in one small nonblinded study.

✅ The LiceGuard Robi Comb is a fine-toothed metal comb that is electrified by a single AA battery. When used on dry hair for 5 to 10 minutes daily for 2 weeks, it is said to eliminate head lice by essentially electrocuting them. No trials have been performed.

✅ **When cosmetically acceptable, head shaving is effective.**

✅ **When one is facing a persistent case of lice, several explanations must be considered,** including misdiagnosis, noncompliance with treatment protocol, reinfestation, lack of adequate ovicidal properties of the treatment product, and resistance to the pediculicide. All household members should be checked for lice, but only those with live lice, or eggs within 1 cm of the scalp, should be treated.

What Not to Do

❌ Do not mistake a hair cast for a nit (which is firmly attached to a hair shaft). Hair casts are freely movable along the hair shaft.

❌ Do not apply pediculicides to wet hair. Water dilutes the product and protects lice, as they reflexively close their respiratory spiracles when exposed to water.

❌ Do not recommend comprehensive cleaning of the whole house. Adult lice cannot survive for more than 1 day if they cannot find a meal of blood.

❌ Do not have the family use commercial sprays (R&C Spray or Li-Ban Spray) to control lice on inanimate objects. Their use is no more effective than vacuuming.

❌ Do not prescribe lindane (Kwell) shampoo. It is an organochloride compound that is absorbed and can be toxic to the central nervous system and cause anemia. In view of reports of lindane resistance and the availability of products with more favorable safety profiles, it is no longer recommended.

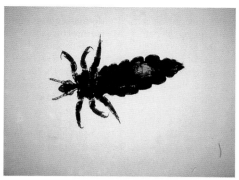

Fig. 176.2 Identifying characteristics of a head louse. (Adapted from Ko, C. J., & Elston, D. M. [2004]. Pediculosis. *Journal of the American Academy of Dermatology, 50, 1–12.*)

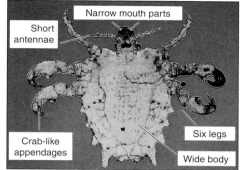

Fig. 176.3 Identifying characteristics of crab louse. (Adapted from Ko, C. J., & Elston, D. M. [2004]. Pediculosis. *Journal of the American Academy of Dermatology, 50, 1–12.*)

 Do not use flammable or toxic substances such as gasoline or kerosene.

 Do not use products intended for animal use.

Discussion

Blood-sucking lice have long been successful obligate parasites of humans. The three major lice that infest humans are *Pediculus humanus capitis* (head louse) (Fig. 176.2), *Pthirus pubis* (crab louse) (Fig. 176.3), and *Pediculus humanus humanus* (body louse). Patients with louse infestation present with pruritus, excoriations, and lymphadenopathy. A hypersensitivity rash, or pediculid, may mimic a viral exanthem.

Head lice infestation crosses all economic and social boundaries. The head louse is the size of a sesame seed, 1 to 2 mm in length. After attaching to the patient, the louse inserts its mouth parts and injects saliva with vasodilatory properties. An inflammatory reaction to injected louse saliva has been suggested as the most likely cause of bite reactions. Transmission in most cases occurs by direct contact with the head of another infested individual. Head lice move by grasping hairs, generally remaining close to the scalp. Head lice can crawl rapidly, traveling up to 23 cm/min. Lice egg cases are referred to as nits. They are firmly cemented to human hair and are thus difficult to remove (Fig. 176.4). Except in very humid climates, lice lay nits (ova within a chitinous case) within 1 to 2 mm of the scalp. Young lice hatch within 1 week and pass through three nymphal stages, maturing to adults over a period of 1 week. Lice must generally

eat every 4 to 6 hours. In most climates, they survive only several hours off the scalp, although they may live for up to 4 days in favorable conditions. In the United States, Blacks have a lower incidence of infestation, possibly because lice are better adapted to grasp the more cylindrical hairs of Whites or Asians.

The diagnosis of head lice is definitive when crawling lice are seen in the scalp hair or are combed from the scalp. Because head lice avoid light and can crawl quickly, the use of louse combs increases the chances of finding live lice. Nits alone are not diagnostic of active infestation, but if the nits are within 1 cm (0.25 inch) of the scalp, active infestation is likely. Hair casts may closely resemble nits stuck to hair shafts. A parent, teacher, or school nurse generally notices them and mistakes them for nits. In contrast to nits, hair casts are freely movable along the hair shaft. Among presumed "lice" and "nits" submitted by physicians, nurses, teachers, and parents to a laboratory for identification, many were found to be artifacts such as dandruff, hairspray droplets, scabs, dirt, or other insects (e.g., aphids blown by the wind and caught in the hair).

The female head louse lives about 3 to 4 weeks and lays approximately 10 eggs a day. The eggs are incubated by body heat and hatch in 7 to 10

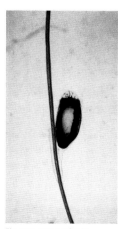

Fig. 176.4 Lice nit firmly cemented to human hair. (Adapted from Ko, C. J., & Elston, D. M. [2004]. Pediculosis. *Journal of the American Academy of Dermatology, 50, 1–12.*)

days. If newly hatched eggs that survived the initial therapy are not retreated, the cycle may repeat itself every 3 weeks. Although there is no proven transmission from fomites, such as brushes, hats, combs, linens, and stuffed animals, head lice and ova have been found on such items; therefore it is probably expedient to eradicate these lice by vacuuming, washing, dry cleaning, or isolating items in sealed plastic bags for 2 weeks. Lice do not hop, jump, or fly. No healthy child should be excluded from or allowed to miss school time because of head lice. "No nit" policies for return to school should be discouraged. Children may return to school after initial and repeat treatments.

Pubic lice are distinct in appearance from head and body lice; they have short crablike bodies. They are challenging to eradicate because they often inhabit several hair areas on an individual patient (Fig. 176.5). A major concern in treating crab lice is the lack of appreciation for their tendency to reside in rectal hairs. If one treats patients with *P. pubis* with topical preparations, one must instruct patients to liberally treat the groin and rectal regions; otherwise, treatment failures will occur. **Some**

dermatologists prefer to treat pubic lice using ivermectin as their first-line therapy. Besides sexual transmission, pubic lice may also be acquired by sharing a bed with an infested person. Children with pubic lice have usually been infected through contact with an adult. Always demand investigation for possible child abuse. Fortunately, head and pubic lice do not transmit systemic disease.

In the United States, **the body louse** has become less common in the general population. Body lice infestation in all developed countries is generally seen among the homeless in urban areas. It also is common among refugees and those who live in crowded conditions or cannot launder their clothing. Worldwide, body lice are important vectors for louse-borne relapsing fever, trench fever, and epidemic typhus, especially among refugees. The body louse and nits are generally found in the clothing seams of a parasitized individual, but the louse grabs on to body hairs to feed. Clothing may be stained with serum, blood, or louse feces. Body lice are eradicated by means of proper hygiene and laundering of clothing. A pediculicide may be helpful to treat any lice adherent to body hairs.

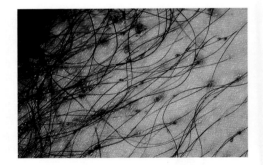

Fig. 176.5 Crab louse nits at the base of lower abdominal hairs. (Adapted from Ko, C. J., & Elston, D. M. [2004]. Pediculosis. *Journal of the American Academy of Dermatology, 50,* 1–12.)

Suggested Readings

Burkhart, C. G., & Burkhart, C. N. (2006). Asphyxiation of lice with topical agents, not a reality…yet. *Journal of the American Academy of Dermatology, 54,* 721–722.

Burkhart, C. G., & Burkhart, C. N. (2004). Oral ivermectin for *Phthirus pubis. Journal of the American Academy of Dermatology, 51,* 1037.

Drugs for head lice. (1997). *The Medical Letter on Drugs and Therapeutics, 39,* 6–7.

Fischer, T. F. (1994). Lindane toxicity in a 24-year-old woman. *Annals of Emergency Medicine, 24,* 972–974.

Frankowski, B. L., & Bocchini, J. A., Jr. (2010). Council on school health and committee on infectious diseases: Head lice. *Pediatrics*, *126*, 392–403.

Huntington, M. K., Allison, J. R., Hogue, A. L., et al. (2019). Infectious disease: Bedbugs, lice, and mites. *FP Essentials*, *476*, 18–24.

Jones, K. N., & English, J. C., III. (2003). Review of common therapeutic options in the United States for the treatment of pediculosis capitis. *Clinical Infectious Diseases*, *36*, 1355–1361.

Pearlman, D. L. (2004). A simple treatment for head lice: Dry-on, suffocation-based pediculocide. *Pediatrics*, *114*, e275–e279.

Resnick, K. S. (2005). A non-chemical therapeutic modality for head lice. *Journal of the American Academy of Dermatology*, *52*, 374.

Steen, C. J., Carbonaro, P. A., & Schwartz, R. A. (2004). Arthropods in dermatology. *Journal of the American Academy of Dermatology*, *50*, 819–842.

Pityriasis Rosea

Presentation

Patients with this rash often seek acute medical help because of the worrisome sudden spread of a rash that began with one local skin lesion. This "herald patch" may develop anywhere on the body, but it is typically on the trunk and appears as an ovoid, 2 to 6 cm in diameter, mildly erythematous and slightly raised scaling plaque with a collarette of scale at the margin (Fig. 177.1). Some patients may be oblivious to the herald patch if it is on the flank or back. There is no change for a period of several days to a few weeks; then the generalized rash appears, composed of crops of small (0.5–2 cm), pale, salmon-colored, oval, raised macules or plaques with a coarse surface surrounded by the same rim of fine scales as the herald patch (Fig. 177.2). The distribution is usually truncal (face, hands, and feet being spared), with the long axis of the oval lesions running in the planes of cleavage of the skin (Langer lines, which are parallel to the ribs), giving it a typical "Christmas tree" appearance and making the diagnosis (Fig. 177.3).

The condition may be asymptomatic or accompanied by varying degrees of pruritus (25% of patients have mild to severe itching). No systemic symptoms typically are present during the rash phase of pityriasis rosea (PR). The lesions will gradually extend in size and may become confluent with one another. By its natural history, the rash persists for 6 to 8 weeks and then completely disappears. Transient worsening of the rash or a second wave of lesions is not uncommon until eventual spontaneous resolution of the eruption. Recurrence of the condition later in life is rare.

Pityriasis rosea can have a distinctly different appearance on patients with brown or dark skin. The herald patch, as well as the diffuse rash that follows, may have a gray, dark brown, or even black appearance. There may be either hypopigmented or hyperpigmented areas visible after the lesions resolve.

What to Do

✓ **Ater performing a careful history and physical examination, reassure patients about the benign self-limited nature of this disease.** Be sympathetic and let them know that it is understandable how frightening it can seem. **Inform them that the rash will last for 6 to 8 weeks.** In addition, inform them about the need to contact their physician if the rash or pruritus lasts more than 3 months.

✓ **Encourage sun exposure** because it hastens resolution of individual lesions.

✓ **Acyclovir may be effective in the treatment of PR, especially in patients treated within the first week of onset of the generalized rash; however, the evidence supporting this is**

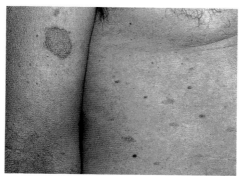

Fig. 177.1 Herald patch on the arm with a collarette of scale at the margin. (From White, G., & Cox, N. [2006]. *Diseases of the skin* [2nd ed.]. St. Louis, MO: Mosby.)

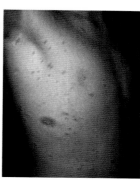

Fig. 177.2 Pityriasis rosea with herald patch and subtle smaller spots on trunk.

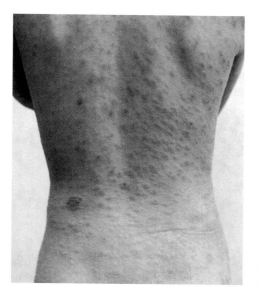

Fig. 177.3 Typical "Christmas tree" pattern of pityriasis rosea. (From Leung, A. K. S., Wong, B. E., & Chan, P. Y. H. [1997]. Pediatrics review. *Resident and Staff Physician, 43*, 109.)

not strong. Prescribe acyclovir (Zovirax), 800 mg given five times daily for 7 days, especially in cases that are particularly severe. This dosage hastened the clearance of lesions in one placebo-controlled study. A single patient has been reported, however, who developed PR while taking low doses of acyclovir. Treatment with acyclovir of patients with severe pruritus was recommended in a 2016 position statement by the European Academy of Dermatology and Venereology.

✅ **Early high doses of acyclovir should probably be prescribed in pregnancy** to prevent miscarriage or premature births, especially when PR develops during the first weeks of gestation, when the lesions have an unusual extension and long duration, and when constitutional symptoms are present. At the moment, however, there is not strong evidence to support this recommendation.

✅ Phototherapy has also been recommended for severe cases, although additional studies are needed to confirm this. There is low-quality to moderate-quality evidence suggesting that erythromycin probably reduces itch more than placebo does.

✅ **If the diagnosis is uncertain, especially if the palms and soles are affected and the patient is sexually active, draw blood for serologic testing for syphilis** (e.g., rapid plasma reagin [RPR], Venereal Disease Research Laboratory [VDRL]). Secondary syphilis can mimic PR. These patients will require close follow-up and treatment if the results are positive.

✅ **Microscopy with potassium hydroxide (KOH) preparation may be helpful to distinguish a herald patch from a tinea infection.**

✅ **Provide relief from pruritus** by prescribing hydroxyzine (Atarax), 25 to 50 mg every 6 hours, or an emollient, such as Lubriderm. Tepid cornstarch baths (1 cup in half-full tub of water) may also be comforting.

What Not to Do

❌ Do not have a biopsy performed when findings are typical for pityriasis rosea. A biopsy is not indicated.

❌ Do not routinely use topical or systemic steroids. These are effective only in the most severe inflammatory varieties of this syndrome. Topical steroids may cause the eruption to generalize to erythroderma.

❌ Do not send off a serologic test for syphilis without ensuring that the results will be seen and acted on.

Discussion

Pityriasis rosea (PR) is a common, acute exanthem of uncertain cause. PR most commonly affects adolescents, with a concentration of cases in the age range of 10 to 35 years, peaking in persons 20 to 29 years of age. Female-to-male ratio is 1.5:1. PR occurs in pregnancy more frequently than in the general population (18% vs 6%, respectively).

The diagnosis of PR can usually be made based on the appearance of the lesions and the history. It has been described in the medical literature for more than 200 years but was given its current name by Camille Gilbert in 1860. Viral and bacterial causes have been sought, but convincing answers have not yet been found. PR shares many features with the viral exanthemas of childhood, and cases tend to cluster in the fall and winter.

Studies have focused on human herpesvirus 6 (HHV-6) and HHV-7 as causative agents. The skin lesions would not be a result of a direct infection of skin cells, but rather would occur as a reactive response to the systemic HHV-6 and HHV-7 replication, alone or through the interaction with other viruses. The higher proportion of pregnant women with PR is probably related to the altered maternal immunity, the innate proinflammatory immune responses being tightly regulated to prevent immunologic rejection of the fetal allograft. In fact, HHV-6 reactivation seems common during pregnancy, and this fact may be one of the causes of spontaneous abortions. The vague link with herpesviruses is enhanced by results of a systematic review showing that treatment with acyclovir improves the rash but does not seem to help with itching.

Up to 69% of patients with PR have a prodromal illness before the herald patch appears. Malaise, nausea, loss of appetite, headache, difficulty in

Discussion continued

concentration, irritability, gastrointestinal and upper respiratory symptoms (up to 69%), joint pain, swelling of lymph nodes, sore throat, and mild fever are often, although inconsistently, reported.

The herald patch often is misdiagnosed as eczema. PR is difficult to identify until the appearance of the characteristic smaller secondary lesions. When these secondary lesions are not on the patient's back, where they form the typical "Christmas tree" pattern, the lesions follow the cleavage lines in the following patterns: transversely across the lower abdomen and back, circumferentially around the shoulders, and in a V-shaped pattern on the upper chest.

The "herald patch" may not be seen in 20% to 30% of cases, and there are many variations from the classic presentation described. Atypical cases make up 20% of the total and occur more commonly in children. Lesions can exhibit urticarial, vesicular,

pustular, or purpuric characteristics. Infrequently, oral lesions will accompany the skin rash and resolve along with it: these include punctate hemorrhages, erosions, ulcerations, erythematous macules, annular lesions, and plaques. There are no noninvasive tests that confirm the diagnosis of PR. Other diagnostic considerations besides syphilis include tinea corporis, seborrheic dermatitis, guttate psoriasis, and tinea versicolor. Numerous drugs have been implicated in a severe prolonged exanthem that resembles PR. Some of the medications that have been associated with a PR-type rash include bismuth, bacillus Calmette–Guérin (BCG) vaccine, captopril, clonidine, diphtheria toxoid, gold, isotretinoin, ketotifen, metronidazole, and omeprazole. Persistence of a rash beyond 3 months should prompt a clinician to reconsider the original diagnosis, to consider biopsy to confirm the diagnosis, and to check for the use of medications that may cause a rash similar to PR.

Suggested Readings

Brangman, S. A. (2004). Appearance of pityriasis rosea in patients with dark skin (letter). *American Family Physician*, *70*, 821.

Contreras-Ruiz, J., Pternel, S., Jimenez Gutierrez, C., et al. (2019). Interventions for pityriasis rosea. *Cochrane Database of Systematic Reviews*, *10*.

Drago, F., Broccolo, F., & Alfredo Rebora, A. (2009). Pityriasis rosea: An update with a critical appraisal of its possible herpesviral etiology. *Journal of the American Academy of Dermatology*, *61*, 303–318.

Drago, F., Vecchio, F., & Rebora, A. (2006). Use of high-dose acyclovir in pityriasis rosea. *Journal of the American Academy of Dermatology*, *54*, 82–85.

Eisman, S., & Sinclair, R. (2015). Pityriasis rosea. *BMJ*, *351*, h5233.

Habif, T. (1996). *Clinical dermatology* (3rd ed.). St. Louis, MO: Mosby-Year Book.

Jones, D. (2003). The young adult: Common inflammatory skin disorders. *Clinics in Family Practice*, *5*, 627–652.

Point of Care. (2020). *Pityriasis rosea*. Amsterdam, Netherlands: Elsevier BV.

Wolfrey, J. D., Billica, W. H., Gulbranson, S. H., et al. (2003). Pediatric exanthems. *Clinics in Family Practice*, *5*, 557–588.

Pyogenic Granuloma or Lobular Capillary Hemangioma

(Proud Flesh)

Presentation

Often there is a history of a laceration or minor trauma to the skin or mucous membrane several days to a few weeks before presentation, but in most cases there is no apparent cause. The head, neck, and extremities are most commonly involved, especially the lips, oral mucosa, and fingers. An unsightly lesion forms, beginning as an extremely friable red or yellow papule or polyp, bleeding with every slight trauma. Objective findings usually include a crusted, sometimes purulent-appearing collection of erythematous, well-demarcated, red granulation tissue arising from a moist, sometimes hemorrhagic, skin ulceration, often with a collarette of scale at the base. There are usually no signs of a deep tissue infection (Fig. 178.1).

What to Do

✅ **Cleanse the area** with an agent such as hydrogen peroxide or povidone-iodine solution.

✅ **Evaluate whether the lesion is in a location amenable to your interventions, and discuss risks and benefits with the patient. Lesions located on the face, in the mouth, or large lesions on the hands may be most appropriate for referral.**

✅ **Consider whether the lesion in question could be malignant, and document your reasoning.**

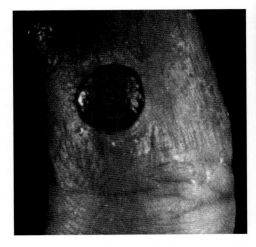

Fig. 178.1 Pyogenic granuloma.

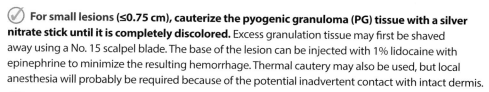 **For small lesions (≤0.75 cm), cauterize the pyogenic granuloma (PG) tissue with a silver nitrate stick until it is completely discolored.** Excess granulation tissue may first be shaved away using a No. 15 scalpel blade. The base of the lesion can be injected with 1% lidocaine with epinephrine to minimize the resulting hemorrhage. Thermal cautery may also be used, but local anesthesia will probably be required because of the potential inadvertent contact with intact dermis.

Dress the wound after applying an antibacterial ointment, and have the patient gently wash and repeat ointment and dressings two to three times a day until healed.

It is not uncommon for secondary cellulitis to develop after the pyogenic granuloma is cauterized. It is therefore reasonable to place a patient on a short course (3–4 days) of a high-dose antibiotic (dicloxacillin or cephalexin, 500 mg four times a day, or cefadroxil, 500 mg twice a day) when the wound is located on a distal extremity or in patients with diabetes or other immune compromise.

For pedunculated lesions, an atraumatic, simple, fast, and cost-effective alternative that does not require anesthesia is to ligate the base of the granuloma using a soft, absorbable, surgical suture material. This maneuver can be facilitated by lifting the pyogenic granuloma with forceps. The tissue is ligated with knots that are as tight as possible. The suture material is then snipped short. This can be covered by a simple wound dressing, and the tumor can be expected to become necrotic and fall off in several days. Inform patients or parents that although uncommon, bleeding could occur, and simple continuous compression for several minutes will control any minor hemorrhage. If the ligature does not reach far enough down to include the nurturing vessel, part of the granuloma may persist. This smaller lesion can then be easily treated with silver nitrate or thermal cautery.

A small study reported in the *Journal of the American Academy of Dermatology* **showed that five patients with pyogenic granuloma were successfully treated with table salt** from a commercially available freshly opened package. White soft paraffin was applied on the perilesional skin to prevent irritation. A pinch of salt enough to cover the entire lesion was applied. The area was occluded with surgical adhesive tape. Patients were instructed to do the same at home daily. It seems reasonable to substitute petroleum jelly for the soft paraffin if that is more readily available. Complete resolution of the lesion was noticed by 7 to 14 days, depending on the size of the lesion. A mild burning sensation was experienced at the time of the first application in two patients who had a raw, bleeding area; however, no other adverse effects were encountered. No recurrence of lesions occurred at 1 month of follow-up.

If this technique is tried, inform the patient and family of the small study that your treatment is based on and make sure they approve of and are comfortable with your simple and inexpensive plan. When practical, it would also be helpful to include the follow-up physician in this uncommon treatment plan.

Another incompletely proven yet simple and noncaustic treatment is the use of topical beta blockers. Timolol is a topical beta blocker that may be very useful to reduce bleeding and tumor size in clinically typical PGs. Timolol 0.5% ophthalmic solution bid under occlusion can be prescribed. A study with one pediatric patient, in follow-up at 4 weeks, showed almost complete resolution. The authors note that timolol has proven to be safe and well tolerated to treat infantile hemangiomas and they believe that represents a worthwhile therapeutic strategy in PG before surgery. Recurrence has been reported although there is limited experience on the use of timolol for the treatment of PG in children.

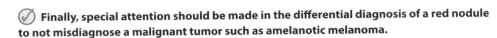

✅ **Finally, special attention should be made in the differential diagnosis of a red nodule to not misdiagnose a malignant tumor such as amelanotic melanoma.**

✅ **Patients with large lesions** can be referred for treatment with a pulsed-dye laser.

✅ **Patients with facial lesions whose scarring might be significant may benefit from debulking by topical beta blocker or imiquimod therapy prior to laser therapy or surgical removal. Such stepwise plans should be initiated by a dermatologist.**

✅ Warn the patient about the potential signs of developing infection and the need to return for treatment.

✅ Patients and parents should also be alerted to the possibility of recurrence after removal.

✅ **Dermatology referral** is recommended if the lesion recurs or multiple satellite lesions occur after excision.

What Not to Do

❌ Do not cauterize or ligate any lesion that by history and appearance might be neoplastic in nature. Only treat clinically obvious cases. Pyogenic granuloma is occasionally confused with amelanotic melanoma, basal cell carcinoma, and squamous cell carcinoma. Periungual malignant melanoma can mimic pyogenic granuloma. Suspicious lesions should be referred for complete excision and pathologic examination.

❌ Do not cauterize a recurrent, large, or extensive lesion. These should also be considered for complete excision.

Discussion

Pyogenic granulomas, also known as lobular hemangiomas, are common vascular tumors of the skin and mucous membranes usually seen in children and young adults. They are usually smaller than 1 cm but can be up to 2 cm. Their cause is unknown, but pyogenic granuloma is a misnomer because it is probably not infectious (pyogenic) in origin. It has been argued to be inflammatory and hyperplastic rather than a true neoplasm. Rapid growth is in response to an unknown stimulus that triggers endothelial proliferation and angiogenesis. They can be solitary or multiple and can arise within preexisting lesions, such as spider angioma and port wine stain.

Although a minority of pyogenic granulomas involute spontaneously within 6 months, most patients seek treatment because of bleeding. Pyogenic granulomas recur if any abnormal tissue remains.

Gingival lesions are common in **pregnant women,** in whom these lesions are called epulis gravidarum. Spontaneous resolution occurs after delivery.

Medical therapy is an active area of research, focused on imiquimod and beta blockers. The idea of using beta blockers for PG stemmed from a 2008 report of two pediatric cardiac patients whose beta blocker therapy seemed to incidentally cause rapid involution of infantile hemangiomas. It was found that infantile hemangiomas avidly express beta-adrenergic receptors—so does PG tissue, but to a lesser degree. Since then many case reports and low-powered studies have replicated the use of topical and systemic beta blocker therapy for treating PG. This practice is still under research but may emerge as a safe alternative to surgical treatment in the emergency department or urgent care center.

It is not uncommon for secondary cellulitis to develop after the pyogenic granuloma is cauterized. It is therefore reasonable to place a patient on a short course (3–4 days) of a high-dose antibiotic (dicloxacillin or cephalexin, 500 mg four times a day, or cefadroxil, 500 mg twice daily) when the wound is located on a distal extremity or in patients with diabetes or other immune compromise.

Suggested Reading

Dany, M. (2019). Beta-blockers for pyogenic granuloma: A systematic review of case reports, case series, and clinical trials. *Journal of Drugs in Dermatology*, *18*, 1006–1010.

Daruwalla, S. B., & Dhurat, R. S. (2020). A pinch of salt is all it takes! The novel use of table salt for the effective treatment of pyogenic granuloma. *Journal of the American Academy of Dermatology*, *83*(2), e107–e108.

Jafarzadeh, H., Sanatkhani, M., & Mohtasham, N. (2006). Oral pyogenic granuloma: A review. *Journal of Oral Science*, *48*, 167–175.

Knöpfel, N., del Mar Escudero-Góngora, M., Bauzà, A., et al. (2016). Timolol for the treatment of pyogenic granuloma (PG) in children. *Journal of the American Academy of Dermatology*, *75*(3), e105–e106.

Scabies

(Human Itch Mite)

Presentation

Patients present for evaluation due to inability to sleep as a result of intense itching. Severe pruritus, which is the hallmark of this disease, is intensified at night for unclear reasons. These patients have skin lesions that include mite burrows, which appear as short (about 2–3 mm in length), elevated, gray, threadlike, serpiginous tracks. A small papule or vesicle may appear at the end of the burrow or may occur independently (Fig. 179.1). These papules and burrows are chiefly found in the interdigital web spaces (Fig. 179.2), as well as on the volar aspects of the wrists, axillae, olecranon area, nipples, waistline, genitalia, and gluteal cleft (Fig. 179.3). Nipple pruritus in females is a useful historical clue. Pruritic erythematous papules on the glans penis are characteristics of scabies infestation in males (Fig. 179.4). The head and neck are usually spared, but scabies lesions can occur anywhere on the body (Fig. 179.5), including the face and scalp. Infants and young children may also have palm and sole involvement with vesicular and pustular lesions. Secondary bacterial infection is sometimes present. Scabies in the elderly may be difficult to diagnose because the cutaneous lesions are often very subtle.

What to Do

✅ **If a microscope is available, attempt to confirm the diagnosis of scabies by placing mineral oil over five or six nonexcoriated suspicious papules or burrows, and scrape or shave them with a No. 15 scalpel blade onto a slide. Examine under low magnification for the mite, its oval eggs, or fecal concretions (scybala). Any one of these findings clinches the diagnosis** (Fig. 179.6). Burrows can be made more visible by first liberally covering the area

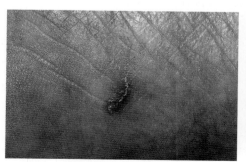

Fig. 179.1 Scabies burrow on the side of the foot. (From White, G., & Cox, N. [2006]. *Diseases of the skin* [2nd ed.]. St. Louis, MO: Mosby.)

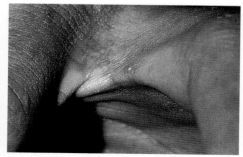

Fig. 179.2 Lesions are commonly found in the interdigital web spaces and the sides of the fingers. (From White, G., & Cox, N. [2006]. *Diseases of the skin* [2nd ed.]. St. Louis, MO: Mosby.)

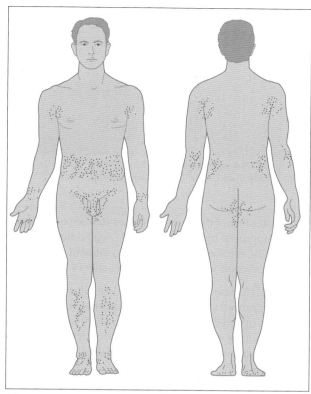

Fig. 179.3   Characteristics of distribution of scabies lesions. (Adapted from Goldstein, B. G., & Goldstein, A. O. [1997]. *Practical dermatology* [2nd ed.]. St. Louis, MO: Mosby.)

with liquid ink and then removing excess ink with an alcohol swab, leaving the burrows stained. If the clinical picture alone is convincing, particularly if there is a close contact (a source) who is itching, treatment should be instituted without the necessity of confirmation, even with negative scrapings.

✅ **Prescribe prescription-strength permethrin 5% insecticidal cream, 60 g, for the patient to massage from the head to the soles of the feet at bedtime, and have the patient leave it on for 8 to 14 hours before washing it off the next morning.** Mites tend to persist in subungual areas. The patient should trim fingernails, scrub beneath them, and then apply the scabicide under the nails. Patients should apply a second treatment 1 week later.

✅ **Oral ivermectin, 0.2 mg/kg as a single oral dose repeated within an interval of 7 to 14 days, is as effective as a single application of 5% topical permethrin cream.** It should be taken on an empty stomach with water. A total of two or more doses at least 7 days apart may be necessary to eliminate a scabies infestation. Ivermectin is currently available in the form of a 3-mg tablet. The safety of ivermectin in children weighing less than 15 kg and in pregnant women has not been established. (Although permethrin is still perhaps the treatment of choice for scabies, this may not be so in future practice. The high cost and extensive surface area of application that is necessary lead to poor compliance, especially in elderly patients.

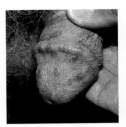

Fig. 179.4 Scabies of the penis causes intense itching and red papules on the glans, which is nearly diagnostic of the disease. (From White, G., & Cox, N. [2006]. *Diseases of the skin* [2nd ed.]. St. Louis, MO: Mosby.)

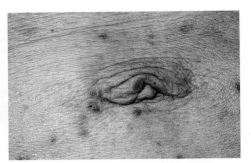

Fig. 179.5 Lesions about the umbilicus. (From White, G., & Cox, N. [2006]. *Diseases of the skin* [2nd ed.]. St. Louis, MO: Mosby.)

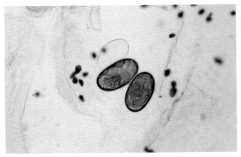

Fig. 179.6 Microscopic examination of burrow scrapings showing two oval eggs and multiple brown feces (scybala). (From White, G., & Cox, N. [2006]. *Diseases of the skin* [2nd ed.]. St. Louis, MO: Mosby.)

Because of this, ivermectin may soon be considered the drug of choice. Currently, it is still not approved by the US Food and Drug Administration [FDA] for treating scabies. Therefore, the US CDC recommends concurrent treatment with permethrin—this ensures that at least one FDA-approved agent is used for the patient's treatment regimen.)

✓ Crotamiton (Eurax) lotion 10% (60 mL, 480 mL) and crotamiton cream 10% (60 g) are approved by the FDA for the treatment of scabies in adults; they are considered safe when used as directed (yet expensive). Massage cream/lotion into entire body from chin down, repeat 24 hours later, and then bathe 48 hours later. Crotamiton is not FDA approved for use in children. Frequent treatment failure has been reported with crotamiton.

✓ Sulfur is the oldest known treatment of scabies, and it is the drug of choice **for infants younger than 2 months of age and for pregnant or lactating women**. It is available as 5% and 10% precipitated sulfur in petrolatum. The cream is applied nightly for 3 consecutive nights and washed off 24 hours later. The major drawback to sulfur treatment is the unpleasant odor and the potential to stain clothes.

✓ **Secondary infection from scratching, such as impetiginized excoriations, can be treated with mupirocin (Bactroban) cream 2%. Folliculitis, abscess formation, lymphangitis, and cellulitis should be treated with appropriate drainage and antibiotics** (see Chapters 165, 168, and 174).

✓ **Advise the patient that the associated pruritis will not go away immediately,** but this does not indicate that treatment was ineffective. Dead mites and eggs continue to cause an immune response but will eventually be eliminated during normal cutaneous turnover.

✓ **An antipruritic agent, such as hydroxyzine, 25 to 50 mg up to four times a day, can be prescribed for comfort. Adding a short course of oral prednisone may be most effective when pruritus is severe.**

✓ **Clothing, bedding, and towels should be washed with hot water or dry cleaned or placed through the heat cycle of a dryer to prevent reinfection.** An alternative method is to place all bedding and clothing that might be infested in sealed plastic bags for at least 72 hours. Thorough cleaning of the patient's room is recommended.

✓ **Family members,** frequent household guests, and close physical and sexual contacts should also be treated simultaneously, whether or not symptoms are present.

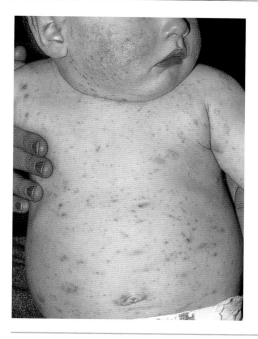

Fig. 179.7 Scabies in an infant involving the face. (From White, G., & Cox, N. [2006]. *Diseases of the skin* [2nd ed.]. St. Louis, MO: Mosby.)

✅ **Patients should be reexamined** 1 to 2 weeks after initiating therapy to ensure that there is no recurrence.

What Not to Do

❌ Do not use lindane on infants, young children, or pregnant women or in widespread Norwegian scabies, because enough of this pesticide may be absorbed percutaneously to produce seizures or central nervous system (CNS) toxicity. For this reason, lindane is generally no longer recommended for any patient with scabies.

Discussion

Scabies should be suspected in any patient with pruritus.

Scabies has been a scourge among humans for thousands of years. The condition is caused by the mite *Sarcoptes scabiei,* var. *hominis.* The adult is barely visible to the naked eye. The organism is an obligate parasite, requiring an appropriate host for survival. The mites subsist on a diet of dissolved human tissue but do not feed on blood. An adult female mite has a tortoise shape and is only about 0.3 to 0.4 mm in size. The male mite is about half the female size. Although mites cannot fly or jump, they can crawl as fast as 2.5 cm/min on warm skin. After mating on the surface of the skin, the gravid female mite dissolves the stratum corneum with proteolytic secretions and then burrows headfirst into the skin. Eggs are laid at a rate of two to three per day. Both male and female mites have a life span of about 1 month. Young mites develop quickly, leaving the burrows to enter hair follicles and skin folds in which to hide and feed. They mature within 10 to 14 days, after which mating takes place, beginning a new cycle. Mites can live only up to 3 days when they are away from a host's body environment.

(continued)

Discussion continued

A delayed hypersensitivity reaction to the mites, their eggs, saliva, and scybala (packets of feces) occurs within approximately 2 to 6 weeks of infestations. This inflammatory reaction is responsible for the intense pruritus (the hallmark of this disease). Although scabietic lesions are uncommon above the neck in children and adults, infants may have involvement of the face (Fig. 179.7). Scabies in an infant usually means that a close adult contact is the source of the infection.

A distinctive highly contagious form of scabies—known as **Norwegian scabies, crusted scabies, or keratotic scabies**—has a predilection for individuals who are immunocompromised, elderly, debilitated, or mentally impaired. The patient becomes infected with thousands to millions of mites, in contrast to the usual case of scabies, where the average infected adult human has 10 to 15 live adult female mites on the body at any given time. Skin manifestations of keratotic scabies are much more severe, but the latter is usually not very pruritic.

Scabies is transmitted principally through close personal contact but may be transmitted through clothing, linens, or towels.

Less than 25% of cases show the characteristic (2–3 mm) serpiginous tracks. Another method of detecting scabies, other than skin scrapings, is video dermatoscopy. This is noninvasive in vivo visualization of the skin at magnifications of up to 600× to detect signs of infestation (mites, eggs, and feces).

Families may acquire **canine scabies** when a puppy is brought into the home. The distribution of lesions on humans infected with dog scabies is distinctively different from that of the human variety. A child who hugs an infested family pet will make greatest contact with the trunk and arms, and most eruptions are thereby seen in this distribution. Canine scabies manifests itself within 24 to 96 hours. It is generally self-limiting in humans because the mites cannot complete their life cycle and therefore do not survive for more than a few days on a foreign host. For those patients who are unwilling to wait for this form of scabies to resolve on its own, 5% permethrin applied topically is the treatment of choice. The assistance of a veterinarian is recommended for treating the pet.

Suggested Readings

Centers for Disease Control and Prevention. (2019). *Parasites—scabies.* http://cdc.gov/parasites/scabies/health_professionals/meds.html.

Huynh, T. H., & Norman, R. A. (2004). Scabies and pediculosis. *Dermatology Clinics, 22*, 7–11.

Madan, V., Jaskiran, K., Gupta, U., et al. (2001). Oral ivermectin in scabies patients: A comparison with 1% topical lindane lotion. *Journal of Dermatology, 28*, 481–484.

Steen, C. J., Carbonaro, P. A., & Schwarz, R. A. (2004). Arthropods in dermatology. *Journal of the American Academy of Dermatology, 50*, 819–842.

Sea Bather's Eruption

(Sea Lice)

Presentation

Patients seek help because of an intense pruritic or painful eruption of red raised welts, sometimes like mosquito bites. They are at times confluent, appearing in areas that had been covered by swimwear (Fig. 180.1). This will occur within a few hours after bathing in the Caribbean or off the coasts of Mexico, Florida, or Long Island during periods when so-called sea lice are active. Exposed areas of skin are spared. Symptoms may have started as a tingling sensation while in the water, with itching and burning becoming more pronounced if a freshwater shower was taken while still wearing the same suit. Symptoms usually resolve spontaneously in a few days; however, some individuals (especially children) experience a more severe delayed hypersensitivity reaction occurring approximately 10 days after exposure. This rash extends to exposed areas of the body not previously affected, and victims may also experience severe itching, fatigue, fever, chills, nausea, and headache. Outbreaks occur between March and August, with a peak incidence in May.

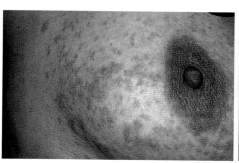

A

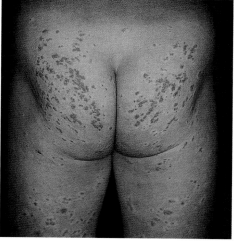

B

Fig. 180.1 Sea bather's eruption with multiple edematous pink papules found in areas previously covered by a bathing suit. (A, From White, G., & Cox, N. [2006]. *Diseases of the skin*. St. Louis, MO: Mosby; B, from Bolognia, J., Jorizzo, J., & Rapini, R. [2003]. *Dermatology*. St. Louis, MO: Mosby.)

What to Do

✅ **At the onset of symptoms, the patient should remove the bathing suit before showering and, if possible, decontaminate the affected areas using papain/urea (spray) 33 mL, unseasoned meat tenderizer with a mildly abrasive pad applicator, or simply vinegar for 30 minutes.**

✅ Inform the patient about the nature of this rash and that it will usually last for 3 to 5 days.

✅ **Prescribe a topical steroid in combination with a topical anesthetic to be applied three to four times per day. Pramosone is a convenient product containing a topical anesthetic and steroid in a cream or lotion 1% and 2.5%, supplied in tubes (1 and 2 ounces) and bottles (2, 4, 8 fluid ounces).**

✅ **Prescribe an oral antihistamine, such as hydroxyzine (Atarax, Vistaril), 25 to 50 mg up to four times a day, to help with itching.**

✅ **If systemic symptoms are present or if the rash is extensive and severe, prescribe 4 to 5 days of a systemic steroid, such as prednisone, 60 to 80 mg once per day (1 mg/kg).**

✅ Because nematocysts may remain in the bathing suit after drying, instruct the patient to wash swimwear in detergent and fresh water and to dry it before wearing it again. Without washing and drying, any unreleased nematocysts can be triggered and discharged, producing lesions without additional exposure to ocean water.

✅ **Instruct the patient about future prevention,** either by avoiding ocean bathing during known outbreaks or by immediately removing swimwear after sea bathing, cleansing the skin with vinegar (to prevent the triggering of nematocysts), and then showering. Showering with fresh water while still wearing swimwear may cause a discharge of nematocysts and worsening of symptoms.

✅ **Safe Sea Sunblock Jellyfish Sting Protective Lotion,** sold by Seavenger (Walnut, CA) reportedly prevents stings from sea lice, stinging corals, and jellyfish. A 4-ounce bottle gives roughly four adult full-body applications, each giving approximately 1 hour of protection. One small randomized controlled study demonstrated a relative risk reduction of 82% (95% confidence interval: 21–96%; $P = .02$). No sea bather's eruption or side effects occurred.

What Not to Do

❌ Do not prescribe systemic steroids for patients in whom there are strong contraindications, as this is a self-limiting condition.

Discussion

Sea bather's eruption typically occurs 4 to 24 hours after exposure, although some persons may develop a prickling sensation or urticarial lesions while still in the water. The larval forms of certain sea anemones and thimble jellyfish, *Linuche unguiculata,* are implicated as the cause. Water flows through bathing suits, trapping the small (2–3 mm) larvae against the skin. The larvae have nematocysts that are discharged into the skin when stimulated by pressure, death,

or fresh water. Lesions also occur on uncovered skin surfaces subjected to friction, such as axillae and inner thighs. Surfers develop lesions on the chest and abdomen that were in contact with surfboards. Children often develop symptoms after sitting on wet bathing suits in vehicles. The term *sea lice* is applied to seabather's eruption as a colloquial term; true sea lice are marine parasites that do not infest humans.

(continued)

Discussion continued

Cercarial dermatitis, or swimmer's itch, is a different condition that occurs sporadically in fresh water as well as ocean water. It occurs on exposed skin rather than under bathing suits. The cause is direct invasion of the skin by various schistosome parasites. For most of these, humans are a dead-end host resulting in no deep tissue invasion. However, human pathogen schistosomes such as *Schistosoma* *mansoni, S. japonicum,* and *S. haematobium* can cause similar skin findings and lead to organ involvement. If cercarial dermatitis is suspected, review the pathogens in the area and refer to an infectious disease specialist if you have concerns about true human pathogen involvement. In either case, supportive care with an over-the-counter topical steroid is helpful.

Suggested Readings

Auerbach, P. S., & DiTullio, A. E. (2017). Envenomations by aquatic invertebrates. In T. A. Cushing, & N. S. Harris (Eds.), *Auerbach's wilderness medicine* (4th ed.). Philadelphia, PA: Elsevier.

Boulware, D. R. (2006). A randomized, controlled field trial for the prevention of jellyfish stings with a topical sting inhibitor. *Journal of Travel Medicine, 13,* 166–171.

Singletary, E. M., Rochman, A. S., Bodmer, J. C., & Holstege, C. P. (2005). Envenomations. *Medical Clinics of North America, 89,* 1195–1224.

Sunburn

Presentation

Patients generally seek help only if their sunburn is severe. There will be a history of extended exposure to sunlight or to an artificial source of ultraviolet radiation, such as a sunlamp. Patients at highest risk typically have fair skin, blue eyes, and red or blond hair. The burns will be accompanied by intense pain, and the patient will not be able to tolerate anything touching the skin. Most exposure is limited to sun-exposed areas of the body (Fig. 181.1). There may be systemic complaints of "sun poisoning" that include nausea, vomiting, chills, and fever. The affected areas are erythematous and are accompanied by mild edema. Erythema develops after 2 to 6 hours and peaks at 12 to 24 hours. The more severe the burn, the earlier it will appear and the more likely that it will progress to edema and blistering. Signs and symptoms usually resolve over 4 to 7 days, often with skin scaling and peeling (Fig. 181.2).

What to Do

✅ **Inquire whether the patient is using a photosensitizing drug** (e.g., tetracyclines, thiazides, sulfonamides, phenothiazines, sulfonylurea hypoglycemic agents, griseofulvin, and vitamin B$_6$); if so, with the prescribing doctor's permission, have the patient discontinue its use and avoid the sun for at least 3 weeks.

✅ **Have the patient apply cool compresses. Cold compresses of skim milk and water or Burrow solution (Domeboro Powder Packets, two packets in 1 pint of water) have all been suggested and can be applied as often as desired to relieve pain. This is the most comforting therapy.** Cool baths or showers will also help. Keep in mind that there is a paucity of evidence regarding which compresses or dressing types are most effective.

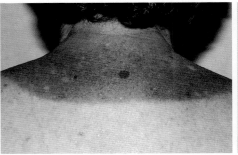 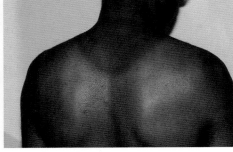

A   B

Fig. 181.1 (A, B) Sunburn on the upper back. Note the sharp cutoff at the line of clothing (A) and the relative sparing further up the neck because of shielding by the hair. (From White, G., & Cox, N. [2006]. *Diseases of the skin* [2nd ed.]. St. Louis, MO: Mosby.)

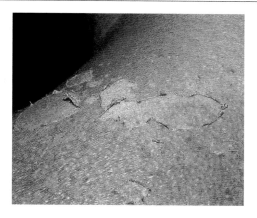

Fig. 181.2 Sunburn typically causes peeling as it resolves, even if frank blistering has not been an early feature. (From White, G., & Cox, N. [2006]. *Diseases of the skin* [2nd ed.]. St. Louis, MO: Mosby.)

✓ **If there is no contraindication, nonsteroidal anti-inflammatory drugs (NSAIDs), such as ibuprofen (Motrin), 400 mg every 6 hours, or naproxen (Naprosyn), 500 mg twice daily, will help reduce pain and inflammation.**

✓ **Suggest an emollient, such as Lubriderm, aloe vera–based gels, or cold cream, for topical treatment. There is a lack of evidence for the use of a topical steroid spray**, such as dexamethasone (Decaspray), or other topic corticosteroids. Most recommend not using them **unless there is coexistent contact dermatitis.** Products with aloe vera are increasingly popular.

✓ **With a more severe burn with significant blistering and systemic symptoms, oral steroids are sometimes prescribed, but they have not been shown to be effective in the few small studies assessing their value. Assess for the use of a photosensitizing drug that might have been the underlying cause. Clean blistered areas with mild soap and water as for any second-degree burn, and apply an appropriate sterile dressing as needed for pain relief.** Add a mild sedative and antipruritic, such as hydroxyzine (Vistaril), 50 mg four times a day.

✓ **Instruct the patient to avoid the sun for a minimum of 3 weeks.**

What Not to Do

✗ Do not advise the patient to use over-the-counter (OTC) sunburn medications that contain local anesthetics (benzocaine, dibucaine, or lidocaine). They are usually ineffective or provide only very transient relief. In addition, there is the potential hazard of sensitizing the patient to these ingredients.

✗ Do not trouble the patient with unnecessary burn dressings. These wounds have a very low probability of becoming infected, and most cases resolve spontaneously with no significant sequelae. Treatment should be directed at making the patient as comfortable as possible.

✗ Do not overlook toxic shock syndrome in the hypotensive patient with fever, diarrhea, vomiting, altered mental status, or abnormal liver functions. The generalized rash looks like sunburn.

✗ Do not forget that sunburns may trigger recurrence of herpes simplex, lupus, porphyria, and other cutaneous disorders. (Being easily sunburned during infancy may indicate a serious underlying disease, such as porphyria or xeroderma pigmentosum.)

Discussion

Sunburn is an acute cutaneous inflammatory reaction that follows excessive exposure of the skin to ultraviolet radiation (UVR).

UVR from the sun that reaches the earth is divided into UVB (290–320 nm) and UVA (320–400 nm). The ratio of UVA to UVB is 20:1. UVR is strongest between 10 AM and 4 PM. The acute response of human skin to UVB irradiation includes erythema, edema, and pigment darkening, followed by delayed tanning, thickening of the epidermis and dermis, and synthesis of vitamin D; chronic UVB effects are photoaging, immunosuppression, and photocarcinogenesis. UVB-induced erythema occurs approximately 4 hours after exposure, peaks around 8 to 24 hours, and fades over a day or so; in fair-skinned and older individuals, UVB erythema may be persistent, sometimes lasting for weeks. To produce the same erythemal response, approximately 1000 times more UVA dose is needed compared with UVB. UVA is more efficient in inducing tanning, whereas UVB is more efficient in inducing erythema and sunburn.

Once the signs and symptoms of sunburn are present, no treatment, including systemic corticosteroids, has unequivocally been shown to be effective.

Prevention is the most effective therapy for sunburn.

Seeking shade and minimizing sun exposure during peak UVR times (10 AM to 4 PM) are recommended. This should be combined with the use of appropriate clothing, a wide-brimmed hat, sunglasses, and broad-spectrum sunscreen to achieve the optimal protection.

Clothing is an excellent photoprotectant. UV protectiveness of fabrics is expressed as "UV protection factor" (UPF), which is analogous to the SPF of sunscreens. Adequate UV protection is provided by a UPF greater than 30. Denim provides a UPF of 1700. Typical summer cotton T-shirts provide a UPF of 5 to 9; when wet, the UPF decreases to only 3 to 4. The introduction of UV-cutting agent (UVCA) compounds, which increase the absorption of UV radiation by the fabrics to which they are applied, has increased the ability of cotton and cotton blend fabrics to protect against the most harmful wavelengths of UV radiation.

SPF-15 sunscreen can filter out 94% of UVB radiation, and SPF-30 sunscreen provides greater than 97% protection. It is known that, in actual use, most people apply less than the amount used in testing (2 mg/cm^2). The overall median application thickness in general is only 0.5 mg/cm^2. **Most sunscreen activity failure is caused by inadequate application and by less-than-adequate frequency of reapplication.** As a rule of thumb, sunscreens provide only 33% of the protection value stated on a label because of this lack of proper compliance. Sunscreen on the skin may shed easily with rubbing, sweating, or water immersion. It has been recommended that sunscreen be applied 20 minutes before sun exposure and be reapplied every 2 to 3 hours or after swimming or sweating. Sensitivity to the sun increases on the second day of exposure; therefore a higher SPF sunscreen is important for individuals who are expected to have multiday sun exposure. **In general, use of a sunscreen with an SPF of 30 is sufficient. Approximately 1 ounce is enough for each application for an average-sized adult in an average-sized swimsuit.** It should be noted that a recent prospective, randomized, double-blind, single-center, split-body/face study of 55 healthy individuals concluded that SPF 100+ was significantly more effective in protecting against UVR-induced erythema and sunburn than SPF 50+ in actual use in a beach vacation setting.

Sunscreen use alone, no matter how substantive or durable the product, should not be trusted to prevent all of the possible harmful effects of sun exposure. For example, most sunscreens offer less protection against UVA, which may be more important in causing melanoma than UVB. Multiple studies demonstrate a major impact of UVA in skin photodamage and emphasize the need for a broad protection covering the entire solar UV spectrum. When they are trusted, it is important to read and follow the label directions on these sunscreen products.

Several preparations combine avobenzone, which blocks UVA, with UVB-blocking agents. They are sold by numerous companies, and patients should be directed to check labels to ensure the presence of a UVA-blocking component. **In 2006, the US Food and Drug Administration (FDA) approved Mexoryl SX. It is the first photostable short-UVA filter in a sunscreen formula to be approved by the FDA.** Mexoryl SX was developed for use in combination with avobenzone and octocrylene for broad-spectrum protection. In this formulation, octocrylene acts to stabilize avobenzone. Mexoryl is the most preferred agent in

Discussion continued

the dermatology literature; it is available in a broad range of SPF levels and in preparations intended for daily or episodic use, but it remains expensive. Mexoryl products are approximately twice the cost of other sunscreens. The product protects against both UVB and UVA.

Photosensitivity reactions occur often with drug ingestion in combination with exposure to the sun. The reaction occurs in sun-exposed areas, primarily of the face, arms, and chest. It resembles sunburn and is usually not pruritic (Figs. 181.3 and 181.4). Reactions are divided into phototoxic and photoallergic. **Phototoxic reactions** are more common and are not truly allergic because previous exposure is not necessary. The severity of the reaction is drug dependent and UVA-dose dependent and usually occurs within hours.

Photoallergic reactions represent delayed-type hypersensitivity and require previous exposure to a drug plus UVA exposure. This reaction is typically pruritic and eczematous and occurs within 1 to 2 days of exposure.

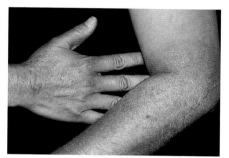

Fig. 181.3 Photodermatitis showing a typical distribution pattern. There is a cutoff from short sleeves, and relative sparing of the ulnar side of the hand and distal fingers. (From White, G., & Cox, N. [2006]. *Diseases of the skin* [2nd ed.]. St. Louis, MO: Mosby.)

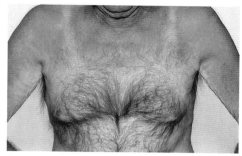

Fig. 181.4 Photosensitivity resulting from a thiazide diuretic, showing sparing under clothing. (From White, G., & Cox, N. [2006]. *Diseases of the skin* [2nd ed.]. St. Louis, MO: Mosby.)

Suggested Readings

Agin, P. P. (2006). Water resistance and extended wear sunscreens. *Dermatology Clinics*, *24*, 75–79.

Eide, M. J., & Weinstock, M. A. (2006). Public health challenges in sun protection. *Dermatology Clinics*, *24*, 119–124.

Faurschou, A. (2008). Topical corticosteroids in the treatment of acute sunburn: A randomized, double-blind clinical trial. *Archives of Dermatology*, *144*, 620–624.

Hatch, K. L., & Osterwalder, U. (2006). Garments as solar ultraviolet radiation screening materials. *Dermatology Clinics*, *24*, 85–100.

Kohli, I., Nicholson, C. L., Williams, J. D., et al. (2020). Greater efficacy of SPF 100+ sunscreen compared with SPF 50+ in sunburn prevention during 5 consecutive days of sunlight exposure: A randomized, double-blind clinical trial. *Journal of the American Academy of Dermatology*, *82*(4), 869–877.

Kullavanijaya, P., & Lim, H. W. (2005). Photoprotection. *Journal of the American Academy of Dermatology*, *52*, 937–958.

Prevention and treatment of sunburn. (2004). *The Medical Letter on Drugs and Therapeutics*, *46*, 45–46.

Yeager, D. G., & Lim, H. W. (2019). What's new in photoprotection: A review of new concepts and controversies. *Dermatology Clinics*, *37*, 149–157.

Tick Bites and Tickborne Illness

Presentation

The patient arrives with a tick attached to the skin (Fig. 182.1) and is often frightened or disgusted and concerned about developing Lyme disease, Rocky Mountain spotted fever (RMSF), or "tick fever." Alternatively, the patient may only have a history of having removed a tick within the past week or so and now has developed a spreading erythematous rash at the previous site of attachment (Fig. 182.2). By this time, systemic signs and symptoms consisting of myalgia, arthralgia, fever, headache, and fatigue may be present.

What to Do

☑ **When there is no tick present,** obtaining a history of tick exposure in the recreational, occupational, and travel history can be essential for diagnosis.

☑ Carefully examine the patient for an individual tick or multiple ticks. Ticks can attach themselves to any part of the body, but certain species appear to prefer particular locations. Dog ticks may favor the head and neck, while the Lone Star tick may favor the lower extremities, buttocks, and groin. Although tick bites can be painful, the ticks are often not detected when they crawl, attach, feed, or depart from human skin.

☑ **When an embedded tick is present, apply protective gloves if available, and promptly remove the tick. Grasp the tick as close to the skin as possible with a pair of narrow-tipped forceps and slowly but firmly pull straight up until the tick mouth parts separate from the skin** (Fig. 182.3). Be careful not to squeeze the tick's body or twist the tick's head. Alternatively, the tick's jaws may be pried away from the skin using a 20-gauge needle tip as a wedge.

☑ **Although not proven, it has been suggested that by injecting and infiltrating lidocaine with epinephrine beneath the attached tick, removal by traction is made easier. Also,** covering the tick with 2% viscous lidocaine has led to spontaneous detachment within 5 minutes in a very small series.

☑ **After removal of the tick, disinfect the attachment site and wash your hands with soap and water. Save the tick in a container of alcohol for future identification or flush it down the toilet after it has been properly identified.**

☑ **If the mouth parts appear to remain embedded, do not make aggressive attempts to remove them,** as the patient's body will expel them spontaneously.

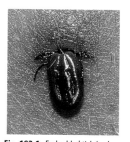

Fig. 182.1 Embedded tick *Ixodes pacificus* (western blacklegged tick). (From White, G., & Cox, N. [2006]. *Diseases of the skin* [2nd ed.]. St. Louis, MO: Mosby.)

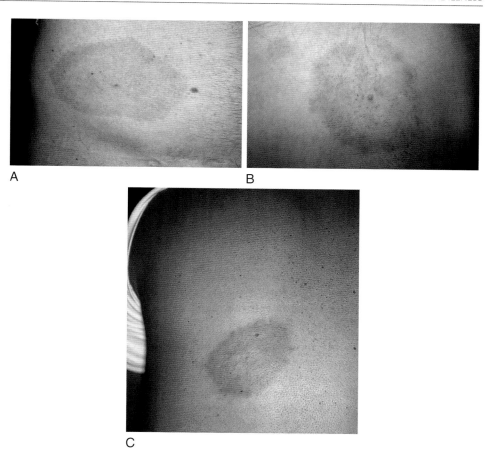

A

B

C

Fig. 182.2 (A–C) Erythema migrans. The causative organism is *Borrelia burgdorferi*. (From White, G., & Cox, N. [2006]. *Diseases of the skin* [2nd ed.]. St. Louis, MO: Mosby.)

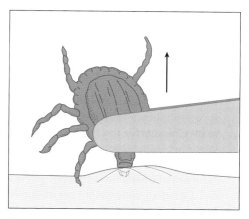

Fig. 182.3 Remove tick with narrow-tipped forceps.

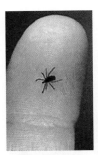

Fig. 182.4 Life-sized deer tick. (From Gorman, C. [1995, July 24]. Deer tick turns deadly. *Time*, 56.)

✅ **If it is an *Ixodes scapularis* or deer tick** (Fig. 182.4) **(or *Ixodes pacificus*)** (see Fig. 182.1), **but it has been attached for less than 72 hours and was not engorged, there is minimal risk for disease transmission. There is no need for prophylaxis.** The patient or family can be reassured, but instruct them to monitor the patient's temperature daily for the next 4 weeks and to notify a physician or return at the first sign of a fever. In addition, over the same time period, instruct the family to watch for an expanding pink patch at the site, which could be the beginning of erythema migrans. Also, if any rash, fever, cranial or peripheral neuropathies, or systemic symptoms such as headache, myalgia, malaise, sweats, chills, or joint pains ("flu symptoms") occur, have them return to evaluate for possible tickborne illness, and initiate treatment as noted later.

✅ **If an *Ixodes* tick has been attached for less than 72 hours, but the tick appears to be engorged with blood, treat prophylactically for Lyme disease with doxycycline, 200 mg orally in one dose. Patients who are at minimal risk for transmission but are very anxious and cannot be reassured may also be given a single preventative dose.**

✅ **If this was an *Ixodes* tick that was attached for more than 72 hours, the patient presents with a focal rash at the site where the tick had been attached, or there are signs and symptoms as noted earlier, prescribe antibiotics to prevent or treat early Lyme disease (see later in this chapter).**

✅ **In a patient with typical erythema migrans, in an endemic area, laboratory confirmation is not required and, in fact, may be misleading, as serology may still be negative. Doxycycline, 100 mg twice daily for 2 to 3 weeks, is the agent of choice.** For nursing women and children younger than 8 years of age, doxycycline is still the agent of choice. The recommended dose for children is 2.2 mg/kg (maximum 100 mg) twice daily. Alternatively, pregnant women can be treated with amoxicillin, 500 mg three times a day for 14 to 21 days; or cefuroxime (Ceftin), 500 mg twice daily for 14 to 21 days; or erythromycin, 250 mg four times a day for 2 weeks.

✅ **If a wood tick (in the western United States) or a dog tick (in the eastern United States) has been removed** (Fig. 182.5), **reassure the patient and family that the likelihood of developing RMSF is very small (1%), and that if it should occur, prompt treatment will be quite effective on development of fever and/or headache.** It is not recommended to give prophylactic antibiotics in an attempt to prevent RMSF. If transmission of infection has occurred, within 1 to 2 weeks after the tick bite, acute onset of fever, chills, severe headache, and myalgias will develop. **Patients should seek immediate care at the onset of their symptoms.** In most patients, fever and severe headache precede the characteristic rash that generally appears on the fourth day, starting on the wrists, ankles, and forearms as blanching red macules that progress to form papules centrally to the arms, thigh, trunk, and face. **Therapy should be started when the disease is suspected and should never be delayed for confirmatory tests. Tetracyclines and chloramphenicol are the only drugs proven to be effective for the treatment of RMSF.** Because of its effectiveness, broad margin of safety, and convenient dosing schedule, **doxycycline is currently considered the drug of choice for nearly all patients, including young children.** The current recommended regimens of treatment with doxycycline are 100 mg per dose given twice daily for adults, and 2.2 mg/kg body weight per dose given twice daily for children weighing less than 45 kg. These recommended doses may be given orally or intravenously, and treatment should

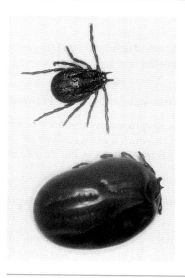

Fig. 182.5 Dog ticks showing normal morphology *(upper photo)* and after being fully engorged with blood *(lower photo)*. (From Bolognia, J., Jorizzo, J., & Rapini, R. [2003]. *Dermatology.* St. Louis, MO: Mosby.)

be maintained for 5 to 7 days. Doxycycline therapy should be continued until the patient is afebrile for at least 3 days and there is clinical improvement. Intravenous therapy is often indicated for hospital inpatients, particularly for those with vomiting, unstable vital signs, and neurologic symptoms. **Doxycycline is now the recommended therapy for RMSF in pregnant women.** Patients treated with **chloramphenicol** seem to have a higher mortality, and this drug **should not be used in any patient population**, except in cases of severe doxycycline allergy when desensitization is not possible. The indicated dose of chloramphenicol is 50 to 75 mg/kg/day, divided into four doses, given for 7 days, or until 3 days after the fever has subsided.

⊘ **Provide information about prevention of tick exposure.** Measures to help prevent tick exposure include avoiding tick-infested areas (especially during the summer months); avoiding the grassy, overgrown areas favored by ticks; staying to the center of a trail while hiking; and avoiding sitting on logs or leaning against trees. Other measures include wearing long pants and tucking pant legs into socks, using tick repellents containing diethyltoluamide (DEET) for exposed skin and permethrin (Duranon) for clothing, and using bed nets sprayed with permethrin when sleeping on the ground or camping. Wearing light-colored clothing and checking the skin carefully at the end of the day for ticks (especially the head, scalp, and genital area ["tick checks"]) will help in spotting a tick before it bites. Special graspers for removing ticks are available and can be handy in the field (e.g., Tick Nipper).

What Not to Do

Ⓧ Do not use heat, occlusion, or caustics to remove a tick. Many techniques have been promoted, but they are generally ineffective and may increase the chance of infection or may potentially do harm.

Ⓧ Do not contaminate your fingers with potentially infected tick products.

Ⓧ Do not mutilate the skin by attempting to remove the tick's "head." Usually what is left behind is cementum secreted by the tick, which is easily scraped off. Retained mouth parts can produce local inflammation or minor bacterial infection, but they do not transmit Lyme disease.

Ⓧ Do not prescribe prophylactic antibiotics for potential RMSF.

Ⓧ Do not prescribe prophylactic antibiotics for Lyme disease if its prevalence is very low in your geographic area.

Ⓧ Do not initiate serologic testing in the asymptomatic patient in whom a tick is removed or early in the course of Lyme disease. It is costly, inaccurate, and unnecessary. Serologic testing may be more useful in later stages of the disease when sensitivity and specificity of the test are improved.

Discussion

Ixodes scapularis (previously *I. dammini*), the tiny deer tick of the eastern United States, and *I. pacificus* of the western United States (Pacific Coast states) can transmit the infectious agents that cause babesiosis, ehrlichiosis, anaplasmosis, Powassan virus, and Lyme disease. **Most patients presenting in the summer with a viral syndrome have just that; however, there are other important considerations. Tickborne diseases may present in this fashion. The clinician must consider the diagnosis in the appropriate epidemiologic setting. Treatment with doxycycline is indicated for RMSF, Lyme disease, ehrlichiosis, and anaplasmosis. In patients with clinical findings suggestive of tickborne disease, empirical treatment should not be delayed. The same tick may harbor different infectious pathogens and may transmit several with one bite.**

Ticks are divided into three families, only two of which are capable of causing infection: soft ticks (Argasidae) and hard ticks (Ixodidae), the latter being responsible for most tick-related diseases. Tickborne diseases in the United States include Lyme disease, RMSF, ehrlichiosis, tularemia, babesiosis, Colorado tick fever, and relapsing fever.

Lyme disease is the most common vectorborne disease in the United States. It has been reported in 49 of the 50 US states, but most cases occur in the Northeast to Midwest and North Central regions of the United States. The highest reported incidence tends to be in New England. The etiologic agent is the slow-growing, motile spirochete *Borrelia burgdorferi,* which is transmitted by ticks. Deer tick nymphs appear to be the most important vector for transmission of Lyme disease. This nymph stage is when they are tiny and likely to be missed. A minimum of 36 to 48 hours of attachment of the tick is required for transmission. Most cases occur between May and August, which corresponds with increased outdoor human activity and nymphal activity. The risk for developing Lyme disease after a tick bite is low, even in endemic areas. It should also be noted that less than half of affected patients recall receiving a tick bite because of the small size of the tick.

The incubation period is typically 1 week, but the rash might develop as late as 16 weeks after the tick bite. In early localized disease, a rash develops with or without systemic symptoms. The rash is

Discussion continued

erythematous, annular, well-demarcated plaque **(erythema migrans)** and has a median diameter of 15 cm. Typically, it is oval or round in shape, with a morphology that usually consists of a flat erythema. The phenomenon of central clearing, previously emphasized, occurs in only a minority of cases. The rash is usually painless but may "burn" or itch and may feel warm to touch. The color may be uniform or centrally darker. Rarely, the center is necrotic or vesicular in nature.

Within days to a few weeks after the infection, hematogenous and lymphatic dissemination of the spirochete to distant sites commonly occurs (early disseminated disease). Other annular plaques develop in up to half of patients. The most common neurologic feature is unilateral or bilateral facial paralysis (unilateral paralysis mimicking Bell palsy (see Chapter 5). Other findings include peripheral neuropathy, meningitis, atrioventricular (AV) block (sometimes fluctuating in degree), and myopericarditis among other cardiac and neurologic manifestations. Late-stage disease can occur months to years after the initial infection. The most common finding in this stage is arthritis, although neurologic phenomenon that consist primarily of a mild to severe encephalopathy, a polyneuropathy, and profound fatigue can occur. Encephalopathy is thought to occur in 9 of 10 patients and is often characterized by subtle disturbances in mood, memory, and sleep.

The diagnosis of Lyme disease is usually based on the history of a tick bite in an endemic area, with characteristic clinical findings. Serology using enzyme-linked immunosorbent assay (ELISA) is the most common laboratory test to screen for antibodies; however, the test is not standardized, and false negatives, especially with active or recent infections (or, more commonly, false positives), are common. When a positive or equivocal test is obtained using ELISA, a Western blot (immunoblot) test should be performed on the same serum sample. If the immunoblot is negative, the ELISA is likely a false positive; if the immunoblot is positive, a diagnosis of Lyme disease can be confirmed in a patient with clinical evidence of Lyme disease.

One bout of Lyme disease will not confer immunity to future infections.

RMSF, the most common acute rickettsial infection in the United States, is caused by *Rickettsia rickettsii*. In the United States, the disease is most commonly seen in the Southeast, West, and South-Central states. The infection typically occurs in spring and summer, and the exposure is usually in rural or suburban areas. Primary offenders in the western United States are the wood tick *(Dermacentor andersoni)*, and, in the eastern United States, the dog tick *(D. variabilis)*. The diagnosis of RMSF is based largely on clinical presentation in a patient with history of tick exposure. **Various serology tests are available to confirm the diagnosis. When administered early in the disease, doxycycline (orally and intravenously) is extremely effective.** The use of doxycycline in the treatment of tickborne rickettsial diseases in children was controversial in the past because of the risk of permanent tooth discoloration. Today there is a consensus that doxycycline is the drug of choice for treating presumptive or confirmed RMSF in children of any age. A prospective study reported that children treated with doxycycline for RMSF did not show substantial discoloration of permanent teeth compared with those who had never received the drug.

Ehrlichieae are a group of small, gram-negative, obligate intracellular pleomorphic bacteria that are closely related to rickettsiae. In the United States, ehrlichiosis (formally referred to as human monocytic ehrlichiosis [HME]) has been seen mainly in the Mid-Atlantic, South Central, and Southeast states as well as in New England. *Amblyomma americanum* (Lone Star tick) and *I. scapularis* are the primary vectors. Most cases occur during summer and autumn, and more than 80% of patients have a history of tick exposure. The clinical manifestations of ehrlichiosis are similar to those of RMSF, with a lesser likelihood of rash. In general, the treatment of choice for ehrlichiosis is a doxycycline. Anaplasmosis (formerly called human granulocytic ehrlichiosis [HGE]) has been reported in the Northeast, the upper Midwest, and regions of northern California. Principal vectors are *I. scapularis* (northeastern America) and *I. pacificus* (western United States). The clinical presentation for anaplasmosis is indistinguishable from HME, and the treatment is similar. Both anaplasmosis and ehrlichiosis can lead to multiorgan failure and death if untreated.

Tularemia is caused by *Francisella tularensis,* a short, gram-negative, nonmotile coccobacillus. In the United States, the disease is most commonly seen in central and western states. Inoculation of

Discussion continued

organisms into the skin most frequently occurs from bites of deer flies or ticks and from direct contact with infected animals, primarily wild rabbits, especially after skinning their hides. The tick in the Southeast and South Central United States is *A. americanum* (Lone Star tick), and in the West it is *D. andersoni* (wood tick); the most widely distributed is *D. variabilis* (dog tick). Tularemia has several presentations, ranging from a primary dermatologic presentation (ulceroglandular) with fever to a primary pulmonic presentation that is characterized by a viral-type prodrome followed by high fever, dry cough, and chest pain. The typical incubation period is 3 to 5 days. The most common clinical presentation is the ulceroglandular type, which begins at the site of the tick bite, as a papule or nodule that rapidly ulcerates. A lymphatic spread occurs with painful regional lymphadenopathy, usually inguinal or femoral, which might progress to ulceration. Streptomycin given intramuscularly is the treatment of choice and the course is 10 days. Alternatives include gentamycin, tetracyclines (only if less clinically ill and requires a 14-day treatment), and fluoroquinolones (although they are not FDA approved for this indication).

Babesiosis is a malaria-like disease caused by an intracellular parasite that invades red blood cells. The major endemic areas in the United States are Massachusetts (Martha's Vineyard, Nantucket), New York (eastern and southern Long Island), Connecticut, and other offshore islands of the Northeast. The causative agent is *Babesia microti*, which is transmitted by the larvae of *I. scapularis* (deer tick). The illness usually occurs in older patients or in asplenic or immunocompromised patients. Symptoms may occur weeks or months later and may recur if a patient becomes immunosuppressed. The classic clinical presentation is high fever, drenching sweats, myalgias, and hemolytic anemia. Blood smear may be confusing: The tetrad of merozoites of babesiosis can be confused with the ring forms of *Plasmodium falciparum*–induced malaria. A concomitant course (7–10 days) of atovaquone *and* azithromycin OR quinine *and* clindamycin are used most commonly to treat the infection.

Colorado tick fever is caused by a ribonucleic acid (RNA) orbivirus transmitted by the *D. andersoni* wood tick. It is predominantly found in the Rocky Mountain region. Influenza-like symptoms usually begin within 1 week after inoculation. The disease usually lasts 7 to 10 days. Treatment is supportive, but at the onset of symptoms most patients will be treated empirically with doxycycline to cover other tickborne diseases.

Tickborne relapsing fever is caused by the spirochete within the genus *Borrelia*. It is transmitted by species of the soft tick genus *Ornithodoros*. The tick species capable of transmitting the disease in the United States tends to exist in remote undisturbed settings in most regions. After an incubation period of 1 week, the disease is characterized by acute onset of high fever with chills, headache, myalgias, tachycardia, arthralgias, and malaise. If untreated, the primary episode lasts 3 to 6 days; rapid-spreading erythematous rash, defervescence, followed by drenching sweats marks resolution of disease. If left untreated, a second shorter course and as many as three to five relapses per year can occur. Tickborne relapsing fever warrants treatment with either tetracycline or penicillin for 5 to 10 days.

Tick paralysis rarely occurs in humans; when it does, it usually affects children. Most cases in the United States occur in the Northwest in the spring or summer months, and the ticks usually attach to the scalp or neck. In the United States, most cases are attributed to wood ticks, dog ticks, Lone Star ticks, and deer ticks. Paralysis usually occurs 4 to 7 days after attachment of the tick and is caused by the production of a neurotoxin secreted in the saliva of the tick. An acute ascending lower motor neuron paralysis develops, beginning in the legs and sparing sensory function. Definitive therapy is simply to remove any ticks attached to the patient's body. However, symptoms can progress after tick removal. In general, improvement is much faster in cases in North America than in Australia. Normally, once the tick is removed in the former setting, symptoms begin to rapidly resolve within hours and are completely resolved 24 hours later. Patients who are minimally symptomatic can be observed for several hours and discharged if no progression occurs. In Australian cases, where symptoms can dramatically progress after the tick is removed, patients should be observed for a longer period, until the clinical course is clearly steadily and unequivocally improving.

In summary, fever and a rash following a tick bite can signify a true medical emergency. Most tickborne illnesses respond readily to doxycycline therapy. In the case of RMSF, therapy should be started when the disease is suspected and should never be delayed for confirmatory tests. Accurate identification of tick vectors can help establish a diagnosis and guide preventive measures.

Suggested Readings

Aberer, E. (2009). What should one do in case of a tick bite? *Current Problems in Dermatology*, *37*, 155–166.

Bratton, R. L., & Corey, G. R. (2005). Tick-borne disease. *American Family Physician*, *71*, 2323–2330.

Clark, R. P., & Hu, L. T. (2008). Prevention of Lyme disease and other tick-borne infections. *Infectious Disease Clinics of North America*, *22*, 381–396 vii.

Dantas-Torres, F. (2007). Rocky Mountain spotted fever. *The Lancet Infectious Diseases*, *7*, 724–732.

Dedeoglu, F., & Sundel, R. P. (2004). Emergency department management of Lyme disease. *Clinical Pediatric Emergency Medicine*, *5*, 54–62.

Edlow, J. A., & McGillicuddy, D. C. (2008). Tick paralysis. *Infectious Disease Clinics of North America*, *22*, 397–413 vi.

Elston, D. M. (2010). Tick bites and skin rashes. *Current Opinions in Infectious Disease*, *23*, 132–138.

McGinley-Smith, D. E., & Tsao, S. S. (2003). Dermatoses from ticks. *Journal of the American Academy of Dermatology*, *49*, 363–392.

Needham, G. R. (1985). Evaluation of five popular methods for tick removal. *Pediatrics*, *75*, 997–1002.

Ross Russell, A. L., Dryden, M. S., Pinto, A. A., et al. (2018). Lyme disease: Diagnosis and management. *Practical Neurology*, *18*, 455–464.

Singh-Behl, D., La Rosa, S. P., & Tomecki, K. J. (2003). Tick-borne infections. *Dermatology Clinics*, *21*, 237–244.

Smith, R. P., Schoen, R. T., & Rahn, D. W. (2002). Clinical characteristics and treatment outcome of early Lyme disease in patients with microbiologically confirmed erythema migrans. *Annals of Internal Medicine*, *136*, 421–428.

Treatment of Lyme disease. (2005). *A Medical Letter on Drugs and Therapeutics*, *47*, 41–43.

Volovitz, B., Shkap, R., & Amir, J. (2007). Absence of tooth staining with doxycycline treatment in young children. *Clinical Pediatrics*, *46*(2), 121–126.

Tinea Pedis, Tinea Cruris, Tinea Corporis

(Athlete's Foot, Jock Itch, Ringworm)

Presentation

Patients usually seek medical care for athlete's foot, jock itch, or ringworm when pruritus is severe or when secondary infection causes pain and swelling. Worrisome spreading of the rash, along with an unsightly and annoying appearance, will also motivate these patients to seek medical treatment.

Tinea Pedis

There are three general clinical presentations: interdigital, moccasin, and vesicobullous. Interdigital disease is most common. Often there is fissuring, scaling, and maceration of the interdigital or subdigital areas, particularly the fourth-to-fifth toe web space (Fig. 183.1A and B). Moccasin-type tinea is characterized by fine silvery scales, with underlying pink to red skin that most commonly affects areas of the soles, heels, and sides of the feet (moccasin distribution) (see Fig. 183.1C). Vesicobullous tinea pedis is the least common form. There may be acute and highly inflammatory vesicular or bullous lesions that are pruritic and commonly found at the instep of the foot; however, inflammation may spread over the entire sole (see Fig. 183.1D).

Tinea Cruris

This is a dermatophyte infection of the inguinal folds, inner thighs, perineum, and buttocks that usually spares the scrotum and penis (unlike *Candida intertrigo*). There is an erythematous scaling eruption that is often annular in appearance (Fig. 183.2). Pruritus is a common symptom, and pain may be present if the involved area is moist and macerated or secondarily infected. More commonly seen in men, tinea cruris often occurs in patients with tinea pedis and onychomycosis (dermatophyte infection of the toenails) and is thought to spread to the groin from contaminated underpants.

Tinea Corporis

This dermatophyte infection of the glabrous (hairless) skin elsewhere on the body typically presents as an erythematous, scaling, annular eruption with central clearing on the extremities or trunk (Fig. 183.3). The classic ringworm pattern is a flat, scaly area with a raised border that advances circumferentially. Vesicles or pustules may form as the lesion becomes inflamed.

What to Do

✅ **When microscopic examination of skin scrapings in potassium hydroxide (KOH) is readily available,** definite identification of the lesion can be made by looking for the presence of hyphae or spores. Using a No. 10 scalpel blade, scrape flakes or scales from the active leading edge of the lesion (or from the web space) onto a glass slide. Sweep the particles toward the center of the slide and

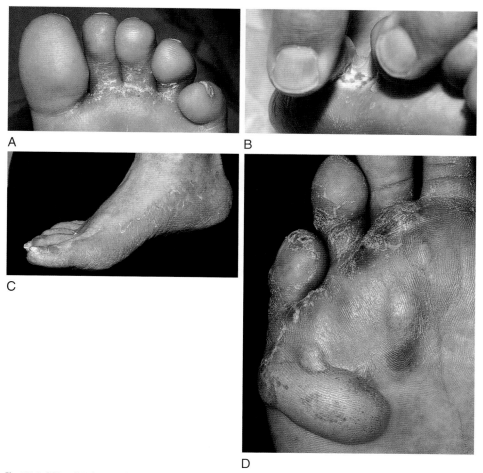

Fig. 183.1 (A) Interdigital tinea pedis. (B) White macerated web between fourth and fifth toes. (C) Moccasin distribution of tinea pedis. (D) Bullous tinea. (From White, G., & Cox, N. *Diseases of the skin* [2nd ed.]. St. Louis, MO: Mosby.)

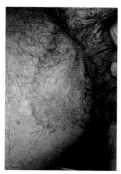

Fig. 183.2 Tinea cruris. (From Bolognia, J., Jorizzo, J., & Rapini, R. [2003]. *Dermatology*. St. Louis, MO: Mosby.)

add a drop of 10% to 20% KOH and a cover slip. Warm with a flame, and then view under low (100×) magnification with the microscope light condenser lowered. **Branching fungal filaments (hyphae and myceliae) identify superficial dermatophytes (Fig. 183.4).** Budding cells and pseudohyphae (spaghetti and meatballs–like appearance) suggest yeast, particularly *Candida* organisms. Fungal cultures are rarely necessary for acute uncomplicated lesions. Treatment can be started presumptively when microscopic examination is not easily accomplished, but **always consider alternative diagnoses** such as the so-called herald patch of pityriasis rosea (see Chapter 177), nummular dermatitis, secondary and tertiary syphilis, lichen planus, seborrheic dermatitis, psoriasis, impetigo (see Chapter 174), and neurodermatitis in the differential diagnosis.

⊘ **When tinea is diagnosed or strongly suspected, treat with terbinafine (Lamisil AT cream or spray), clotrimazole (Lotrimin or Lotrimin Ultra 1% cream, solution, or lotion), or miconazole (Micatin) 2% cream, spray, lotion, or powder, or alternatively with butenafine (Mentax) 1% cream applied once or twice daily. They are available over the counter and can**

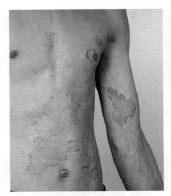

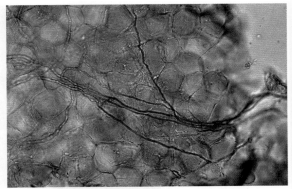

Fig. 183.3 Tinea corporis. (From White, G., & Cox, N. *Diseases of the skin* [2nd ed.]. St. Louis, MO: Mosby.)

Fig. 183.4 Potassium hydrochloride (KOH) preparation of a dermatophyte demonstrating branching hyphae. (From Bolognia, J., Jorizzo, J., & Rapini, R. [2003]. *Dermatology.* St. Louis, MO: Mosby.)

most effectively be applied twice a day. Naftifine (Naftin 1% cream applied once daily or 1% gel applied once to twice daily) requires a prescription and is very expensive. If applied to the rash, they will cause involution of most superficial lesions within 1 to 2 weeks but may need to be continued for up to 4 weeks. They should be continued for 7 to 14 days beyond symptom resolution to prevent relapse. **Advise the patient to apply the topical medication 2 cm past the border of the skin lesion.**

✅ **Sertaconazole nitrate (Ertaczo) cream 2% possesses both fungicidal and fungistatic properties, and it even exhibits anti-inflammatory and antipruritic effects.** Unfortunately, it also is very expensive. Apply twice a day (not approved for children <12 years of age).

✅ Rarely, **more severe or extensive lesions** can be treated with oral antifungals. Terbinafine (Lamisil), 250 mg daily for 2 weeks; ketoconazole (Nizoral), 200 mg daily for 4 weeks; or fluconazole (Diflucan), 150 mg weekly for 2 to 4 weeks, can be used. Be aware of the potential for serious side effects when prescribing systemic antifungals.

✅ **With signs of secondary infection, begin treatment first with wet compresses of Burow solution (2 packets Domeboro powder in 1 pint water) for 30 min every 3 to 4 hours. Use mupirocin (Bactroban) 2% cream for superficial bacterial infections (impetigo). With signs of deep infection (cellulitis, lymphangitis),** begin systemic antibiotics with streptococcal coverage, such as cephalexin (Keflex) or dicloxacillin (Dynapen), 250 to 500 mg four times a day 7 to 10 days. **Always consider coverage for community-acquired methicillin-resistant *Staphylococcus aureus* (CA-MRSA) if it is prevalent in your area** (see Chapter 168).

✅ **With inflammation and weeping lesions, a topical antifungal and steroid cream combination, such as Lotrisone in addition to the wet compresses, will be most effective.** Warn patients that this medication has a potent steroid that can lead to skin atrophy or striae if used for an extended period, especially in the groin. **An alternative is to use the recommended antifungals and add Burrow solution (1% aluminum acetate or 5% aluminum subacetate) wet dressings two or three times a day (for 15–20 min at a time).**

✅ **For tinea pedis,** instruct patients to wear nonocclusive footwear, such as sandals, that allow the foot to breathe. Have them put on socks before underwear to avoid spreading the

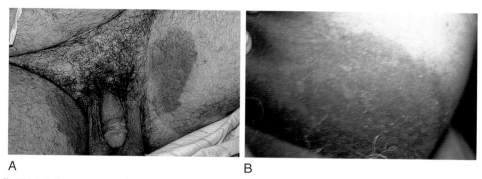

Fig. 183.5 Erythrasma appears as red-brown patches of the groin or axilla that fluoresce coral-pink under Wood light examination. (From White, G., & Cox, N. *Diseases of the skin* [2nd ed.]. St. Louis, MO: Mosby.)

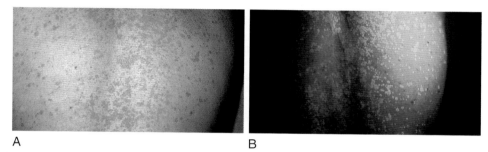

Fig. 183.6 (A) Tinea versicolor on the upper back of a young adult. (B) Wood light examination of the same patient. (From White, G., & Cox, N. *Diseases of the skin* [2nd ed.]. St. Louis, MO: Mosby.)

fungus from feet to groin. **A gel formulation of naftifine may be helpful for moist web spaces.**

✓ **For tinea cruris,** suggest loose undergarments made of absorbent materials, such as cotton, rather than synthetics. Skin should be dried well with a towel or hair dryer. Absorbent powders and drying agents, such as Zeasorb-AF and Drysol, can be applied lightly.

✓ **To prevent reinfection when onychomycosis is present,** nail infections should be treated (see later, this chapter).

What Not to Do

✗ Do not attempt to treat fungal infections of the scalp (tinea capitis) with local therapy. A boggy swelling (tinea kerion) or patchy hair loss with inflammation and scaling requires systemic antifungals, such as griseofulvin.

✗ Do not use nystatin, a drug familiar for its usefulness against *Candida* infections, to treat tinea. Tinea infections are not killed by this drug.

✗ Do not treat with corticosteroids alone. They will reduce signs and symptoms (tinea incognito) but allow increased fungal growth.

Discussion

Tinea infections are caused by superficial fungi known as dermatophytes, which are true saprophytes that take all their nutrients from dead keratin in the stratum corneum of the skin and the keratinized tissue of hair and nails. They cannot invade live epidermis. Some of these infections cause circular lesions that result from the inflammatory reaction, forcing the dermatophytes outward to an inflammation-free area. As long as the infection persists, so does the outward migration.

Tinea pedis, or athlete's foot, is the most common fungal infection. It is seen most in those who wear occlusive footwear because shoes promote warmth and sweating, which encourage fungal growth. Tinea must be differentiated from allergic and irritant contact dermatitis (see Chapter 162). **In several studies, application of the allylamine terbinafine twice daily resulted in a higher cure rate than twice-daily application of the imidazole clotrimazole, and at a quicker rate (1 week vs 4 weeks).**

All superficial dermatophytes of the skin, except those involving the scalp, beard, face, hands, feet, groin, and nails, are known as **tinea corporis**, or ringworm of the body. Contact with pets is often the source of the infection. Systemic diseases (e.g., diabetes, leukemia, acquired immunodeficiency disease [AIDS]) predispose patients to tinea corporis.

Candidiasis and erythrasma may resemble tinea cruris, but candidal lesions are usually more moist, red, and tender (see Chapter 167). Pustules may be seen within the indistinct border, and satellite lesions may be scattered over adjacent skin. Candidiasis also may involve the scrotum or penis, which are usually spared by tinea. *Candida* **organisms may be treated topically with naftifine (Naftin), ciclopirox (Loprox), or clotrimazole (Lotrimin, Mycelex).**

Erythrasma is a skin infection caused by *Corynebacterium minutissimum*, a gram-positive bacterium. The rash characteristically consists of asymptomatic, reddish-brown, superficial dull patches with well-defined margins and no central clearing. The peripheral edge is not usually any more raised than the center (Fig. 183.5A). When illuminated with an ultraviolet Wood lamp, the infected skin glows with coral-pink fluorescence (see Fig. 183.5B). **Erythrasma is treated with oral erythromycin, 250 mg four times a day for 14 days.**

Tinea versicolor is a misnomer, because it is not caused by a dermatophyte fungus but by lipophilic yeast. Pityriasis versicolor is the more correct name. It is asymptomatic, and its presentation to an acute care facility usually is incidental to some other problem. There is, however, no reason to ignore this chronic superficial skin infection, which causes cosmetically unpleasant irregular patches of varying pigmentation that tend to be lighter than the surrounding skin in the summer and darker than the surrounding skin in the winter. Wood light examination sometimes reveals a white or yellow fluorescence (Fig. 183.6).

Differential diagnosis includes tinea corporis, pityriasis alba, pityriasis rosea, vitiligo, leprosy, and secondary syphilis.

Prescribe a 2.5% selenium sulfide lotion (Selsun) to be applied as lather, leave on 10 to 15 minutes, then wash off daily for 10 to 14 days and then every night at bedtime monthly, or use three to five times weekly for 2 to 4 weeks (which also should be followed with monthly retreatments). Alternatively, use terbinafine 1% solution (spray) twice daily for 1 week or ketoconazole (Nizoral) cream 2% daily for 2 weeks, or ketoconazole or fluconazole (Diflucan) as a single 300-mg oral dose to be repeated in 4 weeks. Also, itraconazole can be taken 200 mg four times a day for 3 to 7 days. Superficial scaling should resolve in a few days, and the pigmentary changes will slowly clear over a period of several months. Tinea versicolor has a recurrence rate of 80% after 2 years; patients are therefore likely to need periodic retreatment or preventive maintenance.

Tinea capitis is mainly a disease of infants, children, and young adolescents. Tinea capitis presents variably as scales, papules, pustules, plaques, or nodules on the scalp. Inflammation and superinfection lead to secondary processes, such as alopecia, erythema, exudate, and edema (Fig. 183.7). A kerion forms as a result of increased cell-mediated immune response, demonstrated by an inflamed, exudative, nodular, boggy swelling with associated hair loss and cervical lymphadenopathy (Fig. 183.8). Tinea capitis can be diagnosed on KOH examination of extracted hair. Culture must involve the extracted hair, not simply scales.

Oral antifungals are the mainstay of treatment for tinea capitis. Griseofulvin is the only drug approved by the US Food and Drug Administration (FDA) for use in children, although other medications have been used. Terbinafine (Lamisil) is now considered the primary drug of choice for the treatment of tinea

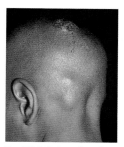

Fig. 183.8 Kerion with swollen regional lymph nodes. (From White, G., & Cox, N. *Diseases of the skin* [2nd ed.]. St. Louis, MO: Mosby.)

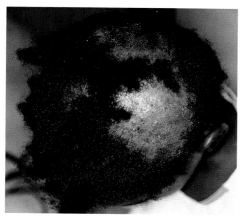

Fig. 183.7 Tinea capitis. (From Bolognia, J., Jorizzo, J., & Rapini, R. [2003]. *Dermatology*. St. Louis, MO: Mosby.)

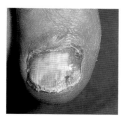

Fig. 183.9 Tinea unguium or subungual onychomycosis. (From White, G., & Cox, N. *Diseases of the skin* [2nd ed.]. St. Louis, MO: Mosby.)

Discussion continued

capitis. **In adults prescribe 250 mg daily for 4 to 8 weeks. Prescribe 6 to 12 mg/kg/day to 8 weeks for children. Griseofulvin is given as 20 to 25 mg/kg/day once daily for 8 weeks (or 2 weeks beyond cure), or liquid microsized griseofulvin (Grifulvin V), 15 to 25 mg/kg every day for 8 weeks. Ketoconazole shampoo and cream can be used to reduce fungal shedding.** To prevent spread to other family members, contaminated combs and brushes should be cleaned, and family members can use selenium sulfide lotion or shampoo for 5 to 10 minutes (then rinse) three times per week.

Onychomycosis (also known as tinea unguium) is an infection of the nail plate or nail bed that interferes with normal nail function (Fig. 183.9). Patients with this infection often have concomitant fungal infections at other sites. Because onychomycosis requires expensive prolonged therapy (6 weeks for fingernail infections and 12 weeks for toenail infections), the diagnosis should be confirmed before treatment is initiated. This can be achieved by clipping off the distal edge of the affected nail, placing it in formalin along with attached subungual debris, and sending it for periodic acid–Schiff staining with histologic examination in a hospital or reference laboratory.

Terbinafine, at a dosage of 250 mg per day for 6 weeks (fingernails), 12 weeks (toenails), has a better mycologic cure rate than pulse therapy, in which 500 mg of terbinafine is given once daily for 7 days of each of 2 months (fingernails) or 4 months (toenails). It should be noted, though, that follow-up must be arranged with a patient's primary doctor or dermatologist. Long-term dosage with this drug has caused some significant liver disease. Terbinafine is considered the drug of choice for dermatophyte onychomycosis, with greater mycologic cure rates, less serious and fewer drug interactions, and a lower cost than continuous itraconazole therapy. Adjunct débridement may improve the clinical and complete cure rates compared with terbinafine alone.

Newer oral antifungal agents have greatly improved the management of dermatomycoses, but not without consequence. Some are very expensive, have side effects and organ toxicity that may or may not be tolerable, and have significant adverse drug interactions. Laboratory monitoring is recommended during treatment with all oral antifungal medications. Liver function tests for itraconazole should be done at baseline, at 1 month, and if any signs or symptoms of liver dysfunction present. Terbinafine use warrants liver function tests at baseline, at 6 weeks, if signs or symptoms are present, and then 4 weeks later. In general, one should monitor patients more closely if taking other medications that impair renal or hepatic function.

Suggested Readings

Alter, S. J., McDonald, M. B., Schloemer, J., Simon, R., & Trevino, J. (2018). Common child and adolescent cutaneous infestations and fungal infections. *Current Problems in Pediatric and Adolescent Health Care, 48*, 3–25.

Fleece, D., Gaughan, J. P., & Aronoff, S. C. (2004). Griseofulvin versus terbinafine in the treatment of tinea capitis. *Pediatrics, 114*, 1312–1315.

Gupta, A. K., Chaudhry, M., & Elewski, B. (2003). Tinea corporis, tinea cruris, tinea nigra, and piedra. *Dermatology Clinics, 21*, 395–400.

Gupta, A. K., Chow, M., Daniel, C. R., et al. (2003). Treatments of tinea pedis. *Dermatology Clinics, 21*, 431–462.

Gupta, A. K., Cooper, E. A., & Montero-Gei, F. (2003). The use of fluconazole to treat superficial fungal infections in children. *Dermatology Clinics, 21*, 537–542.

Hainer, B. L. (2003). Dermatophyte infections. *American Family Physician, 67*, 101–108.

Janniger, C. K., Schwartz, R. A., Szepietowski, J. C., et al. (2005). Intertrigo and common secondary skin infections. *American Family Physician, 72*, 833–838.

Lipner, S. R., & Scher, R. K. (2019). Onychomycosis: Clinical overview and diagnosis. *Journal of the American Academy of Dermatology, 80* 835–351.

Loo, D. S. (2007). Onychomycosis in the elderly drug treatment options. *Drugs & Aging, 24*, 293–302.

Martin, E. S., & Elewski, B. E. (2002). Cutaneous fungal infections in the elderly. *Clinics in Geriatric Medicine, 18*, 59–75.

Nandedkar-Thomas, M. A., & Scher, R. K. (2005). An update on disorders of the nails. *Journal of the American Academy of Dermatology, 52*, 877–887.

Patel, G. A., Wiederkerh, M., & Schwartz, R. A. (2009). Tinea cruris in children. *Cutis, 84*, 133–137.

Ribotsky, B. M. (2009). Sertaconazole nitrate cream 2% for the treatment of tinea pedis. *Cutis, 83*, 274–277.

Vander Straten, M. R., Hossain, M. A., & Ghannoum, M. A. (2003). Cutaneous infections. *Infectious Disease Clinics of North America, 17*, 101–108.

Warshaw, E. M., Fett, D. D., Bloomfield, H. E., et al. (2005). Pulse versus continuous terbinafine for onychomycosis. *Journal of the American Academy of Dermatology, 53*, 578–584.

Toxicodendron (Rhus) Allergic Contact Dermatitis

(Poison Ivy, Oak, or Sumac)

Presentation

The patient is troubled with an intensely pruritic rash that often consists of raised lesions that develop into vesicles and are usually formed in a streaked or linear pattern. Eventually there is a weeping, honey-colored crust, confluence of vesicles, and (sometimes) large bullae (Fig. 184.1). If involvement is severe, there may be marked edema, particularly on the face, periorbital areas (Fig. 184.2), and genital areas. The thick protective stratum corneum of the palms and the soles generally protects these areas. Inflammation usually peaks in 5 days, evolving into a subacute phase in which the swelling and blistering subside, replaced by drier crust and scaling. Redness and itching persist. Secondary bacterial infection can develop, often caused by the patient's scratching.

The patient is often not aware of having been in contact with poison ivy, oak, or sumac but may recall working in a field or garden from several hours to 4 days before the onset of symptoms. In general, the shorter the reaction time, the greater the degree of the individual's sensitivity, which decreases with age. Most cases of *Toxicodendron* dermatitis begin to dissipate after 10 to 14 days.

What to Do

✅ **If it is available, have the patient cleanse all affected areas with Zanfel Poison Ivy Wash** (www.zanfel.com)**, a moderately priced over-the-counter (OTC) product that can actively bind the allergen, reduce its load in the skin, and provide some relief from the itching.**

✅ **To reduce pruritus, have the patient apply cool or cold compresses of aluminum subacetate (Burow solution; Domeboro Powder Packets [2 packets in 1 pint of water]) for approximately 20 minutes every 3 to 4 hours (more often if needed for comfort). Anything that cools the skin, including ice, will reduce itching.**

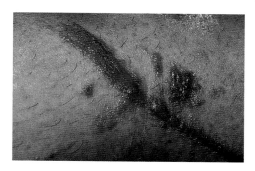

Fig. 184.1 Classic *Toxicodendron* allergic contact dermatitis demonstrating linear streaking of vesicles and bullae. (From White, G., & Cox, N. [2006]. *Diseases of the skin* [2nd ed.]. St. Louis, MO: Mosby.)

813

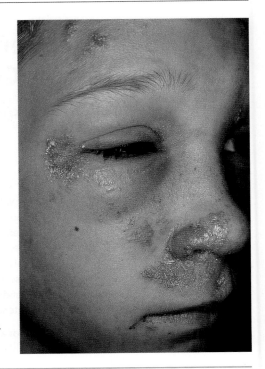

Fig. 184.2 In addition to crusted and weeping plaques, there is periorbital edema in this case of acute allergic dermatitis to poison ivy. (From Bolognia, J., Jorizzo, J., & Rapini, R. [2003]. *Dermatology*. St. Louis, MO: Mosby.)

✅ **Small areas on the trunk or extremities can be treated with potent topical steroids, such as fluocinonide (Lidex) or desoximetasone (Topicort) 0.05% cream or gel, two to three times per day,** after using cool compresses. Topical steroids can be enhanced at night with an occlusive plastic wrap dressing, such as Saran food wrap. These severe reactions may require 2 days of application before itching subsides significantly. These agents must be continued for 2 weeks or the dermatitis will reappear.

✅ Diphenhydramine (OTC, Benadryl) or hydroxyzine (Atarax, Vistaril), 25 to 50 mg orally every 6 hours, may help mild itching between application of compresses but will probably provide nothing more than a soporific effect. There is no evidence to support the efficacy of nonsedating antihistamines.

✅ **Tepid tub baths with Aveeno colloidal oatmeal (1 cup in half-full bathtub) or cornstarch and baking soda (1 cup each in half-full bathtub) will provide soothing relief for more extensive lesions.** To prevent ground oatmeal from caking in plumbing, place it in a tied sock before dropping it into the bathtub.

✅ **When there is involvement of the face, eyes, hands, or genitalia; when there are severe generalized reactions or a history of severe reactions; or when the patient's livelihood is threatened, early and aggressive treatment with systemic corticosteroids should be initiated. Prednisone (60–80 mg [approximately 1 mg/kg] per day, tapered over 2 to 3 weeks) will be necessary to prevent a late flare-up or rebound reaction. One 40-mg dose of triamcinolone acetonide (Kenalog) intramuscularly will be equally effective.** For pediatric patients, use prednisolone syrup, 15 mg/5 mL (Prelone), 1 mg/kg per day, tapered over 2 to 3 weeks.

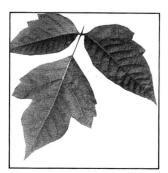

Fig. 184.3   Poison ivy. (From Cruz, P. D. [2003]. *Toxicodendron* dermatitis. Paper presented by Extension Services in Pharmacy, School of Pharmacy, University of Wisconsin–Madison.)

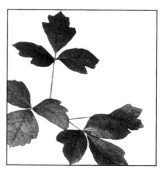

Fig. 184.4   Poison oak. (From Cruz, P. D. [2003]. *Toxicodendron* dermatitis. Paper presented by Extension Services in Pharmacy, School of Pharmacy, University of Wisconsin–Madison.)

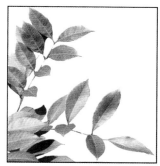

Fig. 184.5   Poison sumac. (From Cruz, P. D. [2003]. *Toxicodendron* dermatitis. Paper presented by Extension Services in Pharmacy, School of Pharmacy, University of Wisconsin–Madison.)

✓ **Avoidance of the offending agent is the key to prevention. Instruct patients regarding how to recognize poison ivy and its close relatives** (Figs. 184.3, 184.4, and 184.5). Also have them cover up in the future with long pants, a long-sleeved shirt, vinyl gloves, and boots. They should wash with water (and soap if available) immediately after suspecting contact with a *Toxicodendron* sap. After 10 minutes, only 50% can be removed; after 15 minutes, only 25%; after 30 minutes, only 10%; and after 60 minutes, none of the urushiol can be removed using soap and water. However, washing even 2 hours after exposure has been shown to decrease the likelihood and the severity of the reaction. **After 60 minutes, Zanfel may be the only cleansing agent that can effectively bind and remove *Toxicodendron* sap from the skin.**

✓ **Inform patients about preventing future exposures** by using IvyBlock, an OTC lotion containing bentoquatam 5%, which binds with plant allergens, preventing them from penetrating the skin. This is of no use for patients who already have a rash.

✓ **Treat secondary infections** with antibiotics such as dicloxacillin, 500 mg four times a day, or cephalexin, 500 mg three times a day, for 10 days along with the cool compresses noted earlier. When appropriate, provide coverage for community-acquired methicillin-resistant *Staphylococcus aureus* (CA-MRSA) (see Chapters 168 and 174).

✓ Although hyperpigmentation can occur in dark-skinned individuals and may last a few weeks after resolution of the dermatitis, patients can usually be reassured that even severe lesions will not leave any visible skin markings when healing is complete. Scarring occurs only if scratching leads to damage beneath the epidermis.

What Not to Do

✗ Do not have the patient use heavy-duty skin cleansers, alcohol, or other strong solvents to remove any remaining antigen. This would be ineffective and may do harm. Strong soap and scrubbing merely irritate the skin and are not more effective than mild soap and gentle washing.

✗ Do not try to substitute prepackaged steroid regimens (Medrol Dosepak, Aristopak). The course is not long enough and may lead to a flare-up.

(X) Do not allow patients to apply fluorinated corticosteroids, such as fluocinonide, for more than 3 weeks to the face or intertriginous areas, where they can produce thinning of skin and telangiectasias. A course of 10 to 14 days should not be a problem. Any significant involvement of the face should be treated with systemic corticosteroids.

(X) Do not institute systemic steroids in the presence of severe secondary infections, such as cellulitis or erysipelas. Also, do not start steroids if there is a history of tuberculosis, peptic ulcer, diabetes, herpes, or severe hypertension without careful monitoring and/or specialty consultation.

(X) Do not rely on OTC topical steroid preparations. They are not potent enough to be effective.

(X) Do not prescribe topical steroids if systemic steroids are being given. They should no longer be necessary.

(X) Do not recommend the use of topical antihistamines (which do not reduce itching) or topical benzocaine because of the added risk for the development of a second allergic contact dermatitis. Topical antibiotics with neomycin should be avoided for the same reason.

Discussion

Poison ivy is the most ubiquitous of the four species of the *Toxicodendron* genus of the Anacardiaceae plant family, which also includes poison sumac and two species of poison oak. In the United States, these four species of plants are responsible for more cases of allergic contact dermatitis than all other contact allergens combined. The strongly sensitizing allergen of *Toxicodendron* plants is urushiol, a catechol derivative found in the plants' sap. It is also found in the Japanese lacquer tree, mango rinds, cashew shell oil, and the seed coat of the ginkgo tree. When exposed to oxygen, urushiol easily oxidizes and, after polymerizing, becomes a shiny black lacquer. Urushiol is found not only in the leaves but also in vines (aerial roots), stems, and root systems.

In an area where *Toxicodendron* grows, *Toxicodendron* dermatitis should be suspected in anyone with severe acute allergic contact dermatitis. In the summer, any contact dermatitis of unknown cause should be considered *Toxicodendron* dermatitis until proven otherwise.

This is an allergic contact dermatitis that is T-cell mediated and develops in genetically susceptible individuals following skin contact with urushiol. This allergen induces sensitization in more than 70% of the population, may be carried by pets, and is frequently transferred from hands to other areas of the body that may, unfortunately, include the genital area. Broad areas of redness and dermatitis are generally the result of rubbing. There is always pruritus, which most often is intense. **If there is no itching, it is almost certainly not *Toxicodendron* dermatitis.**

The gradual appearance of the eruption over a period of several days is a reflection of the amount of antigen deposited on the skin and the reactivity of the site, not an indication of any further spread of the allergen. The vesicle fluid is a transudate, does not contain antigen, and will not spread the eruption to elsewhere on the body or to other people. The rash only seems to spread because different areas of the body have different thicknesses of stratum corneum, leading to different rates of absorption of antigen and therefore different rates of eruption. The allergic skin reaction usually runs a course of about 2 weeks, sometimes longer, and is not known to be shortened by any of the previously mentioned treatments (except possibly in the case of Zanfel). The aim of therapy is to reduce the severity of symptoms. It is not currently clear whether we are able to shorten the course of this reaction. Those skin areas with the greatest degree of initial reaction tend to be affected the longest. **In a dry environment, the allergen can remain under fingernails for several days and on clothes for longer than 1 week.**

Urushiol is degraded by soap and water. Once urushiol touches the skin, however, it begins to penetrate in minutes. It is completely bound to the skin within 8 hours and is probably no longer

Discussion continued

affected by normal soap and water after 1 to 2 hours. Zanfel Poison Ivy Wash is an OTC soap mixture of ethoxylate and sodium lauryl sarcosinate surfactants that is claimed, by its manufacturer, to render urushiol totally inactive by complementing the polarity of the urushiol to form a micelle. This is said to allow the urushiol to be rinsed away with water at any point during the dermatitis cycle. During the first 3 days, multiple washings may be necessary. Small clinical trials showed efficacy in postexposure treatment, shortening the course of dermatitis. A 1-ounce tube costs approximately $40 and is supposed to be enough for 15 applications to an area the size of an adult forearm. The manufacturer also claims that often Zanfel will eliminate the itching of *Toxicodendron* dermatitis with no further treatment. Zanfel is specific for urushiol; it does not work on other causes of allergic contact dermatitis.

Washing skin immediately after exposure can abort the rash. Washing clothes in a standard washing machine will inactivate the antigen remaining on the patient's clothing, as long as they have no black lacquer deposits causing visible staining. Shoes, tools, and sports equipment may require separate cleansing and can be the source of late spread. They should at least be rinsed with copious amounts of water. Pets suspected of harboring urushiol should be bathed.

Poison ivy dermatitis can sometimes be confused with **phytophotodermatitis**, which is a nonallergic skin reaction to psoralens, which react with ultraviolet (UV) light to cause blister formation and burning pain in the skin rather than pruritus. The most common causes include lime juice, weeds, or plants of the Apiaceae family (parsley, celery, parsnip) and other members of the Rutaceae family (includes citrus fruits). Redness, swelling, blisters, and bizarre configurations appear 24 hours after contact with the psoralens and UV light from the sun or a tanning booth. **Within 1 to 2 weeks, patients will develop dark streaks wherever the initial rash occurred.** This color will last for months to years, and the involved skin will often remain very sensitive to UV light.

Suggested Readings

Cruz, P. D. (2003). *Toxicodendron dermatitis*. Paper presented by extension Services in Pharmacy, School of Pharmacy. University of Wisconsin–Madison.

Davila, A., Laurora, M., Fulton, J., et al. (2003). A new topical agent, Zanfel, ameliorates urushiol-induced *Toxicodendron* allergic contact dermatitis. *Annals of Emergency Medicine, 42*, 98.

Froberg, B., Ibrahim, D., & Furbee, R. B. (2007). Plant poisoning. *Emergency Medical Clinics of North America, 25*, 375–433.

Kim, Y., Flamm, A., ElSohly, M. A., et al. (2019). Poison ivy, oak, and sumac dermatitis: What is known and what is new? *Dermatitis, 30*, 183–190.

Mark, B. J., & Slavin, R. G. (2006). Allergic contact dermatitis. *Medical Clinics of North America, 90*, 1–5.

Saary, J., Qureshi, R., Palda, V., et al. (2005). A systematic review of contact dermatitis treatment and prevention. *Journal of the American Academy of Dermatology, 53*, 845–855.

Stankewicz, H., Cancel, G., Eberhardt, M., & Melanson, S. (2007). Effective topical treatment and post exposure prophylaxis of poison ivy: Objective confirmation (abstract). *Annals of Emergency Medicine, 50*, S26–S27.

Uticaria (Hives), Acute

Presentation

The patient is generally very uncomfortable with intense itching. There may be a history of similar episodes and perhaps a known precipitating agent (bee or fire ant sting, food, or drug). More often, the patient will have only a rash. Sometimes this is accompanied by nonpitting edematous swelling of the lips, face, hands, and/or genitalia (angioedema). In the more severe cases, patients may have associated abdominal pain and vomiting (especially if an offending allergen was ingested), wheezing, laryngeal edema, and/or frank cardiovascular collapse (anaphylaxis).

Lesions may occur anywhere on the body. The urticarial rash consists of sharply defined, slightly raised wheals surrounded by erythema and tends to be circular or appear as incomplete rings (Figs. 185.1, 185.2, 185.3, and 185.4). Each eruption is transient, lasting no more than 8 to 12 hours, but may be replaced by new lesions in different locations. It is not unusual to see these characteristic wheals appear or disappear from areas on the patient's body, even during a brief encounter. The edematous central area can be pale in comparison with the erythematous surrounding area. These eruptions may occur immediately after exposure to an allergen, or they may be delayed for several days. Allergic reactions to foods or medications are self-limited,

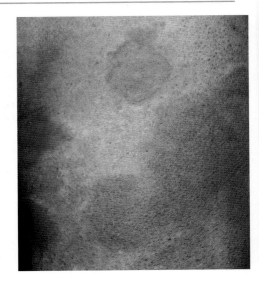

Fig. 185.1 Hives. The most characteristic presentation is uniformly red edematous plaques surrounded by a faint white halo. (From Habif, T. [2004]. *Clinical dermatology* [4th ed.]. St. Louis, MO: Mosby.)

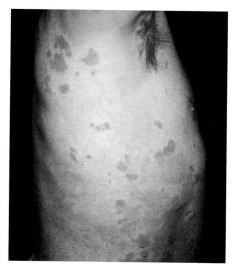

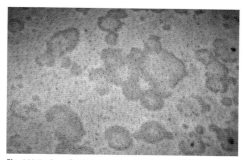

Fig. 185.3 Superficial hives vary in color. (From Habif, T. [2004]. *Clinical dermatology* [4th ed.]. St. Louis, MO: Mosby.)

Fig. 185.2 Hives. Urticarial plaques in different stages of formation. (From Habif, T. [2004]. *Clinical dermatology* [4th ed.]. St. Louis, MO: Mosby.)

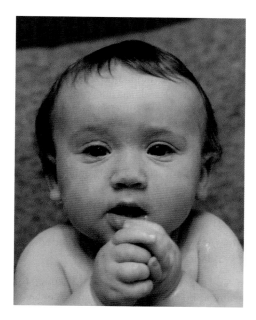

Fig. 185.4 Acute urticaria and periorbital edema secondary to an ingested allergen. Photo taken 15 minutes after the child's first exposure to peanut butter at age 10 months. (Courtesy Kurt Eifling, MD.)

typically 1 to 3 days, but will recur with repetitive exposures to cross-reactive substances. Urticaria can sometimes last for 1 to 3 weeks with some drug reactions.

Contact urticaria (in which contact of the skin with an allergen, such as latex, causes hives at the site of contact) may be complicated by angioedema and even severe anaphylaxis (see Chapter 162).

What to Do

✅ **If the respiratory tract is involved,** the first priority must be to secure the airway, which occasionally may require intubation. Administer oxygen and establish an intravenous (IV) line. **For these and other severe systemic reactions, administer intramuscular (IM) epinephrine (adrenaline) to reduce the edema. A dose of 0.3 to 0.5 mg of epinephrine (0.3-0.5 mL, 1:1000 dilution) should be given IM every 10 to 15 minutes until symptoms subside, and normal saline or lactated Ringer solution should be given IV in generous boluses to correct hypotension.** Diphenhydramine (Benadryl), 50 mg, should be given IV (or IM if there is no venous access) to alleviate itching. Methylprednisolone (Solu-Medrol), 40 mg, given IV will not provide immediate relief but may reduce the possibility of relapse, although the literature to support this is weak. Patients with severe angioedema should be admitted for at least 24 hours of observation and further treatment as required. Glucagon may have a role in refractory anaphylaxis when the patient is taking a β-blocker, although supportive data are again weak. The recommended dose is 1 to 5 mg IV over 5 minutes.

✅ H_2 blockers, such as famotidine (Pepcid), 20 mg IV, may be useful in some patients (responders are unpredictable), and IV epinephrine can be given on very rare (vascular collapse) situations.

✅ **In all cases, attempt to identify a precipitating cause, including stings, drugs, or foods.** Obtain the patient's medical history, focusing on a history of allergy, asthma, or any other preexisting atopic conditions (i.e., allergic rhinitis and atopic dermatitis). Especially in pediatric patients, acute infections (bacterial, viral, and parasitic) can cause urticaria. **Question patients about their use of all drugs, especially penicillin and sulfa drugs and their derivatives, aspirin (which they may not think of as a drug or which may be hidden in Alka-Seltzer or other over-the-counter [OTC] remedies),** oral contraceptives, herbal and vitamin supplements, and foods or drugs containing tartrazine (FD&C yellow dye #5), nitrates, nitrites, sulfites, monosodium glutamate, and aspartame (NutraSweet), among others. **Inquire about the foods eaten 6 to 12 hours before developing the rash. Pay particular attention to tree nuts, peanuts, shellfish, eggs, soy, dairy products, and fish, as well as fresh fruits (e.g., kiwi fruit, banana, avocado, strawberries, and tomatoes).**

✅ **If the cause is identified, it should be removed or avoided. In food or drug hypersensitivity, future avoidance is critical.**

✅ Perform a general physical examination, with special attention to the skin, to determine the location of lesions and their morphology. Urticaria should present as nontender erythematous cutaneous elevations that blanch with pressure.

✅ **For immediate relief of severe pruritus, especially if accompanied by systemic symptoms, such as wheezing or hoarseness (although not life threatening as noted previously), give 0.3 mL of epinephrine (1:1000) IM; this may need to be repeated. If the lesions do not clear with epinephrine,** the patient most likely does not have urticaria.

Because of the potential for unpleasant side effects, **epinephrine use can be omitted for most urticarial reactions that are less intense.**

✓ **For relief of rash and itching, administer H$_1$ blockers—diphenhydramine (Benadryl), 25 to 50 mg IV, or hydroxyzine (Vistaril, Atarax), 50 mg orally or IM stat—followed by a prescription for 25 to 50 mg orally four times a day, or cyproheptadine hydrochloride (Periactin), 4 mg orally three times a day (all of which can be sedating). Alternatively, give nonsedating cetirizine (Zyrtec), 10 mg daily or fexofenadine (Allegra), 60 mg (going up to 180 mg if necessary) twice daily for the next 48 to 72 hours.** Patients might prefer nonsedating antihistamines during the day and sedating antihistamines at night to help with sleep.

✓ **Adding H$_2$ blockers to H$_1$ antagonists may result in improved clearing of urticaria. Combine one of the antihistamines mentioned with cimetidine (Tagamet), 400 mg IV/IM/PO or famotidine (Pepcid), 20 mg twice daily. Follow this with a prescription for cimetidine, 400 mg four times a day, or famotidine, 20 mg twice daily, for the next 48 to 72 hours.**

✓ **Prednisone, 60 mg PO stat, followed by 20 to 50 mg daily for 4 days, can be added to the previous treatments, but there is scant evidence to support its efficacy. When possible, avoid systemic corticosteroids in patients with diabetes, active peptic ulcers, or other steroid risks.**

✓ **In chronic resistant cases, the tricyclic antidepressant doxepin (Sinequan) can be used** in doses of 10 to 50 mg every night before bedtime. This drug has activity against both H$_1$ and H$_2$ histamine receptors and is 700 times more potent than diphenhydramine. Sedation is common. **Leukotriene modifiers,** such as montelukast (Singulair), 10 mg daily, and zafirlukast (Accolate), 20 mg twice a day, **in combination with antihistamines may also provide additional benefit in chronic cases.**

✓ **Inform the patient that the cause of hives cannot be determined in most cases.** Let the patient know that the condition is usually of minor consequence but can at times become chronic and, under unusual circumstances, is associated with other illnesses. Therefore, with recurrent symptoms, the patient should be provided with elective follow-up care, preferably by an allergist.

✓ **Patients with suspected food allergies can be referred to the Food Allergy and Anaphylaxis Network at (800) 929-4040 (**www.foodallergy.org**).**

✓ **Patients who experience a more severe reaction** should be given a prescription for injectable epinephrine (EpiPen or EpiPen Jr., Ana-Kit), which should be available to them at all times, and they should be advised to wear a medical alert bracelet inscribed with this information.

✓ **When angioedema of the lips, tongue, pharynx, and larynx is the predominant finding and pruritic urticaria is absent,** consider angiotensin-converting enzyme (ACE) inhibitors [e.g., captopril (Capoten), enalapril/enalaprilat (Vasotec), benazepril (Lotensin), lisinopril (Zestril)] as the precipitating cause. For a patient who is not taking ACE inhibitors, consider hereditary angioedema (see Chapter 60).

✓ **If the urticarial lesions are tender and accompanied by fever or arthralgias,** consider an underlying infection or illness (e.g., collagen vascular disease with vasculitis, viral infections of children and adolescents, anicteric hepatitis, cytomegalovirus, or infectious mononucleosis).

What Not to Do

(X) Do not perform a comprehensive medical and laboratory investigation in simple straightforward cases of acute urticaria. These studies are expensive and unnecessary. Even with chronic idiopathic urticaria, the evaluation should generally be limited to a complete blood count (CBC), erythrocyte sedimentation rate (ESR) or C-reactive protein (CRP), thyroid testing, and liver function tests.

(X) Do not let the patient take aspirin or consume excessive alcohol. Some patients experience precipitation or worsening of their symptoms with the use of aspirin, other nonsteroidal anti-inflammatory drugs (NSAIDs), or alcohol. Morphine and codeine as well as certain food additives, such as azo food dyes, tartrazine dye, and benzoates, are often allergens or potentiate allergic reactions and should probably also be avoided.

(X) Do not recommend or prescribe topical steroids, topical antihistamines, or topical anesthetic creams or sprays. They are ineffective and have no role in the management of systemic urticaria.

(X) Do not overlook the possibility of an urticarial vasculitis when the presenting rash is more painful than itchy and there are systemic symptoms, such as purpura, arthralgias, fever, abdominal pain, and nephritis. Obtain an ESR, consider the diagnosis of systemic lupus erythematosus or Sjögren syndrome, and consult specialists appropriately.

(X) Do not restrict the use of iodinated contrast media for patients with a history of seafood allergy. There is no evidence that seafood allergy is a specific contraindication to use of ionic contrast. Most events occur randomly.

Discussion

Urticaria, also referred to as hives or wheals, is a common and distinctive skin reaction pattern that may occur at any age.

Urticaria present for less than 6 weeks is classified as acute, greater than 6 weeks is considered chronic. Simple urticaria affects approximately 20% of the population at some time. Most cases are acute. This local skin reaction is the result, at least in part, of the release of histamines and other vasoactive peptides from mast cells following an IgE-mediated antigen-antibody reaction. This results in vasodilatation and increased vascular permeability, with the leaking of protein and fluid into extravascular spaces. The heavier concentration of mast cells within the lips, face, and hands explains why these areas are more commonly affected. The edema of urticaria is found in the superficial dermis. The edema in angioedema is found in the deep dermis or subcutaneous/submucosal tissues. Angioedema is more common in children and young adults. Chronic urticaria is more common in middle-aged women. Acute urticaria is often allergic in origin; in the event that a

particular cause can be identified, symptoms resolve rapidly after avoidance and do not recur without further exposure. **The ideal treatment for allergic urticaria is identification and elimination of its cause.** Because the cause is often obscure, however, only symptomatic treatment may be possible. The spontaneous resolution of symptoms obviates the need for an extensive evaluation.

It is well established that food allergies are common causes of acute urticaria. Although virtually any food can act as a food allergen, it is remarkable that most type I (IgE-mediated) food allergies are caused by a rather limited number of food categories. Specifically, milk (dairy), egg, wheat, legumes (including peanut, soybean, and pea), tree nuts, and seafood (fish, crustacean, and mollusk) account for more than 95% of all food allergies. It is also common for acute symptoms to have no obvious cause and spontaneously resolve over the course of a few weeks.

(continued)

Discussion continued

Chronic urticaria and angioedema, on the other hand, usually remain symptomatic for months to years, with periodic remissions and relapses. Although they look like an allergic reaction, they are rarely the result of an allergic process and instead are considered to be caused by an autoimmune or idiopathic mechanism. A significant proportion of chronic urticaria is triggered through particular physical stimuli. Most common among these is **dermographism**, in which mast cell degranulation is caused by minor skin trauma (e.g., simple scratching). **Cold-induced urticaria** is another relatively common form of chronic physical urticaria.

Urticarial vasculitis should be considered if a single urticarial lesion (rather than being short lived) lasts longer than 24 to 36 hours, if lesions are burning or painful, if they are more common in the lower extremities, or if they leave an area of hemosiderin pigment after they have resolved. Infection, drug sensitivity, serum sickness, chronic hepatitis, and systemic lupus erythematosus may cause urticarial vasculitis. These patients should be referred to a dermatologist for punch biopsy, further evaluation, and management.

The overall incidence of **ACE inhibitor–induced angioedema** is reported to be approximately 0.1% to 0.2% and is five times more common among black than among white patients. Although angioedema most typically occurs during the first week of therapy, some patients may have taken the ACE inhibitor without any problem for weeks or months before angioedema develops. Because of this, ACE inhibitors are often overlooked as a cause of angioedema, and this may lead to the unfortunate continuation of the edema-producing drug, along with more severe attacks. **A clue to the underlying cause is angioedema without urticaria.** Because of the risk for relapse and airway compromise and the slow response to standard therapy, some authors recommend that all of these patients should be admitted to a hospital for overnight observation. However, others believe that if patients experience significant improvement and are comfortable after treatment, it is reasonable to consider them for discharge. A minimum of 6 hours of observation is always warranted. Symptoms tend to resolve within 24 to 48 hours of cessation of the ACE inhibitor, although the course may be more variable. **The use of fresh frozen plasma to replenish ACE stores has been used for the treatment of life-threatening angioedema, especially when it is resistant to other treatments.**

A plan for airway management should be made before emergent intubation is required. This may involve alerting other specialists to the patient's condition.

Fresh frozen plasma has also been used to treat hereditary angioedema. In addition to fresh frozen plasma two other therapeutic options for both forms of angioedema include icatibant and ecallantide. All three of these therapeutics have been used successfully to treat **hereditary angioedema** but with variable results in treating ACE inhibitor–induced angioedema. Thus, with the ACE inhibitors, these treatments are not currently recommended. Therefore their use should first be discussed with an appropriate consulting physician. Experts do agree on the discontinuation of the causative drug.

In general, angiotensin II receptor antagonists are tolerated by patients who have reacted to ACE inhibitors.

Suggested Readings

Alper, B. S. (2000). Soap: Solutions to often asked problems. Choice of antihistamines for urticaria. *Archives of Family Medicine, 9*, 748–751.

Alsrabi, M., & Shikh, A. (2007). A comparison of international guidelines for the emergency medical management of anaphylaxis. *Allergy, 62*, 838–841.

Depetri, F., Tedeschi, A., & Cugno, M. (2019). Angioedema and emergency medicine: From pathophysiology to diagnosis and treatment. *European Journal of Internal Medicine, 59*, 8–13.

Dibbern, D. A. (2006). Urticaria: Selected highlights and recent advances. *Medical Clinics of North America, 90*, 187–209.

Horan, R. F., Schneider, L. C., & Sheffer, A. L. (1992). Allergic skin disorders and mastocytosis. *Journal of the American Medical Association, 268*, 2858–2868.

Kaplan, A. P., & Greaves, M. W. (2005). Angioedema. *Journal of the American Academy of Dermatology, 53*, 373–388.

Kemp, S. F., Lockey, R. F., Wolf, B. L., et al. (1995). Anaphylaxis: A review of 266 cases. *Archives of Internal Medicine, 155,* 1749–1754.

Lin, R. Y., Curry, A., Pesola, G. R., et al. (2000). Improved outcomes in patients with acute allergic syndromes who are treated with combined H1 and H2 antagonists. *Annals of Emergency Medicine, 36,* 462–468.

Pollack, C. V., & Romano, T. J. (1995). Outpatient management of acute urticaria: The role of prednisone. *Annals of Emergency Medicine, 26*(5), *547–551.*

Schaefer, P. (2017). Acute and chronic urticaria: Evaluation and treatment. *American Family Physician, 95,* 717–724.

Schlifke, A., & Geiderman, J. M. (2003). Medical mythology: Seafood allergy is a specific and unique contraindication to the administration of ionic contrast media. *Canadian Journal of Emergency Medicine, 5,* 166–168.

Thomas, M. (2005). Glucagon infusion in refractory anaphylactic shock in patients on beta-blockers. *Emergency Medicine Journal, 22,* 272–273.

Warts

(Common and Plantar)

Presentation

Patients generally seek medical care when a wart has become painful, partially avulsed, cosmetically unacceptable, or otherwise annoying.

Common warts usually appear as one or more dome-shaped hyperkeratotic verrucous papules on the hands but may occur anywhere on the body. Plantar warts occur on the soles of the feet, interrupting the normal skin lines and frequently occurring at points of maximum pressure, such as over the heads of the metatarsal bones or on the heel. Plantar warts do not have a verrucous or cauliflower appearance but are surrounded by a thick painful callus that impairs walking. Both types of wart contain black dots within their substance, which represent thrombosed capillaries (Figs. 186.1 and 186.2).

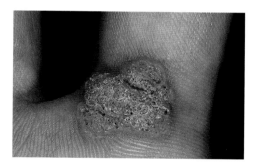

Fig. 186.1 A common wart with black dots on the surface. (From Habif, T. [2004]. *Clinical dermatology* [4th ed.]. St. Louis, MO: Mosby.)

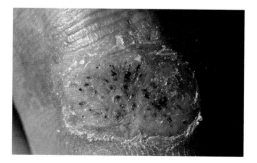

Fig. 186.2 Thrombosed black vessels are trapped in the cylindric projections. (From Habif, T. [2004]. *Clinical dermatology* [4th ed.]. St. Louis, MO: Mosby.)

These lesions may appear at any age but commonly occur in children and young adults. Their course is highly variable; most resolve spontaneously in weeks or months, and others may last years or a lifetime.

What to Do

✓ Confirm the diagnosis by obtaining a typical history, along with noting classic physical findings, which include the obscuring of normal skin lines. Shaving off the overlying hyperkeratotic surface with a No. 15 or No. 10 surgical blade may also reveal the typical black dots of thrombosed vessels, along with a uniform mosaic surface pattern. (The pattern can be seen with a hand lens.)

✓ **Inform patients that warts often require several treatments before a cure is realized and that, in general, the more rapid the wart removal technique, the more likely the process will cause pain.**

✓ **Nonpainful techniques can be used on patients of any age. Duct tape occlusion therapy may be more effective than cryotherapy for common warts.** The patient completely covers the wart and the area around the wart with common duct tape. This is left on for 6 days; the wart is then soaked in warm water until its surface is softened; then the surface is scraped off using an emery board or pumice stone. After 12 hours, the patient puts on a new piece of tape for another 6 days and then repeats the process for 2 months or until the wart is gone. This technique is effective approximately 85% of the time. When the skin lines are reestablished, the warts are gone.

✓ **More traditional keratolytic therapy (40% salicylic acid plasters—Mediplast and others) can also be used on both common and plantar warts.** Shave excessive tissue from the surface of the wart using a No. 15 or No. 10 scalpel blade. Have the patient cut a piece of the salicylic acid plaster to a size and shape that will fit over the entire wart. (This is particularly useful for treating large plantar warts.) The sticky surface is applied to the wart and then secured with tape. The plaster is removed after 48 hours, and the white keratin is scraped off as described, using an emery board or a pumice stone. Another plaster is immediately applied, and the process is repeated every 2 days for many weeks or until the wart is completely gone.

✓ **Salicylic acid liquid (DuoPlant gel, Occlusal-HP liquid and many others that are now available over the counter [OTC]) is also effective** but is more likely to cause inflammation and soreness.

✓ **One single-blinded clinical trial performed on 60 patients with common hand warts compared cryotherapy with the application of an 80% phenol solution (which is a caustic agent).** Thirty patients were treated with cryotherapy and 30 patients were treated with 80% phenol, on a once-weekly basis until complete clearance of the lesions or a maximum duration of 6 weeks occurred. Complete clearance of warts after 6 weeks was observed in 70% of patients who were treated with cryotherapy, and 82.6% of patients in the 80% phenol group; there was no statistically significant difference between the two methods ($P = 0.14$). This study showed that 80% phenol and cryotherapy were both effective and simple treatments for common warts of the hands, and patients do not experience any pain during the phenol treatment.

✓ **For resistant lesions, the immunomodulating drug imiquimod 5% cream can be used in combination with a keratolytic agent.** It is essential to débride the thick scale before applying imiquimod. The patient applies the cream daily before bedtime and covers the area with tape (for ≥12 hours). This may be used 3 days per week for 10 to 16 weeks. **This treatment is quite expensive, costing from $200 to $250.**

✓ **The most rapid but most painful treatment for common warts is cryotherapy.** The hyperkeratotic surface is reduced using a scalpel blade; then liquid nitrogen is applied to the wart using a cotton-tipped applicator until a 1-mm to 2-mm zone of frozen tissue is created and maintained around the lesion for about 5 seconds. The area is then allowed to thaw. A second or third freeze during the same treatment session may increase the cure rate. Severe pain may develop and last for minutes to hours; appropriate analgesia should be provided. Inform the patient that a small blister that is sometimes hemorrhagic will develop under the wart. If the wart does not completely resolve, freezing may be repeated in 2 to 4 weeks. **One small randomized controlled trial provided evidence to support the use of cryotherapy over salicylic acid treatment for common warts only. For plantar warts, they found no clinically relevant difference between cryotherapy, salicylic acid treatment, and a wait-and-see approach after 13 weeks. It should also be noted that one study demonstrated that OTC refrigerants did not achieve results equivalent to liquid nitrogen when used for treating warts.**

✓ **Recalcitrant warts or periungual warts** that may be difficult or painful to remove should be referred to a dermatologist. **Carbon dioxide (CO_2) laser vaporization and pulsed-dye laser treatments** may be used under certain circumstances, and they have a 51.1% to 90% success rate.

What Not to Do

✗ Do not mistake corns (clavi) that form over the metatarsal heads for plantar warts. After paring warts with a No. 15 blade, they will reveal centrally located black vessels (dots) that will sometimes bleed with additional paring. Corns, on the other hand, have a hard, painful, well-demarcated translucent central core (Fig. 186.3). Lateral pressure on a wart causes pain, but pinching a plantar corn is painless.

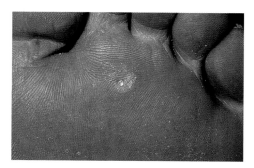

Fig. 186.3 A pared corn shows a translucent core. (From White, G., & Cox, N. [2006]. *Diseases of the skin* [2nd ed.]. St. Louis, MO: Mosby.)

Discussion

Warts are common and usually benign. They are caused by human papillomaviruses. The virus infects keratinocytes, which proliferate to form a mass that remains confined to the epidermis. There are no roots that penetrate the dermis. Wart-causing papillomaviruses are transmitted simply by touch. Plantar warts may be acquired from moist surfaces in communal swimming areas.

Diagnosis is usually made by history and simple examination of these familiar-appearing growths. Some warts respond quickly to routine therapy, whereas others are resistant. Subungual and periungual warts are more resistant to treatment than are warts located in other areas. There may

be more to these warts than meets the eye, with a portion of the wart being hidden under the nail. Because warts are confined to the epidermis, they can usually be removed with little, if any, scarring.

It should be noted that suggestive therapy can sometimes work for children through the age of 10 years. A banana peel, a potato eye, or a penny applied to the skin and covered with tape for a period of 1 to 2 weeks has been effective in young children. Another technique is to draw the body part on a piece of paper and then draw a picture of the wart on the diagram. Finally, crumble the pictures and throw them away.

Suggested Readings

Banihashemi, M. (2008). Efficacy of 80% phenol solution in comparison with cryotherapy in the treatment of common warts of hands. *Singapore Medical Journal, 49*, 1035–1037.

Bruggink, S. C. (2010). Cryotherapy with liquid nitrogen versus topical salicylic acid application for cutaneous warts in primary care: Randomized controlled trial. *Canadian Medical Association Journal, 182*, 1624–1630.

Burkhart, C. G. (2007). An in vitro study comparing temperatures of over-the-counter wart preparations with liquid nitrogen. *Journal of the American Academy of Dermatology, 57*, 1019–1020.

Park, H. S. (2008). Pulsed dye laser treatment for viral warts: A study of 120 patients. *Journal of Dermatology, 35*, 491–498.

Sanfilippo, A. M., Barrio, V., Kulp-Shorten, C., et al. (2003). Common pediatric and adolescent skin conditions. *Journal of Pediatric and Adolescent Gynecology, 16*, 269–283.

Sterling, J. (2016). Treatment of warts and molluscum: What does the evidence show? *Current Opinion in Pediatrics, 28*, 490–499.

Veitch, D., Kravvas, G., & Al-Niaimi, F. (2017). Pulsed dye laser therapy in the treatment of warts: A review of the literature. *Dermatologic Surgery, 43*, 485–493.

Complete Eye Examination

What to Do

✓ Record visual acuity, using a Snellen (wall) or Jaeger (handheld) chart, first without and then with the patient's own corrective lenses. If glasses are not available, a pinhole will compensate for most refractory errors.

✓ Wearing gloves and using a bright light, inspect the lids, conjunctivae, sclera, cornea, iris, extraocular movements, and pupillary reflexes.

✓ Use a 10× magnification slit lamp to further examine the cornea and anterior chamber; look for any injection of ciliary vessels at the corneal limbus, which indicates iritis. When the slit lamp is stopped down to a pinhole, look for light reflected from protein exudate or suspended white cells in the normally clear aqueous humor of the anterior chamber (a late sign of iritis). Look for red cells (hyphema) or white cells (hypopyon) settling to the bottom of the anterior chamber after the patient has been sitting up for 15 minutes. The ophthalmoscope can be used to evaluate the optic nerve and retina.

✓ Demonstrate the integrity of the corneal epithelium with fluorescein dye, which is taken up by exposed stroma or nonviable epithelium and glows green in ultraviolet or cobalt blue light.

✓ Note the depth of the anterior chamber with tangential lighting.

Digital Block

It is necessary to provide complete anesthesia before treatment of most fingertip injuries. Many techniques for performing a digital nerve block have been described. The following technique is effective and rapid in onset. This type of digital block provides complete anesthesia distal to and including the distal interphalangeal joint, the site that most often demands a nerve block.

What to Do

✓ Cleanse the finger and paint the area with povidone-iodine (Betadine) solution or equivalent antiseptic.

✓ **Using a 27- to 30-gauge needle, slowly inject 1% lidocaine (Xylocaine) warmed to body temperature and buffered 10:1 with sodium bicarbonate (Neut) midway between the dorsal and palmar surfaces of the finger at the midpoint of the middle phalanx.**

✓ **Inject straight in along the side of the periosteum;** then, pull back without removing the needle from the skin and fan the needle dorsally.

✓ **Advance the needle dorsally and inject again.** Pull the needle back a second time and, without removing it from the skin, fan the needle in a palmar direction.

✓ **Advance the needle and inject the lidocaine in the vicinity of the digital neurovascular bundle** (Fig. B.1).

✓ With each injection, instill enough lidocaine to produce visible soft tissue swelling.

✓ **Repeat this procedure on the opposite side of the finger.** This can be made less painful if, while injecting on the initial side of the finger, you inject across the dorsum of the digit to initiate anesthesia on the opposite side, thereby eliminating the sensation of the second needlestick.

✓ **For anesthesia of the proximal finger as well,** a similar block may be performed as far proximally as the middle of the metacarpal (a metacarpal block) with a dorsal approach. The connective tissue is looser there, and the needle need not be fanned into digital septa as described earlier. Be prepared to use larger amounts of lidocaine and to wait 3 to 10 minutes for adequate anesthesia.

✓ **With fractures, burns, crush injuries, or other conditions in which the pain will be prolonged** or when the procedure itself will be prolonged, substitute bupivacaine (Marcaine), 0.25% to 0.5%, for the lidocaine.

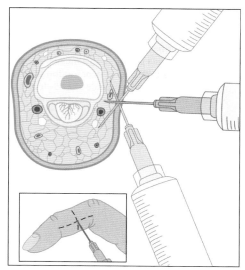

Fig. B.1. Needle insertion points for a digital block.

What Not to Do

(X) Do not use lidocaine with epinephrine routinely. Although this combination has been shown to be safe, it causes more pain on injection, and it is usually unnecessary when there has been adequate infiltration with plain lidocaine. This mixture should not be used for injuries involving vascular compromise or in patients with peripheral arterial disease. The use of lidocaine with epinephrine can be better justified when performing a metacarpal block or when a tourniquet is required for a bloodless field but is unavailable. Use 1% to 2% lidocaine and 1:100,000 or 1:200,000 epinephrine.

Discussion

Digital nerve blocks are often described as being injected at the base of the proximal phalanx, but it is not necessary to block the whole digit when only the distal tip is injured. The first technique described here provides anesthesia faster than the traditional technique. **Toes** are difficult to separate, and it may be easier to perform a modified ring block at their base (Fig. B.2).

For injuries over the dorsum of the proximal phalanx and proximal interphalangeal joint, the connective tissue is loose enough for direct infiltration of anesthetic with minimal discomfort, and a digital block is not required.

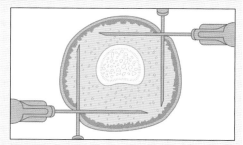

Fig. B.2. Needle insertion for a modified ring block. (Courtesy Mary Albury-Noyes. From Gillette, R. D. [1998]. Practical management of ingrown toenails. *Postgraduate Medicine, 84,* 145–146.)

Discussion continued

Some studies have demonstrated adequate digital anesthesia by injecting 2 mL of buffered lidocaine directly into the flexor tendon sheath, using a 25- or 27-gauge needle at a 45-degree angle at the distal palmar crease of the hand.

Allergy to amide anesthetics such as lidocaine (Xylocaine) and bupivacaine (Marcaine) is rare, and when it does occur, it is usually caused by the preservative methylparaben. One way to circumvent a potential allergic reaction is to use preservative-free lidocaine, which is available in single-dose vials. History of an allergy to an ester anesthetic, such as procaine (Novocain) or tetracaine (Pontocaine), is not a contraindication to the use of lidocaine or bupivacaine because they are chemically different, and cross reaction is rare.

An alternative for avoiding any possibility of an allergic reaction is to use benzyl alcohol or benzyl alcohol with epinephrine as a substitute for both the amide and ester anesthetics.

Suggested Readings

Achar, S., & Kundu, S. (2002). Principles of office anesthesia: Part I. Infiltrative anesthesia. *American Family Physician*, *66*, 91–94.

Chowdhry, S., Seidenstricker, L., Cooney, D. S., et al. (2010). Do not use epinephrine and digital blocks: Myth or truth? Part II. A retrospective review of 1111 cases. *Plastic Reconstructive Surgery*, *126*, 2031–2034.

Denkler, K. (2001). A comprehensive review of epinephrine in the finger: To do or not to do. *Plastic Reconstructive Surgery*, *108*, 114–124.

Wilhelmi, B. J., Blackwell, S. J., Miller, J. H., et al. (2001). Do not use epinephrine in digital blocks: Myth or truth? *Plastic Reconstructive Surgery*, *107*, 393–397.

Fingertip Dressing, Simple

To provide a complete nonadherent compression dressing for an injured fingertip, first cut out an L-shaped segment from a strip of oil-emulsion (Adaptic) gauze. Cover the gauze with antibiotic ointment to provide occlusion and prevent adhesion to the wound surface, as well as making it possible for the gauze to stick to itself.

What to Do

⊘ Place the tip of the finger over the short leg of the gauze and then fold the gauze over the top of the finger (Fig. C.1) (See Video Appendix C.1).

⊘ Take the long leg of the gauze and wrap it around the tip of the finger.

⊘ For absorption and compression, fluff a cotton gauze pad and apply it over the end of the finger.

⊘ Cover with roller or tube gauze and secure with adhesive tape.

What Not to Do

⊗ Do not place tight circumferential wraps of tape around a finger, especially if swelling is expected. Such a wrap may act as a tourniquet and lead to vascular compromise. For the same reason, use caution applying tight layers of tube gauze—three or four layers will suffice.

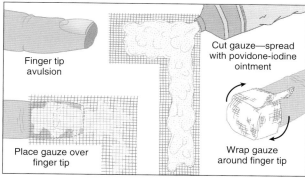

Fig. C.1. Simple fingertip dressing.

Discussion

With small fingertip injuries or partially healed injuries, for convenience, the patient can apply a simple homemade fingertip dressing. Instruct the patient to use the two halves of an adhesive strip bandage cut lengthwise. One half is crossed over the fingertip, the adhesive portions of the cut strip being placed along the long axis of the finger. The second half of the cut strip is then placed at a right angle to the first, thereby covering the entire end of the finger. Finally, instruct the patient to encircle the distal phalanx with a second uncut strip bandage to provide full fingertip coverage (Fig. C.2) (See Video Appendix C.2).

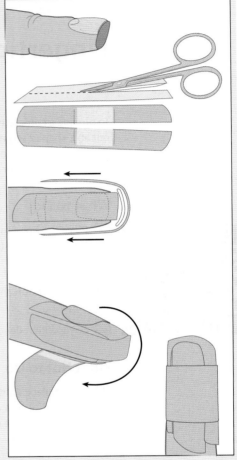

Fig. C.2. Homemade fingertip dressing using two adhesive strip bandages.

Oral Nerve Blocks

What to Do

(✓) **An inferior alveolar nerve block** provides anesthesia and rapid relief of pain in all teeth on one side of the mandible, the lower lip, and the chin via the mental nerve (Fig. D.1).

(✓) **Stand on the side of the patient opposite the side you are injecting.** Palpate the retromolar fossa with your gloved index finger and identify the convexity of the mandibular ramus.

(✓) Hold the syringe parallel to the occlusal surfaces of the teeth so that its barrel is in line between the first and second premolars on the opposite side of the mandible.

(✓) **With your nondominant hand, retract the cheek laterally and find the pterygomandibular triangle posterior to the molars.** Leave your noninjecting thumb in the coronoid notch, on the anterior surface of the mandible.

(✓) **Puncture in this triangle 1 cm above the occlusive surface of the molars, ensuring that the needle passes through the ligaments and muscles of the medial mandibular surface (~1–2 cm).**

(✓) **Stop advancing the needle when it reaches the mandibular bone, withdraw it a few millimeters, aspirate to be sure the tip is not in a vein, and deposit 1 to 2 mL of local anesthetic** (e.g., lidocaine 1% with epinephrine, bupivacaine 0.5%). Inject 3 to 5 mL if the needle is placed suboptimally.

(✓) **A supraperiosteal block (apical block)** provides intraoral local anesthesia for pain arising from maxillary teeth. It is best suited for anesthesia of a single tooth or of a circumscribed portion of the maxilla.

(✓) **First, the mucosa of the upper lip is pulled downward and out.** (The distraction technique of shaking the lip may decrease the pain of injection.) **The mucobuccal fold is then punctured with a 27-gauge needle. Hold the bevel of the needle toward the bone and aspirate the area; then, if you are not in a vessel, inject 1.5 to 3 mL of anesthetic near the apex of the affected tooth.** This technique usually produces full anesthesia in 5 to 10 minutes. For best results, inject as close as possible to the tooth-bearing maxillary bone (Fig. D.2).

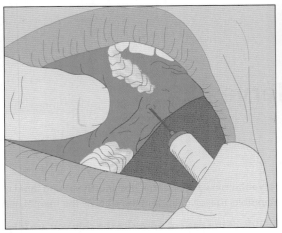

Fig. D.1 Needle placement for an oral nerve block.

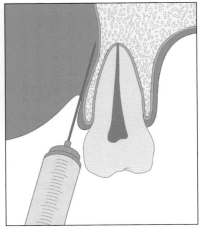

Fig. D.2 Schematic illustration of supraperiosteal injection. (From *Manual of local anesthesia in dentistry*. New York: Cook-Waite Laboratories, Inc. Reprinted courtesy Eastman Kodak Company.)

Discussion

See Appendix B for a discussion of allergy to infiltrative analgesics.

For video examples of multiple mandibular nerve blocks, go to http://www.youtube.com/watch?v=eCK6K0YrjEQ&feature=related.

For video examples of multiple maxillary nerve blocks, go to http://www.youtube.com/watch?v=3haklcbCWmw&NR=1.

Suggested Reading

Crystal, C. S., & Blankenship, R. B. (2005). Local anesthetics and peripheral nerve blocks in the emergency department. *Emergency Medicine Clinics of North America, 23*, 477–502.

Procedural Sedation and Analgesia

Daniel Wolfson

The very nature of emergency medicine has led to emergency physicians (EPs) becoming experts in the control of pain for emergency department (ED) procedures. From children to seniors, EPs must be adept at minimizing pain, relieving anxiety, and providing cooperation for diagnostic studies. **Effective procedural sedation and analgesia not only help the patient but also make it much easier for any qualified clinician to successfully complete a procedure.**

No single procedural sedation and analgesia (PSA) policy is appropriate for every institution. It is well worthwhile for any department to design a specific policy that addresses its unique staffing, credentialing, monitoring, and formulary characteristics. **As a very general rule, every PSA case will require a minimum of two individuals, one to perform the procedure and one to monitor the patient.**

Procedural sedation begins with a focused history and physical examination, with particular attention paid to the oral pharynx and respiratory tract. An American Society of Anesthesiologists (ASA) classification status should be assigned and documented for the patient. Most institutions now require a formal pause or "time out" before beginning any procedure. Regardless of how trivial you may believe this process to be, it has clearly been shown to reduce errors and complications for all procedures. In the ED setting, this is an excellent time to be certain all of the proper supplies are in place and functional. This should include all airway and suction equipment, supplies for the particular procedure, and monitoring equipment, including a pulse oximeter, cardiac monitor, and blood pressure device.

There are many procedural sedation options, and no single agent is appropriate for every clinician or every patient. As such, anyone performing PSA should be familiar with multiple options for any procedure. **All procedural sedation agents have unique pharmacologic characteristics, and the clinician using them should be familiar with them before their use. The following agents have all been used successfully in ED and ambulatory settings.**

Medication	Dose	Maximum Unit Dose	Duration	Precautions
Fentanyl (Sublimaze)	Ped 1-3 yr, 2-3 µg/kg IV 3-12 yr, 1-2 µg/kg IV Adult 0.5-1 µg/kg IV given slowly over 1-2 min, titrate to effect	200 µg	0.5-1 hr	Rigid chest, vomiting Decrease dose in infants
Methohexital (Brevital)	Adult 0.5-1 mg/kg IV Ped 18-25 mg/kg PR	100 mg	20-60 min	Respiratory depression Respiratory depression Avoid all barbiturates in children with porphyria
Midazolam (Versed)	0.05-0.2 mg/kg IV or 1 mg IV slowly q2 min up to 5 mg	5 mg	1-2 hr	Respiratory depression Agitation with low dose
Propofol* (Diprivan)	0.5-1 (mg/kg) slow IV bolus 1-3 mg/kg/hr; adult <55 yr, give 40 mg IV q10 sec, titrate to effect, maintain with infusion 100-200 µg/kg/min	100 mg	6-10 min	Respiratory depression
Remifentanil (Ultiva)	0.15 µg/kg/min drip	0.2 µg/kg/min	5 min	Same as with fentanyl
Etomidate (Amidate)	0.1-0.3 mg/kg IV	300 mg	15-20 min	Myoclonic jerks
Ketamine* (Ketalar)	3-5 mg/kg IM 1-2 mg/kg IV		1-2 hr 0.5-1 hr	Airway secretions, avoid with URI
Naloxone (Narcan)	0.005-0.01 mg/kg (partial reversal), 0.1 mg/kg (total reversal); give 0.4-2 mg q2-3 min	10 mg	20 min	Opiate antagonist
Flumazenil (Romazicon)	0.01 mg/kg; give 0.2 mg IV over 15 sec, then 0.2 mg q1 min prn up to 1 mg total	1 mg	30 min	Local irritation can occur following vein extravasation

Ped, Pediatric; *URI*, upper respiratory infection.

*Propofol and ketamine may be combined in single syringe as ketofol, given IV with a dosage of ketamine 0.5 mg/kg and propofol 0.5 mg/kg, followed by propofol 0.5 mg/kg every 2 minutes, titrated to the desired depth of sedation. This combination produces slightly faster recoveries while also demonstrating less vomiting and higher satisfaction scores (with similar efficacy and airway complications) than either agent used alone. Another approach is to combine both drugs in the same syringe as a 1:1 mixture. The combination is then administered intravenously, beginning as 0.5 mg/kg of propofol and 0.5 mg/kg of ketamine and titrating up to a maximum dose of 1 mg/kg of each drug.

The advantage to giving ketamine separately as an IM injection is that, in children, it avoids any painful struggle in attempting to start an IV line before any analgesia and sedation has been provided. If administering ketamine IM, establish IV access after the child is sedated in case additional dosing is needed.

Many procedural sedation cases require a combination of both a sedative and an analgesic. The most commonly used analgesic is fentanyl, which is generally combined with either midazolam or propofol. When using these combinations, the fentanyl is generally administered first, followed by the sedative.

Remifentanil is another new agent that is as potent as fentanyl but has a duration of action of only 5 minutes. It is administered as a continuous infusion of 0.15 µg/kg/min.

Reversal agents are available for both the narcotics (naloxone) and the benzodiazepines (flumazenil).

What Not to Do

(X) Do not ignore proper monitoring. Almost all adverse events from procedural sedation are associated with inadequate monitoring. Proper monitoring begins before the procedure and ends only when the patient is awake and back to baseline, not simply when the procedure is complete.

Discussion

The most common and potentially most serious complications of PSA are adverse respiratory events, such as diminished pulse oximetry levels, hypoventilation, and apnea. Appropriate monitoring with pulse oximetry and a bedside observer, such as a nurse or technician, will identify these problems before any patient complications occur. **The most current consensus recommends that capnometry should be used in all episodes of procedural sedation.**

Most respiratory problems result from airway obstruction and can be resolved with simple maneuvers, such as head repositioning or jaw thrusts. **More severe problems** may require bag valve mask ventilations and/or administration of a reversal agent.

Preoxygenation or use of oxygen during the procedure can avoid hypoxic episodes resulting from respiratory depression.

Adverse events from procedural sedation generally occur within minutes of administration of the medications; however, delayed problems have been documented.

With ketamine, provide a quiet area with dim lighting for recovery and advise the parents not to stimulate the patient prematurely.

Often, sedative medications alone will be adequate for performing brief painful procedures. When significant pain relief is required, add an analgesic agent, such as morphine or fentanyl. Morphine is preferred rather than fentanyl when more prolonged pain relief is anticipated.

Intravenous isotonic saline solution can be administered to prevent or treat potential cardiovascular preload reduction and subsequent hypotension.

Suggested Readings

Agrawal, D., Manzi, S. F., Gupta, R., et al. (2003). Preprocedural fasting state and adverse events in children undergoing procedural sedation and analgesia in a pediatric emergency department. *Annals of Emergency Medicine, 42*, 636–646.

Burton, J. H., Bock, A. J., Strout, T. D., et al. (2002). Etomidate and midazolam for reduction of anterior shoulder dislocation. *Annals of Emergency Medicine, 40*, 496–504.

EMSC Grant Panel. (2004). Clinical policy: Evidence-based approach to pharmacologic agents used in pediatric agents used in pediatric sedation and analgesia in the emergency department. *Annals of Emergency Medicine, 44*, 342–377.

Green, S. M. (2003). Fasting is a consideration—not a necessity—for emergency department procedural sedation and analgesia. *Annals of Emergency Medicine, 42*, 647–650.

Green, S. M., Rothrock, S. G., Lynch, E. L., et al. (1998). Intramuscular ketamine for pediatric sedation in the emergency department: Safety profile in 1022 cases. *Annals of Emergency Medicine, 31*, 688–697.

Mace, S. E., Brown, L. A., Francis, L., et al. (2008). Clinical policy: Critical issues in the sedation of pediatric patients in the emergency department. *Annals of Emergency Medicine, 51*, 378–399.

McGlone, R. G., & Howes, M. C. (2004). The Lancaster experience of 2.0 to 2.5 mg/kg intramuscular ketamine for pediatric sedation. *Emergency Medicine Journal, 21*, 290–295.

Newman, D. H., Azer, M. M., Pitetti, R. D., et al. (2003). When is a patient safe for discharge after procedural sedation? *Annals of Emergency Medicine, 42*, 627–635.

Roback, M. G., Bajaj, L., Wathen, J. E., et al. (2004). Preprocedural fasting and adverse events in procedural sedation and analgesia in a pediatric emergency department: Are they related? *Annals of Emergency Medicine, 44*, 454–459.

Sacchetti, A., Senula, G., Strickland, J., et al. (2007). Procedural sedation in the community emergency department: Initial results of the ProSCED registry. *Academic Emergency Medicine, 14*, 41–46.

Shah, A., Mosdossy, G., McLeod, S., et al. (2011). A blinded, randomized controlled trial to evaluate ketamine/propofol versus ketamine alone for procedural sedation in children. *Annals of Emergency Medicine, 57*, 425–433.

Treston, G. (2004). Prolonged pre-procedure fasting time is unnecessary when using titrated intravenous ketamine for paediatric procedural sedation. *Emergency Medicine Australasia, 16*, 145–150.

Rabies Prophylaxis

Presentation

A possibly contagious animal has bitten the patient, or the animal's saliva has contaminated an abrasion or mucous membrane. There may have only been a questionable exposure to a bat, but the nature of the contact (if there was any contact) is unknown.

What to Do

✓ **Clean and débride any wound thoroughly.** Irrigate with soap and water, with povidone-iodine, or with 1% benzalkonium chloride, and rinse with normal saline or tap water. Provide tetanus prophylaxis and provide appropriate treatment for bite wounds (see Chapter 142).

✓ Know the local prevalence of rabies or ask someone who knows (e.g., local health department).

✓ **If the offending animal was an apparently healthy dog or cat and is available for observation, arrange to have the animal confined for 10 days.** During that period, an animal infected with rabies will show symptoms. If the animal has symptoms of rabies, it should be euthanized and examined using a fluorescent rabies antibody (FRA) technique. **If the FRA test is positive for rabies,** the patient must be treated with rabies immune globulin (RIG) and human diploid cell vaccine (HDCV) or another rabies vaccine.

✓ **If the animal is not available for observation, the decision whether to provide rabies prophylaxis depends on the local prevalence of rabies in domestic animals, rodents, and lagomorphs.** It should be noted that international travelers to areas where canine rabies is still endemic have an increased risk for exposure to rabies.

✓ **An unprovoked attack is more likely than a provoked attack to indicate that the animal is rabid.** Bites inflicted on a person attempting to feed or handle an apparently healthy animal should generally be regarded as provoked.

✓ **If the patient has been bitten by a wild animal (e.g., bat, coyote, fox, opossum, raccoon, skunk) capable of transmitting rabies, the animal should be caught, killed, and sent to the local public health department for brain examination with FRA. If the animal did not appear to be healthy or if the bite is on the patient's face,** the patient should be started on RIG and HDCV in the meantime. Treatment should be stopped only if the FRA test is negative.

✓ **If the offending wild animal is not captured,** no matter how normal appearing it was, assume that it was rabid and provide a full course of RIG and HDCV.

✓ **Postexposure prophylaxis should be considered when contact with a bat or a bite from a bat is possible but uncertain, such as when a bat is found near a sleeping person or a previously unattended child and the animal is unavailable for testing.** In the United States, bats have been the most common source of rabies among humans.

When Postexposure Prophylaxis Is Required

✓ **Provide passive immunity with 20 IU/kg of RIG (Imogam Rabies-HT, HyperRAB).** Infiltrate around the wound (if anatomically feasible) as much as possible and administer the remainder intramuscularly in the gluteus. Give two separate injections if the remaining volume is greater than 5 mL. This passive protection has a half-life of 21 days.

✓ **Begin immunization with human rabies vaccine, rabies human diploid cell (Imovax), 1 mL IM in the deltoid (or the anterolateral thigh in children), at a site distant from the immune globulin.**

✓ **Make arrangements for repeat doses of rabies vaccine at 3, 7, and 14 days postexposure, and a fifth dose should be administered on day 28 for immunosuppressed patients. Obtain an antibody level after the series.**

What Not to Do

✗ Do not treat patients who were only petting a rabid animal or only came into contact with blood, urine, or feces (e.g., guano) of a rabid animal. Because the rabies virus is inactivated by desiccation and ultraviolet irradiation, in general, if the material suspected of containing the virus is dry, the virus can be considered noninfectious.

✗ Do not treat the bites of rodents and lagomorphs (e.g., hamsters, rabbits, squirrels, rats) unless rabies is endemic in your area. To date, rodent and lagomorph bites have not caused human rabies in the United States.

✗ Do not defer prophylaxis because there has been a delay in seeking care for a documented or likely exposure unless clinical signs of rabies are present. Incubation periods of greater than 1 year have been reported.

✗ Do not omit RIG from treatment. Treatment failures have resulted from giving rabies vaccine alone.

✗ Do not withhold treatment because **the exposed patient is pregnant.** Although a theoretical risk exists for adverse effects from rabies immune globulin and killed rabies virus vaccines, several studies assessing the safety of this treatment have failed to identify these risks. Indeed, the consensus is that pregnancy is not a contraindication to rabies postexposure prophylaxis (PEP).

Discussion

Previously, the Advisory Committee on Immunization Practices (ACIP) recommended a five-dose rabies vaccination regimen with HDCV or PCECV. Their new recommendations reduce the number of vaccine doses to four. The reduction in doses recommended for PEP was based in part on evidence from rabies virus pathogenesis data, experimental animal work, clinical studies, and epidemiologic surveillance. These studies indicated that four vaccine doses in combination with RIG elicited adequate immune responses and that a fifth dose of vaccine did not contribute to more favorable outcomes.

The older (but still feared by some patients) duck embryo vaccine (DEV) for rabies required 21 injections and produced more side effects and less of an antibody response than the new HDCV. Sometimes, neurologic symptoms would arise from DEV treatment, raising the agonizing question of whether the symptoms represented early signs of rabies or side effects of the treatment and thus whether treatment should be continued or discontinued.

Currently, it is much easier to initiate immunization with HDCV and provide follow-through, because side effects are minimal and antibody response is excellent. Approximately 25% of patients experience redness, tenderness, and itching around the injection site, and another 20% experience headache, myalgia, or nausea. The newer rabies vaccine that is prepared in purified chick embryo cell culture appears to be as effective as HDCV but does not cause the serum sickness–like hypersensitivity reactions, which include generalized urticaria, sometimes accompanied by arthralgia, arthritis, angioedema, and vomiting.

Patients with immunosuppressive illness or those taking immunosuppressive medications, corticosteroids, or antimalarials may have an inadequate response to vaccination. For such persons, PEP should continue to comprise a five-dose vaccination regimen (the fifth dose on day 28) with one dose of RIG.

Recommendations for standard preexposure prophylaxis remain unchanged, with four doses of vaccine administered on days 0, 3, 7, and 14 post exposure.

The incubation period of rabies varies from weeks to months, roughly in proportion to the length of the axons on which the virus must propagate to the brain, which is why prophylaxis is especially urgent in facial bites.

Suggested Readings

Abazeed, M., & Cinti, S. (2007). Rabies prophylaxis for pregnant women. *Emerging Infectious Diseases, 13*, 1966–1967.

Grace S. Hwang, Elsie Rizk, Lan N. Bui, Tomona Iso, & Emily I. Sartain. Adherence to guideline recommendations for human rabies immune globulin patient selection, dosing, timing, and anatomical site of administration in rabies postexposure prophylaxis, *Human Vaccines & Immunotherapeutics,* Volume 16, 2020 - Issue 1, Published online: 01 Aug 2019.

Human rabies prevention—United States. (1999). Recommendations of the Advisory Committee on Immunization Practices (ACIP). *MMWR, 48*(RR-1), 1–21.

Kauffman, F. H., & Goldmann, B. J. (1986). Rabies. *American Journal of Emergency Medicine, 4*, 525–531.

Noah, D. L., Drenzek, C. L., Smith, J. S., et al. (1998). Epidemiology of human rabies in the United States, 1980 to 1996. *Annals of Internal Medicine, 128*, 922–930.

Rupprecht, C. E., Briggs, D., Brown, C. M., et al. (2010). Use of a reduced (4-dose) vaccine schedule for postexposure prophylaxis to prevent human rabies. *MMWR Recommendations and Reports, 59*(RR-2), 1–9.

Tetanus Prophylaxis

Presentation

The patient may have stepped on a nail or sustained any sort of laceration, abrasion, or puncture wound when the question of tetanus prophylaxis arises.

What to Do

✅ Always provide appropriate wound care with adequate cleansing, débridement, irrigation, and antibiotics when indicated.

✅ **Determine tetanus immunity status by asking if the patient has ever received a series of primary tetanus shots (or attended primary school in the United States or has been in the military), and if and when the patient received any booster shots since then.**

✅ **If the patient's tetanus immunization is up to date, no prophylaxis is required.**

✅ **If the patient has not had tetanus immunization in the past 5 years, give adult tetanus and diphtheria toxoid (Td) or reduced diphtheria toxoid and acellular pertussis (Tdap), 0.5 mL intramuscularly (IM). For clean minor wounds,** Td or Tdap is not required unless it has been more than 10 years since the last booster. **Give pediatric diphtheria and tetanus toxoid (DT), 0.5 mL, to children younger than 7 years of age if their history of previous immunization is unknown or includes less than three doses of DT;** otherwise, no prophylaxis is necessary.

✅ **Individuals 19 years of age or older who never have received tetanus-diphtheria-pertussis vaccine (Tdap),** now receive a *one-time* dose of Tdap, **regardless of the interval since the most recent tetanus or diphtheria-containing vaccine. Then boost with Td or Tdap every 10 years thereafter.**

✅ **Administer a one-time dose of Tdap to adults aged less than 65 years who have not received Tdap previously or for whom vaccine status is unknown,** to replace one of the 10-year Td boosters, and, as soon as feasible, to all (1) postpartum women, (2) close contacts of infants younger than age 12 months (e.g., grandparents and childcare providers), and (3) health care personnel with direct patient contact.

✅ **Adults aged 65 years and older who have not previously received Tdap** and who have close contact with an infant aged less than 12 months also should be vaccinated. Other adults aged 65 years and older may receive Tdap.

✅ **If there is any doubt whether the patient has had the original series of three tetanus immunizations, add tetanus immune globulin (TIG; Hyper-Tet), 250 mg IM, and make arrangements to complete the full series with additional immunizations at 4 to 8 weeks**

and 6 to 12 months. Administer the first two doses at least 4 weeks apart and the third dose 6 to 12 months after the second. If incompletely vaccinated (i.e., less than three doses), administer the remaining doses. Substitute a one-time dose of Tdap for one of the doses of Td, either in the primary series or for the routine booster, whichever comes first. (For children <7 years of age, give boosters 2 to 8 weeks after the first dose, 4 to 8 weeks after the second, and 6 to 12 months after the third.) **Some experts advise using TIG plus a tetanus toxoid booster (or Tdap) for all patients older than age 65 years with a tetanus-prone wound, regardless of their known immunization status. TIG is also appropriate in individuals with immune deficiency.**

⊘ **If a woman is pregnant**, she should receive one dose of Tdap during each pregnancy, irrespective of their history of receiving the vaccine. Tdap should be administered at 27–36 weeks' gestation, preferably during the earlier part of this period, although it may be administered at any time during pregnancy. If a tetanus toxoid–containing vaccine is indicated for wound management in a pregnant woman, Tdap should be used.

⊘ **If there is a history of true hypersensitivity to tetanus toxoid,** provide passive immunity with TIG, but instruct the patient that there is no protection against future exposure. TIG has had no reported adverse effect in pregnant patients but is classified as a category C drug in pregnancy. Consequently, it is recommended for pregnant women only if clearly indicated.

⊘ **Provide the patient with written documentation of the immunizations given.**

What Not to Do

⊗ Do not assume adequate immunization. **The groups most at risk in the United States today are immigrants from outside of North America and Western Europe, patients older than 70 years, and particularly those of lower socioeconomic status without education beyond grade school. Persons with human immunodeficiency virus (HIV) infection, injecting-drug users, and those undergoing cancer therapy may also be at risk.** Many patients incorrectly assume that they were immunized during a surgical procedure. Although it occurs rarely, surviving tetanus does not confer immunity. Children attending school in the United States and active military personnel tend to be well protected against tetanus. Veterans usually have been immunized.

⊗ Do not give tetanus immunizations indiscriminately. Besides being wasteful, too-frequent immunizations are more likely to cause reactions, probably of the antigen-antibody type. (Surprisingly, the routine of administering toxoid and immune globulin simultaneously in separate sites does not seem to cause mutual inactivation or serum sickness.) Most tetanus cases occur in individuals who are unvaccinated or whose history of vaccination is not known.

⊗ Do not believe every story of allergy to tetanus toxoid (which is actually quite rare). Is the patient actually describing a local reaction or a reaction to older, less pure preparations of toxoid? The only absolute contraindication is a history of immediate hypersensitivity (urticaria, bronchospasm, or shock or neurologic complications), polyneuropathy, Guillain-Barré syndrome, or encephalopathy. Tetanus toxoid and Tdap are safe for use in pregnancy.

(X) Do not give pediatric tetanus and diphtheria toxoid (DT) to an adult. DT contains eight times as much diphtheria toxoid as Td and can cause adult patients to become very ill.

Discussion

The estimated worldwide incidence of tetanus is between 700,000 and 1 million cases annually. Tetanus is caused by the exotoxin of *Clostridium tetani,* a gram-positive, spore-forming anaerobic rod. Spores of *C. tetani* are ubiquitous in the soil and in the feces of animals. They are highly resistant to destruction and can survive on almost any surface for long periods of time. Once these spores enter a break in the skin, they germinate and begin to secrete the toxin tetanospasmin, a very potent neurotoxin. Spores become vegetative only in an anaerobic environment such as occurs in necrotic tissue and poorly vascularized areas. The incubation period for the disease averages 8 days, with a range of 24 hours to several months. A shorter incubation period corresponds to more severe disease.

Tetanospasmin irreversibly binds and blocks the release of inhibitory neurotransmitters, resulting in unrelenting muscle spasms, also known as tetany. Masseter muscle contractions cause trismus, also referred to as lockjaw, or the classic grinning expression, called risus sardonicus (the sardonic smile). Progression leads to diffuse muscle rigidity and autonomic dysfunction, resulting in death in up to 45% of cases.

There continue to be 50 to 100 cases of tetanus in the United States each year. From 1995 to 1997, puncture wounds were the major type of disease-producing injury, with 15% of all tetanus patients having stepped on a nail. Lacerations and abrasions comprised the great majority of the remaining cases. Other forms of inoculation include self-performed body piercing and tattooing, animal bites, insect bites, and splinters. About 18% of cases occurred in intravenous (IV) drug users, half of whom report a wound, such as an abscess, at the injection site.

The Centers for Disease Control and Prevention (CDC) recommends that everyone older than 7 years of age should receive Td or Tdap every 10 years, but somehow physicians and patients alike forget tetanus prophylaxis except after a wound. Because tetanus has followed negligible injuries, spontaneous infections, and chronic wounds, the concept of the "tetanus-prone wound" is not helpful. The CDC recommends including a small dose of diphtheria toxoid (Td), but because this is more apt to cause local reactions, it is reasonable to

revert back to plain tetanus toxoid in patients who have complained of such reactions. Adverse side effects of tetanus toxoid administration may include local tenderness, erythema, swelling, flulike illness, low-grade fever, Arthus-type sensitivity reaction, and (rarely) anaphylaxis. Other severe reactions may include Guillain-Barré syndrome and acute relapsing polyneuropathy.

Passive immunization using human TIG involves the administration of a bolus of antibody that becomes available immediately. Although the protection is temporary, it remains within the protective range throughout the time frame necessary to protect against tetanus related to a recent wound. TIG is generally associated with a lower incidence of adverse effects than tetanus toxoid is. It is highly protective when given in a dose of 250 U IM, but if the wound is very high risk, including those that are more than 24 hours old and those that may have happened in areas with a very high level of bacterial contamination (such as barns or sewers), a higher dose of up to 500 U may be warranted.

For routine immunization, pediatric diphtheria-pertussis-tetanus vaccine is given at 2, 4, and 6 months, with a fourth dose at 12 to 18 months (6 months after the last dose), and a fifth dose at 4 to 6 years. Thereafter, tetanus toxoid with a reduced dose of diphtheria (Td) is given every 10 years, and boosters are given within 5 years for tetanus-prone wounds, which the CDC guidelines define as wounds contaminated with dirt, feces, or saliva; puncture wounds; tears; and wounds from bullets, crushing, burns, and frostbite.

During the October 2019 meeting of ACIP, the organization updated its recommendations to allow use of either Td or Tdap where previously only Td was recommended. These situations include decennial (every 10 years) Td booster doses, tetanus prophylaxis when indicated for wound management in persons who had previously received Tdap, and for multiple doses in the catch-up immunization schedule for persons aged ≥7 years with incomplete or unknown vaccination history. Allowing either Tdap or Td to be used in situations where Td only was previously recommended increases provider point-of-care flexibility.

Suggested Readings

Alagappan, K., Rennie, W., Kwiatkowski, T., et al. (1996). Seroprevalence of tetanus antibodies among adults older than 65 years. *Annals of Emergency Medicine*, *28*, 18–21.

Alagappan, K., Rennie, W., Kwiatkowski, T., et al. (1997). Antibody protection to diphtheria in geriatric patients: Need for ED compliance with immunization guidelines. *Annals of Emergency Medicine*, *30*, 455–458.

Alagappan, K., Rennie, W., Narang, V., et al. (1997). Immunologic response to tetanus toxoid in geriatric patients. *Annals of Emergency Medicine*, *30*, 459–462.

Centers for Disease Control and Prevention (CDC). (2020). Use of Tetanus Toxoid, Reduced Diphtheria Toxoid, and Acellular Pertussis Vaccines: Updated Recommendations of the Advisory Committee on Immunization Practices— United States, 2019. Vol. 69(3), 77–83.

Fernandes, R., Valcour, V., Flynn, B., et al. (2003). Tetanus immunity in long-term care facilities. *Journal of the American Geriatric Society*, *51*, 1116–1119.

Gergen, P. J., McQuillan, G. M., Kiely, M., et al. (1995). A population-based serologic survey of immunity to tetanus in the United States. *New England Journal of Medicine*, *332*, 761–766.

Giangrasso, J., & Smith, R. K. (1985). Misuse of tetanus immunoprophylaxis in wound care. *Annals of Emergency Medicine*, *14*, 573–579.

Halperin, S. A., Sweet, L., Baxendale, D., et al. (2006). How soon after a prior tetanus-diphtheria vaccination can one give adult formulation tetanus-diphtheria-acellular pertussis vaccine? *Pediatric Infectious Disease Journal*, *25*, 195–200.

Kruszon-Moran, D. M., McQuillan, G. M., & Chu, S. Y. (2004). Tetanus and diphtheria immunity among females in the United States: Are recommendations being followed? *American Journal of Obstetrics and Gynecology*, *190*, 1070–1076.

Macko, M. B., & Powell, C. E. (1985). Comparison of the morbidity of tetanus toxoid boosters with tetanus-diphtheria toxoid boosters. *Annals of Emergency Medicine*, *14*, 33–35.

MMWR. (2011). Recommended adult immunization schedule. *Morbidity and Mortality Weekly Report*, *60*, 1–4.

MMWR. (2011). Updated recommendations for use of tetanus toxoid, reduced diphtheria toxoid and acellular pertussis (Tdap) vaccine from the Advisory Committee on Immunization Practices. *Morbidity and Mortality Weekly Report*, *60*, 13–15.

Talan, D. A., Abrahamian, F. M., Moran, G. J., et al. (2004). Tetanus immunity and physician compliance with tetanus prophylaxis practices among emergency department patients presenting with wounds. *Annals of Emergency Medicine*, *43*, 305–314.

IUD removal

IUD removal consists of speculum exam to visualize strings coming from the cervical os. Grasp stings with a clamp and apply gentle traction to remove the device. Expect some minor discharge or bleeding from the os. Patients may experience some mild cramping after removal.

Index

Note: Page numbers followed by *b* indicate boxed material, page numbers followed by *f* indicate figures, and page numbers followed by *t* indicate tables.